PHYSICIAN ASSISTANTS

POLICY AND PRACTICE

THIRD EDITION

Roderick S. Hooker, PhD, PA, MBA

Department of Veterans Affairs and
Adjunct Professor
University of North Texas
School of Public Health
Fort Worth, Texas

University of Texas Southwestern Medical Center
Department of Medicine
Dallas, Texas

James F. Cawley, MPH, PA-C

Professor and Vice Chair, Department of Prevention and Community Health
School of Public Health and Health Services
Professor of Health Care Sciences
School of Medicine and Health Sciences
The George Washington University
Washington, DC

David P. Asprey, PhD, PA

Professor and Program Director
Physician Assistant Program
Assistant Dean for Students and Curriculum
Carver College of Medicine
University of Iowa
Iowa City, Iowa

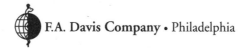
F.A. Davis Company • Philadelphia

F. A. Davis Company
1915 Arch Street
Philadelphia, PA 19103
www.fadavis.com

Printed in the United States of America

Last digit indicates print number: 10 9 8 7 6 5 4 3 2 1

Senior Acquisitions Editor: Andy McPhee
Manager of Content Development: George W. Lang
Developmental Editor: Liz Schaeffer
Art and Design Manager: Carolyn O'Brien

As new scientific information becomes available through basic and clinical research, recommended treatments and drug therapies undergo changes. The author(s) and publisher have done everything possible to make this book accurate, up to date, and in accord with accepted standards at the time of publication. The author(s), editors, and publisher are not responsible for errors or omissions or for consequences from application of the book, and make no warranty, expressed or implied, in regard to the contents of the book. Any practice described in this book should be applied by the reader in accordance with professional standards of care used in regard to the unique circumstances that may apply in each situation. The reader is advised always to check product information (package inserts) for changes and new information regarding dose and contraindications before administering any drug. Caution is especially urged when using new or infrequently ordered drugs.

Library of Congress Cataloging-in-Publication Data

Hooker, Roderick S.
   Physician assistants : policy and practice / Roderick S. Hooker, James F. Cawley, David Asprey. — 3rd ed.
      p. ; cm.
   Rev. ed. of: Physician assistants in American medicine / Roderick S. Hooker, James F. Cawley. 2nd ed. c2003.
   Includes bibliographical references and index.
   ISBN-13: 978-0-8036-1812-1
   ISBN-10: 0-8036-1812-3
   1. Physicians' assistants—United States. I. Cawley, James F. II. Asprey, David P. III. Hooker, Roderick S. Physician assistants in American medicine. IV. Title.
   [DNLM: 1. Physician Assistants—United States. 2. Interprofessional Relations—United States.
3. Professional Role—United States. W 21.5 H784pa 2010]

   R697.P45H66 2010
   610.69′5302373—dc22
                        2009031311

FOREWORD

New ideas about healthcare delivery and education were among the sweeping changes that affected American society after World War II. The steady growth of hospitals, the trend toward medical specialization, the rapid spread of employer-based health insurance, and steady attrition of the general practitioner combined to create huge new demands for clinical care. By the 1960s, physicians, patients, and policy makers all agreed that the nation suffered from a doctor shortage. At about the same time, battlefield medicine in Vietnam demonstrated that the team concept of a doctor, nurse, and corpsman could improve outcomes dramatically and that medical corpsmen could perform at advanced clinical levels with relative independence. When these veteran corpsmen re-entered civilian life, however, the only jobs open to them were as orderlies—an enormous waste of resources in a clinician-hungry country. In 1965, Eugene Stead, an internist at Duke University, initiated the first formal training program for returned corpsmen and the physician assistant (PA) was born. In this book, more than 40 years later, we have the privilege of reflecting on the birth of a profession.

The early experience of the PA in America was under the radar. Initially viewed as technicians or clinical extenders for busy family practitioners, PA numbers and acceptance grew slowly but steadily. In the 1970s and 1980s, the first cohort of PAs entered practice, typically in rural and medically underserved regions and meeting needs not provided by other clinicians. In the early 1990s, during the debate generated by President Clinton's healthcare reform proposals, PAs gained increasing prominence as important players in the team needed to provide broader coverage to the American people. As the Director in the Bureau of Health Professions during that era, I recognized that PAs had become important contributors to the nation's workforce, but their numbers were still small. Research about the efficiency and acceptance of PAs (often conducted by the authors of this book) was reaching the Bureau, supporting the modest but steady investment of federal funds in expanding PA education.

Four decades into their history, we are privileged to be sitting in the front row of an educational experiment that has proven enormously successful. As of 2010, the number of clinically active PAs is more than 75,000 and still growing. The annual number of PA graduates is more than one-quarter of the number of physician graduates, and they are in practice in every corner of the United States, working as generalists and specialists. The cost of PA education is approximately one-fifth of physician education, and PAs graduate in 26 months as compared to 9 years of education and training for doctors. Their numbers in terms of productivity are substantial, and their ability to manage ambulatory patients may represent almost 15% of the U.S. patient flow (now estimated to be 1.2 billion outpatient visits annually).

The authors are seasoned scholars in history, health services research, medical workforce economics, and education. Coming from diverse backgrounds they have brought together a work that serves policy analysts, scholars, educators, and students alike. *Physician Assistants: Policy and Practice* is the third edition of this book (formerly titled *Physician Assistants in American Medicine*) and represents substantial improvement and change over the previous edition. The book is a unique resource, providing critical information and analysis about the labor dynamics of the PA profession and its role in the healthcare workforce in America and around the world.

As an observer of the medical workforce in North America and abroad, I am intrigued with this book and the movement it represents. A worldwide shortage of doctors is looming in countries as diverse as the United States, Ghana, Australia, and Bangladesh. The 1,900 medical schools around the world are hard pressed to keep up with population growth and clinical demand. The "brain drain"—the trend of the United States relying on doctors from poorer countries to backfill our clinical deficiencies—deprives struggling nations of their scarce intellectual capital. Calling on advanced practice nurses to bolster the flagging number of physicians has limits because nurses and nursing faculty are already in short supply. Using PAs to augment the U.S. clinical workforce allows for an efficient educational model to bring new and flexible talent to the clinical workplace quickly.

As documented in this volume, the PA profession has made major contributions to health care during its brief existence. The model works, and the contributions will only grow with time.

Fitzhugh Mullan, MD
Murdock Head Professor of Medicine and Health Policy
Professor of Pediatrics
The George Washington University
Washington, DC

PREFACE

The concept of the physician assistant (PA) is difficult to capture in print; it is a dynamic process that is constantly in flux, both in the United Sates as well as globally. With this in mind, we had three objectives when we set out to write the third edition of what used to be titled *Physician Assistants in American Medicine*. The first was to provide an updated and interpretative history of PAs and their place in contemporary medicine. A second objective was to provide a central repository for the scholarly work that documents and analyzes the role of PAs. Finally, we trust that this text will serve as a resource for understanding the place of PAs in delivering health care to the many diverse societies globally.

Change is inevitable and this book is no exception. We changed the title from a reference to American medicine to *Physician Assistants: Policy and Practice* to make the book more relevant globally and more focused on policy. Policy guides the practice of PAs and practice produces evidence to adjust the policy. We also added a new member to the author team—the respected PA educator and researcher David Asprey. Dave provides the view of a program director and a springboard for new ideas. In addition, we have transferred the publishing of the text to F. A. Davis. This move was in response to the publisher's sincere interest in advancing the literature relevant to the PA profession. F. A. Davis invited us to be a part of their publishing house early on in the discourse of what we wanted the third edition to look like, and their expertise in developing this new edition is the result you see. We could not be happier.

We think it is important that the overall picture of health care should not overshadow PAs and the contributions they make. When writing the first edition, we identified over 700 documents about PAs and by the second edition we approached nearly 2,000. Since that time, our collection has grown, and now 3,000 articles, books, papers, articles, reports, theses, and dissertations address some aspect of PA care. For our book, we have winnowed this literature to the 975 most current and salient.

In launching this project, it quickly became apparent that the evolution of PAs could not be fully understood without being placed in a broad social and cultural context. We were gratified to learn from the reviewers and users of our first two editions that we got it right. What the third edition has allowed us to do is to go back to many developers of the PA model, of those who are still around, and ask for clarification of the history and other social factors that may have been overlooked.

This book represents collaboration in the truest sense, and no single ownership can be claimed for any chapter. We are fused with a common mission and common ethos to be accurate in our interpretations, and each served as a counterweight to the other's writing. Consequently, we take responsibility for all statements and errors.

Roderick S. Hooker, PhD, PA, MBA

James F. Cawley, MPH, PA-C

David P. Asprey, PhD, PA-C

ABOUT THE AUTHORS

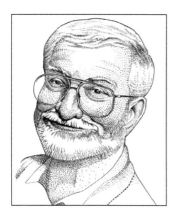

Roderick S. Hooker, PhD, PA, MBA, is the director of rheumatology research at the Department of Veterans Affairs and a clinical rheumatology PA. He is also an adjunct professor in the School of Public Health at the University of North Texas Health Sciences Center and in the Department of Medicine, Division of Rheumatic Diseases, at the University of Texas Southwestern Medical Center in Dallas. His health career began in the 1960s as a hospital corpsman in the U.S. Navy. This period was followed by time as a civilian emergency department technician. He graduated from the University of Missouri with a degree in biology and briefly pursued a career as a tropical biologist. After working as a research assistant in Costa Rica and northern Missouri, he joined the Peace Corps and spent 2½ years as a volunteer in the Kingdom of Tonga working as a biologist, teacher, and health worker. Following a brief period on the Peace Corps staff, he enrolled in the St. Louis University Physician Assistant program in the mid-1970s. After graduating as a PA, Hooker joined Kaiser Permanente in Portland, Oregon, where he worked clinically in rheumatology. A second role was that of a health services researcher with the Kaiser Permanente Center for Health Research. During the two decades in Portland, he obtained a master of business administration degree in healthcare organization and a doctorate in health policy from the Mark O. Hatfield School of Public Administration and Policy at Portland State University. He also was a PA in the U.S. Coast Guard Reserves and retired after 24 combined years of active and reserve duty. In the late 1990s Hooker helped inagurate, as well as teach at, the Pacific University School of Physician Assistant Studies as an adjunct faculty. From there he joined the Department of Physician Assistant Studies at the University of Texas Southwestern Medical Center in Dallas to develop a Division of Health Services Research. In 2003, he joined the Dallas VA Medical Center to organize a rheumatology research division and launch a postgraduate program for PAs in rheumatology.

Hooker likes to think of himself as a health services researcher, examining the role of PAs, NPs, and doctors in an effort to understand how a mix of healthcare workers can improve healthcare organization and delivery. This work has expanded overseas through the International Medical Workforce Collaborative, an organization that exchanges information on how health care can be better managed globally. He has provided consulting roles in Taiwan, Canada, Scotland, the Netherlands, and Australia. At various times, he held visiting professor positions at the University of Queensland and James Cook University. This broad portfolio permits views of how medicine is organized in various settings and identifies predictors of outcomes. In the end, though, he regards himself as an amateur sculptor who finds himself, through force of circumstances, trying to shape health services rather than clay.

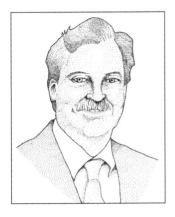

James F. Cawley, MPH, PA-C, is the director of the Physician Assistant/Master of Public Health Program and professor of Health Care Sciences in the School of Medicine and Health Sciences at The George Washington University. He is also professor and vice chair in the Department of Prevention and Community Health in the School of Public Health and Health Services at GWU. A PA educator since 1974, Cawley has held faculty appointments at the Johns Hopkins University, the State University of New York at Stony Brook, and Yale University. He has been on the faculty at George Washington University since 1982.

Cawley earned a bachelor of arts degree in political science from St. Francis University in 1970, a bachelor of science degree and certificate as a PA from Touro College Physician Assistant Program in New York in 1974, and a master of public health degree in infectious disease epidemiology from the Johns Hopkins University Bloomberg School of Public Health in 1979. He has undertaken doctoral work in health policy studies at Johns Hopkins and in the Department of Health Services Management and Leadership at George Washington University. He was coauthor with Gretchen Schafft of *Physician Assistants in a Changing Health Care Environment* (1986). Cawley has authored more than 75 peer-reviewed papers in the biomedical literature on topics spanning the PA profession, PAs in the health workforce, and preventive medicine and epidemiology. In 2003, Cawley was president of the Association of Physician Assistant Programs; other leadership roles include terms as president of the Physician Assistants Foundation, president of the Maryland Academy of Physician Assistants, and commissioner on the National Commission on Certification of Physician Assistants. He serves as a consultant to numerous educational institutions, boards, and government panels. From 1989 to 1995, he served as a member of the U.S. Public Health Service National Coordinating Committee on Clinical Preventive Services. Cawley has also served as HRSA Primary Care Health Policy Fellow and is currently a member of the Federal Advisory Committee on Training in Primary Care Medicine and Dentistry (ACTPCMD).

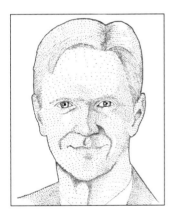

David P. Asprey, PhD, PA, is a professor and the Director of the University of Iowa Physician Assistant Program and Assistant Director of Student Affairs and Curricululm in the Carver College of Medicine, in Iowa City, Iowa. He also holds a secondary appointment in the Graduate Program in Physical Therapy and Rehabilitation Sciences. Initially, Asprey worked clinically as a PA in emergency medicine and pediatric cardiology, then became a faculty member in the PA Program at the University of Iowa, College of Medicine in 1990. In 1998, he became the PA Program Director.

Asprey's academic background includes a bachelor's degree in biology from Bethel College in St. Paul, Minnesota, and a bachelor's degree from the University of Iowa Physician Assistant Program. He also received a master's degree in education in instructional design and technology and a PhD in higher education from the University of Iowa, College of Education. Asprey has been an active member in the profession for more than 20 years at the local, state, and national levels. He has served as the President of the Iowa Physician Assistant Society, President of the Association of Physician Assistant Programs, and a member of the Federal Advisory Committee on Training in Primary Care Medicine and Dentistry (ACTPCMD) including vice-chair. He has authored or coauthored numerous journal articles, book chapters, and texts on topics related to PA education, clinical topics, workforce related issues, rural health issues, and clinical procedures.

REVIEWERS

Meredith Davison, PhD
Associate Dean for Academic Services
Associate Director, Physician Assistant Program
University of Oklahoma College of Medicine
Tulsa, Oklahoma

Matt Dane Baker, PA-C, DHSc
Philadelphia University
School of Science and Health
Philadelphia, Pennsylvania

ACKNOWLEDGMENTS

Numerous observers of medical labor behavior have made suggestions that would improve a new edition of a book on physician assistants (PAs). Some reviewers have offered good ideas and others made useful critiques. Our appreciation goes to all.

We are grateful to a handful of early PA developers who helped us improve the story, set the facts in the right context, and situate them in the historical place they deserve. It is a rare privilege for historians to have the originators of a movement still around to clarify certain events, and we turned to them often. This book has been improved by friendships and discussions with those who have made substantial contributions to the PA profession, including Richard Smith, Thomas Piemme, Alfred Sadler, Reginald Carter, E. Harvey Estes, Jesse Edwards, Archie Golden, and Jack Ott. To them, we express our gratitude and enduring affection for retaining the history and allowing us to appreciate the shared roles you have created in your illustrative careers. You are among the few who are rightly considered to be the important pillars on which this profession stands. Thank you for refining our thoughts and guiding our efforts.

Additional thanks to Marilyn Fitzgerald, Nicole Gara, Nancy Hughes, Steven Lane, Donald Pedersen, Eugene Jones, Justine Strand, Leslie Kole, Sarah Zarbock, Jeff Heinrich, Steve Crane, Richard Rohrs, Ron Nelson, Dennis Blessing, Richard Dehn, Randy Danielsen, Bert Simon, Tony Miller, Ruth Ballweg, Michael Rackover, Nish Orcutt, Michael Powe, Glen Combs, Anita Glicken, Walt Eisenhauer, Robert McNellis, and Greg Thomas. We also appreciate the help of fellow health workforce policy buffs including Richard "Buz" Cooper, Fitzhugh Mullan, Kevin Grumbach, Eric Larsen, Perri Morgan, and Ed Salsberg.

We owe a special debt of gratitude to the American Academy of Physician Assistants, especially, Bill Leinweber, Howard Glassroth, Ann Davis, Marilyn Fitzgerald, and Kevin Bayes, for sharing with us select photographs and documents. Officials from the other PA organizations were also very generous in providing up-to-date information; these persons include Janet Lathrop, John McCarty, and Timi Barwick.

Aside from our individual dedications, we want to single out the talented Liz Schaeffer for her extraordinary work in editing our book and at times arbitrated with a good eye as to what our readers would want the most. A note of thanks also goes to Andy McPhee, our publisher at F. A. Davis, for his insight and assistance in developing this book. Through his unstinting support, our faith has been restored in the author-publisher relationship scholars so much need.

Although much of the research and writing was done on personal time, the three of us are full-time academicians, and, as such, we are grateful to our deans and department chairs, who provided the atmosphere and indirect support to undertake such work.

CONTENTS

A TIME LINE OF THE PROFESSION

1650 Feldshers, originally German military medical assistants, are introduced into Russian armies by Peter the Great in the 17th century.

1778 Congress provides for a number of hospital mates to assist physicians in the provision of patient care modeled after the "loblolly boys" of the British Royal Navy.

1803 Officiers de santé are introduced in France by René Fourcroy to help alleviate health personnel shortages in the military and civilian sectors. They are abolished in 1892.

1891 The first company for "medic" instruction is established at Fort Riley, Kansas.

1898 The practicante is introduced in Puerto Rico (circa). The role is phased out in 1931.

1930 First "physician assistant" (PA) in the United States (urology) at Cleveland Clinic is described in the literature.

1940 Community health aids are introduced in Alaska to improve the village health status of Eskimos and other Native Americans.

1959 U.S. Surgeon General identifies shortage of medically trained personnel.

1961 Charles Hudson, in an editorial in the *Journal of the American Medical Association*, calls for a "midlevel" provider from the ranks of former military corpsmen.

World Health Organization begins introducing and promoting healthcare workers in developing countries (e.g., médecin africain, dresser, assistant medical officer, and rural health technician).

1962 Dr. Henry McIntosh, cardiologist at Duke University, trains local firemen in emergency procedures for the community; in exchange, off-duty firemen staff the cardiac catheterization laboratory. Former Navy hospital corpsmen are hired for similar roles and are classified as *physician's assistants* by Duke's payroll department, which is considered the first formally recognized use of the name.

1965 First PA class enters Duke University.

White House Conference on Health discusses the use of former military corpsmen/medics as *assistant medical officers*.

1966 Barefoot doctors in China arise in response to Chairman Mao's purge of the elite and intellectual. This action sent many physicians into the fields to work, leaving peasants without medical personnel.

The child health associate program begins at the University of Colorado, which serves as the origin of the nurse practitioner (NP) profession and PA specialty.

Allied Health Professions Personnel Act (Public Law 751) promotes the development of programs to train new types of primary care providers.

1967 First PA class graduates from Duke University.

1968 American Academy of Physician Assistants (AAPA) is established.

Health Manpower Act (Public Law 90-490) funds the training of a variety of healthcare providers.

Physician Assistants, Volume 1, the first journal for PAs, is published.

First conference on PA education is held at Duke University. This even precedes the Association of Physician Assistant Programs (APAP).

1969 First class graduates from the University of Colorado's Child Health Associate PA program.

1970 Kaiser Permanente becomes the first health maintenance organization (HMO) to employ a PA.

First class graduates from the Medex Northwest program at the University of Washington.

American Registry of Physician's Assistants is founded by Robert Howard, MD, at Duke University.

1971 American Medical Association (AMA) recognizes the PA profession and begins work on national certification and codification of its practice characteristics.

Comprehensive Health Manpower Training Act (Public Law 92-157) contracts for PA education and deployment. Congress includes $4 million for establishing new PA educational programs in 1972 (Health Manpower Educational Initiative Awards).

First class graduates from the University of Washington Medex Northwest program.

Essentials of an Accredited Educational Program for the Assistant to the Primary Care Physician, the minimum standards for PA program accreditation, are adopted by the AMA.

1972 *The Physician's Assistant: Today and Tomorrow,* by Alfred Mitchell Sadler, Blair L. Sadler, and Ann A. Bliss, is published; the first book written about the PA profession.

The Association of Physician Assistant Programs (APAP) is established.

Alderson-Broaddus College's first 4-year program graduates its first class.

"The Essentials" accreditation standards for PA programs are adopted, and the Joint Review Committee on Education Programs for the Physician Assistant (JRC-PA) is formed to evaluate compliance with the standards.

Federal support for PA education is enacted by the Health Resources Administration.

The Medex Group is established at the University of Hawaii by Richard Smith. International PA-type programs in the Pacific, Asia, Africa, and South America begin development.

1973 First AAPA Annual Conference is held at Sheppard Air Force Base, Texas, with 275 attendees.

AAPA and APAP establish a joint national office in Washington, DC.

National Commission on Certification of Physician Assistants (NCCPA) is established.

National Board of Medical Examiners administers the first certifying examinations for primary care PAs.

First postgraduate program for PAs is started at Montefiore Hospital by Richard Rosen, MD

1974 AAPA becomes an official organization of the JRC-PA. The committee reviews PA and surgeon assistant programs and makes accreditation recommendations to the Committee on Allied Health Education and Accreditation.

The American College of Surgeons becomes a sponsoring organization of the JRC-PA.

From 1974 to 1977, 150 PAs are recruited to work on the Alaska pipeline—the largest scale employment of PAs in the private sector.

1975 *The Physician Assistant: A National and Local Analysis,* by Ann Suter Ford, is published.

1976 Federal support of PA education continues under grants from the Health Professions Educational Assistance Act (Public Law 94-484).

1977 *The New Health Professionals: Nurse Practitioners and Physician's Assistants,* by Ann Bliss and Eva Cohen, is published.

The Physician's Assistant: A Baccalaureate Curriculum, by Hu Myers, is published.

AAPA Education and Research Foundation (later renamed the Physician Assistant Foundation) is incorporated to recruit public and private contributions for student financial assistance and to support research on the PA profession.

Rural Health Clinic Services Act (Public Law 95-210) is passed by Congress, providing Medicare reimbursement of PA and NP services in rural clinics.

Health Practitioner (later renamed *Physician Assistant*) journal begins publication; the publication is later distributed to all PAs as the official AAPA publication.

1978 *The Physician's Assistant: Innovation in the Medical Division of Labor,* by Eugene Schneller, is published.

AAPA House of Delegates becomes the policy-making legislative body of the academy.

U.S. Air Force begins appointing PAs as commissioned officers.

1979 Graduate Medical Education National Advisory Council estimates a surplus of physicians and nonphysician providers in the near future.

1980 The AAPA Political Action Committee is established to support candidates for federal office who support the PA profession.

Formation of the Veteran's Caucus of the AAPA.

1981 *Staffing Primary Care in 1990: Physician Replacement and Cost Savings,* by Jane Cassels Record, documents that PAs in HMO settings provide 79% of the care of a primary care physician, at 50% of the cost.

1982 *Physician Assistants: Their Contribution to Health Care,* by Henry Perry and Bena Breitner, is published.

1984 *First Annual Report on Physician Assistant Educational Programs in the United States,* by Denis Oliver, PhD, and the APAP, is published.

Alternatives in Health Care Delivery: Emerging Roles of Physician Assistants, by Reginal D. Carter, is published.

1985 AAPA's first Burroughs Wellcome Health Policy Fellowship for PAs is created.

Membership of the AAPA surpasses the 10,000 mark. Membership categories are expanded to include physicians, affiliates, and sustaining members.

University of Colorado PA program awards a master's degree to their graduates, the first master's for PA education.

1986 AAPA succeeds in legislative drive for coverage of PA services in hospitals and nursing homes and for coverage of assisting in surgery under Medicare Part B (Omnibus Budget Reconciliation Act [Public Law 99-210]).

1987 National PA Day, October 6, is established, coinciding with the anniversary of the first graduating class of PAs from the Duke University PA program 20 years earlier.

The AAPA national headquarters in Alexandria, Virginia, is dedicated.

AAPA publishes the *Journal of the American Academy of Physician Assistants (JAAPA)*. The editor selected is the first PA hired as AAPA professional staff.

Additional Medicare coverage of PA services (in rural underserved areas) is approved by Congress.

1991 U.S. Navy PAs are commissioned.

AAPA assumes administrative responsibility of the Accreditation Review Committee on Education for the Physician Assistant (ARC-PA) (formerly the JRC-PA).

Clinician Reviews debuts, the first clinical journal to target PAs and NPs. The publication is created, owned, and managed by PAs.

1992 U.S. Army and Coast Guard PAs are commissioned.

The Canadian National Forces inaugurates a Canadian PA.

1993 A total of 24,600 PAs are in active practice in 50 states, territories, and the District of Columbia.

1995 *Physician Assistants in the Health Workforce, 1994* (report of the Advisory Group on Physician Assistants and the Workforce), which develops the current definition of the PA, is published.

1996 The AMA grants observer status to the AAPA in the AMA House of Delegates.

1997 Passage of the Balanced Budget Act of 1997 (Public Law 105-33) changes level of reimbursement of PA services under Medicare.

1998 Mississippi becomes the last state to pass PA enabling legislation.

The APAP Research Institute is founded.

1999 *Perspectives on Physician Assistant Education* becomes a peer-reviewed indexed journal.

Manitoba creates legislation for the introduction of PAs.

2000 The APAP determines that the master's degree is the appropriate degree for PA education.

The ARC-PA becomes the independent accrediting agency for PA educational programs.

Louisiana becomes the 47th state to pass PA prescribing legislation.

NCCPA converts the Physician Assistant National Certification Examination (PANCE) and the Physician Assistant National Recertification Examination to computer-based administration.

2001 A record 4,267 PAs sit for the PANCE (91.5% pass rate).

2002 The 35th anniversary of the first graduation of PAs is chronicled in a special edition of *JAAPA*.

The AAPA estimates that there are approximately 45,000 clinically active PAs in American medicine.

The APA celebrates its 30th anniversary. The number of accredited PA programs is 134.

2003 PAs are introduced in England.

The Centers for Medicare and Medicaid Services (CMS) expands the ability of PAs to have an ownership interest in a practice under the Medicare program.

A PA program at Base Borden in Ontario becomes the first accredited PA program in Canada.

The Netherlands starts three PA programs.

2004 The number of clinically practicing PAs in the United States reaches 50,121.

Two PAs, Karen Bass of California and Mark Hollo of North Carolina, become the first PAs to be elected to state legislatures.

PA organizations draft shared definition of PA competencies. The participating organizations are the AAPA, APAP, ARC-PA, and NCCPA.

The 33rd annual PA Conference in Las Vegas, Nevada, boasts the largest attendance to date, with a total attendance of more than 10,500.

2005 The Association of Physician Assistant Programs (APAP) changes its name to the Physician Assistant Education Association (PAEA) and relocates to offices separate from the AAPA in Alexandria, Virgina.

The Netherlands graduates its first class of PAs.

University of Herfordshire, England, inaugurates first PA program in the United Kingdom.

Eugene Stead, MD, a founder of the PA profession, dies at age 96.

2006 Rear Admiral Mike Milner becomes the first PA flag officer.

ARC-PA issues the third edition of accreditation Standards.

The State of Ohio passes legislation allowing PAs to prescribe, meaning 49 states, the District of Columbia, and Guam allow PAs to prescribe.

Scotland introduces 12 PAs as a pilot program.

2007 The United States celebrates the 40th anniversary of the U.S. PA movement. An estimated 65,000 U.S. PAs are clinically active.

The PAEA celebrates its 35th anniversary.

The Society for the Preservation of Physician Assistant History, Inc. becomes a supporting organization of the AAPA.

HealthForceOntario, an initiative by the Ontario Ministry of Health, begins a pilot program introducing PAs in the province.

Indiana passes legislation allowing PAs to prescribe. All 50 states, the District of Columbia, and Guam now allow PAs to prescribe.

The AAPA, PAEA, NCCPA, and ARC-PA joined representatives from the National Human Genome Research Institute, and other genomics experts to define how PAs could introduce genomics in patient care.

2008 Manitoba begins the first civilian Canadian PA program.

ARC-PA awards initial accreditation to its first two postgraduate PA programs—the University of Texas M. D. Anderson Cancer Center PA Postgraduate Program in Oncology (Houston), and the Johns Hopkins Hospital Postgraduate Surgical Residency for PAs (Baltimore).

The Bureau of Labor Statistics identifies the PA profession as one of 30 occupations expected to grow fast over the next decade.

Number of PAs in active practice in the United States exceeds 70,000.

William Leinweber is appointed the sixth Executive Director of the AAPA.

2009 The number of U.S. PA graduates is approximately 5,640.

The AAPA and the PAEA hold a Summit Meeting on the PA clinical doctorate, and declare their opposition to the entry-level doctorate degree for PA education.

Australia begins the first PA program at the University of Queensland.

The number of PA programs in the world totals 160: 145 in the United States, 1 in Australia, 4 in England, 3 in Canada, 4 in the Netherlands, and 3 in South Africa.

The NCCPA announces that it will offer specialty certification examinations in five clinical specialties by 2011.

2010 The estimated number of clinically active PAs: United States, 75,000; Australia, 15; Canada, 100; Great Britian, 80; the Netherlands, 200.

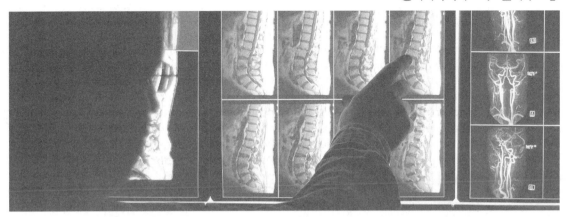

INTRODUCTION AND OVERVIEW
OF THE PROFESSION

RODERICK S. HOOKER ■ JAMES F. CAWLEY ■ DAVID P. ASPREY

ABSTRACT

In October 1967, three graduate physician assistants (PAs) began their careers. By years end 2009, the PA profession boasted more than 90,000 U.S. graduates (with 86% of them still active in the workforce) and 300 or so graduates in other countries. The United States has 145 PA programs, and 13 PA programs are in other countries (with more in development). The United States, Canada, Great Britian, Australia, the Netherlands, and South Africa enable PAs to work under the supervision of a doctor. Three-fifths are female, the average age is 42 years, and the majority have a graduate degree. Spanning four decades PA education has stayed the course in teaching primary care, although the majority are employed outside primary care. Along the way the role of the PA has evolved, the educational level has advanced, and professional organizations have become established, indicating the stability and maturity of the profession. This book is a journey through PA development and current practice. It includes policy analysis and recapitulation of historical events that shaped the profession. We are privileged observers and report our findings in 19 chapters, 6 appendices, and include an extensive bibliography.

THE PHYSICIAN ASSISTANT PROFESSION

The concept of the physician assistant (PA) emerged in the 1960s as a strategy to cope with a shortage of primary care physicians. Giving impetus to idea, what spawned was a handful of graduates and a new profession. From humble beginnings the new profession struggled to survive, grow, and become recognized. It was not an easy task. Prior to the creation of the PA, the domain of the doctor had never really been challenged. For more than 100 years, the laws and policies in place favored the doctor over any other professional licensed to practice medicine. But history repeated itself; a few charasmatic doctors, having been in the right place at the right time with the right credentials, prevailed. The fact that this historical phenomenon occurred at least half a dozen times in the late 1960s suggests that the ground was fertile for almost any seed of change to take root.

With more than four decades of growth, the PA profession is a mature and capable component of the medical workforce in America and budding as well as other countries. It appears that the United States and the health systems of other countries have come to the conclusion that PAs are an important and effective component of the healthcare workforce. Collectively, the PA profession can claim more than 90,000 U.S. graduates, a strong and stable set of educational programs, and a growing importance within healthcare systems globally. For the United States, in the decades following the origin of the PA profession, there were many debates about the need for PAs and other nonphysician clinicians. These debates came during a prediction about a surplus of doctors and nurses by the end of the 20th century. Despite these predictions, the PA profession survived, if not prospered. Why then has this profession flourished, and will its success and growth continue along with the new century? The answers to these and other questions about PAs were less clear when previous editions of this book were written. Now, with roots extended beyond the United States and the concept affirmed in multiple systems, PAs are part of the wide and varied healthcare system that wraps around the world. The labor that went into the planting is bearing fruit in unexpected ways. As policy analysts, we point to continued growth and success for this young profession because the demand continues to exceed the supply in a wide variety of societies that value choice, diversity, quality, and availability. It is also a world with looming shortages of doctors and other healthcare workers. In fact, in 2005 the U.S. Bureau of Labor Statistics identified the PA profession as the third fastest growing profession, with a projected 49% increase between 2002 and 2012. For the forseeable future, the cost benefits for employers appear to favor the PA over other medical personnel.

EVIDENCE REVIEWED: SUCCESS OF THE CONCEPT

The startling growth and success of the PA concept from its origins in the 1960s probably could not have occurred in the absence of ferment and change in the U.S. medical system and in society. The 1960s were a time of transformation in America. A driving force of the change was the existence of social inequities that many members of society believed needed to be addressed if not fixed. Consumers of health care, existing professions, governments, bureaucratic hierarchies, educational institutions, and accrediting bodies were all involved in the transformation. All implicitly, if not explicitly, aided in the process by creating a positive political climate. Cultural revolution was in the air and a desire to reengineer the social wrongs of the previous 100 years seemed at hand.

The PA innovation was born in the 1960s following two decades of scientific breakthroughs, development of new medical specialties, and overgrowth of hospitals and hospital services. Young doctors, exposed early to this exciting display of technical power, were flocking to academic-based specialties. For the generalist physician, education and training had shrunk after the Korean War. Once the foundation of the medical workforce, the single-year, intern-trained generalist was becoming an anachronism; the new graduates of medical schools were not replacing the general practitioners who were retiring. New graduates immediately headed into 3 to 5 years of postgraduate education, and from this trend a number of specialities arose. The consequences of this lack of general practitioners were not so obvious in cities with good hospitals and a strong cadre of newly trained specialists. However, in small towns and rural areas, the impact of this trend was devastating. Towns that had always enjoyed having their own local doctor suddenly had none.

Setting the Stage

Thus the stage was set for entry of alternative providers who promised improved access to health care for small towns and rural areas. The country's leaders were aware of inequities in the distribution of medical services, and most were convinced that the problem was one of inadequate numbers of medical care providers. A series of federal and state actions aimed to correct this problem. The most notable ones were the advent of the PA profession, the development of the nurse practitioner

(NP), and the reintroduction of the nurse mid-wife. However, other actions were undertaken in the 1970s:

- Medical schools increased class size.
- New medical schools were established.
- The generalist physician was "revived" in the form of a new general specialty: family medicine.
- Special offices to promote medical practice in underserved areas were created in many states and in the federal government.
- Dispersed medical educational systems (area health education programs) were created.
- Wellness and prevention had taken on a new dimension with immunization advances, epidemiology, new technology in diagnostics, and safety.

Catalysts for Change

When significant social transformation occurs, it is rarely dependent on one circumstance—an observation made by sociologists, anthropologists, political scientists, and historians. Yet a single, significant catalyst for change can occur, and when coupled with other events, a chain reaction can take place. Explaining why the PA innovation occurred in America and elsewhere requires documenting the events and identifying the factors leading up to this change.

One contributing factor was that the war in Southeast Asia was reaching its tragic conclusion in the late 1960s and early 1970s. Yet there was an upside to this conflict—the advancement of trauma management science. Military medical care had significantly improved by using trained medical care teams operating in combat areas. Physicians, nurses, medics, and corpsmen were returning home with knowledge of these improvements and the key roles played by members of these medical teams. The highly integrated team of doctor, nurse, and corpsman was pivotal in saving lives in forward-positioned battalion aid stations; yet when they returned home, the corpsman was absent from that critical triumverate because the constraints of the existing healthcare system did not recognize this type of provider in

its educational or credentialing systems. Many recognized that a highly skilled member was missing.

Another factor was the social climate within the country. The War on Poverty had brought to public attention the substandard conditions and deprivation of some people within the bounds of the "richest country on Earth." President Lyndon Johnson's Great Society program brought an optimism that solutions might be found for these chronic social ills. The burden of social inequities had reached a critical point, and righting wrongs were required if Americans were going to be a nation of "We the people . . ."

In retrospect, it is easy to understand why this era was a favorable time for PAs to enter the health workforce stage. State and federal governments were willing to support some of the most far-reaching social programs seen to that time to increase access to health care. The fact that this innovation tapped the newly available source of returning military corpsmen was serendipitous.

Intertwined with these circumstances were events more directly related to the PA profession. In 1961, a prominent leader of the American Medical Association (AMA) proposed the idea of using military trained personnel as assistants to physicians (Hudson, 1961). A White House conference called for a medical auxillary tapping returned veterans. In the mid-1960s, Dr. Richard Smith, then a deputy director of the Office of Equal Health Opportunity, moved into a new role in which he proposed to create a new source of healthcare providers for rural areas. At this same time, a prominent academic pediatrician, Dr. Henry Silver, with Dr. Loretta Ford, a nurse educator, began to develop a new type of nonphysician practitioner at the University of Colorado.

At Duke University, the first PA program began with four ex-Navy corpsmen under the direction of Dr. Eugene Stead and Dr. E. Harvey Estes, Jr. As an academic physician leader, Dr. Stead had been impressed by the need for new personnel in the medical center and in the rural areas of his state. His previous experience with military personnel convinced him that the training period for assistants in a new program could be much shorter than that for medical students, and that close supervision by their physician employers would ensure competence and further development of skills in practice. Additionally, Dr. Stead noted that a prominent generalist in a rural town had trained a highly skilled assistant. Influenced by this prototype PA, the concept of extending the services of physicians in rural practices emerged. Shortly after the inauguration of the first PA educational track, Dr. E. Harvey Estes, a respected internist and academic at Duke, took the reins and further developed the PA movement.

The specific histories of the University of Colorado program, the Duke program, and the Medex program—another model of PA education—are discussed in detail in later chapters. At this point, various features of the PA conceptual model need recognition. Two have already been mentioned: the relatively brief history of the PA concept and the role of the employing physician as supervisor. Additionally, all of the PA programs were patterned after the familiar medical model: a period of basic science education followed by clinical skill development under medical instructors. The prospective PA would be trained to take a medical history, document symptoms, develop diagnoses, examine the patient, and take over some medical management tasks. Complicated cases or procedures were to be referred to the supervising physician. Although it was expected that the new personnel might spend more time with patient education and preventive interventions, the activities and skills would be similar to those of the physician, with the assistant assuming many, but not all of the physician's tasks.

Another feature of the PA model, as each developer envisioned it, was the clear intention to train a generalist assistant, whose training and skill development were adequate to serve as a platform for further education and further skill development by the physician employer. The generalist assistant could work with a rural doctor, gaining further insights and skills with time, but could also work with a highly focused specialist, who would add another layer of expertise to the general education of the PA.

As might have been predicted, state and federal governmental attention was quickly achieved by three of the model PA programs: Duke University, University of Washington, and University of Colorado. Soon the government developed an interest in the regulation of this new category of healthcare provider. The Department of Health, Education, and Welfare sponsored a study and a series of conferences at Duke University on the regulation of practice of PAs. This activity, under the direction of Martha Ballenger, JD, and Dr. Estes, resulted in model regulatory laws that were enacted by many states and prepared the way for the 1971 Health Manpower Act. This legislation provided funds for medical schools to increase the number of students to meet the perceived shortage of medical personnel. It also included funding for PA training programs. The availability of funding quickly increased the number of training sites, and 50 such programs were active by 1974.

In 1971, the AMA recognized the new profession and lent its name and resources to the process of national certification process, accreditation of educational programs, and codification of practice laws. This recognition, however, did not ensure acceptance by all physicians. Occasional roadblocks to acceptance and scope of practice persisted within state medical practice acts all the way up to 2007. Even the AMA did not fully endorse the PA concept until the 1990s, and this endorsement was spurred on by the decision of the NP movement to maintain its independence of medicine. (NPs are an extension of nursing and, therefore, fall under the state-specific nurse acts.)

Physician Assistants Today

The PA of the new century differs from the predecessor four decades ago. Much of what we know comes from the United States, but new information is emerging from other countries. Following is an overview of the PA of today:

- **Graduates:** In the beginning of 2009 there were more than 73,500 PAs in active clinical practice globally, although the United States dominates with the most graduates (Exhibit 1-1). The stability and dedication of this workforce to the profession are demonstrated by the fact that this number represents almost 88% of all persons formally trained as PAs since the first class graduated in 1967. The annual attrition rate is less than 8%.

■ **PA characteristics:** The mean age of PAs is 42 years; 64% are women. The age reflects the relative youth of the profession and the shift in gender. The early predominance of men in the profession (related to the male gender of the former military students of the early years) has gradually changed, and women represent a majority of the profession.

■ **Deployment:** Forty-two percent of U.S. PAs practice in communities with a population smaller than 50,000, and 20% practice in communities smaller than 10,000 (a much higher percentage than physicians). Twelve percent of PAs work in inner-city clinics.

■ **PA educational programs:** Globally, there were 158 PA programs in 2009, with more in development. U.S. programs are accredited by the Accreditation Review Commission on Education for the Physician Assistant (ARC-PA). Canadian programs are accredited by the Canadian Medical Association Conjoint Commission on Accrediation. The Dutch

EXHIBIT 1-1
Physician Assistant Movement, 2009

Country	Number of Clinically Active PAs	Number of PA Programs
Australia	20	2
Canada	150	3
Netherlands	200	4
United Kingdom	75	4
United States	73,500	145
South Africa	Unknown	2
Total (estimated)	>73,945	160

PA programs are accredited by a governmental agency. PA Programs in the United Kingdom are accreditated by the Department of Health. The typical PA program is 26 months long and usually requires a college degree and some healthcare experience before admission. As the 22nd Annual Report on PA Educational Programs in the United States, 2005–2006 reports, 74% of the U.S. programs award a master's degree, a number that continues to increase.

■ **Students:** In the United States, more than 11,000 students are enrolled in PA programs at any one time. In 2009, more than 5,500 new graduates passed the national certification examination and became eligible to practice.

■ **Prescribing:** All 50 U.S. states, the District of Columbia, and Guam have enacted laws that authorize PA prescribing. Prescribing legislation is under development in other countries.

■ **Income:** The mean total income from the main employer for PAs who are not employed by the federal government or who are not self-employed and who work full time (at least 32 hours per week) is $89,897 (standard deviation, $21,901); the median is $85,710. The comparable mean for PAs who are recent graduates is $76,232.

■ **Legislation:** Fifty states plus the District of Columbia and Guam have laws or regulations recognizing PA practice. All require graduation from an accredited PA program and national certification. Canadian provinces, Australian states, and the central governments of other countries are working through these issues.

■ **Certification:** U.S. PAs receive their national certification from the National Commission on Certification of Physician Assistants (NCCPA). All states require this certification for licensure. Canadians are certified by a commission involving the Canadian Association of Physician Assistants.

■ **Ethnicity:** According to 2008 census data from the American Academy of

Physician Assistants (AAPA), the U.S. PA profession has 16.7% of its members from underrepresented groups. Of those in active clinical practice, 6.2% are African Americans, 5.0% are Hispanic/Latinos, 4.6% are Asian/Pacific Islanders, and 0.9% are American Indian/Alaskan Natives. The remaining 83.3% are white or do not choose to identify their racial/ethnic origin.

PAs practice in all the types of clinical settings where physician services are traditionally offered: urban neighborhoods, rural communities, hospitals, and public and private medical offices. They serve as commissioned officers in all U.S. and Canadian military branches and in the U.S. Public Health Service. In clinical practice, most PAs spend their time in medical offices or clinic settings, but some work in hospitals and divide their time among the wards and the operating and delivery rooms. In addition to roles in all the primary care specialties, PAs can be found in most nonprimary care specialties. They are

underrepresented in nursing home care, home health care, pathology, radiology, and some of the surgical and medical subspecialties.

During the formative years of the profession, the distribution of PAs reflected the federal and state initiatives and the interest of the medical profession in extending primary care into areas of need. Early recruits were individuals with experience that enabled them to practice with minimal supervision. As the capability of PAs to fit into specialties outside primary care has become known, and as their ability and productivity have been confirmed, physicians in these specialties have successfully "outbid" the primary care specialties for their services. In comparison with physicians, PAs remain more likely to be found in primary care practice (34% of PAs, 33% of physicians) and in rural and other medically underserved areas. However, there are many influences on PA selection for a career, and these influences vary at different times. Exhibit 1-2 illustrates how the primary care specialties have traded off with the nonprimary care influences.

EXHIBIT 1-2
Estimated Percent Distribution of Practicing Physician Assistants by Specialty: Selected Years 1984–2009*

Specialty	1984	1989	1990	1992	1994	1996	2000	2002	2009
PRIMARY CARE[†]	55.8	49.3	45.9	472.8	45.2	50.8	47.9	43.1	34.2
Family Medicine	54.5	37.9	33.0	31.4	33.7	39.8	36.5	32.1	24.9
General Internal Medicine	9.2	7.8	9.0	8.9	9.2	8.3	8.8	8.4	6.9
Pediatrics	4.1	3.6	3.0	2.5	2.3	2.7	2.6	2.6	2.4
NONPRIMARY CARE[‡]	44.2	50.7	55.0	57.2	48.5	49.2	52.1	56.9	57.6
Obstetrics/Gynecology	3.1	4.6	4.0	3.3	2.9	3.0	2.7	2.7	2.4
Surgical Subspecialties	9.0	7.5	9.0	9.8	10.5	8.8	10.4	10.0	19.5
General Surgery	9.2	7.9	8.0	8.0	7.7	3.1	2.7	2.5	2.5
Internal Medicine Subspecialties	4.8	3.8	6.0	7.1	6.3	5.8	8.1	9.4	11.3
Pediatric Subspecialties	0.0	1.0	2.0	1.2	1.2	2.1	1.5	1.5	1.6
Emergency Medicine	6.4	6.2	7.0	8.0	8.7	7.0	9.7	10.2	8.7
Othopedics	4.1	5.6	6.0	7.6	7.8	6.9	7.3	9.2	9.5
Occupational Medicine	4.1	5.8	5.0	3.9	3.4	3.0	3.4	3.0	2.1
Other Specialties[§]	3.5	10.3	8.0	8.3	6.3	9.5	6.3	8.4	—

*Practicing physician assistants are figured at 85% of total graduates.

[†]Primary care includes internal medicine, family/general practice, and pediatrics.

[‡]Includes general medicine.

[§]Includes correctional medicine, neurology, geriatric medicine, psychiatry, and industrial medicine.

Data from authors and from the American Academy of Physician Assistants, Alexandria, VA.

Primary care is defined as comprising family medicine, general internal medicine, and general pediatrics. In some reporting, the AAPA also considers obstetrics/gynecology as primary care, and as such raises the percentage of PAs in the primary care specialties to 37%.

The medical model of PA education has been confirmed by the adaptability of PAs to new roles in the medical and surgical specialties. In the primary care and the specialty care roles of the PA, the relationship between the PA and the supervising doctor remains constant—a functional team. This relationship has been characterized as "negotiated performance autonomy," reflecting the continually evolving delegation of medical tasks from physician to PA based on a mutual understanding and trust in their respective professional roles. Schneller and Weiner (1978) proposed that this mutual evolution was a major determinant of clinical practice effectiveness of the PA and was advantageous to both types of providers.

The recognition and acceptance of this association is key to understanding the durability between the PA and physician. It is also key to understanding the official stance of the profession: that it does *not* desire autonomy from physician supervision. The creators' early recognition of this principle is reflected in their prediction that PAs would gain greater freedom and growth from delegation by wise physician supervisors who share the benefits of this growth than from legislated autonomy. Further proof of the beauty of this concept that allows PAs to have functional autonomy within the dependent role is the high degree of job and career satisfaction.

Delegation of tasks from doctors to PAs is also contained in the basis of the legal and regulatory authority granted to PAs in most state laws. Model legislation proposed as a result of the Duke conferences on this topic in the late 1960s permitted PAs to work in the full range of clinical practice areas: office, clinic, hospital, nursing home, or patient's home. This wide latitude was considered essential for a full range of services and effectiveness. The model legislation recognized the authority of physicians to delegate medical tasks to qualified PAs

while holding them legally responsible through the doctrine of "respondeat superior." North Carolina, Colorado, and Oklahoma were among the first states to amend their medical practice acts and Mississippi the last.

Developed state-by-state over 40 years, these practice regulations and the supervisory relationship have led to the striking versatility among the practice roles of PAs. As a result, PAs are permitted to assist the physician in any task or function within the scope of the physician's practice but with the recognition that the responsibility and legal liability for this delegation remain with the physician. This delegation is not limited to the immediate presence of the physician, but it can be extended to locations from which the supervising physician can be readily contacted for consultation and assistance, such as through various telecommunication means.

Although there has been a steady increase in the demand for PAs and growing acceptance of their roles, added emphasis on cost-effectiveness has greatly augmented the importance of the profession in health delivery. Managed care organizations quickly found PAs to be capable of providing primary care at a lower cost than physicians and to be willing to move into areas in which it would not be cost-effective to place a doctor. Later, physicians, particularly those in specialty groups, recognized the favorable economic advantages that PAs brought to private practices and hospitals. The development and demand for PAs in these settings have caused a shift of PAs away from primary care. In addition, to some degree, PAs have been willing to move into various other settings that have not been popular with physicians, such as correctional health systems, substance abuse clinics, occupational health clinics, and geriatric institutions. Patient acceptance has remained high, disproving critics predicting patient rejection.

The Physician Assistant Defined

The benefits of using generalist assistants, capable of mastering new skills and enlarging their roles under responsible supervision of a physician partner, continues to be confirmed. In fact, the original PA concept has been modified and enlarged so much that the AAPA periodically developed new definitions of the profession. The current definition was adopted by the AAPA House of Delegates in 1995. This definition addresses the versatility of the profession, its distribution in all geographic locations, and the various nonclinical roles that PAs might pursue.

PAs are health professionals licensed to practice medicine with physician supervision. PAs are qualified by graduation from an accredited PA educational program and/or certification by the National Commission on the Certification of Physician Assistants. Within the physician–PA relationship, PAs exercise autonomy in medical decision-making and provide a broad range of diagnostic and therapeutic services. The clinical role of PAs includes primary and specialty care in medical and surgical practice settings in rural and urban areas. PA practice is centered on patient care and may include educational, research, and administrative activities.

Some interpretation of this definition of PAs may be required. The Professional Practices Council of the AAPA provides the following explanations.

Physician assistants are health professionals . . .

This statement recognizes the scope of PA practice, the advanced knowledge required to be a PA, the PA's use of discretion and judgment in providing care, the PA's use of ethical standards, and the PA's orientation toward service.

. . . licensed to practice medicine with physician supervision.

This part of the definition may be of concern to PAs accustomed to the terms *certified* and *registered*. Examination of accepted definitions of occupational regulation, however, reveals that PAs are subject to *de facto* licensure regardless of terminology used by the state.

Registration is the least restrictive form of regulation. It is the process of creating an official record or list of persons; for example, voter registration. The main purpose of registration is not to ensure the public of quality but to serve as a record-keeping function.

Under a certification system, practice of an activity or occupation is not directly restricted, but limits are placed on the use of certain occupational titles. The label *certified* publicly identifies persons who have met certain standards but does not prevent uncertified practitioners from engaging in the activity.

Under licensure, which is the most restrictive method of regulation, persons have no right to engage in a particular activity without permission to do so by the state. Such permission is generally conditioned on stringent requirements, such as certain educational qualifications and passage of an examination.

Because PAs must meet such standards and may not practice without state approval, *licensed* is the most appropriate way to describe the control exercised by states over PA practice. PAs are qualified to practice by graduating from an accredited PA educational program and/or by certification by the NCCPA. (For qualification standards for PAs employed by the federal government, see Chapter 17.)

Within the physician–PA relationship, PAs exercise autonomy in medical decision-making and provide a broad range of diagnostic and therapeutic services. This role reinforces the concept of team practice while emphasizing the ability of PAs to think independently when making diagnoses and clinical decisions.

The clinical role of PAs includes primary and specialty care in medical and surgical practice settings in rural and urban areas. PA practice is centered on patient care and may include educational, research, and administrative activities. This book addresses the versatility of the PA profession, the distribution of the profession in all geographic regions, and the nonclinical roles that PAs may pursue.

What has emerged from defining the role of the PA is a template for a PA body to move within the tangles of state, provincial, and federal government rules and regulations. Not all countries have the same definition of a PA, but those who have a PA-like entity have crafted an assistant that stands alongside the doctor employer or doctor in charge. New PA definitions will emerge, and new policies will be created for the governance of PAs. However, we are confident that these policies will be created with the interests of society in mind. What is significant in these instances is that these other countries have adopted the concept of the PA.

PHYSICIAN ASSISTANT: THE NAME

The name *physician assistant* has a historical base, and this history is outlined in Chapter 2. The name has been used since the concept originated but has not always been embraced. Nor is it embraced today because the word "physician" means different things in different countries. "Physician" in the United Kingdom and former British Commonwealth countries refers to an internal medical specialist—an internist. This fact was ignored when the name was coined by U.S. doctors. Many have speculated what the term should be and what it would have been had PAs themselves been asked.

The original PA concept was of an assistant who would be able to handle many aspects of a doctor's work. Initially, the focus was on the education process, not the name. PA was not a copyrighted term such as *physical therapist* or *psychologist*, but it generally conveyed what U.S. doctors thought should be conveyed. Other names were proposed and continue to be proposed (Exhibit 1-3). For example, the term *medical care practitioner* was considered in England because of the inaccuracy of the word *physician*; however, the term *physican assistant* has now been selected for use there. Scotland decided to forego any discussion on a name not ensconced in the literature, and said *physician assistant* was what it was. Shortly after these decisions, a 2006 survey in England found that patients did not care if the name was *physician assistant* as long as their needs were being met.

It was evident that the PA's role filled a healthcare delivery need, but before long the movement was growing and taking on new dimensions. However, confusion arose about the label *PA*, which, after coming to public attention, was sometimes misused to describe a variety of individuals, including support personnel from physicians' offices (Fasser, Andrus, & Smith, 1984).

The title *PA* is not a legally recognized term either nationally or internationally. However,

National Physician Assistant Day (October 6) is observed in most states. It is up to the states to protect the public health, safety, and welfare by determining how the term *PA* is used. Generally, this means setting minimum standards and regulations to practice using a certain health profession or occupation. In the United States, state statutes or regulations define PAs as individuals who have graduated from an accredited program and/or passed the NCCPA examination. Although these statutes or regulations have not prevented some imposters from occasionally emerging, the known incidences are rare, and the checks and safeguards in place in most states seem sound.

From a historical standpoint, PAs themselves did not determine the title by which they would be known. Instead, educators, physicians, regulators, and advocates of the concept made the first suggestions for a name. Later, PAs exerted some influence in the drive

EXHIBIT 1-3
Historical List of Proposed Names for Assistants to Physicians

Physician assistant (PA)
Physician's assistant, physicians' assistant
Physician associate, physician's associate
Medex (Mx)
Child health associate (CHA)
Surgeon's assistant (SA)
Anesthesia assistant and associate
Clinical associate
Community health aide
Community health medic
Medical services assistant
Medical care practitioner
Ophthalmic assistant
Orthopedic physician's assistant
Pathologist's assistant
Primex (Px)
Radiology physician's assistant
Syniatrist
Urologic physician's assistant
Flexner
Osler

toward title uniformity when state laws were being enacted, accreditation and certification mechanisms were being established, and professional organizations were being founded. It was at this point that Eugene Stead observed, "The time has come to consider a new name for the product produced by Duke and other similar programs." Although he favored the title *physician's associate*, Stead (1971) concluded, "Agreeing on a name is the important step. What name is adopted is secondary." A number of names were advanced, including *Medex*, coined by Dr. Richard Smith at the Medex Northwest Physician Assistant Program at the University of Washington in Seattle (Smith, 1974).

Although *PA* has become the dominant title, some believe that the term *assistant* is demeaning and inconsistent with the level of responsibility and autonomy involved in the role. They argue that the term leaves the impression that PAs are mere helpers or auxiliary personnel who facilitate the work of their superior or function in a subordinate position. Inclusion of the word *assistant* leads people to draw parallels with medical assistants and nurses' aides.

Another argument for changing the title is that it does not accurately describe what PAs do. The scope of medical services and the level of care that PAs provide go beyond assisting physicians. In many underserved areas, PAs are the main primary providers of health care. Even if the term at one time appropriately described PA practice, it is no longer accurate. The AAPA describes PAs as "practicing medicine with physician supervision."

A third point made by advocates for change is that the title is not readily understood. The word *assistant* implies entry-level knowledge, on-the-job training, or trade school education. Confusion of physician assistant with medical assistant is, to PAs, an insulting and demeaning confusion. It fails to reflect PAs' substantial clinical and didactic education and the fact that many have earned graduate degrees (Mastrangelo, 1993). Patients may be confused and may sometimes ask when the PA plans to attend medical school. Other healthcare providers such as nurses resist taking orders from PAs because they do not understand the PA's role, although that is now an increasingly uncommon occurrence. The title—although not universally recognized and understood, which leads to problems with insurers, employers, and others—is now familiar to most individuals in the healthcare sector and the public. A 2008 public opinion poll conducted by the AAPA revealed that two-thirds of all Americans were familiar with (had heard of) the PA.

Proponents of a name change tend to favor the term *physician associate* because they believe it more accurately reflects the PA–physician relationship, avoids comparison with medical assistants, and is less confusing to the public. In other parts of the world *doctors' assistants* and *physician's assistants* are well-defined terms for people who support general practitioners (Fischer, 1995). Advocates point to the change from *Medex* to *PA* that occurred easily and say a change could occur again, given the relative simplicity of changing the word from *assistant* to *associate*. Other suggestions include the terms *medical practitioner, physician practitioner, clinical practitioner, assistant physician, clinical associate*, and *associative physician*.

Defenders of the title *PA* argue that replacing the term *assistant* with *associate* does not guarantee greater respect. Respect and self-esteem are gained by practicing with excellence and skill and by providing the best possible medical care to patients. These defenders find little or no dissatisfaction with the current title. For them, the title correctly conveys the dependent nature of the relationship with their supervising physician.

For some, the issue is one of semantics. Clerks and telemarketers may be called *sales associates*, whereas high government officials hold the title *special assistant to the president*; in academics, assistant professors are still referred to as *professors*. Supporters of the current name say that time and growth, not a new name, will produce more recognition. The lack of universal recognition occurs because the profession is small and has a relatively brief history, but this situation is changing. The profession has already made an enormous investment in educating the patients and the public about the true meaning of the title *PA*. State laws define the qualifications of those who use a particular title, and once the profession abandons the title *PA*, it could be awarded to another category of healthcare provider, such as unlicensed medical graduates (Anthony, 2000; Cornell, 1998).

Another important observation is that the laws of all legislative jurisdictions and the federal government could not be changed simultaneously. A period of years would pass during which many different individuals would reap the benefits achieved by the PA profession by assuming the name and calling themselves PAs. In addition to the changes required by the state legislatures, licensing boards, and the federal government, other agencies would be required to make changes. Educational institutions, state and national PA organizations, and the accrediting and certifying agencies would need to be persuaded to change. Many of these organizations would have to bear significant administrative and financial costs to make the change.

The argument most strongly expressed by opponents of change is that this debate draws time and effort away from issues that demand urgent attention. The PA profession is at a crossroads and is faced with unprecedented opportunities to define and influence its future. The name has been adopted in some countries; in others, a euphemism for PA has been derided. The options are varied. One observer says, "it is time for PAs to dedicate themselves to achieving the greatest benefit for the greatest number of people by becoming advocates for health promotion and preventive medicine" (Tiger, 1993).

Physician Assistant-Certified

U.S. PAs who have passed the Physician Assistant National Certification Examination (PANCE) have the option of putting the word *certified* behind the title *PA: PA-certified* (PA-C). The intent of using *PA-C* is to distinguish formally trained PAs who are nationally certified from PAs who are informally trained and not eligible to sit for the PANCE. In the 1970s and 1980s this distinction was thought to be important because the percentage of noncertified PAs was small but significant, and formally trained PAs felt they should have some way to show the public the difference. It is not recognized across all states and is considered superfluous by some. But by 2008, the designation *PA-C* has become commonplace and reflects the fact that well over 90% of practicing PAs hold active certification through the NCCPA. Yet, as the profession becomes global this designation is likely to be cast aside.

Many PA observers feel that the identification of *PA-C* is unnecessary and probably confuses more people than it reassures. It is simply an indication that one has passed a test, a fact known for the most part only by the profession. The accomplishment is debatable and pales in light of other more commonly recognized letters such as *MPH*, *PhD*, and *MBA*. Adding additional letters such as *R* for *registered*, as in *RPA-C*, which is done in New York, tends to confuse people even further. The *R* in this instance means that the PA has registered with a New York state health regulatory agency. Physicians must be licensed but do not place initials after *MD* or *DO* (e.g., *MD-L*). Nurses who have passed their boards do not use *RN-B* (Begely, 1993). If other countries adopt the term *PA*, as has Canada, the certified portion may become more divisive than intended.

Generic Terms for Nonphysician Providers

One of the more confusing evolutions of names has been the effort on the part of health services workers and medical sociologists to develop a generic term that encompasses PAs and other workers who fill traditional physician roles, such as NPs and certified nurse-midwives (CNMs). One term used in the early 1970s was *new health professionals*. Once this was the most frequently used term for PAs and NPs. Other terms that came into vogue were *physician extenders* and *midlevel practitioners*. These terms were never defined and remain largely meaningless: midlevel between whom?

What does it mean to extend a physician? Another term carelessly used is *allied health. Allied health providers* is a term used rather restrictively to indicate only those occupations that are allied with the medical profession through their cooperative scheme of accreditation and certification organizations. This term has a fairly precise definition and is usually reserved for those occupations that support physician services, such as x-ray technicians, physical therapists, and medical laboratory personnel. Most in the PA profession are uncomfortable being lumped under the umbrella terms of allied health professionals. Nurses are in an occupation that is not considered part of allied health personnel, so it is not appropriate to refer to advanced practice nurses such as NPs and CNMs as allied health, and it is not appropriate to refer to PAs as allied health.

One attempt to encompass both PAs and NPs has been the advancement of the term *affiliated clinician.* It was suggested that somehow the two professions, PAs and NPs, should merge under one title (Mittman, 1995). Not unlike the term *affiliated staff* used at Group Health Cooperative in Seattle, this effort was to counter the otherwise seemingly negative-sounding term *nonphysician provider.* The response from readers to an editorial in *Clinician Reviews* on the term *affiliate clinician* was one of disapproval. The term *nonphysician provider* was introduced in 1988 in the public health literature and seems to have been largely adopted and used by medical sociologists and the federal government. More recently, *nonphysician clinician* (NPC) has emerged in the health services research literature (Cooper, Hendersen, & Dietrich, 1998; Cooper, Laud, & Dietrich, 1998; Mullan & Frehywot, 2007). For now, the easiest practice seems to be to use the terms *PAs* and *NPs* and to leave the search for a generic term for another time.

THE EVOLVING ROLE

During the formative years of the PA profession, many arguments were put forth about why this new health occupation was not needed or would fail. Among these arguments was the idea that PAs would be frustrated in their role and leave the field for greener pastures. The source of frustration envisioned by these critics was the stress and strain of being an "almost doctor" without the intrinsic or extrinsic rewards that our society provides for physicians. For others, the intrinsic rewards of professional autonomy in clinical practice would not be available because of the need for close supervision by a physician (Perry, 1989).

For more than four decades the PA occupation has helped to fill a health sector niche with highly skilled professionals. These clinicians are capable of carrying out responsibilities that in the past had been within the physician's domain. Given the degree of formal training involved, the PA profession offers highly challenging and satisfying work.

Job Satisfaction

The demand in the medical sector for PAs continues to exceed the available supply, and this demand has been unabated for more than 20 years (Cawley, 2000; Hooker, 1997). The legal and bureaucratic obstacles preventing a broader scope of responsibilities in diagnosis and treatment have largely been overcome during the first two decades. The initial view held by some that PAs would be frustrated because of a narrow and limited professional role is now untenable. The intrinsic rewards are there, and the job satisfaction of PAs remains high.

A career as a PA is an attractive alternative to the years of competition, pressure, long hours, and expense required to enter and complete medical school and to finish residency training. Even 30 years ago it was recognized that "The career as a PA is also an alternative to the narrower scope of work and lower pay available to the nursing profession" (Perry, 1989).

PAs have the responsibility and independence most could reasonably expect. Role frustration is certainly present but does not appear to be a dominant problem (Freeborn & Hooker, 1995). Although salary levels and career advancement opportunities may be less than optimal, they are certainly not problematic enough to cause a significant exodus from the PA profession. There is a greater demand for graduates of PA programs than there are applicants entering the PA training programs (Rubeck et al, 2007).

In the first decade of the PA movement (1965 to 1975), there was considerable interest in exploring the characteristics of this new healthcare profession. As the profession matures, we expect to see renewed vigor for research that will shed new light on our understanding of this group of highly motivated, well-trained, compassionate healthcare providers. This work is expected to emerge from concentrated efforts around the world. Such research should help the PA profession to become an even more dynamic force in the improvement of the quality and availability of health care for all people.

Qualification for Practice and Legal Parameters

Federal, state, and provincial medical practice statutes and regulations define the scope of practice activities, delineate the range of diagnostic and patient management tasks permitted, and set standards for professional conduct. Qualification for entry to practice as a PA in most areas requires that individuals possess a fairly uniform set of characteristics. These requirements usually include a certificate of completion verifying graduation from a PA educational program accredited by some national body and/or proof of having sat for and obtained a passing score on a national examination. In the United States, the PANCE is a standardized test of competence in primary care medicine administered annually by the NCCPA and is assembled and scored through the National Board of Medical Examiners.

The clinical professional activities and scope of practice of PAs are regulated by federal, state, and provincial licensing boards, which are typically boards of medicine but in some instances comprise a separate PA licensing board. The PA profession appears to be comfortable with its dependent practice role and has not wavered in that stance since its inception. In contrast, NPs have articulated a position of practice independent from physicians. Statements by professional nursing organizations have stirred debate with physician groups on the national level regarding the turf of primary care and related legal practice barriers and regulations. Although NPs are professionally autonomous in the performance of nursing care functions, most state medical and nursing practice regulations require that NPs work in collaboration with a physician practice, recognizing that their extended roles encompass medical diagnostic and therapeutic tasks. Thus, in providing medical care tasks, most NPs work closely with physicians in a majority of clinical settings.

In contrast, the legal basis of PA practice is centered on physician supervision. Doctors are ultimately responsible for the actions of the PAs, and state laws typically require that physicians clearly delineate the practice scope and supervisory arrangements of employed PAs. However, wide latitude exists within the physician's practice for the PA to exercise levels of judgment and professional autonomy in medical care decisions.

It has been noted that the level of acceptance and integration of PAs in American medicine is related to the profession's continued adherence to this position and to the PA's willingness to practice in settings, locations, and clinical care areas that physicians deem to be less preferable. Observers believe that PA use will continue as long as it extends the medical care services of physicians without competing for or challenging physician authority and autonomy.

PHYSICIAN ASSISTANTS: POLICY AND PRACTICE—THE BOOK

This book is written by and for PAs. It is also written for academics, scholars, policy analysts, historians, sociologists, economists, and students—to name a few. It is written with one foot firmly planted in the historical development and the other in the future of this novel profession. Because the authors wear the hats of academics, analysts, historians,

PAs, futurists, and lifetime learners, this book is molded for the global audience of today and tomorrow. Finally, the authors hope that PA students and their faculties find this book useful in pursuing medical workforce and organizational research.

The chapters of the book are written as stand-alone reports, and each can be referenced separately. At the same time, each chapter follows the other in a logical manner. This book was written to be fluid and subject to modifications and change; recognizing that the moment it was published it was outdated.

Chapter 1: Introduction and Overview of the Profession

The introduction is an overview of PAs and sets the stage for all other chapters to unfold. It prepares the reader for the rest of the book and offers some navigating tips. Even if you read no other chapter, you will still have a sense of what this book intends to reveal.

Chapter 2: Development of the Profession

All entities have a beginning; this entity is no exception. The historical roots of the PA profession are recorded with an eye on preserving it. For this endeavor, the authors identified the national and sociocultural trends that led to the emergence of the PA profession in the United States and elsewhere.

Chapter 3: Current Status: A Profile of the Physician Assistant Profession

This chapter provides a broad update and overview of the contemporary PA profession, including where PAs work, what they do, how well they do it, and how they are part of financing policies, the public domain, and private enterprises.

Chapter 4: Entry-Level Physician Assistant Education

The origins of PA education and its evolution are detailed in this chapter. Creative use of the classroom and the effectiveness of curricula set the stage for the deployment strategies

used for PAs. A major practice role for the PA has been—and continues to be—primary care; the educational origins of this philosophy are probed. A profile of PA programs, students, graduates, and faculty is included.

Chapter 5: Postgraduate Physician Assistant Education Programs

One of the educational evolutions in the PA profession is the development of postgraduate training programs. Seen originally as a means for addressing a shortage of skilled and economical labor in hospitals, the development of dozens of specialized residencies and fellowships for PAs has slowly emerged as an educational pathway for some PAs.

Chapter 6: Physician Assistants in Primary Care

Chapter 6 examines the bedrock of PA practice: primary care. The United States and most other coutries have selected primary care as the foundation for PA education. It is the generalist model that is largely thought to be one of the key factors for their success. We describe PAs' accomplishments and activities in various primary care settings.

Chapter 7: Physician Assistant Specialization: Nonprimary Care

After four decades of role delineation, the PA is slowly evolving away from primary care and into nonprimary care roles. The diversity of roles is as broad as the types of doctors today. Most of the major specialities and subspecialities are examined.

Chapter 8: Physician Assistants in Hospital Settings

Another key practice area for PAs is in the hospital setting. This chapter describes the multiple roles that continue to evolve for PAs in inpatient settings in the United States, the Netherlands, and elsewhere.

Chapter 9: Physician Assistants in Rural Health

All countries have populations that live outside urban areas. Many define these areas as rural. The authors created a chapter for this body of knowledge knowing that PAs are providing care in underserved and rural areas throughout the world.

Chapter 10: Other Professional Roles for Physician Assistants

Whereas most PAs work as clinicians, a number of PAs have elected to direct their careers toward nonclinical areas. This growing assortment of occupations and subfields continues to expand as PAs seek to use their training in areas related to medicine, such as management, publishing, politics, and the law. PAs are managers, directors, professors, researchers, chief executive officers, and entrepreneurs. For many, being a PA serves as a springboard or provides the credentials needed to function outside a clinically defined role.

Chapter 11: Economic Assessment of Physician Assistants

If PAs were not, in part, an economical alternative to doctors, then they probably would not survive. How they produce an economic benefit through efficient educational strategies are important aspects to PA development and success.

Chapter 12: Physician Assistant Professional Relationships

Like politics, relationships with other professional entities would be untenable if not cultured and nurtured. These relationships start with patients and include doctors, nurses, pharmacists, and organized medicine. PAs have developed special relationships with physicians in certain specialties, such as family medicine, and have a history with other groups, such as international medical graduates and NPs.

Chapter 13: Legislation and Policy

The legal basis of the PA profession in the United States is grounded in practice and codified in laws. Such laws that address the conduct of doctors and other health professionals are evolutionary and their historical roots are anchored over a period of 100 years.

This body of laws spells out what a doctor may do and to whom he or she may delegate medical authority. All 50 states enable PAs to work, to prescribe, and to be reimbursed for their services. That accomplishment came about through legal activism, concern for public safety, coordinated political action, and professionalism.

Chapter 14: Legal Issues of Physician Assistant Practice

One of the primary aspects of using PAs is supervision. State, provincial, and federal systems have put into place regulatory and contractual arrangements in which a doctor is obligated to properly supervise the PA. This chapter discusses the legal basis of and liabilities involved in PA practice. Common legal issues, such as malpractice and tort reform, are also addressed.

As the PA profession developed, the U.S. legal system has needed to address this type of healthcare provider.

Chapter 15: Professional and Workforce Issues

Issues related to the professional practice of medicine as a PA and the practice dynamics associated with the workforce tend to shape policy and governance. Factors that impact the culture and environment of the PA's practice have the potential to influence core issues such as job satisfaction, scope of practice, and role delineation. Although these professional and workforce issues may be viewed as peripheral to the clinical practice of medicine, they do influence the behavior of PAs.

Chapter 16: Physician Assistant Professional Organizations

In this chapter we describe the major organizations that represent PAs. Reflecting the brisk growth in size and scope of the PA profession, the major PA organizations are identified as playing separate, distinct, and important public roles in the advancement of the profession.

Chapter 17: Physician Assistants in the Federal Workforce

PAs employed in federal service are a growing and important entity as the United States moves toward a greater national role in healthcare service delivery. There are deep military roots in the PA profession, and their presence remains strong in the traditional uniformed branches. Moreover, there has been expansion and increased recognition of PAs in other areas of federal services, such as the Bureau of Prisons, the Department of State, and the Department of Transportation.

Chapter 18: Global Expansion of the Physician Assistant Concept

The PA is no longer an American product, and the world has improved on this entity. This chapter examines where the PA profession is occurring. It is a global undertaking and the countries with PAs are described. In addition to those with PAs, many countries have nonphysician clinicians that are emerging as PAs.

Chapter 19: Future Directions of the Physician Assistant Profession

In the concluding chapter, we gaze into the future and analyze the likely trends and forces that will influence the future direction of PAs.

Appendices

The expansion of this section reflects the need for this book to serve as a directory and reference for vital documents about PAs.

SUMMARY

For over 40 years there has been continual evolution and enlargement of the PA, both in development and role. As for employment, the 15-year future appears rewarding for new graduates of this profession. What pitfalls the distant future contains can be anticipated but only to a limited degree. A worldwide shortage of doctors and medical schools portends permanent shortages for two-thirds of the globe. This book begins with an overview of what has occured and ends with what the future holds. The authors have tried to be broad in their vision and seek scholarly views to be informative and produce the most contemporary information about this novel movement. However, they suffer the frailties of being human and encumbered with inherent biases. It is hoped that this book makes a small contribution to the scholarship of a new labor body. The PA profession is a lively one that could not have been foreseen even a few years ago; we are privileged viewers.

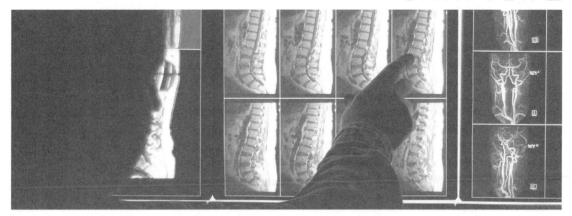

CHAPTER 2

DEVELOPMENT OF THE PROFESSION

JAMES F. CAWLEY ■ RODERICK S. HOOKER ■ DAVID P. ASPREY

ABSTRACT

The history of the physician assistant (PA) involves a series of events that eventually gave rise to the model of today. Early prototype PAs included the barber surgeon's assistant and the *feldsher*, who marched with Peter the Great in Russia in 1650. This model was followed by the *officier de santé* in 19th century France, the *practicante* of Puerto Rico, and later, the American Hospital Corpsman/Medic of the Vietnam War—the inspiration for the modern PA. Other examples abound. The development of the PA profession was not happenstance. The combination of charismatic leaders, cataclysmic events of a society seeking to redress the injustice of centuries, the fading presence of the generalist doctor, and medical care shortages produced an assistant who could reliably and safely function as an extension of the doctor. No one person is credited with this movement; instead, several experiments arose almost simultaneously, survived, merged, and prospered. From this epoch a series of planners and leaders helped to solidify the profession. What follows discusses the various eras of the PA movement, from the first tenuous early experiments to the globalization of the PA profession.

INTRODUCTION

When physician assistants (PAs) were introduced into medical practice in the United States in the 1960s, the major expectation was to create a new type of clinician to assist physicians because of evolving changes in the medical practice environment. Most observers of the health system held the perception that there was a shortage of doctors. An exacerbating factor was the demise of the general practitioner and the rise of the specialist physician. Organized around and continuously engaged in the early development of the PA profession, these elements combined to prompt their introduction as an appropriate, timely, and useful strategy for improving health care in underserved communities. The PA was envisioned as a new type of medical generalist, one whose role could build on prior medical background and experience, one who could be trained in a reasonably short period, and one who could be rapidly deployed to practice locations in medically needy areas.

The idea of using practitioners who are not physicians to provide medical care in a health system is far from new. Doctors have informally and formally trained and used a wide range of assistants and associates throughout the history of medicine. Over the past two centuries, healthcare providers who were not physicians, or *nonphysician clinicians* (a modern term), have and continue to play important roles in meeting medical service needs in many nations (Roemer, 1977; Terris, 1977; Mullan & Frehywot, 2007).

Circumstances leading to the need for new types of health workers include sociocultural changes such as an undersupply or maldistribution of doctors. These circumstances prompt societal reassessment of the roles of physicians and other providers. The use of nonphysician health professionals has been shown to be an effective health workforce measure in improving medical care delivery in the health systems of several countries in the 20th century (Rousselot, Beard, & Berrey, 1971; Storey & Roth, 1971; Roemer, 1977). In fact, the nonphysician clinician concept appears to have achieved global recognition with the institution of PAs and nurse practitioners (NPs) in the health systems of many nations by the first decade of the 21st century (Cawley & Hooker, 2003).

The development of various types of healthcare professionals and occupations is an ever-evolving phenomenon in most societies' health systems. However, in the 20th century, the medical systems of most countries typically regarded physicians (those who hold the MD, DO, or MBBS degrees) as the "captains of the ship." For many, the status of doctors is thought of as the "gold standard" among healthcare professionals. Because nonphysician clinicians are assuming increasing medical practice roles similar to doctors, the two roles often overlap considerably.

The development of nonphysician clinicians occurred in several countries after times of turmoil, such as war and revolution. In some parts of the world, nonphysician clinicians have established well-accepted niches in the health system. Since the mid-1960s, two new types of nonphysician professions (PAs and NPs) have emerged in the United States and a third reemerged (nurse-midwives). These new roles involve a broad range of medical practice activities and varying levels of autonomy. In this chapter, we describe the forces that led to the creation and development of the PA profession over the past half century.

Creation of New Healthcare Providers

Broadly speaking, nonphysicians have fewer years of formal training than physicians, may have a regulated or physician-linked practice status, and may have roles largely defined by technology. In the case of PAs, a key rationale was to create providers who could supplement and extend the delivery of medical services in a typical doctor's office. The clinical roles of PAs were founded on a strong base of medical-model education, but also include perspectives imported from other health paradigms and disciplines. As a result, PA practice may not merely be substitutive of physician functions but may be expanded to encompass services that may be termed *physician complementary*, for example, health and medical services not performed by physicians.

The developmental experience of the PA in American medicine is in many ways unique, but with similarities to nonphysicians used in other countries and in other eras. International experience with clinicians who are not doctors parallels the formation of the PA and within the new century is expanding in other countries. In analyzing the emergence of the PA, it is instructive to note the characteristics, natural history, and experiences of nonphysicians in the United States as well as other countries.

PREDECESSORS OF PHYSICIAN ASSISTANTS

For centuries, and all over the world, individuals who are not fully trained doctors have been involved in the delivery of medical care. Known by various names, given differing clinical prerogatives by societies, and discharging different functions, these types of care providers play important roles in delivery systems, often in primary care. For the most part, nonphysician providers and their functions are a product of the systems and nations that have fostered their development and incorporated their roles (Golden & Cawley, 1983; Hooker, Hogan, & Leeker, 2007; Mullan & Frehywot, 2007).

Whereas the role of doctor as chief minister to the person who is ill has existed since time immemorial, the role of the physician is a more recent incarnation. In the United States, physicians were in practice in colonial times; some were better trained than others. By the mid-1800s, the establishment of the U.S. medical profession was based on a profound European influence in training and role, the incorporation of newly developing scientific advancements, and a propensity to exert political and economic strength to define and protect professional prerogatives (Starr, 1982). During the last part of the 1800s, a number of rivals popular with patients competed with allopathic physicians for acceptance and legal recognition (e.g., osteopathy, homeopathy, chiropractic, and naturopathy). Allopathic physicians prevailed based largely on adherence to a philosophical and scientific approach and their ability to convince state regulatory boards to grant them authority to perform medical diagnosis and treatment, commonly as the sole authority.

In the early part of the 20th century, physicians commonly trained assistants at various levels and used them in their practices. One of the earliest documented descriptions was written by George Crile, a surgeon at the Cleveland Clinic, who described the "world's first physician assistant," an informally trained surgical provider in urology working at that institution during the 1930s and 1940s (Crile, 1987). The activities of his assistant would be a role model for a urology PA today.

Another predecessor of PAs was the surgical laboratory assistant, Vivian Thomas, who for decades helped the famous Hopkins' surgeon Alfred Blalock. Thomas worked closely with Blalock in perfecting techniques of open-heart surgery and training several generations of world-class cardiovascular surgeons. Blalock worked in the operating room and

clinics and Thomas supervised the surgical laboratories. Thomas was a major contributor in the development of operative techniques and the design of surgical equipment, and he supervised the surgical laboratories at Hopkins for more than 35 years. In 1976, he was appointed instructor in surgery at the Johns Hopkins University School of Medicine, and in 1979, upon his retirement, he became instructor emeritus of surgery. In 1976, he was awarded the honorary doctorate by the Johns Hopkins University (Thomas, 1997).

These predecessors are examples of healthcare providers who performed medical and surgical tasks that in some societies were exclusively in the domain of physicians. Such tasks include performing physical examinations, diagnosing common illnesses, performing minor surgical procedures, and knowing and dispensing basic medications. Countries in Africa, Asia, Oceania, and North, South, and Central America continue to employ these types of providers mainly to increase healthcare delivery to poorly served regions (Mullan & Frehywot, 2007).

Various objectives underlie strategies to incorporate nonphysicians into medical systems: the need for general health care, the need for medical assistance in times of doctor shortages, and the need for trained personnel to staff developing technology (Fulop & Roemer, 1982). Sometimes the incorporation of nonphysicians into a nation's healthcare system appears to be connected to social strife, and a type of healthcare provider emerges to fill specific health workforce policies (Exhibit 2-1) (Cawley & Golden, 1983).

Loblolly Boys

The roots of the contemporary PA movement are in the military. What is underappreciated about this history is that the PA-military connection dates to the 18th century. A Navy rating, or specialty, was established in 1799 when an Act of Congress mandated that all Navy ships provide an area where sick and injured men could be brought to and cared for by other crew members. The term *loblolly boy* was mentioned for the first time in Navy regulations

EXHIBIT 2-1
Nonphysician Clinicians in Select Countries*

Name	Country	Time
Midwife	Universal	More than 10,000 years ago to present
Feldsher	Russia, Eastern Europe	1600s–present
Officier de santé	France	1803–1892
Behdars	Iran	Early 1900s
Practicante	Puerto Rico	1866–1931
Apothecaries	Ceylon	1900s
Assistant medical officer	Oceania, Tanzania	1950–1998
Clinical assistant	Kenya, elsewhere	1900s
Nurse-midwife	United States, Europe, others	1900–present
Village health worker	Developing countries, Alaska	1940–present
Barefoot doctor	China	1966–present
Physician assistant	United States, Canada, the Netherlands, Australia, South Africa, Taiwan, Great Britain	1965–present
Nurse practitioner	United States, Canada, Great Britain, Australia	1966–present
Community health technician	Colombia, Mexico, Peru, Guyana	1970s

*Many names denote healthcare workers who were modeled after the barefoot doctor. These nonphysician providers were introduced and promoted by the World Health Organization in many developing countries: dresser, medical auxiliary, health assistant, paramedic, medical aide, assistant medical officer, me'dicin Africain, and rural health technician.

in 1814. These individuals were crewmembers who were assigned to carry gruel to the sick sailors aboard ship and to assist the ship's surgeon when needed. John Wall was the first U.S. loblolly boy on record. He signed aboard the USS Constellation on June 1, 1798.

Many duties associated with the loblolly boy were considered bleak but nonetheless had to be carried out in preparation for battle. The loblolly boy had to provide the cockpit with empty containers to collect amputated limbs and provide containers of coal to heat tar, which was used to cauterize. These usually elderly sailors also provided the surgeon with buckets of sand to ensure that the surgeon did not slip on blood while trying to perform his duties. They were also expected ". . . to do anything and everything that was required—from sweeping and washing the deck and saying 'amen' to the chaplain, down to cleaning the guns and helping the surgeon to make pills and plasters and to mix medicine" ("Loblolly boys," 2004; "History of the navy corpsman," 2006).

The *surgeon's steward* replaced the loblolly boy in 1842. This enlisted rate for this new

position was first seen on Navy pay charts in 1841. Surgeon's stewards, like loblolly boys, served on large ships and were trained in basic medicine. However, they were more capable of providing support to the surgeons than loblolly boys. The Department of the Navy changed the term once more in 1842, deciding that surgeon's stewards should be called *apothecaries*.

In 1898, President William McKinley signed a bill into law establishing the Hospital Corps as a recognized member of the Medical Department. With the passage of this bill, the designation of *apothecary* changed to *hospital steward*, (Chief Petty Officer), a *hospital apprentice first class*, (Hospital Corpsman Third Class) and finally, a *hospital corpsman apprentice* (Weiner, 2006).

Frontier Nursing Service

Founded in 1925 by Mary Breckinridge, the Frontier Nursing Service (FNS) began as a demonstration project and used nurse-midwives to provide needed maternal and child health care in rural areas of Kentucky.

Breckinridge decided, following the death of her two children, to devote her life to the health care of children in remote areas. She acquired her basic nursing education at St. Luke's Hospital in New York City, and then served as a volunteer with the American Committee for Devastated France following World War I. It was in France that Mrs. Breckinridge met a British nurse who was also a midwife and realized that the nurse-midwife had unique qualifications for work in rural, medically underserved areas. Breckinridge studied midwifery at the British Hospital for Mothers and Babies in London and spent some time with the Highlands and Islands Medical and Nursing Service in Scotland to observe the kind of decentralized health care that would become the model for the FNS. After the war, Breckinridge studied public health nursing at Columbia University, where she formulated two goals: improving the health of children and pioneering a system of rural health care that could serve as a model for healthcare systems serving the most remote regions of the world.

When the FNS was founded, the nurse-midwifery profession was not established in the United States, so the service employed British nurses who were already qualified as midwives. Additionally, American nurses were sent to Great Britain for graduate training. When World War II began, however, a number of the British members of the FNS staff returned home, and it was no longer possible to send American nurses to Great Britain for training. In response to these events, the Frontier Graduate School of Midwifery was established in 1939. The school has been in continuous operation since that time. As part of its legacy, it has graduated more than 1,700 nurse-midwives and family nurse practitioners.

In the late 1960s, when nursing roles began to expand, the FNS developed the first certificate program to prepare family NPs. In 1970, the name of the school was changed to the Frontier School of Midwifery and Family Nursing (FSMFN). This program existed until 1990. The Community-Based Family Nurse Practitioner (CFNP) education program was reestablished in 1999 and grants MSN degrees using a distance education model (see the website of the Frontier Nursing Service: http://www.frontiernursing.org/History/HowFNSbegan.shtm).

Practicante

Puerto Rico had a PA prototype called a *practicante*. As recently as the first half of the 20th century, Puerto Rico had many isolated areas that were difficult to reach because of a lack of roads. Care of the poor fell to another type of provider who worked under the auspices of physicians—the practicante. During the period when Puerto Rico was a colony of Spain, in 1866 the practicante was authorized. Practicante duties included making diagnoses, providing treatment, suturing wounds, and setting fractures. Major practicantes had responsibilities to "minor practicantes" and, in turn, both reported to doctors who were located in urban areas. The *Practicante Manual* empowered the practicante to ". . . treat the sick and injured as soon as they arrive at the hospital and if the [level of injury] requires it, involving the surgeon by notifying him of the diagnosis and treatment you have provided" (Strand, 2006).

The practicante continued to exist after the U.S. government took over the country (and the regulation of medicine) in 1899, but the position was phased out in 1931. In 1945, a law establishing a role of *surgical technical auxiliary* (surgical technician) was created, which subsumed some aspects of the practicante's scope of practice (Strand, 2006).

France: The Officier de Santé

In 1803, shortly after the French Revolution, the scientist and educator René Fourcroy submitted a report to the legislature outlining plans for a major reorganization of the French medical care system. Among his proposals was the creation of a new independent grade of health officers who would help alleviate healthcare personnel shortages in the military and the civilian sector, particularly in rural areas. These providers were called *officiers de santé* (health officers).

Qualifications for the grade of officier de santé in the French healthcare system required a 6-year apprenticeship with a physician, a 5-year period either in a hospital, or 3 years in medical school. To fully qualify as a physician, one had to complete 6 years of medical school. The officiers de santé had a far-reaching independent but ultimately limited scope of practice. They could not perform major operations, but they could suture, perform minor surgical procedures, prescribe medications, and practice medicine to a large degree on an independent basis. For activities within their practice scope, officiers de santé were legally liable for malpractice. In Flaubert's classic novel, *Madame Bovary,* the heroine's husband Charles was an officier de santé.

The practice of officiers de santé stirred substantial opposition from physicians. The officiers de santé came under attack from the medical profession soon after their inception and remained so almost constantly until their abolition in 1892. As French social, medical, and economic conditions improved throughout the 19th century, opposition to the officier de santé created a clamor from physicians to reestablish a single qualifying degree in medicine. The argument of the entrenched doctors to the French legislature was bolstered by the reluctance of officiers to practice in rural areas. The grade of officier was attacked by physicians as sustaining "second-class practitioners" and after 1850 was considered by French physicians to have outlived its usefulness. After several legislative measures had reduced their practice privileges, officiers de santé were abolished in 1892. The introduction of second-class practitioners who were "good enough for the troops and the country folk" had not fulfilled the original expectations. In the end, it had done little to remedy the maldistribution of medical care between town and country. The problem of this imbalance is still with us today, affecting developed and developing countries alike in varying degree (Heller, 1978).

Russia: Feldshers

The *feldsher,* historically, represented a link between the eras of folk cures and modern medicine. Originally, feldsher was the name for medieval barber-surgeons who were German military assistants to the barber-surgeons of the 17th century. They worked as army field surgeons for the German and Swiss Landsknecht until real military medical services were established by Prussia in the early 18th century. The term was then exported with Prussian officers and nobility to Russia.

Following military service, early feldshers served as civilian clinicians and, in many cases, were the only available providers for the rural peasant population. Typically, they were apprenticed to doctors for some time and provided low-cost health care for much of the Russian countryside well into the 20th century (Sidel, 1968; Sidel, 1969; Sidel, 1972).

For many years, feldshers were used by the armies of several eastern European countries, but eventually more highly trained personnel replaced them. In pre–Soviet Russia and throughout the existence of the Soviet Union, feldshers were used as primary care providers, mainly in rural areas. In these settings, they were commonly the only type of trained medical personnel available and typically functioned in a semi-independent manner (Knaus, 1981; Storey & Roth, 1971).

For a time after the 1917 Bolshevik Revolution, it was determined that each Soviet citizen should be treated by his or her own physician. The concept of *feldsherism* was considered second-class medicine and a short-term solution to health personnel strategies. As the years went by, feldshers retained their role as the enormity of the healthcare needs of the newly formed Soviet Union, then the largest country in the world, became apparent. In 1936, the Soviet government reinstituted formal training for feldshers, and by the mid-1970s, Russia was training approximately 30,000 feldshers annually (Condit, 1977).

At first, feldshers practiced in the rural and underserved regions of Russia and entrenched themselves as an important personnel link in the healthcare system: the delivery of primary care. Inevitably, as the supply of physicians began to grow in Russia, feldshers were perceived as expendable practitioners. Policymakers regarded feldshers practicing in rural areas as necessary, but only to the degree that they could be replaced by physicians (Knaus, 1981; Terris, 1977). However, an abundance of physicians did not change the distribution of medical care, and the rural areas continued to suffer limited access to health care.

The role of the feldsher is twofold: (1) as personnel serving in the urban areas as side-by-side assistants to physicians (similar to PAs and NPs in the United States), and (2) as alternatives to physicians in underserved regions. Like PAs, doctors supervise feldshers in their clinical activities when available.

At one time, an estimated 1 million feldshers were in practice (Kenyon, 1985). There have been reports that feldshers are on the wane because of the breakup of the Soviet Union and restructuring of health care in these countries. Although there may be an oversupply of physicians in several of the eastern European countries, feldshers remain a type of healthcare personnel in the healthcare systems of the former Soviet Union. They play an intermediary role in medical labor with capacities in primary medical care and the ability to assume technical and specialized roles. In the estimation of one historian, the PA profession is a "classic 'semiprofession' that is, an occupational group lacking in one or more of the traits required for society to grant full professional status. They did not have exclusive mastery of an esoteric and socially vital body of knowledge nor did they have autonomy over their own practice. By definition, they stood in the physician's shadow" (Ramer, 1996).

Although the early developers of the PA concept did not have the feldsher specifically in mind, there is some parallel between the feldsher and the American PA. With an adequate supply of doctors in the former Soviet Union, many believe the occupation of feldsher is becoming obsolete. The health systems of Russia and other countries of the former Soviet Union are now plagued by problems of too many physicians, many of them specialists, and a lack of professionalism among physicians resulting from the state-enforced breakup of professional associations. Poorly trained primary care doctors, limited inpatient and outpatient diagnostic capacity, too many hospital beds, excessive use of services (particularly inpatient care), and the obsolete and poor condition of capital stock are among the litany of problems faced by the healthcare systems of many of these countries. In 1994, the physician-to-population ratios varied from 2.1 physicians per 1,000 population in Tajikistan to 3.8 in Russia, with a six-country average of 3.3. These findings compare with an average of 2.5 in Western countries. Since 1994, these ratios have fallen slightly in all six countries except Uzbekistan. Nonetheless, the ratios throughout are still well above the European average. Because many former Soviet bloc countries have significant healthcare system problems, it is likely that the need for feldshers in some form as an adjunct to other medical personnel will remain.

Whereas a nurse's function consists mostly of comforting the patient and carrying out physician's orders, feldshers are commonly independent practitioners who are trained to perform certain diagnostic and therapeutic procedures, frequently without physician supervision. Feldshers typically receive between 1 and 3 years of medical education after graduation from secondary school. Length of training depends on the specialty the feldsher elects: general feldsher, 2 years; midwife, 2.5 years; feldsher laborer, 2 years; and sanitarian feldsher, 1 to 1.5 years. Candidates usually enter directly from secondary school. Tuition is free, stipends and living expenses are provided, and positions are guaranteed at the completion of training.

Reportedly, the upper 10% of graduate feldshers are encouraged to go on to medical school. Otherwise, they can take evening study at medical school after 3 years of clinical service.

Once admitted, these students are eligible for advanced placement. At one time as many as 25% to 30% of doctors in the former Soviet Union were initially trained as feldshers. As the number of doctors grows, feldshers may become less needed. However, in urban areas, emergency medicine is a field in which feldshers are still used (Gaufberg, 2007).

China: Barefoot Doctors

The Chinese barefoot doctor is a health worker once described as a "poor cousin of the Russian feldsher" and was overly romanticized in many quarters in the 1970s (Terris, 1977). A type of nonphysician, barefoot doctors are more like village aides than feldshers, PAs, or NPs. The levels of function and training are very basic. Armed with only 3 to 6 months of medical education, barefoot doctors were created to increase the basic level of primary care delivered to China's enormous and expanding population. Most barefoot doctors were farmers who worked in rural villages in the People's Republic of China to bring health care to rural areas where urban-trained doctors would not settle. They promoted basic hygiene, preventive health care, and family planning, and treated common illnesses.

Barefoot doctors emerged from the social cataclysm that marked the 1966 Cultural Revolution in China. During that period, drastic reductions in medical education took place under a campaign against medical and professional elitism. This anti-intellectual movement led to a massive reorganization of the system of medical education. Many medical schools were closed, with a reduction in the length of physician training and a dispersal of faculty to the rural villages. The Chinese leader Mao Ze-Dong attacked the medical status quo with a vengeance and called for the formation of a legion of primary healthcare workers based in the villages of China who, when not providing health care, would tend the rice fields (Wen & Hays, 1975). Mao's enthusiasm regarding barefoot doctors diminished the influence of the Weishengbu, China's health ministry, which was dominated by Western-trained doctors.

Barefoot doctors received less than 6 months of on-the-job training in the villages in which they would serve. Their roles were oriented to enforcing public health measures and preventing common diseases. *A Barefoot Doctor's Manual* was the guiding book for their care delivery (Exhibit 2-2).

In the ensuing years, several million barefoot doctors were trained and deployed throughout China. As the fervor of the Cultural Revolution waned, the system of medical training was restored, and China has worked steadily to rebuild its system of medical education and increase its supply of physicians (Blendon, 1979). Policy assessments of the introduction of barefoot doctors note that

EXHIBIT 2-2
A Barefoot Doctor's Manual

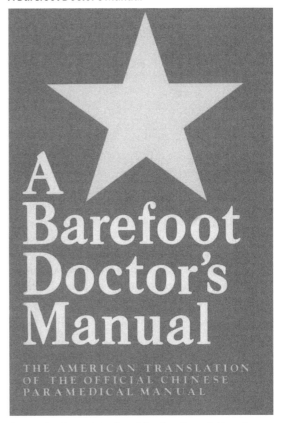

Reprinted with permission from A Barefoot Doctor's Manual, *Copyright © 1990, 2002 by Running Press Book Publishers, Philadelphia and London, http://www.runningpress.com.*

"the program has not been a panacea; the usefulness of the barefoot doctor lies in there being a stopgap measure rather than a long-term solution to the shortage of physicians." About one-fifth of the barefoot doctors later entered medical school (Hsu, 1974).

Barefoot doctors comprised a basic first tier of Chinese medicine and were the entry point to the system for peasants seeking curative services. Their numbers have declined somewhat from a high of more than 2 million in the late 1970s to about 1.2 million in 1984 (Hsiao, 1984). The roles of barefoot doctors changed as economic reforms occurred in China, resulting in a decline in the cooperative medical system. Today the barefoot doctor, a vestige of 1960s Cultural Revolution ideology, is still present, although the practice configuration has changed. In modern times, as the old Cooperative Medical System collapsed, the barefoot doctor became unemployed. They abandoned their roles in providing public health functions and turned to private, fee-for-service practice and charging for medications, which has driven up the price of drugs in China (Yuanli et al, 1995). A lack of educational or practice standards for barefoot doctors continues, and their clinical capabilities have been questioned (Blumenthal & Hsaio, 2005). This reduction in public health service coincided with economic reforms in China, resulting in a decline in the cooperative medical system, the last vestige of the Cultural Revolution ideology. Soon farmers demanded better medical services as their incomes increased, bypassing the barefoot doctors and going straight to the commune health centers or county hospitals.

Canada

For a time, Canada followed the U.S. model by promoting the development of the NP concept. Unfortunately, steady pressure from doctors over time eroded the effectiveness of NPs in the system. In the early 1980s, organized medicine in Canada effectively abolished the NP concept and the number of NPs steadily dwindled (Spitzer, 1984). However, in 2000 the NP reemerged, reviving the concept.

In 1992, Canadian Forces developed a PA role that is similar to the U.S. version. These PAs are career medical assistants who receive advance training at the Canadian military base in Borden, Ontario, and then are deployed with the various services in the Canadian Forces. As of 2008, approximately 100 PAs are in uniform and a few dozen retired military members work in the mining or oil drilling industry in remote areas and formally in Ontario. The Canada Association of Physician Assistants is in the early stages of development and actively working with the Royal College of Physicians and Surgeons and the Canadian Medical Association to determine how to best integrate into Canadian society (Hooker, MacDonald, & Patterson, 2003; Talbot, 1994). In 2008, two Canadian PA programs started, and other programs are planned. An initiative in Manitoba and Ontario to recruit and train PAs has begun in earnest. Other provinces are observing this development with interest.

Other Developed Countries

A number of other developed countries faced with the trends of increasing physician specialization and demand for primary care services have adopted different approaches in medical education to meet health workforce requirements and encourage primary care deployment. A major policy thrust in some industrialized countries has been to place limitations on the numbers of physicians who can become specialists. This fundamental determination in personnel ensures that a country's healthcare system has an adequate supply of primary care providers and precludes the need for a nonphysician provider in this role. By 2008, the PA concept was growing in Canada, the United Kingdom, Australia, South Africa, Taiwan, Liberia, and the Netherlands. Germany and Japan have expressed interest in the concept.

Nonetheless, in some countries in Europe, the use of nonphysicians to provide primary care in rural areas or similar types of healthcare providers in urban tertiary care centers is unheard of. Fully trained doctors deliver medical generalist services to most of the population and access to specialists is controlled. Roles are also expanding for advanced practice nursing such as NPs and nurse-midwives in several countries, England being the most noted.

In the medical systems of most developed countries, such as Sweden, healthcare personnel and primary care staffing are well established and planned by governments and key groups. In addition, the homogeneity of individual European countries' societies, the common belief that health care is a fundamental right, the smaller geographic areas of these nations, and the less entrepreneurial approach to health services' delivery systems are major reasons that most European countries have not adopted the nonphysician healthcare personnel concept. In Latin American countries, most healthcare systems avoid using nonphysicians of any type; some countries in Latin America, as in Europe, have an oversupply of physicians, particularly in urban areas.

Developing Countries

The incorporation of nonphysician health providers into the health system depends fundamentally on the extent of the needs of that country for medical services. In many developing countries, where the supply of physicians is lacking, various types of practitioners are employed to ensure delivery of essential primary care services such as prenatal care, immunization, and disease screening. In the latter half of the 20th century, many countries have successfully used nonphysicians, propelled by the increasing demand for healthcare services, the emphasis on primary care, and the World Health Organization (WHO) policy of "Health for All by the Year 2000" (WHO, 1980; Fulop & Roemer, 1982; WHO, 1987a; WHO, 1987b).

Throughout many countries of the world, particularly in Africa (Algeria, Sudan), Asia (Burma), South America (Venezuela), and Oceania (Micronesia, Melanesia, and Polynesia), healthcare workers were known by many different titles. These were (and in some instances still are) known as *health officers, community health aides* (CHAs), *medical auxiliaries, health assistants, village health workers, adjoint medicaux de lasante, medical assistants,* and *auxiliar de enfermeria* (Expert Committee on Professional and Technical Education of Medical and Auxillary Personnel [WHO], 1968). Historically, they provided health care in small communities and in rural areas. These healthcare providers vary greatly in their backgrounds and level of clinical function (Smith, 1978). Health workers of various sorts were present in sub-Saharan Africa during the colonial era; the British, in particular, trained health workers known as *apothecaries,* who dispensed medicines and assumed clinical duties. In Uganda, an African Native Medical Corps was formed in 1918, with training programs at the government hospital. In Kenya, beginning in the 1920s, health workers known as *dressers* and *dispensers* were trained to provide basic surgical and medical care. *Agents sanitaire* were trained in the Congo and elsewhere in French-speaking colonial Africa (Mullan & Frehywot, 2007). Some of these auxiliaries have been done away with and others converted to more contemporary nonphysician clinicians, in both title and action.

The WHO has provided leadership in health personnel activities in developing countries with the aim of improving primary care and other basic healthcare services. In the 1980s, a major WHO objective in healthcare personnel was total population coverage for healthcare services. Only a rapid expansion of programs incorporating use of multipurpose auxiliary healthcare personnel would help developing countries achieve this goal (Fulop & Roemer, 1982; Storms & Fox, 1979; WHO, 1980; WHO, 1987b).

The Pan American Health Organization has promoted other types of providers with roles similar to those of PAs. Peru trains and approves healthcare providers with professional status; this training is provided by a specialized high school education leading to a bachelor's degree in health (Acuna, 1977a; Acuna, 1977b). In the 1970s, Colombia and Mexico started several experimental training programs for community health technicians—with components of clinical and preventive medicine, public health, and community practice—that involved postsecondary education. The modalities may vary, but the principle of incorporating the PA in the healthcare team was gaining acceptance (Acuna, 1977a).

In the 1970s, Guyana took a further step by approving the training of a full-fledged PA with characteristics and functions similar to those of the U.S. version. Experience there has attracted the interest of neighboring countries (Acuna, 1977a). More recently, Mullan has documented the rather extensive number of nonphysician healthcare workers that make up the health workforce in a large number of countries in Africa (Mullan & Frehywot, 2007). Most of these workers are not comparable to American PAs with regard to their length of training and level of function.

FELDSHERISM AS A WORKFORCE POLICY

Public health activist and physician Victor Sidel (1968, 1972) wrote several important papers on the use of nonphysicians in various countries. These articles reflected the then widespread medical interest in new types of healthcare providers and in experiments with new forms of the division of medical labor. He used the term *feldsherism* to denote a country's policy of using clinicians who are not doctors to provide primary care health services (Sidel, 1968). Many countries have used the feldsherism policy as a strategy to deal with personnel shortages, particularly when healthcare needs are great and physicians are in short supply. The acceptance of feldsherism depends in large part on the system of healthcare organization and the needs of the population. In developing countries, increasing the numbers of primary care workers is essential (Smith & Hendersen-Andrade, 2006); their level of skill in areas of high technology may be irrelevant. Most needed are providers who can deliver basic health services referent to the acute needs of the populations of these countries, and not the advanced skills of the physician. Specifically, clinicians with knowledge of

infectious diseases and their treatment, immunization, fluid-replacement therapy, prenatal care, cancer screening, surgical and orthopedic procedures, and health education regarding environmental health hazards are essential in providing healthcare services to these populations (WHO, 1987a; WHO, 1987b).

In developed countries generalist doctors, rather than nonphysicians, are the principal providers of primary care. Roemer (1977) notes that this was the prevailing personnel policy in countries such as Belgium, Norway, Canada, and Australia, where directions focused on increasing the proportion of generalists, limiting specialization, and giving priority to primary care. He suggests that the U.S. policy, coming on the worldwide trend of experimentation in health workforce in the 1960s, was a hasty expedient to shortages in primary care in America. Roemer (1977) states:

> In the world's most affluent nation, there would hardly seem to be economic justification for the use of physician extenders for primary care. U.S. policies in the 1970s were based on an unwillingness to impose social obligations on the physician (e.g., location in areas of need) and to train adequate numbers of primary care doctors. Such policies were an unfortunate acknowledgment of failure by medicine to fulfill its social mission.

In America, PAs have emerged as primary care providers. They are recognized as such by the Institute of Medicine along with NPs as important providers of primary care services (Donaldson et al, 1996a; Donaldson et al, 1996b).

Historically, *feldsherism* was commonly thought of as term or policy for interim healthcare personnel. This view assumes a fully trained doctor best delivers primary care, an assumption that has been challenged by the success of the American PA and NP. And, indeed, a key observation in the experience of the PA and NP professions in America is that nonphysicians can provide a large amount of primary care services. It is a poor use of medical talent to suggest that a physician needs to be present to deal with every human infirmity. The Western system of medical education is akin to putting all bus drivers through astronaut training, the point being that most physicians are overtrained for the role of the primary care generalist.

In a number of countries where nonphysicians have been used for long periods, roles have changed with advances in healthcare delivery and policy shifts. Eastern European feldshers were employed for many years on the front lines of primary care in much of the countryside. As the medical system in the country became more sophisticated, and as the supply of physicians came into balance with the medical needs of the population, policymakers and citizens sometimes viewed *feldsherism* as sustaining second-class care to those already relegated to second-class health care in the system. Although the PA is not (yet) formally recognized in most countries of Western Europe, the countries of the Pacific Basin, or Central or South America, in nearly all of these countries there are many discussions regarding incorporating nonphysician healthcare providers as key additions to healthcare personnel for the future.

The use of nonphysicians has been championed as an attack on medical elitism and the professional establishment. However, others, such as Dr. Eugene A. Stead, Jr., a key player in the development of one of the first PA programs at Duke University, suggested that the medical profession has been arrogant in its stance toward entry policies and pathways leading to medical licensure. According to Stead (2001), PAs have demonstrated high levels of patient acceptance and have been shown to function on a high level with shorter training than physicians. Although early critics of PAs and NPs said they represented a second tier of medical care, nonphysicians have been shown to augment the delivery of primary care to certain populations, such as the poor, those in medically underserved areas, and other disadvantaged members of society, in proportions greater than physicians. The employment of nonphysicians in various roles, spanning most primary care functions, as well as a wide swath of technical and public health and preventive medicine duties, appears to be an appropriate niche in the systems of many countries.

THE IDEA

Charles Hudson, the president of the National Board of Medical Examiners in 1961, first suggested the concept of new types of healthcare personnel to extend physician services in the United States. In a speech to the House of Delegates of the American Medical Association (AMA) and in a subsequent article in *JAMA*, Hudson articulated the rationale for new healthcare personnel based on changing medical labor, hospital staffing personnel demands, and advancing technology. His idea for a new type of health practitioner was to "extend the usefulness" and experience of Army and Navy corpsmen as efficient assistants who "would not be expected to exercise medical judgment, but . . . might well develop considerable technical skill which could be a source of satisfaction" (Hudson, 1961). Hudson (1961) believed "a curriculum could be devised, consisting of 2 or 3 years of college work with certain prescribed courses" that paralleled medical school, and that these new health providers should be called *externs* in a broader sense than just *medical students*.

Hudson felt that reaction to his proposal was generally favorable, but for years he believed that this proposal had died in some AMA committee. In the early 1980s, Hudson said that he was amazed at how the PA concept exceeded his imagination. Although Hudson theorized that the "goals of nursing could be redefined as part-nursing and part-medicine," thus allowing the nursing workforce to fill the role of the *externe*, he believed, correctly, that nurse leaders would frown on "the proposal of a medicine-nursing hybrid" (Hudson, 1961).

Assistant Medical Officer

In the early 1960s, considerable interest was generated around training a new category of allied health worker in the United States, modeled after the U.S. Navy corpsman and U.S. Army medic. Like other initiatives of the time, this interest was centered on doctor shortages and pressing demand for access to healthcare services. During a 1965 White House Conference on Health, the possibility of such a health worker was raised. The concept of a medical officer assistant was mentioned a number of times during this meeting. References to interest in this activity were presented in the Summary of Panels of the White House Conference in 1965. As Rosinski and Spencer wrote, neither an appropriate nor an adequate title had been given to this "proposed new auxiliary."

> Although an adequate title is elusive, the duties of such a person are even more nebulous. What an auxiliary like this would *not* be can be predicted. He would *not* be a qualified physician, but might assume some of the duties of a physician. He would *not* be in competition with a physician, but might serve as his ranking assistant. He would *not* be a nurse, but might be more highly trained than a nurse. One of the reasons why it is difficult to affix a title to this individual and describe his responsibilities is that there has not been a counterpart for such a health worker in the United States. (Rosinski & Spencer, 1967)

The authors used the name *assistant medical officer (AMO)* to describe this type of healthcare worker. The title was not original and the authors identified countries where such assistants were performing medical services, "although it must be reported they are not always accepted with enthusiasm" (Rosinski & Spencer, 1967). Examples included *behdars* in Iran, *apothecaries* in Ceylon, *public health workers* in Ethiopia, *clinical assistants* in Kenya, and *AMOs* in Fiji and Papua-New Guinea. Because the AMO they defined was serving as the "doctor" to millions of persons throughout the world, it was their intent to adopt this name and prototype for the United States. However, supervision of AMOs would be one of the chief difficulties the two authors mention in this and other reports (Rosinski & Spencer, 1965; Rosinski & Spencer, 1967; Rosinski, 1971; Rosinski, 1972).

The postscript on this effort remains unwritten. The work that Rosinski and others did apparently was not lasting. Some of their work may have been eclipsed by the individuals moving forward with their own decentralized plans for what ultimately became the PA. Historians have yet to link the efforts of Hudson with any of the work by Rosinski and Spencer, although it seems coincidental that both ideas were developed independently.

THE FIRST PHYSICIAN ASSISTANT PROGRAMS

The transition from technician and assistant to what is a formal PA occurred over a few decades. Some of this is documented and others are not well known. For many years preceding the first formal primary care PA, there were technicians in various specialties who were taught to assist the doctor. The formally trained PA that is delegated to take over many of the routine tasks of a doctor is where the contemporary PA story begins.

Duke University

The period from 1961 through 1965 was one of thought and formulation regarding the PA concept. At this time, Dr. Eugene A. Stead, Jr. was intensely engaged in an effort to convince persons within Duke University and elsewhere that his notion to create a new type of medical practitioner was a worthy one. From 1962 through 1964, Stead's failed attempt to create a PA-like practitioner built on the model of the nurse was a frustration and a set back (Holt, 1998). However, Stead's initial efforts to work toward the goal of establishing some form of medical education program would improve the circumstances of healthcare delivery in North Carolina. Of particular interest is not only the story of Stead's unsuccessful attempt to establish a PA program using nurses as the training template, but also the interplay between organized medicine and nursing in the struggle to create the PA.

In the 1960s, Stead was a towering figure in academic medicine. He received his undergraduate and medical education at Emory University in Atlanta and interned at the Peter Bent Brigham Hospital in Boston. He was a resident at the Cincinnati General Hospital and held a faculty position at Harvard and the Boston City Hospital prior to becoming the youngest person to chair the Department of Medicine at Emory University in 1942. In 1946, Stead was named Dean of the School of

Medicine at Emory, but he left after 1 year to become Professor of Medicine and Chairman of the Department of Medicine at Duke University. After 20 years, he relinquished his Duke chair to explore other avenues of research and medical care. Stead was widely recognized as a leading clinical scientist, educator, and administrator, and over the years a substantial number of his former students went on to become department chairmen and leading medical educators and researchers throughout the United States (Exhibit 2-3).

Over his 3-year period of educating physicians at Emory and overseeing Grady Hospital's residents and medical students during the Second World War, Dr. Stead was convinced that physicians learn best by applying their knowledge to meet patient care needs. As a result, Stead became interested in new and more efficient modes of medical education. An opportunity presented itself to Stead when he met Thelma Ingles, a senior nurse at Duke, who initiated a discussion with him related to advancing the training of nurses.

The story of Stead and Ingles began when Stead encouraged Ingles to use her sabbatical to spend a year in the medical school. After a series of negotiations, she agreed. During that year, "she operated much as a medical student in a clinical clerkship. She selected patients in the hospital in whom she had taken an interest, investigated their conditions, and met with Stead daily to determine what instruction she needed." If Stead was not prepared to provide her with instruction in a particular area of biology or pathology, he would collect some "green stamps" from somebody who owed him a favor and Ingles would receive instruction with the willing or begrudging assistance of other Duke medical professors. Stead admired Ingles because of her willingness to undertake what amounted to medical training in spite of the disapproval of her nursing peers (Stead, 1968a; Stead, 1968b).

After her sabbatical year, Ingles returned to the Duke Nursing School and created a master of science in nursing program based in large part on her experience in the medical school. The program contained structured clinical rotations on medical services and included physician instructors from the medical school. Although the program was approved by Duke University, the National League for Nursing (NLN) denied accreditation for the program, citing poor structure and, importantly, the use of physician instructors in the program (Holt, 1998). Opposition also came from the director of nursing at Duke Medical Center. After several attempts, the NLN refused to accredit the program.

Stead was frustrated and disappointed over the rejection of the nursing hybrid program—particularly with the nursing education establishment. He would later recount in his various debates with Luther Christman, a nurse educator and leader, that nursing leaders were antagonistic to innovation and change and had misconstrued his original notion for a greater and more responsible role for nurses who sought advanced levels of skills in patient care. Stead believed that the leaders of the NLN had overreacted without

EXHIBIT 2-3
Eugene A. Stead, MD

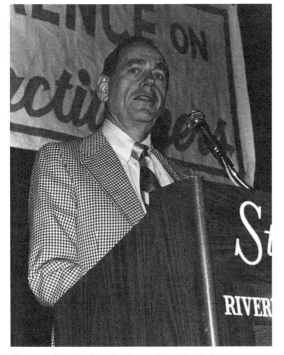

Courtesy of the American Academy of Physician Assistants.

adequate discussion to what he considered a reasonable and progressive approach to nursing educational advancement and enrichment (Christman, 1998).

Duke colleague, Dr. E. Harvey Estes, Jr., affirmed that if the master's degree program started by Ingles had been successful, "we would never have had a PA program." He confirmed, "once it failed, Gene Stead washed his hands of contact with the nursing profession" (Holt, 1998).

Much later, Christman, who debated Stead on several occasions regarding the nurse and the PA, admitted that nursing may indeed have missed an opportunity by rejecting the Stead and Ingles hybrid program (Christman, 1979; Christman, 1998). After noting that "from its inception, the physician assistant role, as constructed, has rankled many nurses and has tended to create another gulf between physicians and nurses," he then quotes Stead as saying that (as a result of the attempt to initiate the nursing hybrid program), "I became very angry at both nurses and women. I concluded that nursing leaders were interested primarily in maintaining the status quo. I decided to do the program without women" (Christman, 1998).

Although the hybrid nurse program was considered dead, Stead remained determined to advance the notion of developing a program to train PAs. His thinking shifted to the notion of basing the PA on the model of the military corpsman. The idea was not entirely without precedent. Duke physicians had been in the military and many were in the Reserves or were consultants in the major military hospitals in the area. In those hospitals, they had observed corpsmen and medics working with physicians in direct patient care and in technical areas of diagnosis and treatment. Former military corpsmen also worked in special clinical units at Duke Hospital and other hospitals in the region (Carter & Strand, 2000). The technological advances in medicine had put pressure on hospitals for well-trained technicians. Many of these veterans were able to assume a large portion of these tasks with little or no additional training.

In 1964, Stead wrote letters to Dr. Elliot Finkelstein of the U.S. Public Health Services and Robert L. Ballentine of the U.S. Department of Labor indicating his intentions to train PAs and seek outside financial support to initiate a training program. Stead asked Finkelstein, who headed the Neurological and Sensory Disease Service Program, if the program would have any interest in the PA program, especially if PAs could be trained to care for stroke victims. His letter to Ballentine stressed the need for PAs to meet growing demands in the health system: "The economic potential for physician-assistants is good. They will be immediately used by all segments of the medical profession and will make an immediate contribution to general medical care." Stead finished his letter by asking whether "the Manpower Development Act can offer financial support for such a project" (Stead, 1969). Although specific support was not forthcoming from these agencies, Stead was able to garner external support for his new program, first from private philanthropy and later from private and federal sources.

During this time Stead developed, and Duke University sponsored, a Continuing Medical Education (CME) Program for physicians living in the region. Unfortunately, the CME program failed because of lack of attendance. Many physicians were interested in such a program but could not attend because their patient loads and the intensity of their practices were too demanding. Stead reasoned that if the physicians had well-trained assistants, they would be able to leave their practices for a day or two to attend CME programs (Howard, 1969).

Stead's idea of an assistant found encouragement from Dr. Amos H. Johnson, a solo general practitioner in Garland, a small rural town in North Carolina. Dr. Johnson was able to maintain his practice and keep up with his CME programs. In addition to these activities, he accepted professional appointments, such as the presidency of the American Academy of General Practice (1965 to 1966), because he had an assistant. The assistant, Henry "Buddy" Treadwell, had been trained by Johnson for his practice needs and functioned in many ways like a contemporary PA, assuming many tasks such as diagnosing and treating (Gifford, 1987a; Gifford 1987b).

In the spring of 1965, with encouragement from Stead, the Vice Provost for Medical Affairs at Duke University appointed an ad hoc committee to evaluate the existing programs and personnel needs at Duke's hospital. The committee concluded that two types of medical personnel were needed: one, a very highly skilled technician limited to a specific medical discipline or specific area and the other, a more advanced specialist with a broad and basic knowledge of medicine (Lewis, 1975). This committee, chaired by Dr. Andrew Wallace, met on several occasions throughout the spring of 1965 and made the following observations:

- The need for extensive numbers of highly trained technical personnel existed inside and outside of the medical center.
- Two types of allied health personnel were needed: one highly skilled and limited to a specific area, the other more advanced with a broad and sophisticated background.
- There existed a need for a core curriculum to provide a means for academic advancement and variation in careers.
- There must be an attempt to define specific needs necessary to resolve various individual manpower problems.

The committee decided a method of attracting qualified applicants and providing them with a functional and compact curriculum was needed:

> The proposal to be outlined calls for the definition of a new member of the health team called a physician's assistant. The PA is seen as a new category within the structure of the health field, designed to provide a career opportunity for men functioning under the direction of doctors and with greater capabilities in growth potential than informally trained technicians. (Lewis, quoting the Wallace Report, p. 23, 1975)

For Stead, the Wallace Report provided the needed impetus to initiate his new version of the PA program. A memo about the program was spread throughout the Duke Medical Center. Around this time, Herbert Saltzman, a physician at Duke, applied for a National Institutes of Health (NIH) grant seeking support for training chamber operators in hyperbaric medicine. He cited a need for "paramedical technicians to provide the doctors with support needed in their clinical and research endeavors" (Lewis, 1975). Saltzman's concept of the type of personnel needed was consistent with Stead's concept of the PA. Before 1965, the National Heart Institute had not funded "nonprofessional" training programs, but Stead had recently served on the institute's study section and its members were aware of this thinking (Exhibit 2-4).

When the NIH grant was approved in April 1965, the successful piggybacking of the PA concept with this grant provided the initial source of funding for Stead's experiment in medical education and established the foundation for the first PA educational program in the United States. Recruits for this first PA program were sought from the ranks of the medical center's employees. The four members of the first class started class on October 6, 1965—Stead's 57th birthday. This date has been memorialized by the profession as National PA Day.

When the PA program first started, the new concept received nationwide publicity; *Reader's Digest* produced a series of articles entitled "Where the Jobs Are" (Velie, 1965). Even before the curriculum for the first class was planned, the *Digest* announced to its readers that the Duke faculty hoped the program would help make up for the dwindling number of rural doctors. Halfway through the training the program was portrayed in a September 6, 1966 article in *LOOK* magazine. This article, "More Than a Nurse, Less Than a Doctor," had a substantial impact and was the first airing of the concept to the public. The article began with a paragraph implying that the social change taking place in providing the public increased access to healthcare services would be accomplished through "the use of mid-level providers" (Berg, 1966).

It was widely accepted at that time that the nation was experiencing a demand for physicians. The article asserted:

> There is a shortage of doctors, and it's getting worse. With the demand for medical care

EXHIBIT 2-4
Duke University PA Leaders [From left, Reginald Carter, PhD, PA-C; Joyce Copeland, MD; Eugene A. Stead, Jr., MD; E. Harvey Estes, Jr. MD; Jay Skyler, MD; and Michael Hamilton, MD, at the occasion of the 25th Anniversary of the founding of the Duke PA program (1990)]

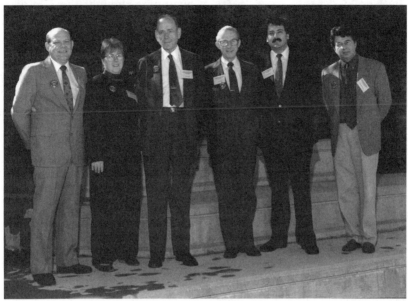

Courtesy of the American Academy of Physician Assistants.

swelling and treatment itself growing more complex daily, the supply of physicians cannot keep up with the need for their skills. Although plans are under way to build more medical schools and expand existing ones, the experts figure it takes almost ten years from the time a medical student drops into one end of the funnel and a practicing physician emerges from the other. Sick people can't wait that long. (Berg, 1966)

In 1967, three students graduated as PAs from this new program. For 2 years they used the house staff's television lounge in the medical center hospital as their classroom, and their graduation ceremony was held in a small barbecue restaurant in Durham. Within such inauspicious environments these prototype PAs began formulating a new role, one as yet uncharted.

The Duke program began to expand. In September 1967, just before the first class graduated, the training program moved from the Department of Medicine to the Department of Community Health Sciences. In 1969, Stead retired from active professional duties at Duke and the PA program was moved to the Department of Family and Community Medicine. The chair of the department, Dr. E. Harvey Estes, Jr., essentially oversaw the development of the Duke program and the dissemination of the PA concept and educational programs throughout the country (Exhibit 2-5). Under the leadership of Estes the Duke program continued to grow, increasing its number of students, adding the first female student, and improving its physical facilities. From the house staff television lounge the program moved to a small white trailer purchased by the newly formed American Academy of Physician Assistants (AAPA).

Under the leadership of E. Harvey Estes, Jr., the Duke PA program and the concept of the PA grew. In many ways Estes was the major factor in the program's success, particularly in terms of acceptance by organized medicine. The Duke program represented the academic, medical center program that eventually became the model for other PA programs. Medical center-based PA programs quickly

EXHIBIT 2-5
E. Harvey Estes, Jr., MD

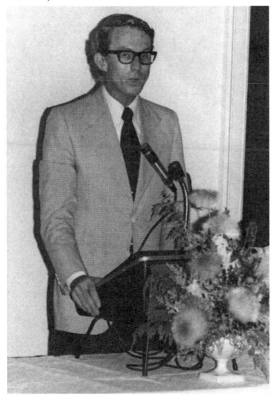

Courtesy of the American Academy of Physician Assistants.

emerged at centers where resources and needs were similar. These included programs at Wake Forest, the University of Oklahoma, Baylor, the University of Texas Southwestern Medical Center, Yale, the University of Alabama, George Washington University, Emory, St. Louis University, and the Johns Hopkins University.

One interesting aspect of the Duke program was the program's idea of what the role of the PA as a dependent practitioner should be. Those at Duke initially held the view that the PA would enter the medical decision-making process before and after the stages of diagnosis and prescription, but the final diagnosis and prescription would be reserved for the physician (Schneller, 1978). E. Harvey Estes, Jr., chair of the Duke University Department of Community Health Sciences

in 1968, explained that in practice the new assistant would take no part in traditional doctor functions (Estes, 1968a; Estes, 1968b). Thus, although Estes and colleagues in the beginning thought the role of the PA would consist of purely technical tasks, before long the PA role came to include diagnosis and patient management functions.

Medex and the University of Washington

Although credit is given to Stead and Estes at Duke for initiating PA education, other pioneering physicians were concurrently involved in designing and developing PA training programs. Prime among them was Richard A. Smith, MD, MPH (1932–), who founded the Medex concept. The Medex program, started by Smith at the University of Washington, was an innovative approach to health professions education, one that perhaps was a bit more radical in its departure from traditional medical education, and one with a strong sense of social purpose (Smith, 1969; Smith et al, 1971).

Dr. Smith's interest in medicine was stimulated in 1951 during a college summer work camp in pre-Castro Cuba where he worked in the cane fields and observed a nurse running a rural clinic. At that time, he decided that he wanted to become a medical missionary and train large numbers of people to provide basic, life-maintenance health services in underserved areas.

Smith attended undergraduate and medical school at Howard University, receiving his MD in 1957 (Exhibit 2-6). He did a residency in public health/preventive medicine while attending the School of Public Health at the University of Washington. Like Stead, Smith had his early ideas regarding medical training and personnel denied at first. In 1960, he requested his church mission board to allow him to work overseas as a trainer of new healthcare providers but was turned down. Undaunted, he had England's Archbishop of Canterbury present his plan to the World Council of Churches' meeting in New Delhi in 1961. Once again, however, his plan to be able to "multiply my hands" (R. Smith, personal communication, 2008) by training other

EXHIBIT 2-6
Richard A. Smith, MD

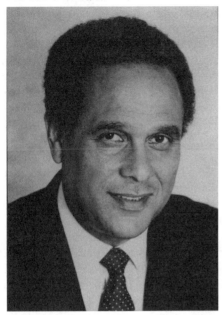

Courtesy of the American Academy of Physician Assistants.

healthcare providers on a large scale was turned down.

When Smith joined the U.S. Public Health Service, he was assigned to the Indian Health Service in Arizona in the early 1960s. This was followed by 2 years in the Peace Corps in Nigeria. While overseas, Smith validated the need for and the appropriateness of training nonphysician providers to meet healthcare needs in underserved areas. Some of his ideas were formed as a result of visiting the notable missionary Albert Schweitzer at Lambaréné Hospital in Gabon, West Central Africa. Schweitzer did not think that anyone less than a doctor could be in charge of medicine. Not to be discouraged, Smith decided he needed to further develop his ideas. Upon returning to the United States, he accepted a government position.

From 1965 to 1968, Smith worked in the Surgeon General's office in Washington DC, eventually becoming the Deputy Director of the Office of International Health. During this period, he began to refocus his development interests domestically. It was also during this time that Smith accepted the assignment from the Surgeon General to lead the effort to desegregate hospitals in the South. Smith, an African American, was the federal representative who had the unenviable task to inform hospitals that if they did not stop segregationist practices they would be ineligible for Medicare subsidies.

It was during the 1960s when Smith became acquainted with the same Dr. Amos Johnson from Garland, North Carolina, who had influenced Eugene Stead to seek acceptance for his PA concept. Johnson, a country doctor, was a dominant figure in North Carolina medical politics at that time. He was president of the American Association of Family Practice and an influential figure in the AMA. He had heard of Smith's ideas, knew of Stead's work, and introduced Smith to the leadership in the AMA. Johnson often mentioned the relationship he had with his assistant, Buddy Treadwell, and wanted Smith to develop a similar type of assistant (R. Smith, personal communication, 2000).

The Medex PA concept was centered on an individual with an enriched medical background and one willing to serve in primary care settings in rural and medically underserved areas. Smith was a physician with broad vision, a curious mind, and a wealth of experience in medical care in the Third World as well as in the United States. During his time in the Peace Corps in the early 1960s, he was exposed to the French African Medical Officer and an Asian counterpart (the Officier Medecin Indochinois). Smith returned to the United States in the mid-1960s as International Health Planning Director for Surgeon General William Stewart. During that time, he was assigned to the U.S. delegation to the annual World Health Organization Assembly in Geneva where he further explored use of new health providers with health officials from other countries. He continued to nurture the idea of the creation of a new category of healthcare professional, one who could work with doctors and perform tasks associated with the majority of the routine care that a physician provided (Ballweg, Hooker, & Cawley, 2006).

The Medex concept (a contraction of the words MEDicine and EXtension) involved a collaborative model of healthcare development, one that actively involved health professions' schools, local and national medical organizations, rural and urban communities, and overworked practicing physicians. These collaborating partners participated in introducing and supporting the PA concept as an appropriate, timely, and useful tool for improving health care in underserved communities. The concept's most important feature was the element of deploying clinicians to rural and remote areas.

Smith wanted his Medex program to be more than a demonstration project that was typically underwritten by the federal government and then forgotten a few years later. Believing that he could sell his concept to physicians in a conservative state, he chose to start his program at the University of Washington. Because Smith had earned his master's in public health at this institution and had worked in Washington state, he believed he understood the local medical politics.

In 1968, the Medex Demonstration Project, as the program was originally called, was jointly sponsored by the University of Washington and the Washington State Medical Association and was funded by the National Center for Health Services Research. One year later, the first Medex class of 15 former military medical corpsmen was selected and began training. The program was initially a 1-year program, but later increased to 15 months, and then further extended to 24 months. The first class graduated in 1970. Graduates referred to themselves as Medex, and put Mx after their names. In 1971, as a result of Smith's work with organized medicine, an amendment to the Washington State Medical Practice Act was passed, allowing PAs to practice medicine under the supervision of a licensed physician.

The Medex program differed from the Duke model in that entering students needed to have considerable medical knowledge. Coursework was built on background health experience and introduced concepts of medicine. Students received most of their training through "on-the-job" preceptorships with selected physicians in rural areas of the Pacific Northwest. Often these sponsoring physicians became employers (Ballweg, Hooker, & Cawley, 2006).

Within a few years, eight Medex programs were established nationally (Exhibit 2-7). The curriculum consisted of 3 months of intensive didactic work in basic and clinical sciences at the university medical center, followed by a preceptorship with a practicing primary care physician for 9 to 12 months. Medex programs were widely distributed from the inner city of the Watts district of Los Angeles at Drew University, to rural areas such as Alabama, North Dakota, and Hershey, Pennsylvania. Programs also emerged at the University of Utah, the University of South Carolina, and Dartmouth University. On completion of the preceptorship, the student received a certificate (Smith, 1969).

Smith's efforts were not solely domestic. Under Dr. Smith's leadership, the Medex Group produced the Medex Primary Health Care Series, a 7,000-page, 35-book resource used for training and managing thousands of health personnel in 88 countries (in 33 languages) to improve basic health services. Elected to membership in the Institute of Medicine of the National Academy of Sciences, Dr. Smith is currently a member of two World Health Organization expert committees on human resource development (Physician Assistant History Center, 2008).

Some Medex programs evolved over time from Smith's original conceptualization to a more "conventional" configuration. Most Medex programs changed their educational philosophy to a more academic medical center model configuration. There were also several Medex PA programs that, after a successful beginning, closed. The programs at Dartmouth, the Medical University of South Carolina (MUSC), and Penn State University were among those that closed due to loss of federal funding (however MUSC reopened later as a Duke model program). From a historical and policy standpoint, the Medex movement was one of the notable and successful models in physician assistant education; one that had superior records in terms of graduate

EXHIBIT 2-7
Medex Programs

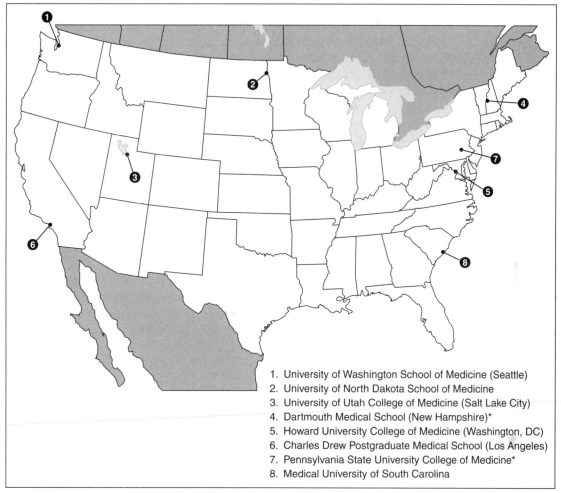

1. University of Washington School of Medicine (Seattle)
2. University of North Dakota School of Medicine
3. University of Utah College of Medicine (Salt Lake City)
4. Dartmouth Medical School (New Hampshire)*
5. Howard University College of Medicine (Washington, DC)
6. Charles Drew Postgraduate Medical School (Los Angeles)
7. Pennsylvania State University College of Medicine*
8. Medical University of South Carolina

*Defunct programs.

deployment into primary care specialties and into medically underserved areas. The Medex model was also important in that its centerpiece was the apprenticeship experience, because in the 1960s there was a resurgence of the preceptorship approach as the model for education. In the Millis report, "The Graduate Education of Physicians," John Millis commented on the relationship between demonstrated effectiveness of apprentice-type training and the efficiency of academic preparation. He noted that the weakness of the apprentice approach is that the apprentice might become as good as the master. The weakness of the academic approach relates to the manipulation of abstract symbols that stand imperfectly in the place of real-world phenomena. Millis' conclusion was that some mix of the abstract and concrete, appropriately articulated with undergraduate medical education, would be required to assume competent medical providers (Millis & Council on Medical Education, 1966).

Child Health Program at the University of Colorado

The third pioneering model of PA education was at the University of Colorado where the Child Health Associate Program began in 1968. In the early and mid-1960s, Henry Silver and colleagues recognized that there were many children not receiving medical care. They developed three programs to address this problem, including the Pediatric Nurse Practitioner (PNP) Program (1968), the Child Health Associate Program (1968), and the School Nurse Practitioner program (1970). (The University of Colorado PNP program is generally recognized as the basis for the entire NP profession.)

Dr. Henry Silver, a well-respected professor of pediatrics at the University of Colorado, with Loretta Ford, RN, EdD, Professor and Chair of Public Health Nursing, recruited nurses and other applicants with diverse backgrounds for a 5-year (later reduced to 3 years) training program to assist pediatric physicians (Glicken, Merenstein, & Arthur, 2007). The program drew applicants from nursing and became the progenitor of the NP movement. Originally, the mission was to supply preventive and routine care to children and it began as an NP program. The NP program opened in 1965 at the University of Colorado's Schools of Medicine and Nursing with Susan G. Stearly, MS, enrolled as the first student. In 1968, Dr. Silver launched the Child Health Associate Program at the University of Colorado Medical Center (Silver, 1971b). Individuals with 2 to 3 years of college education enrolled in the 3-year training program to become PAs who would provide primary healthcare services to children.

Silver was born in Philadelphia, Pennsylvania, and attended college and medical school at the University of California San Francisco (UCSF). He was an Assistant Professor of Pediatrics at UCSF before he moved to Yale University School of Medicine where he rose to the rank of associate professor (Exhibit 2-8). In 1957, he moved to the University of Colorado School of Medicine as Professor and Vice Chair of Pediatrics. Silver directed the CHA program (now called the Child Health Associate/Physician Assistant) from 1968 to 1991. As a recognized expert in general pediatrics, pediatric endocrinology, and growth, he coined the term "the Silver Syndrome," a condition of failure to grow. He was one of the early pioneers in the recognition of child abuse and neglect, recognizing

the implications these syndromes had on normal growth in children. Among Dr. Silver's many awards is the prestigious Institute of Medicine Gustav O. Lienhard Award for outstanding achievement in improving health and services in the United States.

In a letter dated November 1, 1981, Dr. Stead acknowledged Dr. Silver's important contributions that led to the establishment of the PA profession. He said, "Your statement about the chronology is correct. The demonstration that you could effectively use nurse practitioners was one of the happenings that led to the establishment of the Duke PA Program." Dr. Silver succeeded where Dr. Stead had failed in the late 1950s to provide nurses with advanced clinical training so they could assume greater roles in patient care.

The CHA/PA Program was the first (and remains the only) PA program to focus on the healthcare needs of children. Henry Silver recognized the need to document the educational, legal, and healthcare ramifications of

EXHIBIT 2-8
Henry Silver, MD

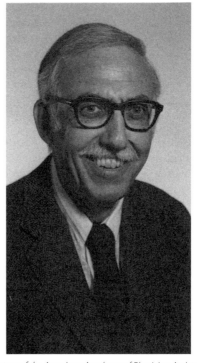

Courtesy of the American Academy of Physician Assistants.

these new professions. He and his colleagues published multiple articles on these topics, as well as documenting the competency, efficiency, and effectiveness of the CHA/PA (Dungy, 1975; Dungy & Sander, 1977; Dungy & Silver, 1977; Ott et al, 1974). This program was later expanded to cover almost all areas of pediatric primary care and enrolled non-nurses (Fisher & Horowitz, 1977). For a number of years, graduates of this program put CHA after their names, but they now take the Physician Assistant National Certifying Examination (PANCE) and are certified as pediatric PAs (Physician Assistant History Center, 2008). The CHA/PA Program was also the first PA program to offer the master's degree in 1975.

University of Alabama Birmingham

The first surgical assistant (SA) program was founded by Dr. John Webster Kirklin at the University of Alabama Birmingham (UAB) in 1967. Kirklin was chairman of the university's Department of Surgery and an internationally renowned pioneer in cardiac surgery. He started the program to train SAs, or surgical PAs, to assist in the surgical care of patients (Byrnes, 1991). The decision to train nonphysician providers to assist in the preoperative, intraoperative, and postoperative care of surgical patients was the culmination of Kirklin's years of work in medical education. He and his wife, Dr. Margaret Kirklin, recognized the value of a trained professional assistant who was not a physician but who could provide competent continuity of care (Condit, 1992).

Dr. Kirklin was born in Muncie, Indiana, in 1917. At the age of 8 he moved with his family to Rochester, Minnesota, because his father, a radiologist, was recruited to the Mayo Clinic. After finishing his undergraduate training at the University of Minnesota, he attended medical school at Harvard University, graduating magna cum laude in 1942. After interning at the University of Pennsylvania, he returned to the Mayo Clinic for a residency in surgery in April 1943. In mid-1944, at the peak of World War II, he was inducted into the Army where he trained in and practiced military neurosurgery until

August 1946. He returned to the Mayo Clinic and completed his surgical residency there in October 1950. His residency included spending 6 months under Dr. Robert Gross at Children's Hospital, Boston. While on the faculty at the Mayo Clinic during the 1950s, he modified the Gibbon heart-lung bypass machine and performed the first series of successful operations with it. Kirklin became Professor of Surgery in 1960 and Chairman of the Department of Surgery at the Mayo Clinic in 1964.

In September 1966, the UAB recruited Kirklin to chair their Department of Surgery. He started the SA training program in 1967, and recruited his wife to be the program's first academic director. Kirklin's SA concept was based on his contention that physicians were maldistributed by region and by specialty. He believed that doctors were overtrained for many of the tasks they performed, and he envisioned qualified assistants, properly trained and supervised, performing some of the more routine tasks traditionally performed by physicians. The SA program was typical of the two dozen programs that tried to develop a type of PA who could assist a physician in either primary care or some specialized service. It was a 2-year program, patterned after the Duke model, except that the clinical phase emphasized in-depth training in general and cardiothoracic surgery and surgical subspecialties.

However, as policy directives were shaping the PA healthcare workforce in the early 1970s, there was much debate over the role of the PA in surgery. This debate centered on whether surgeons should use nonsurgeons as first assistants. In 1973, the American College of Surgeons (ACS) issued its statement on SAs, in which they supported the concept. This support was published in *Essentials for the Educational Training Programs of Surgeon's Assistants* (1973).

There were initially four students in the program—three of whom remained at UAB for the rest of their careers. As a general surgical resident in his research year, Dr. John J. Gleysteen recalls being asked in 1973 to teach medical physiology to SA students. He found that it was all he could do to stay one chapter ahead of these eager students as they navigated through Arthur Guyton's *Textbook of Medical Physiology.* Jacqueline Hall was one of the first graduates of the program and was recruited to be the program's director in 1978.

Kirklin remained UAB's Chairman of the Department of Surgery until 1982. He continued his cardiovascular surgery practice as director of that division until 1989. Afterward, he continued as editor of *The Journal of Thoracic and Cardiovascular Surgery* (Physician Assistant History Center, 2008).

Military and Federal Physician Assistant Programs

As previously discussed, the roots of PA education run deep and include not only military programs but programs that emerged from other uniformed services. Federally sponsored PA programs, including the military PA programs, were among the first to be established in the United States. A number of federally sponsored programs emerged from existing federal, usually military, medical training courses and were transformed into PA programs as the concept grew and expanded in the civilian sector. Military programs are based on the 2-year university model and have contractual arrangements with universities to award an academic degree. The configuration of most of the early military PA programs was essentially the same as programs located in university medical centers, at least in terms of their curricula and educational approach. PA educational programs sponsored by the military emerged in the very earliest stages of the development of the concept. Enlisted members with broad military medical backgrounds were selected.

One of the first PA programs (and an example of a PA program that sprung from an existing medical training program) was the purser mate-training program. During World War II, more than 800 *purser mates* were trained by the U.S. Coast Guard. This 4-month course supplied the Coast Guard with medical corpsmen-like personnel aboard ships. In 1966, the Coast Guard began certifying graduates of the U.S. Public Health Service Purser Mate Training Program, which replaced the old Staff Officers' Association of America Pharmacist Mate Program. The program was based at the Public Health Hospital in Staten Island, New York. The designation of the graduates was changed to *marine physician assistant* in 1970. Initially a 9-month training program, it derived influences from the Duke model and expanded its length of training to 2 years in the early 1970s (Perry & Breitner, 1982).

Another example of a federally sponsored PA program was based in the federal Bureau of Prisons (BOP). Since the 1930s, former military corpsmen had been recruited to serve as medical personnel in the federal prison system (Perry & Breitner, 1982). Formal training for personnel to serve as PAs started as a 2-year model at the U.S. Medical Center for Federal Prisoners in Springfield, Missouri, in 1968.

The Indian Health Service (IHS) also opened a 2-year training program for PAs in Gallop, New Mexico (DeMaria, Cherry, & Treusdell, 1971; Hughbanks & Freeborn, 1971; Wakerlin, Stoneman, & Rikli, 1972). Another IHS PA Program was based in the Indian Hospital in Phoenix, Arizona.

The civilian sector and the military were experiencing shortages of physicians in the 1960s. Shortfalls in recruiting doctors for any form of federal service were made difficult by the unpopular war in Vietnam, for which the draft ended in 1973. By 1970, with the popularity of the PA concept growing, the Department of Defense began to form physician assistant training programs within the military branches. PA programs were instituted by the Air Force, Army, and Navy in 1971 and were based initially at military medical installations at Sheppard Air Force Base in Wichita Falls, Texas and at Ft. Sam Houston in San Antonio, Texas. In 1972, the Army began a 2-year medical center model PA training program at Ft. Sam Houston with an affiliation with Baylor University to grant the bachelor's degree. The PA program sponsored by the Air Force began in 1972 with 25 students accepted into a 2-year medical center model program at Sheppard Air Force Base.

The Navy's PA program began in 1972 at the Sheppard Air Force Base with an affiliation with George Washington University (Sadler, Sadler, & Bliss, 1972). Later, a trilateral arrangement was made with Sheppard Air Force Base (Wichita Falls, Texas), the University of Nebraska, and the Navy to award the bachelor's degree to trainees in the Navy and Air Force training programs. In 1973, the program was required to accept a small number of civilian "overflow" enrollees from the University of Nebraska PA Program—up to five per class. Then in 1974, the Sheppard program also began accepting Air Force nurses and training them as NPs (although it was purely a PA curriculum with no "theory of nursing" courses).

The small numbers of Navy PAs allowed to attend Sheppard Air Force Base (up to 10 per class, with classes commencing three times per year) was insufficient to meet Navy operational needs. In 1978, the first Navy PA Program at the Naval School of Health Sciences, San Diego, California, commenced with academic sponsorship from George Washington University. The first PA program director there was Robert (Bob) Glen Stephenson, Jr. P. Eugene Jones, PA, was ordered to relieve him as program director in 1981, but shortly thereafter, the Navy decided to close the San Diego program and move it to the Naval School of Health Sciences, Portsmouth, Virginia. The last San Diego Navy class graduated in 1983, and the Portsmouth program commenced in 1984. Following the move to Portsmouth, the Navy started sending students to the then Army PA Program (which evolved into the current interservice program) at Ft. Sam Houston in San Antonio, Texas (Salyer, 2002).

The curricula of the military programs involved intensive didactic preparation in the medical sciences. This was termed "Phase I" training and consisted of the typical basic sciences, clinical medicine, clinical assessment, and related biomedical medical courses. The typical model was 2 years, with the Phase I (didactic) year held at the major training centers such as Ft. Sam Houston, Naval School of Health Sciences. Prior to 1996, the Navy program trained students in one annual class in

San Diego. The Air Force educated 75 students in three matriculated classes annually and the Army had 50 students in two classes annually. The Coast Guard relied on recruiting civilian PAs or sending enlisted personnel to civilian PA programs. In 1990, the Air Force School of Health Care Sciences began to train Coast Guard PAs.

In 1996, all military PA training was consolidated into a single program at the Army Medical Department Center and School at Ft. Sam Houston, Texas. The Interservice Physician Assistant Program (IPAP), Academy of Health Sciences, Ft. Sam Houston, Texas, educates uniformed personnel to become PAs in the uniformed services. IPAP incorporates a mixed faculty of PAs from the various branches for didactic and clinical instruction. As the largest PA program in the world, it enrolls more than 250 students in the didactic year and 250 in the clinical year and intends to grow to 300 per year. A master's degree is awarded by the University of Nebraska. Nonmilitary students from other federal agencies have attended IPAP (Exhibit 2-9). Between 1996 and May 2002, the IPAP graduated 535 PAs (94 in the Air Force, 42 in the Navy, 381 in the Army, 13 in the Coast Guard, 2 in the Department of Defense, and 3 in the Federal Bureau of Prisons). Most students enter as enlisted grade and graduate with a PA certificate, an academic degree, and an officer's commission (Colver, Blessing, & Hinojosa, 2007).

The IPAP enrolled its first class in August 1996, which graduated in September 1998. Because it is considered a joint military operation, the program's directorship rotates every 4 years between the Army, Navy, and Air Force. Assigned more than 40% of the slots, the Army has the largest number of PA students each year (including National Guard), with the Air Force, Navy, and the Coast Guard the remainder.

The early PAs who had been trained in the military were from the enlisted and warrant officer ranks. Originally, military PA programs awarded only certificates of completion because the PA programs were viewed as advanced coursework that utilized the experience of

EXHIBIT 2-9
Major Brian Burk Instructing the Entering Class 3-08 of IPAP at Ft. Sam Houston

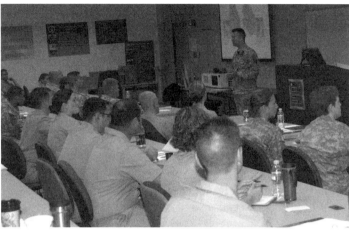

Courtesy of Colonel William Tozier, Director, Interservice PA Program, Ft. Sam Houston.

existing military corpsmen/medics. As they developed, military programs formed affiliations to award a bachelor's degree. Currently, military PA graduates receive a certificate that makes them eligible to sit for the PANCE. They also receive an academic degree from a sponsoring university. Military PA programs grant a certificate because if the sponsoring institution's accreditation status should become an issue, graduates of these programs would retain their eligibility to sit for the PANCE.

Military PAs principally work in primary care and family medicine, but their skills are broad, encompassing public health, preventive medicine, and sanitation. They also work in emergency medicine and in other specialty settings such as aviation medicine, orthopedics, cardiovascular perfusion, education, bone marrow transplantation, occupational medicine, oncology, head and neck surgery, and general surgery. Eighty percent of Army PAs are assigned to combat or field maneuver units; the remainder being deployed to outpatient care facilities at military hospitals or to administrative posts (Chitwood, 2008). In 2005, approximately 1,100 PAs were in the uniformed services. Because of the major role that military PAs provide, they are considered the gatekeepers of the Department of Defense's health system. The Air Force was the first branch to commission PAs as officers, doing so in 1978. The Navy followed in 1989, the Army in 1992 (Hooker, 1991a; Hooker, 1991b; Hooker, 2008).

Alderson-Broaddus College

In 1963, 2 years after Dr. Hudson's article calling for the training of doctor's assistants, and 2 years before Dr. Stead started the Duke University Physician Assistant Program, Dr. Hu C. Myers conceived of a PA program. Myers, a local general practice physician, approached the administration of Alderson-Broaddus College, a small private college in rural Phillippi, West Virginia, with a proposal to establish a new type of healthcare provider training program. The college's board of trustees approved the proposal in 1967, but the board had three caveats. First, Myers had to get the approval of organized medicine. Second, he had to obtain adequate funding from alternative sources. Finally, the faculty had to approve the completed program. Undaunted, Myers promoted his concept, formed advisory councils, and worked with leaders from the AMA, the West Virginia Society of Medicine, and the State Nursing Association to win their support.

As was the case with most of the pioneering PA programs, the development of the Alderson-Broaddus program was supported by grants from the Commonwealth Fund, the Robert Wood Johnson Foundation, and the Department of Health, Education, and Welfare (Myers, 1978). All the necessary pieces came together, and in the fall of 1968 the first PA class enrolled at the college. Myers was appointed professor, and later, Chairman of the Department of Medical Science in 1971.

Alderson-Broaddus was the first PA program to offer a 4-year curriculum that awarded a bachelor's degree upon completion. Unlike the Medex, Duke, and Colorado programs, Alderson-Broaddus PA students entered training directly from high school, and students were not required to have previous healthcare experience. Alderson-Broaddus established that PA education could be undertaken at a liberal arts college and not at a medical school. By the time the first class graduated in 1972, Alderson-Broaddus College joined four other PA programs in gaining full accreditation by the AMA (Perry & Breitner, 1982).

Johns Hopkins University

An underappreciated chapter in the early development of the PA profession was the contribution of the School of Health Services at the Johns Hopkins University in 1972. Established by faculty primarily from the School of Public Health, the School of Health Services had a progressive and to some extent nonmedical tone, which would serve as its lasting and dooming characteristic. Hopkins established in 1969 the Office of Health Care Programs and a Health Services Research and Development Center. Two clinical practices were inaugurated: one at the Columbia Plan, a suburban health maintenance organization (HMO), and the East Baltimore Plan, an urban HMO. At these sites, Hopkins faculty and researchers experimented with varied staffing patterns for delivering health care and evaluated PA employment. In 1970, the Center for Allied Health Careers was created under the direction of Dr. Dennis Carlson and charged

with developing programs for the education and training of new types of health professionals. A component of the intended role for the School of Health Services would be the continuation of nursing education (although 2 years earlier, the University had closed the 81-year-old School of Nursing). The School of Health Services at Hopkins was intended to be the educational sponsor for the continuation of nursing education, ideally on the graduate level.

In 1972, Malcolm Peterson, the Director of the Health Services Research and Development Center, was appointed dean of the new School of Health Services. Several types of PA programs were within the school. For example, the Health Assistant Program was an associate's degree program sponsored in collaboration with Essex Community College. At the same time, Archie Golden, a pediatrician who had experience in designing training programs for a variety of community health outreach initiatives while working for Project Hope in South America, founded the Hopkins Health Associate Program in the Johns Hopkins School of Health Services in 1972. In 1973, with a $3 million grant from the Robert Wood Johnson Foundation, the school started the Health Associate Program, a bachelor's degree PA program.

Johns Hopkins University dropped its sponsorship of the Health Assistant Program in 1977 and transferred the program to Essex Community College. The Health Associate Program closed with the closure of the School of Health Services in 1979. The curriculum was designed to be distinctly different from the medical model, which was well established in the adjacent Hopkins School of Medicine. This curriculum was captured in a book, *The Art of Teaching Primary Care*, authored by the faculty of the School of Health Services (Golden, Hagan, & Carlson, 1981).

The Hopkins School of Health Services was short lived. Steven Mueller, the president of the Johns Hopkins University, announced in 1978 that it would close the following year, indicating that the school was begun as "an experiment" and left the impression that the experiment had not succeeded. He did note, however, that the Hopkins commitment to nursing (the school also contained an NP program) was "absolute" and would resurface in some form in the future. That commitment proved to be true when the Hopkins School of Nursing was reestablished some years later.

Alaska Community Health Aides

The Alaska Community Health Aides (CHAs) program trains local residents to provide emergency and primary care services in villages that are often hundreds of miles away from the nearest physician. Most Alaska natives live in small villages isolated by mountain ranges, glaciers, and stretches of tundra, impassable river systems, and vast distances. These CHAs use procedures set forth in an easy-to-read manual and consult by telephone or radio with a hospital-based physician. The foundation for a CHA program was laid in the 1940s and 1950s when, in response to tuberculosis epidemics, the federal government used village volunteers to dispense medicine in remote villages. These volunteers, mostly women, generally act as intermediaries between patients and hospital-based physicians. The title CHA was chosen to show the position's link to the community and to emphasize that the person in this role did not practice independently of a physician. In 2006, CHAs were in 230 villages, serving about 45,000 Alaska natives and handling more than 253,000 patient encounters. Although the program's effects have not been measured by rigorous study, available data indicate that the program has achieved substantial acceptance among the population it serves and has played a major role in improving the health status of Alaska natives. The federal government assumes responsibility for medical malpractice claims against services provided by CHAs (General Accounting Office, 1993).

One of the important developments of the CHA from the PA standpoint is the pathway that is created for them to apply to and matriculate through a PA program. The Medex Northwest PA Program actively recruits and educates CHAs to return to their villages to serve as PAs for a region. Over a dozen have

done so and more are being given the appropriate education to allow them to qualify for PA application (R. Ballweg, personal communication, February 2008).

OTHER LEADERS OF PHYSICIAN ASSISTANT EDUCATION

The pioneering ideas developed by Eugene Stead, Richard Smith, Hu Myers, and Henry Silver were major elements of the larger movement to produce new types of healthcare providers. Because of the leadership of these individuals, the "new health practitioner" movement gained strength as dozens of training programs developed during the late 1960s and early 1970s. In 1970, according to one survey, there were 36 programs listed by the U.S. Bureau of Health Manpower Education; 10 of these programs trained personnel such as clinical technicians and emergency medical technicians, 10 were apprenticeship programs rather than formal educational experiences, and 16 were formal educational programs training PAs or NPs (Bureau of Health Manpower Education, 1971). Often, these programs were considered experimental and were begun primarily because federal grant support was available to support such efforts. Typically, these training programs were 1 to 2 years in length, but sometimes they were shorter, technically oriented, and designed to deploy providers quickly to alleviate what was considered then to be a physician shortage. Most of these training programs involved the creation of clinicians who had extensive nursing and/or military medical backgrounds. They went by many different names: *health assistant, health associate, Primex, Medex, physician assistant, physician associate, nurse practitioner, surgeon assistant, syniatrist, child health associate, clinical associate,* and many others. Somehow, from all of this experimentation with new provider education, two lasting models emerged: the PA and the NP.

Although Stead, Smith, Myers, and Silver are generally given credit for founding the first PA educational programs, the job was not finished in 1970. Other distinguished physicians carried the nascent PA profession into the medical mainstream. Dr. Alfred Sadler founded the Yale Physician Associate Program, which emerged from the Yale Trauma Program. Sadler was the first president of the Association of Physician Assistant Programs (APAP) in 1972, and with his twin brother, Blair (a lawyer), and Ann Bliss (a nurse), co-authored *The Physician's Assistant: Today and Tomorrow*, the first book on the PA profession (Sadler, Sadler, & Bliss, 1972; Bliss & Cohen, 1978). In 1973, Sadler left Yale to join the Robert Wood Foundation.

Among the many other significant accomplishments of Dr. Sadler was his work to draft the Uniform Anatomical Gift Act in 1968, which was adopted by all 50 states during the next 3 years and provided the legal underpinning for the national network of organ sharing we have today. While working for the Assistant Secretary for Health and Scientific Affairs, he was involved in preparing a position paper on the credentialing of PAs and NPs. Sadler was also a founding fellow of the Institute of Society, Ethics, and Life Sciences (Hastings Institute) in 1969.

Dr. Thomas Piemme was Chairman of the Department of Health Care Sciences at the George Washington University Medical Center and founded the PA program at George Washington University. Piemme used his position as a member of the Goals and Priorities Committee of the National Board of Medical Examiners (NBME) to define the profession's educational standards and practice qualifications. Additionally, while serving on the board of advisors of the AAPA, Piemme arranged for the formal incorporation of the AAPA and the APAP.

Sadler and Piemme were significant forces in establishing PA licensing and certification systems and national PA organizations. They went to New York and successfully appealed to three foundations for funding to establish a joint national office in the District of Columbia. When funding was secured, Dr. Piemme worked closely with the two national organizations to recruit Donald W. Fisher, PhD, to serve as executive director of the AAPA and the APAP.

Inheriting Henry Silver's creation, Dr. John E. Ott directed the Child Health Associate Program at the University of Colorado and performed many of the early health services research studies on CHA performance. Ott later succeeded Piemme as chair of the Department of Health Care Sciences at George Washington University and served as the medical director of their PA program for many years.

Another key figure who deserves special mention in the annals of pioneering PA educators is Denis Oliver of the University of Iowa (Exhibit 2-10). A biochemist, Oliver was among those who developed the Iowa PA program and instituted a number of health services research studies demonstrating the effective deployment of Iowa graduates in rural and medically underserved counties in that state. Oliver was also responsible for instituting the Annual Surveys of Physician Assistant Education in the United States. The survey began in 1985 and is administered annually by the APAP (now the Physician Assistant Education Association [PAEA]). The standardized questionnaire allows for tracking of trends within PA education. In its 24th version, this annual report is regarded as the primary source of information on PA educational programs.

At Johns Hopkins University in 1972, Malcolm Peterson, who became the first chairman of the Joint Review Committee, was

EXHIBIT 2-10
Denis Oliver, PhD

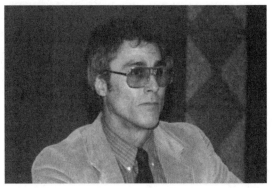

Courtesy of the American Academy of Physician Assistants.

appointed dean of a new School of Health Services. This program in turn sponsored the Health Assistant Program, in collaboration with Essex Community College and the Health Associate Program.

Prominent figures were agents of change for PA education and development. Dr. J. Rhodes Haverty was Dean of Allied Health at Georgia State University, and a driving force in the establishment of the NCCPA. Thomas Gallager, MD, and Jesse Edwards, MS, were the founders of the PA program at the University of Nebraska. Hal Wilson, MD, started programs at the University of Kentucky and later at Wake Forest University. Richard Rosen, MD, Chairman of Surgery at Montefiore Medical Center in the 1970s, first utilized PAs in inpatient surgical units and founded the first PA postgraduate program. Fran Horvath, MD, a pediatrician at the St. Louis University founded the PA program at that institution and was a leader in the development of the Joint Review Committee and the PA program accreditation system. Joseph Hamburg was a Dean of Allied Health at the University of Kentucky during the 1970s and was responsible for the institution of the PA Program at that institution. Other physician leaders included Robert Howard and Michael Hamilton at Duke University, Ashutosh Roy of the University of California at Los Angeles, David Lawrence and Robert Harmon at the University of Washington, and Katherine Anderson at Wake Forest University.

These and other leaders were pioneers in medical education; they took what had been learned to the next level. Their focus differed from those whose values were in traditional medical education, which stressed biomedical research and mechanistic approaches. PA education emerged with a philosophy of training practitioners to meet specific societal needs—increasing the supply and distribution of primary healthcare providers. Thus, there was a strong community orientation and service focus in these leaders and the programs they created. As physicians and leaders, they were strong and creative individuals who urged traditional institutions to start PA educational programs and to participate in the grand experiment with new types of healthcare providers. Often, they developed curricula from scratch or with minimal resources. Their work was mission-driven and practical focused. Moreover, they would be called upon frequently to describe and justify the role of the PA to legislators, health regulators, and skeptical medical groups. The job could be summarized as one where the educators need to be both an internal as well as external ambassador for the PA concept, in addition to being a teacher in the classroom and clinic, an administrator, a counselor and advisor, a curriculum designer and educational researcher, and community service provider. These include Suzanne Greenberg who founded the Physician Assistant Program at Northeastern University in 1970 and later became a president of APAP. Harriet Gayles founded the program at what was then Mercy College in Detroit. David Lewis inaugurated the PA program at the University of Florida. Don Fisher founded the defunct program at the University of Mississippi and became the first executive director of the American Academy of Physician Assistants. David Glazer began his career as faculty at the Emory University PA Program and went on to head the NCCPA for many years.

NURSING AND THE EVOLUTION OF THE PHYSICIAN ASSISTANT CONCEPT

In the 1960s, organized nursing was not interested in expanding its role to one that included the medical model. What became the PA concept was less appealing to nurses because organized medicine had suggested it. Beginning with the initial proposal of Stead and Ingles in 1964, and later in 1969 when the AMA suggested the recruitment of nurses to be trained as PAs, the American Nurse's Association (ANA) flatly rejected these ideas. The rejection was based on the view that nursing was unwilling to be subordinate to physicians in performing professional duties and served as a reminder to medicine that it is not the prerogative of one profession to speak for another (Holt, 1998).

Ultimately, the position of the ANA became, "If physicians want additional assistance, they can have it but nurses should not supply the manpower [sic]" (Holt, 1998). In spite of this attitude on nursing's part, Loretta Ford, RN, and Henry Silver, MD, started the first NP program at the University of Colorado (Silver, 1971a). Ironically, when this occurred physicians were quick to suggest that NPs were practicing medicine, whereas nursing leaders claimed that NPs had left nursing to become handmaidens to physicians. Later, nursing leaders suggested that the NP role had done much to invigorate nursing as a whole (Christman, 1998; Holt, 1998).

The AMA proposed the PA profession as an opportunity for nurses to leave their field to gain more responsibility and pay. Referencing the fact that most PAs were men and earned salaries equal to or higher than more formally educated nurses, the ANA retorted by characterizing the new role as a bit of "government supported male chauvinism." What leaders at the respective organizations did not know was that the PA concept was the result of nearly a decade's work by Stead and others. These leaders were exploring options for training healthcare professionals—nurses among them—for advanced clinical role. The AMA and the ANA's dialogue on the PA were often characterized by sharp language and strong debate over the new profession. It is becoming axiomatic that miscommunication and misunderstanding between medicine and nursing caused their respective professional organizations to hinder rather than promote collaborative endeavors (Holt, 1998).

Stead had great respect for nursing experience in patient care. After creating a prototype advanced medical training program for nurses at Duke, he concluded that nurses "were very intelligent and they learned quickly, and at the end of a year we had produced a superb product, capable of doing more than any nurse I had ever met" (Stead, 1979). This program could have initiated the NP movement, but was refused accreditation as an educational program by the NLN, the agency for degree-granting nursing programs, because the NLN determined that delegating medical tasks to nurses was inappropriate (Fisher & Horowitz, 1977). This early foray into an advanced practice nursing program was eventually phased out. Ingles left Duke for the Rockefeller Foundation, and Stead was left with a conviction that people with varied backgrounds can deliver high-quality patient care if adequately trained (Christman, 1998), which led to the historic development of the first PA program at Duke University.

EARLY PROFESSIONAL CHALLENGES

A major challenge for the new PA profession was how to obtain legal recognition within the medical regulatory system while avoiding seeking licensure for the PA to perform any specific task. It was determined, however, that the features of physician dependency and exclusion from the diagnostic and prescriptive process were consistent with an assistant role and did not require licensure (Ballenger, 1971; Ballenger & Estes, 1971). An even more interesting fact is that the PA role now includes considerable diagnostic and therapeutic management responsibilities.

If the idea of the PA concept was a gleam in the eye of its creators, its success also rested squarely on the shoulders of its first students. The first PA students recall thinking that if any of them did poorly, it could be the early demise of the concept. Additionally, some physicians coolly received the idea of a PA, and only a few were initially willing to engage in the novel experiment of a formally trained assistant for doctors. Ken Ferrell, from the first Duke class, recalls that some of the physicians who would have benefited most from assistants were quite resistant to the idea. They were reluctant to relinquish any of their responsibilities, even though they were overworked (Mastrangelo, 1993).

SPECIALTY PHYSICIAN ASSISTANT MODELS

Movements in specialization took place in the late 1960s as well, including a surge of new programs to train nonphysician providers in specific areas of care. Examples include the orthopedic assistant and the urologic PA; 2-year programs designed to train personnel to work directly for specialists. A 4-month "health assistants" training program sponsored by Project Hope in Laredo, Texas, was launched in 1970. The program was intended to improve Hispanic health care. The only requirement for entry was that the student had to be 18 years of age. Of the 11 students who entered the first class, eight lacked high school equivalence but were able to earn their General Equivalency Diploma (GED) certificate on completion of the program (Sadler, 1975).

Other specialty programs included gastroenterology, allergy, dermatology, and radiology. In fact, the radiology program at the University of Kentucky and the pathology program at Duke University lasted longer than most specialty programs. By 1971 more than 125 programs in 35 states announced they were training "physician support personnel" (Bureau of Health Manpower Education, 1971). Yet, it is interesting to note that the concept of the primary care PA became consolidated in the early years. By 1975 the PA concept was anchored in primary care and survived; at the same time most of the specialty programs expired.

Most primary care-based programs flourished. A number of these programs were sponsored by academic health centers. By 1972 a total of 31 programs were in operation: 21 of the programs were federally supported by agencies such as the Office of Economic Opportunity, the Model Cities Program, the Veterans Administration, the Public Health Service, the Department of Defense, and the Department of Labor, whereas the remainder were financed by private foundations and institutional sources (Fisher & Horowitz, 1977). Throughout the 1970s, private philanthropy from the Robert Wood Johnson Foundation, the Macy Foundation, and the Brunner Foundation provided start-up support for a number of PA educational programs.

STANDARDIZING THE PHYSICIAN ASSISTANT

In 1970, the National Congress on Health Manpower (sponsored by the AMA's Council on Health Manpower) sought to develop uniform terminology for the many emerging PA programs. Congress concluded that *physician's assistant* was too general to be adopted as the single generic term because PAs were receiving varied levels of training. They decided that *associate* would be a preferred term for healthcare workers who assume a direct and responsible role in patient care and act as colleagues to physicians, rather than as technical assistants. Congress noted that the PA terminology is often confused and used interchangeably with the established *medical assistant*, the title for the nonprofessional office helper who functions in a clerical and technical fashion (Curran, 1972). However, the AMA's House of Delegates rejected the *associate* terminology in the belief that *associate* should be applied only to physicians working in collaboration with other physicians. (This criticism ignores the "'s," which denotes that the *associate* is not another physician.) Thus, no consistent position emerged from organized medicine (Sadler, Sadler, & Bliss, 1972).

In the United States, the nonphysician practitioner concept initially embodied multiple types of healthcare providers, including PAs. Educational curricula designed to train a variety of PA-style healthcare providers were becoming abundant in the late 1960s. In 1970, the Institute of Medicine of the National Academy of Sciences (NAS) unsuccessfully attempted to classify various types of PAs according to the degree of independent function in exercising medical judgment. The board report identified three levels of PAs: Type A assistants, Type B assistants, and Type C assistants.

Type A assistants are capable of collecting patient history and physical data and organizing and presenting them so the physician can visualize the medical problem and determine appropriate diagnostic or therapeutic steps.

The assistant can assist the physician by performing diagnostic and therapeutic procedures and coordinating the roles of other more technical assistants. Functioning under the general supervision and responsibility of the physician, the assistant may practice under defined rules without the immediate surveillance of the physician. The assistant is qualified to integrate and interpret clinical findings on the basis of medical knowledge and to exercise a degree of independent judgment.

Type B assistants, although not equipped with general knowledge and skills relative to the entire range of medical care, possess exceptional technical expertise in a clinical specialty or in certain procedures within such a specialty. Within a specialty area, this provider may have a degree of skill beyond that of a Type A assistant and perhaps that normally possessed by physicians who are not engaged in the specialty. Because Type B assistants' knowledge and skill are limited to a particular specialty, they are less qualified for independent action.

Type C assistants are capable of performing a limited number of medical care tasks under the more direct supervision of a physician. These providers may be similar to the Type A assistants in the areas in which they can perform, but they cannot exercise the degree of independent synthesis and judgment.

Initially, the NAS classification of PAs using the Type A, B, and C system appeared to help define the nature of the relationship and division of duties between physicians and PAs, but it was soon discarded because it tended to create confusion within the hierarchy of emerging models of PA providers. The leaders of Medex programs were unhappy with this concept; their graduates were assigned a Type C rating, whereas Duke graduates were assigned a Type A rating—designations based on perceptions of formal training rather than on past healthcare experience. Although this system was changed and refined, eventually the entire NAS classification scheme lost relevance in attempting to capture the emerging nature of the PA-physician relationship and was abandoned (Estes & Howard, 1970).

FEDERAL POLICY

The critical role of the federal government in nurturing the development of new healthcare practitioners in general, and the PA in particular, came about through specific legislation. The Comprehensive Health Manpower Training Act called for the Bureau to provide support for educational programs for PAs and other nonphysicians. This act established the education grants program that was administered by the Bureau of Health Manpower under the Health Resources Administration, Department of Health, Education, and Welfare, mandated by Section 774a of the Public Health Service Act as Public Law 93-157.

Shortly thereafter assistance for 24 of the then 31 existing programs and contracts with 16 developing programs was initiated. Federal support represented an investment in health professions programs to test the hypothesis that nonphysician healthcare professionals could provide many physician-equivalent services in primary and continuing care. The Bureau's programs were designed to carry out the intent of Congress to relieve problems of geographic and specialty maldistribution of physicians and the U.S. healthcare workforce. This intent was reflected in the contract process, which required each PA program to emphasize the following three major objectives in its demonstration:

- Training for delivery of primary care in ambulatory settings
- Placing graduates in medically underserved areas
- Recruiting residents of medically underserved areas, minority groups, and women as students for these programs

Each program was free to devise various curricula and methods of instruction, but the preceding three requirements were held constant to carry out the intent of Congress (Fisher & Horowitz, 1977). This factor contributed to the demise of most Type B and C programs. They either folded in a few years because of lack of funding support or converted into primary care programs. The only survivors are the SA, CHA (which teaches primary care, and graduates are eligible for national certification), and pathologist's assistant programs.

NAMING THE PROFESSION

As the PA profession grew, experimentation to identify a more appropriate title also took place. The title *physician's assistant* was problematic because it incorrectly indicated possession by the physician, and the title was not initially well accepted by physicians and PAs alike. Silver suggested a new term, *syniatrist*, from the Greek *syn* signifying "along with" or "association," and *-iatric*, which means "relating to medicine" or a "physician" (Silver, 1971a). He proposed that the syniatrist terminology have a prefix relating to each medical specialty; for example, general practice would be a *general practice syniatrist associate* or a *general practice syniatrist aide* (Sadler, Sadler, & Bliss, 1972). Smith opted for *Medex* and saw his graduates placing the letters Mx after their names as an appropriate and distinct title. Other proposed titles in lieu of PA included *Osler, Flexner,* and *Cruzer* in honor of famous figures in American medical history. The intent of these new names was to be neutral, less controversial, and less demeaning than "PA." Little interest in these names developed, with the exception of Medex. There were no strong advocates for one over the other, and Medex had not reached prominence enough. Thus, the title *physician assistant* remains.

SUPPORT OF ORGANIZED MEDICINE

The PA concept would not have germinated and certainly would not have succeeded without the overt support and active involvement of major physician groups. The AMA in particular contributed substantially to confirming legitimacy and acceptance of the concept and had a strong role in the establishment of standards of PA educational program accreditation and professional credentialing organizations. Support for the development of the PA profession also came from the American College of Surgeons, the American Academy of Family Physicians, the American Academy of Pediatrics, the American College of Physicians, and other medical groups in shaping the infrastructure of the PA profession. These groups worked to build the critical components of the profession's structure, particularly legal and regulatory components. PA practice certification mechanisms were patterned to a large degree on their counterparts in the medical profession. An example of medical collaboration was the creation of the NCCPA, the national credentialing agency for the PA profession that administers the PANCE. Physician and PA groups worked with government agencies, the NBME, the Federation of State Medical Licensing Boards, and members of the public to create the NCCPA, and most of these groups continue to comprise the governance of the organization.

PHYSICIAN ASSISTANT ORGANIZATIONS

The American Academy of Physician Assistants (AAPA) was founded by students at Duke University in 1968, and the Association of Physician Assistant Programs (APAP) was founded by physician faculty from major PA educational programs in 1972. PA programs of all types proliferated between 1965 and 1970. This was a period of unwieldy growth and preceded the development of accreditation standards in 1971 and national certification requirements in 1973. Consequently, many of these programs were highly experimental. The curricula for these "generalist" and "specialist" programs ranged in length from a few weeks to more than 4 years, depending on the background of the student and on the role the "new health practitioner" was to play. Programs were located in medical schools, schools of allied health professions, universities, colleges, junior colleges, hospitals, clinics, and federal facilities.

The first attempt of professional consolidation was the American Registry of Physicians' Associates which was incorporated in North Carolina on May 26, 1970. The Articles were signed by Robinson O. Everett, Martha D. Ballenger, and D. Robert Howard. The first board of directors included Robert Ewer, MD, University of Texas, Galveston; D. Robert Howard, MD, Duke University; and Leland Powers, MD, Bowman Gray School of Medicine. The purpose of the Registry was to encourage training and to promote and regulate the activities of physicians' associates by determining their competence through examinations and investigative studies. It would grant and issue certificates to graduates of approved educational and training programs and to others who demonstrated by examination that they possessed the background and experience to perform satisfactorily as graduates of approved programs.

Duke University and several other programs started using the term *associate* rather than *assistant* to distinguish their programs from the Type B and C programs, and the term *associate* became embedded into the Registry's name. Bylaws were adopted, officers were elected, and other university-based programs soon joined the Registry. Graduates of these programs were eligible to apply to the Registry and be certified as *registered physicians' associates*. Once registered, the graduates were encouraged to place the initials RPA after their names, wear a lapel pin and patch with the Registry's patented insignia on it, and display a signed certificate from the Registry

in their offices. From May 1970 until April 1972, Dr. Howard served as the Registry's first appointed and then elected president until the position was assumed by Alfred Sadler, MD, of Yale University. Dr. Powers served as secretary treasurer until Susanne Greenberg of Northeastern University assumed this role, keeping minutes and handling the organization's finances.

Although a useful focal point for exchange of ideas, the Registry did not meet educators' broader academic needs. In April 1972, at the fourth Duke Conference in Durham, North Carolina, PA educators decided to form the APAP. A meeting of the Registry was held following the Association meeting and the Registry was formally transferred to the AAPA. The Academy's first task was to elect new officers of the Registry. William Stanhope was elected president, Steven Turnipseed secretary, Jeffery Heinrich treasurer, and Gail Spears member-at-large.

Along with the APAP and AAPA, the Registry appeared as a cosponsor on the programs distributed at the first and second National Conference on New Health Practitioners held in 1973 in Wichita Falls, Texas, and in 1974 in New Orleans, Louisiana (Exhibit 2-11). With the administration of a national certifying examination for PAs in

EXHIBIT 2-11
AAPA Leaders with Conference Guest Richard Schweicker, Then Secretary of Health and Human Services, 1981 [From left: Peter Rosenstein, Bruce Fichandler, Jarrett Wise, Then Secretary of Health Richard Schwieker, Dee Dee Alexander, Ron Fisher, and Charles Huntington (circa 1981)]

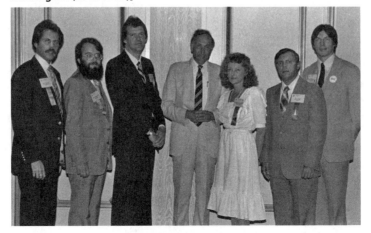

Courtesy of the American Academy of Physician Assistants.

1973 and the development of the National Commission on Certification of Physician Assistants, which became operational in 1975, the need for the Registry disappeared and the organization was liquidated by the AAPA soon thereafter. At its peak, the Registry included 12 member programs and listed over 125 graduates as registered physicians' associates (Carter & Fasser, 2003).

EVOLUTION OF THE PHYSICIAN ASSISTANT PROFESSION

All social movements have periods of evolution, and the development of the PA profession is no exception. To appreciate the evolution of the PA profession, we divide its history into six periods. These periods span the first five decades of the PA profession. As stages in the evolution of the PA profession, the natural history of other nonphysician professions is shown in Exhibit 2-12.

Period 1: Ideology (1960 to 1969)

The PA was envisioned as a new type of medical generalist, one whose role would build on prior medical experiences. As such, PAs would be trained in a short time frame and be deployed to practice locations in medically needy areas. The assistant to the primary care physician in rural and underserved areas was idealized during this time. Concept is put into action, PA programs are inaugurated (independent of each other), and the concept begins to gel.

Period 2: Implementation of the Concept (1966 to 1975)

Charismatic leaders and the federal government provided strong support for the creation and early development of PAs in the healthcare system. Domestic policy in the early 1970s sought to improve citizen access to health services by increasing the development and dispersal of healthcare personnel. Most policymakers believed there was a shortage of physicians overall with a decreasing proportion in general practice. Because organized

medicine had not adequately addressed these issues, a new federal workforce approach was created. This initiation consisted of two major elements:

- expansion of physician supply by expanding medical education and
- promotion of the introduction of new practitioners whose roles would focus on primary care.

The early 1970s was a period of intense activity and evolution for the PA concept. During this period, the key organizations representing the profession were founded: the AAPA in 1968, the APAP in 1971, and the NCCPA in 1973.

Also during this time the mantle of responsibility for the continuation of the development of the PA profession was passed on to the next cadre of progressive-thinking physician educators who had assumed leadership positions in medical education. These individuals were also leaders in medical and regulatory organizations.

Legal and Regulatory Challenges

The introduction of the PA into the American health system brought with it the necessity to consider appropriate legal and regulatory approaches to enable these and other emerging healthcare practitioners to enter clinical practice. Important decision points were the determination of the scope of practice of these new professionals, appropriate levels of state board recognition (licensure, registration, and certification), and stipulations for supervision and prescribing activities (Ballenger, 1971; Ballenger & Estes, 1971).

To support the entry of PAs into clinical practice, the House of Delegates of the AMA in 1970 passed a resolution urging state medical licensing boards to modify health occupations statutes and regulations to permit PAs to qualify as medical practitioners. Among the first states to amend medical acts allowing PAs to practice were Colorado, North Carolina, California, and New York. On the federal level important leadership in the early nurturing of the PA concept was provided by the government in the form of grant support

EXHIBIT 2-12
Stages in the Development of the New Health Professionals

STAGE I—IDEOLOGY
- The existence of an appropriate social, medical, and political climate; medical personnel factors; and educational influences leads to a coherent rationale and expected role necessitating the creation of a new category of health personnel.
- This rationale must gain the acceptance of critical existing stakeholders in the health system (e.g., doctors and nurses, government health policymakers, educational institutions, medical regulators, state legislators, and health administrators).
- The climate in which the conceptualization of new health occupations develops helps set the stage. Stakeholders must perceive a benefit. Public policymakers must be convinced that introduction of a new health profession will benefit society in improving health services, and not directly threaten existing professions.

STAGE II—IMPLEMENTATION
- Key health policy, medical education, and organizational collaboration grow to implement the conceptual framework, educational preparation, and professional regulation of the new profession.
- Critical areas must be defined: length and level of training, curriculum content, scope of practice, legal status and mechanisms of regulation, sponsorship and funding, and credentialing.
- Academic institutions begin to develop educational programs.
- Levels of state recognition (licensure, regulation, or certification) of practice activities for new practitioners entering medical practices are organized. Systems of educational sponsorship, academic recognition and accreditation, professional credentialing, occupational regulation, and definition of practice scope are established.

STAGE III—EVALUATION
- Conduct and evaluation of organized health services research and public policy analysis are designed to measure the levels of clinical performance effectiveness and practice characteristics of the new professional: measurement of levels of acceptance by patients, physicians, and other professionals; content and quality of care; cost-effectiveness; practice deployment; and role satisfaction.
- Studies begin to examine longitudinal trends of provider utilization patterns and professional demographics in the health system.

STAGE IV—INCORPORATION
- Steady growth and acceptance of the new professionals occurs.
- Utilization extends from original generalist/primary care roles to include specialty areas.
- Clinical practice settings include private solo and group medical offices; hospitals, health facilities, and organizations; academic centers; managed care systems; long-term care facilities; and public health clinics.
- Legislation is promulgated in states authorizing in statute for medical licensing boards to regulate the new health professional; regulations are adopted permitting new professionals in health workforce supply and requirements planning; summary policy reports on impact and practice experiences are published.

STAGE V—MATURATION
- Acceptance and institutionalization of the profession among the health occupations occurs.
- The acceptance of educational institutions is evidenced by faculty appointments for PA educators.
- Professional utilization patterns are characterized by steady, ongoing demand for practitioners' services by both patients and physicians, and continuing utilization in a variety of medical care settings.

STAGE VI—GLOBALIZATION
- Growth extends to other governments; these countries modify the model of the nonphysician clinician.
- Program development changes to adapt to the nuances of each country.

for PA educational programs. Legislative initiatives included the Allied Health Professions Personnel Act of 1966 and the Health Manpower Act of 1968. PA programs quickly sprang up in medical centers, hospitals, and colleges; state legislatures and private foundations provided support for education programs as well.

State Regulation

The legal basis of PA practice is codified in state medical practice statutes granting authorization to licensed physicians to delegate a range of medical diagnostic and therapeutic tasks to individuals who meet educational standards and practice requirements. Authority for medical task delegation is based on the legal doctrine of *respondeat superior*, which holds that it is the physician who is ultimately liable for PA practice activities and mandates that doctors who employ PAs appropriately define and supervise their clinical actions. State acts exempt PAs from the unlicensed practice of medicine with the stipulation that they function with physician supervision.

Professional activities and the scope of practice of PAs are regulated by state licensing boards, which are typically boards of medicine, boards of health occupations, or, in some instances, separate PA licensing boards. Laws define PA qualification requirements, practice scope and professional conduct standards, and the actions of the PAs. State laws commonly require physicians to delineate the practice scope and supervisory arrangements of PAs. Medical practice acts define the boundaries of PA practice activities but tend to vary considerably by state, particularly with regard to scope of practice, supervisory requirements, and prescribing authority. This variability has led to barriers in practice effectiveness in a number of states. After 40 years, all of these barriers have been overcome.

As originally envisioned, the role of the PA working with physicians encompassed the full range of clinical practice areas: office, clinic, hospital, nursing home, surgical suite, or in the patient's home. Laws in many states were written to give PAs a practice scope, allowing the physician to delegate a broad range of medical tasks to PAs. This latitude allows PAs to exercise a degree of clinical judgment and autonomic decision-making within the parameters of state scope of practice regulations and the supervisory relationship. Whereas innovation tended to precede legislation, eventually laws and policies were considered essential for PAs to be fully effective in practice. Geographic practice isolation in rural and frontier settings may, by necessity, result in varying degrees of offsite physician supervision and require the PA to exercise some autonomy in clinical judgment, particularly when the PA is the only available onsite provider. Regulatory reluctance to support such physician-PA relationships in satellite and remote clinical settings restricts the PA in extending and providing services that might otherwise be unavailable.

Practice regulations have progressed from a delegatory model achieved by amending medical practice acts to a regulatory/authority model wherein health-licensing boards are explicitly authorized to govern PA practice (Davis, 2002). Typical state regulatory acts establish PAs as agents of their supervising physicians; PAs maintain direct liability for the services they render to patients. Supervising physicians define the standard to which PA services are held are vicariously liable for services performed by the PAs under the doctrine of *respondeat superior*.

Practice Qualification

Over a number of years and by the actions of state legislatures, a standard emerged for PA practice: qualification as a PA requires that individuals be graduates of an accredited PA educational program and pass the PANCE.

Physician Assistant Education

Establishment of formal accreditation standards for PA programs marked an important milestone for the PA profession. Initially established by organizations affiliated with the AMA in 1971, the Council on Education for Allied Health developed standards for PA program accreditation, promulgated as the *Essentials of an Approved Educational Program for the Assistant to the Primary Care Physician.* Authority for PA program accreditation was set within the Commission on Accreditation of Allied Health Education Programs (CAAHEP). In 2000, the Accreditation Review Committee on Education for the Physician Assistant (ARC-PA) became an independent accrediting body for the PA profession, separate and independent of the CAAHEP. Over the years, the accreditation criteria underwent frequent revisions reflecting changes in educational preparation in a rapidly developing field. The *Essentials,* as they were called, were revised and updated in 1978, 1985, 1990, 1997, and 2000. Minor changes are made frequently. Accreditation is necessary for PA programs to receive federal Title VII grant funding and in most states for program graduates to qualify for entry to practice. The *Standards,* as they were later referred to, define the necessary core components of PA educational programs, the nature of institutional sponsorship, the curriculum content, clinical training affiliations, basic and clinical science course offerings, faculty qualifications, and admission and selection guidelines (McCarty, Stuetzer, & Somers, 2001). Early versions of the *Standards* were written to permit PA educational programs a wide degree of latitude to create curricular configurations based on a structure awarding several types of academic degrees.

Period 3: Evaluation and Establishment (1976 to 1980)

The Comprehensive Health Manpower Act of 1973 was an important legislative milestone, marking the inclusion of PA program funding support programs. Since then, federal awards have totaled over $200 million supporting PA educational programs. In fiscal year 2002, programs received $6.4 million; although by 2008, the amount dispensed under Title VII for PA programs declined to about $2 million (Cawley, 2008a).

A great deal of health services research was performed during the 1970s and 1980s examining the impact of PAs when introduced into medical practice. Both the PA and the NP concepts and related advanced practice nursing

programs were novel medical education experiments, and their outcomes were the target of intense social research focus. After a decade of studies, more than 100 research publications revealed that PAs were well accepted, safe, and effective practitioners in medical care delivery. Studies also showed that there was a high degree of patient acceptance of the PA role and that most PAs were in primary care practices in medically needy areas (Hooker, Potts, & Ray, 1997; Office of Technology Assessment, 1986).

PAs can lower healthcare costs while providing physician-equivalent quality of care. Despite that PA cost-effectiveness has not been conclusively demonstrated in all clinical practice settings, substantial empirical and health services research supports this finding. The present increasing use and market demand for PAs in clinical practices would be unlikely if they were not to some degree cost-effective (Hooker, 2002). Evidence also indicates that the organizational setting is closely related to the productivity and possible cost benefits of PA utilization.

Initial PA practice distribution tended to reflect the federal and medical sector intent that PAs assume primary care roles in areas of need. Early recruits to the PA profession typically were individuals with extensive levels of prior healthcare experience (e.g., military medical corpsmen, registered nurses, physical therapists, and emergency medical technicians), factors thought to contribute to their ability to function effectively with a minimal level of physician supervision. Selection of physician preceptors in rural areas was then and remains a goal of many of the programs. After graduation, many PAs selected primary care physicians located in a rural or medically underserved community.

Many of the seminal evaluations of PA use were performed in ambulatory practice and in HMO settings. In such settings, PA clinical performance has been impressive. Their productivity (number of patient visits) has been shown to approach and sometimes exceed levels of primary care physicians (Sox, Sox, & Tompkins, 1973; Hooker, 1993, 2002). Record (1981b) carefully documented PA productivity rates in a large group model HMO. She determined that the physician/PA substitutability ratio, a measure of overall clinical efficiency, was 76%. This assumed a practice environment in which PAs were used to their maximum capacity to perform medical services (consistent with educational competency and legal scope and/or supervision), and that they worked the same number of hours per week as physicians.

By the end of the first decade of practice for PAs, experience and empiric research indicated that U.S. medicine's adoption of the PA had been generally positive (Sox, Sox, & Tompkins, 1973; Scheffler, 1979). PAs were responsive to the public and the medical mandate to work in generalist and primary care roles in medically underserved areas. As their numbers pushed 10,000 in 1980, PAs were gaining recognition as being competent, effective, and clinically versatile healthcare providers (Nelson, Jacobs, Breer et al, 1975; Nelson, Jacobs, Cordner et al, 1975).

An important element in the acceptance and use of PAs was the development of a single pathway to licensure based not only on formal education but also on a nationally standardized certification examination. Recognizing the need for a credentialing body, which would be organizationally separate from the profession, the NCCPA was formed in 1973 and formally chartered in 1975. The NCCPA administered the first PA certifying examination in 1973 and began issuing certificates shortly thereafter. Soon the PANCE became recognized as the qualifying examination for entry to PA practice by a rapidly increasing number of state medical licensing boards. The NCCPA was established with federal and private grant support and assistance from the AMA and was closely linked to the NBME in the development of the PANCE and later the recertifying examinations for PAs. During the late 1970s and early 1980s, the PANCE examination and the NCCPA certification process had become incorporated into the practice acts of most state medical practice statutes. By the 1990s, successful completion of the PANCE became a universal qualification for PA practice.

Period 4: Recognition and Incorporation (1981 to 1990)

In the early 1980s PAs, as well as the other nonphysician health professions (NPs and certified nurse-midwives [CNMs]), had become widely used and accepted. The cumulative results of the past decade of health services research and practical experience with PAs were overwhelmingly positive, with the specific measures being patient and healthcare professional acceptance, quality of care, cost-effectiveness, productivity, and clinical versatility (Cawley & Golden, 1983; Carter, Emelio, & Perry, 1984; Schafft & Cawley, 1987).

For a time it appeared that the sole focus of PA practice would be primary care, although not all demand for PA services was in primary care. The PA role broadened during the 1980s when utilization extended beyond primary care into inpatient hospital settings and specialty areas. The trend toward specialization by PAs was the result, in part, of their clinical versatility and the health workforce demand. Market forces were at work and many medical and surgical specialties realized that the services of a PA could be used on inpatient hospital floors and in various settings. In 1977, the percentage of PAs working in the primary care specialties, defined as family practice, general internal medicine, and general pediatrics, was 77%. In 1981, the percentage had fallen to 62%. From 1981 to 2001, the percentage had settled at 50%. Over the same period, the percentage working in surgery and the surgical subspecialties rose from 19% to 28%; PAs in emergency medicine rose from 1.3% to 10% (and continues to grow).

During the early 1980s, the prediction of the Graduate Medical Education National Advisory Council of a rising number of physicians in the workforce prompted questions of whether there was much of a future for PAs. Yet, after a few years of doubt during which utilization was sluggish and several PA educational programs were closed (e.g., University of Indiana, Johns Hopkins University, and Stevens College), the PA profession continued to evolve and gain ground. On important levels recognition of PAs has occurred. At the federal level during the 1980s, two landmark events signaled incorporation of the occupation into the healthcare workforce mainstream. Perhaps the most significant of these was the congressional passage in 1986 of an amendment to the Medicare law providing reimbursement policies for PA services under Medicare Part B (Omnibus Budget Reconciliation Act, 1986). Recognition by Medicare, the largest health insurance program in the nation, indicated the legitimacy of PA services in medical care.

One event that represented a major landmark for the profession on the national and federal level was the attainment of commissioned officer status among uniformed services in 1988. Although this milestone tends to have little impact on PAs today, it was highly significant during the time and involved efforts on many levels to obtain. Doctors, nurses, physical therapists, and administrators were commissioned. PAs had gradually moved from senior enlisted ranks to warrant officers, but full commissioning was a ceiling that was not breached until the Air Force did away with warrant officers and commissioned their PAs as full officers. Given the rich history between the military and the PA profession, this event was of particular significance and satisfaction to the profession (Hooker, 1991a).

A less obvious, but no less important set of events that occurred during this time, was the increasing number of states passing legislation to update medical practice acts recognizing PA practice. This achievement was incremental, yet the progress in the aggregate was significant. Then (as well as now), many policy changes occurred on the state level. Most of them were enactments or substantial improvements. Good Samaritan laws were enacted to protect PAs. Policies changed to allow PAs to work some distance from the doctor. Reimbursement restrictions were lifted in some states and in others PA programs were inaugurated with tax dollars.

Research on the PA, the behavior of the PA, and how he or she compared to physicians began to appear. More than just anecdotal observations, experiments, manipulation of variables, and hypotheses began to drive the research. The research emerged as credible and critics became less.

On the organizational level, the AAPA headquarters in Alexandria, Virginia, was erected in 1987. The building, modeled in Georgian architecture characteristic of the area, marks the establishment of the PA profession as a permanent member of the health professions on the national organizational level.

Period 5: Maturation and Establishment (1991 to 2001)

By the 1990s, the PA profession had achieved a remarkable degree of integration in U.S. medicine. Over the preceding 30-year period, they achieved acceptance and incorporation in healthcare delivery, federal policies endorsed their presence in society, and they reached a critical mass as a profession.

As a recent entrant, in contrast with other new professions, the PA profession was consolidated in its representative organization early and became well stabilized. Among the notable indicators of further advancement of the profession is how often it is incorporated into national health policy projections and debate. Longevity has added depth to PA roles and status. On the federal level, PAs have been considered relevant players in healthcare reform under various proposals. Significant achievements included the passage of enabling legislation in all states and prescribing in all states. For example, the Balanced Budget Act (BBA) of 1997 better clarified the Medicare policy of PA reimbursement. States have modified their practice acts to enable PAs to practice with few barriers. Together with primary care physicians and NPs, PAs are considered essential members of America's primary care workforce (Donaldson, 1996). During this period, healthcare reform and universal medical care access became a political instrument for politicians. President William J. Clinton was pushing for health reform, as were many legislators. First Lady, Hillary Rodham Clinton, was the keynote speaker at the AAPA convention in 1993. In 1992, Mrs. Clinton convened a working committee to overhaul the federal system of health care and extend the care to all people. To do so, she included PAs, NPs, and CNMs in the mix. Subcommittees were formed to assess the role and responsibilities of PAs (Osterweis & Garfinkel, 1993).

There was much speculation that, if healthcare reform legislation passed, there would be a strong demand for primary care providers to serve the uninsured population. This demand, in turn, would result in a strong demand for PAs and other primary care providers. For the PA profession, this possibility was seen as a potential boom period where the number of programs and graduates would markedly expand. Although the Clinton reform plan did not become law, the expansion of the PA profession indeed occurred. From 1994 to 2001, the number of PA education programs doubled, as did the number of annual program graduates. A number of papers generated from this spurt of activity assessed the role of the PA and NP in managed care organizations, which may have stimulated employment (Hooker & Freeborn, 1991; Hooker, 1992; Hooker 1994; Ballweg, 1998; Freeborn & Hooker, 1995).

The power of marketing came into play in ways unexpected. The award-winning television show *ER* did much to raise the awareness about the role of PAs in healthcare delivery. A bright, personable, intelligent, knowledgeable, and sympathetic figure was found practicing in various PA roles in the hospital and before the camera from one week to the next for a few years.

Period 6: Global Expansion (2001 to present)

For PAs, the new century was heralded in a number of ways. The evolution of enabling legislation was complete with Mississippi being the last state to grant licensure for PAs. In 2007, Indiana became the last state to grant prescription rights to all PAs. More than 40 years of change has taken place: from the first graduates to granting enabling legislation, prescribing rights, and reimbursement nationally. What started as a noble experiment in the back room of a medical school has evolved to a system of healthcare delivery across 50 states and most of the U.S. territories. Countries such as Canada, Great Britain, and the Netherlands are producing their own graduates. Increasingly, the world is recognizing and allowing PAs to work. More than 75,000 people have graduated from formal PA programs, and more than 73,000 are working clinically.

In 2005, APAP changed their name, organization, and address. The more global and encompassing name of Physician Assistant Education Association (PAEA) was selected. The headquarters was moved into new space in Alexandria, Virginia. Such change was heralded by the launch of a new journal, the *Journal of Physician Assistant Education (JPAE)*, a new mission, new staff, and an annual conference of PA educators that would showcase innovations in education.

In 2008, the PA profession encompasses professional practicing in primary care as well as in specialties and subspecialties. As if to add legitimacy, the federal government in the United States (the Department of Veterans Affairs and the military) and Canada (military) are the largest single employers of PAs.

In 2009, the $2.2 trillion cost for health care in America had steeled its citizens to do something in regard to efficiency, organization, and financing. PAs represented an opportunity for change for consumers, purchasers, providers, and insurers. Health care was no longer dominated by a fee-for-service model, and the majority of Americans had been pulled into managed care organizations that were more oriented toward health prevention and wellness instead of illness—a situation ideal for PAs with their training and emphasis on health promotion. The HMOs and preferred provider organizations (PPOs) also attempted to limit "unnecessary care" and offer networks of providers who could deliver a set of healthcare benefits for a fixed fee. Medicine became a corporate endeavor, and the PA was the ideal employee who could assume care for many routine cases of medicine and do it well with little supervision.

The worldwide expansion of the PA concept is perhaps the major landmark of this era.

Globalization of PA development marks it as a stellar profession worthy of being adopted in other cultures and lands. For countries such as Taiwan, the Netherlands, South Africa, the United Kingdom, Australia, and Canada to embrace PAs is testimony that this occupation has merit worth emulating. The policies and practices of these countries means the PA will be redefined and modified in ways not fully anticipated as the developers envisioned. However, it is no longer an American product. Whereas the PA still embodies the role of assistant to the doctor, this role means different things to different governments.

History has a way of repeating itself. Some of the social issues worked out between 1980 and 2000 for inclusion will be struggles for some countries (and may need to be worked out again). Organized medicine may oppose the development and expansion of the PA role in some form. Nurses, especially NPs, may feel threatened and ask why not expand the NP role. Editorials will be written on both sides of the equation drawing support for their views, and debates will take place in many settings. What will most likely prevail is some modification of the assistant to the doctor that emerges as in the best interest of the people whom medicine serves. If the PA movement is found wanting, it will die. On the other hand, the tide is running out and there are not enough doctors. With supply and demand driving the behavior of most, the only alternative beside doubling the cadre of doctors to stem the tide is to expand the presence of the PA (Murray & Wronski, 2006).

ASSESSING THE PHYSICIAN ASSISTANT PROFESSION

The history of the PA profession is a remarkable one from a number of standpoints. Visionaries such as Charles Hudson, Eugene Stead, Richard Smith, Harvey Estes, Henry Silver, Loretta Ford, and others believed that lack of improvements in healthcare delivery demanded transformation. From what became a prime impetus for change, the PA emerged. Instead of the "one great man" theory that often precedes important social movements, the PA profession was founded on a few great people with remarkably similar ideas. Today, the product has exceeded even the boldest imagination of its creators (Hooker & Cawley, 2003; Ballweg, 2008).

In modern medicine, the creation of the PA marked the occurrence of doctors voluntarily deciding to share with another healthcare provider the key intellectual and professional functions of performing medical diagnosis and treatment. These activities were legally and functionally in the sole domain of physicians until the creation of PAs.

Some assert that curriculum revisions to increase primary care experiences for medical students should consider the approaches developed and used in PA educational programs. Innovation has flourished in PA programs partly because of their multidisciplinary design and partly because they have greater latitude in making curricular adjustments. PA programs have been pioneers in incorporating topic areas increasingly recognized as important in medical education: behavioral sciences; communication sciences; the humanities; epidemiology, preventive medicine, health promotion, and disease prevention; geriatrics; and community-based practice and community-oriented primary care. Educators of PAs are also proven innovators in the development of effective strategies in deploying graduates to medically underserved areas and in primary care specialties. The cumulative experiences of PA programs, including those ensconced in academic health centers, teaching hospitals, colleges, and universities, are successful educational endeavors. There are now 145 accredited PA programs in the United States, and over a dozen outside of the United States (along with others in development) that prepare competent and versatile generalist providers capable of handling most patient problems encountered in many settings.

To what degree has the PA profession succeeded in fulfilling a key objective of its creation: service in meeting the needs of medically needy populations? A traditional part of the social mission of medicine has been to provide health services that meet the needs of a nation's population. American medicine continues to be criticized as being overly specialized and unresponsive to the health needs of many citizens. Since the 1980s, the U.S. workforce policy reform debate has centered on policy questions of the accountability of the nation's workforce to meet societal healthcare needs, in particular the needs of the uninsured, the rural citizens, and the medically underserved. Government study groups have concluded that America's present system of health professions education and composition seems ill fit to meet the nation's future needs for healthcare providers (Cawley, 1995). U.S. policymakers remain frustrated with the realization that despite the substantial expansion of physician numbers over the past two decades, as well as the long-standing federal Medicare subsidy of graduate medical education, the number and percentage of physicians who select primary care continues to dwindle. The creation of the PA and the NP professions has helped to alleviate this shortage, but demand for services continues to outstrip supply in rural and underserved areas. America has failed to produce a balanced healthcare workforce and has fallen short of meeting the nation's need for generalist medical care services and universal access to care.

For the creation of the PA to have occurred, the critical issue of practice autonomy had to be addressed. Medical sociologists regard autonomy as the most important defining attribute of a professional within occupations, and particularly the health occupations. Medicine, like law and religion, have long been regarded as the true professions: Doctors possess their own language and distinct body of knowledge, collect direct fees for their services, are autonomous in function, and are largely self-regulated. The dependent-practice role of PAs and their willingness to function within the practice of the doctor and under supervision has been a critical factor in their acceptance, utilization, and success. The decision to establish the role of the PA as a dependent professional role—one characterized by a close practice relationship with a supervising physician—was a product of the collective wisdom of the profession's founders. They recognized that acceptance and use of these new providers held a direct relationship to the perceptions of physicians regarding the threat PAs may present in terms of income and professional domain. Dependent practice for PAs represented the central condition on which physician groups first accepted the PA concept. That PAs practice with supervision has always been the major factor in their acceptance and use.

There is little question that the American experience with PAs is successful. This is due, in large part, to a close educational and practice relationship with physicians, an affiliation that stands them in good stead. Many similarities exist between the medical training approaches of PAs and primary care physicians. They are now well integrated into many medical practices; all working with physicians, nurses, and others on the healthcare team.

Conventionally defined "barriers to practice" clearly affect levels of PA clinical productivity in a broad sense and differences in the delegatory styles of physicians are important determinants of PA practice effectiveness. Formalized barriers to practice effectiveness (e.g., restrictive regulations and payment ineligibility) represent the major limiting factors in PA use. This is manifested in clinical practice style, overlap, and in many instances, scope of practice. Professional domain ("turf") issues arise almost universally between health professionals. Yet, in spite of this, physicians now share more of their medical diagnostic and therapeutic responsibilities with PAs, than was the case in 2000. That they continue to share medical functions is a result of generational shifts, social forces, changing healthcare environments, and the inevitable division of complex labor.

SUMMARY

In the turbulent 1960s, a decade of change in many areas of U.S. society, a fundamental restructuring of the division of medical practice labor evolved. The introduction of the PA and the NP, along with the rebirth of the CNM in North America, represented a major transformation in U.S. medical practice. The role of the PA was created to assume a scope of practice that included medical tasks previously reserved for physicians. The concept developed with a medical and societal expectation focusing on extending the capabilities of doctors in the delivery of primary care, particularly to medically underserved populations or rural areas. With over four decades of existence, PAs have gained widespread recognition in nearly all aspects of medical care delivery in the United States and the concept has extended globally.

In terms of its educational systems, the PA profession has evolved successfully in preparing tens of thousands of PAs for active medical practice. The present model of PA education and certification gives graduates an opportunity to obtain employment in a primary care or generalist area or in a specialty or subspecialty area and to have clinical career-long specialty flexibility. There is strong evidence that PA educational approaches have been successful in preparing healthcare providers for employment in the healthcare system and beyond. The creators of the profession looked at models of nonphysician health personnel such as the European feldsher, the Chinese barefoot doctor, and the military corpsman. This examination gave credence to the notion of developing a more rational structure of healthcare personnel, one that made more efficient use of the training and capabilities of physicians and provided the opportunity to utilize nonphysicians to maximal effectiveness.

The trend toward international utilization of PAs represents a type of coming full cycle in the natural history of these personnel. Now PAs are recognized for their clinical versatility and assist industrialized countries in addressing medical workforce shortages. PAs are particularly valuable in supplementing doctors and replacing doctors in areas of doctor shortage. In some systems, there may be reluctance to create a new category of practitioner—a concern sometimes raised by nurses. However, the PA concept may encourage highly qualified people into the health system who may not otherwise have been attracted.

The use of nonphysicians has at times been championed as an attack on medical elitism and the professional establishment, as was the circumstance with the barefoot doctor. Stead believes that the medical profession has been arrogant in its stance toward entry policies and pathways leading to medical licensure. PAs have demonstrated high levels of patient acceptance and function with shorter training than physicians. Early critiques of PAs were that they represented a second tier of medical care. Yet, nonphysicians have been shown to augment the delivery of primary care to various patient populations, including the poor, those in medically underserved areas, and other disadvantaged members of society, and they do this in proportions greater than doctors. The employment of PAs in various roles, spanning most primary care functions as well as a wide swath of technical and public health and preventive medicine duties, appears to be an appropriate niche in the systems of many countries.

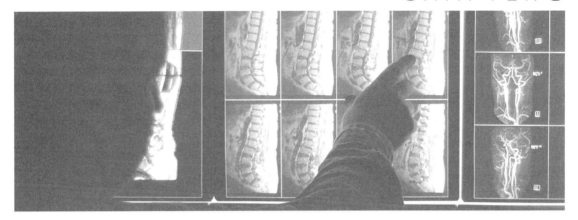

CHAPTER 3

CURRENT STATUS: A PROFILE OF THE PHYSICIAN ASSISTANT PROFESSION

RODERICK S. HOOKER ■ JAMES F. CAWLEY ■ DAVID P. ASPREY

ABSTRACT

The physician assistant (PA) of the new century does not fit any convenient stereotype. No longer just a creation of the United States, the PA profession is a product of a handful of countries and has the capability to acclimatize to any healthcare environment. The PA role has been designed to meet the needs of people around the world by adapting to various medical disciplines and health systems. In the United States alone there are more than 75,000 clinically active PA graduates. Hundreds more PAs are in other countries as expatriates or as graduates of new and emerging educational programs. Practice settings and their characteristics are diverse, ranging from family medicine in urban areas to surgery in rural locations. The demographics of the PA profession have changed dramatically to reflect the new millennium. Female PAs now outnumber males. They enter PA programs as their first chosen careers and tend to graduate in their late 20s. Fewer PAs work in primary care than in nonprimary care specialties. The racial and ethnic mix reflects the United States as a whole more than any other health profession. PAs are distributed into dozens of different medical and surgical specialities and are represented to a lesser extent in psychiatry, anesthesiology, pathology, and radiology. Genetics, one of the newest frontiers for medicine, already has a small but growing cadre of PA experts. Although improving access to care has been one of the principle justifications of developing the PA profession, PAs have proven to be productive as well, often requiring little supervision. The quality of care provided by PAs is as good as that provided by doctors (if care provided by doctors is considered the gold standard), making PAs valuable employees in most healthcare systems. When compared to other professions, the PA role is one of the most career-satisfying jobs in this decade, and the graduates are more likely to remain PAs than in almost any other occupation. Finally, the salary is considered middle to upper middle class—more than adequate to raise a family and afford a comfortable lifestyle.

INTRODUCTION

Describing the characteristics of physician assistants (PAs) requires drawing a profile of PAs incorporating contemporary data regarding their practice activities, distribution, specialties, productivity, and remuneration. The composition of the profession has changed considerably since the graduates of programs even a couple of decades ago. Neither the people nor the role of the PA is static, and healthcare needs are ever changing. With it are the PAs adapting to this change. Although much of the information provided is on the U.S. PA, other countries are portrayed wherever possible.

DISTRIBUTION

At the end of 2008, there were 73,893 PAs in active clinical practice in the United States, an increase of 7.8% from the 68,124 of the previous year. At the same time, there were more than 86,000 individuals eligible to practice as PAs. At the same time, more than 75,000 PAs have graduated from an approved U.S. PA program. Exhibit 3-1 depicts the growth of PAs based on new graduates and the total number of graduates. A rise in the number of PA programs in the 1970s was followed by a decade during which the number of annual graduates remained stable or went down. The 1990s and the 2000s saw a boom in annual graduate outcomes (Exhibit 3-2).

Some decline of the number of annual graduates occurred in the early years; the result of closure of some programs and consolidation of others. For the first few years of PA program development, the number of programs could not be determined with precision because of the difficulty defining and counting them at that time; some merged, some folded, and some converted from specialty to primary care. Outside of the United States, the Canadian military PA program can be considered the first non-U.S. program that graduated PAs beginning in 1992.

The supply of PAs varies considerably from country to country (Exhibit 3-3). The United States, with its more than 40 years of PA development, has the largest number of PAs clinically eligible to practice: 73,893 as estimated by the American Academy of Physician Assistants (AAPA) as of January 2009. Canada has graduated PAs since 1992

EXHIBIT 3-1
Physician Assistant Statistics, 2008

GENERAL	
Ever eligible to practice (1967–2009)	83,345
Clinically active (of those eligible to practice)	73,893 (86.6%)
Female	59.6%
Age (mean years)	43
EMPLOYER TYPE	
Single or multispecialty physician group practice	34%
Hospital	24%
Solo physician practice	12%
Government	9%
WORK SETTING	
Hospital inpatient	19%
Hospital emergency department	10%
Hospital outpatient	8%
PRIMARY SPECIALTY OF THE PRACTICE	
Primary care (family/general medicine, general internal medicine, general pediatrics)	34%
Surgery/surgery subspecialties	23%
Internal medicine subspecialties	7%
INCOME	
Annual income (median total income for more than a 32-hour work week)	$85,710
Annual income (mean total income for more than a 32-hour work week)	$89,297

Data from American Academy of Physician Assistants. (2008a). 2008 AAPA Physician Assistant Census Report. Alexandria, VA: Author.

and as of 2009 has approximately 170 who are clinically active (100 in uniform and 70 in a few provinces). The Netherlands has approximately 200 PAs that are formally trained and working.

In the United States, the number of PAs per state varies considerably. Some of this variation is historical and due to enabling legislation that was slow to evolve (such as in Mississippi) or a surge of demand (e.g., Alaska's need for PAs to care for those working on the Alaskan pipeline in the late 1970s). This patchwork distribution of PAs is represented in Exhibit 3-4, with California and New York accounting for one-sixth of the graduates. New York, Pennsylvania, Michigan, North Carolina, and Florida are among the states with the highest

EXHIBIT 3-2
Physician Assistant Graduates and Education Programs*

Year	New Graduates (United States)	Number in Active Practice (United States)	U.S. PA Programs	PA Programs Outside the United States
1967	3	3	1	—
1968	17	20	2	—
1969	17	37	4	—
1970	46	83	—	—
1971	60	143	—	—
1972	277	420	—	—
1973	730	1,150	—	—
1974	1,116	2,339	—	—
1975	1,375	3,767	—	—
1976	1,552	5,354	—	—
1977	1,600	6,980	—	—
1978	1,352	8,355	—	—
1979	1,415	9,797	—	—
1980	1,437	11,258	—	—
1981	1,539	12,815	—	—
1982	1,400	14,240	—	—
1983	1,365	15,624	—	—
1984	1,228	16,884	—	—
1985	1,175	18,091	53	—
1986	1,158	19,261	51	—
1987	1,097	20,368	49	—
1988	1,051	21,420	50	—
1989	1,156	22,578	51	—
1990	1,232	23,814	51	1
1991	1,308	25,124	55	1
1992	1,565	26,690	54	1
1993	1,647	28,338	56	1
1994	1,901	30,226	63	1
1995	2,188	32,397	63	1
1996	2,570	34,696	68	1
1997	2,866	32,782	84	1
1998	3,704	35,898	94	1
1999	3,856	41,421	105	1
2000	4,668	42,762	116	1
2001	4,750	52,716	128	1
2002	4,925	51,607	132	1
2003	5,125	55,616	134	4
2004	5,125	58,826	136	6
2005	5,225	62,723	136	6
2006	5,410	62,968	137	7
2007	5,004	69,473	139	10
2008	5,217	73,893	142	12
2009	5,600	—	145	14
2010[†]	6,100	—	146	16

*Aggregated data from the American Academy of Physisican Assistants, the Physician Assistant Education Association and based on projections by the authors.
[†]Estimate.

EXHIBIT 3-3
Physician Assistant Education (Non-U.S.)

Country	Number of Graduates	Year Commenced	PA Program
Australia	0	2009	University of Queensland
	0		James Cook University
Canada	150	1990	Canadian Armed Forces
	0	2008	University of Mannitoba in Winnepeg
	0	2008	McMasters University
	0	2010	University of Toronto
England		2005	University of Birmingham
	20	2004	University of Wolverhampton
	20	2005	Kingston and St. George's University
	25	2005	University of Hertfordshire
			Warwick University
			University of Surrey
The Netherlands	100	2001	Academie Gezondheidszorg in Utrecht
	100	2003	University of Arnhem/Nijmegen
	50	2005	University of Gronengen
	50	2006	Amsterdam
South Africa	0	2009	University of Witswaterrand
	0	2009	University of Pretoria

number of annual PA graduates. At the other end of the scale, low-population states such as Arkansas and Wyoming have the fewest number of PAs. Alaska has the highest concentration of PAs per population and Mississippi the lowest.

Although most of the U.S. PAs are distributed throughout the continent, approximately 2% report residencies overseas. These locations include the U.S. territories (e.g., Puerto Rico, Guam, the Virgin Islands, and American Samoa), U.S. military settings (e.g., Iraq, Afghanistan, Europe, Germany, Japan, Korea, and Turkey), private agencies that have medical facilities outside the United States (e.g., Central America, Southeast Asia, and Saudi Arabia), the Department of State, the Central Intelligence Agency, and the Peace Corps.

The PA profession was asked by its early proponents to prove that it could provide quality care to the underserved, reduce the perceived personnel shortage in health care, and make the lives of physicians less harried. All of these goals were achieved in the first 10 years within the confines of the limited number of personnel being trained in relatively small programs. However, the criteria by which effectiveness is judged have changed, and the healthcare context has also shifted radically, raising new questions about the role of PAs.

The annual *AAPA Physician Assistant Census Report* revised its classification scheme regarding the practice location of PAs (Exhibit 3-5). The 2008 census shows that only 1,113, or 4.4%, of practicing PAs work in nonmetropolitan communities that are not adjacent to metropolitan areas; 2,631, or 10.6%, work in nonmetropolitan areas that are adjacent to metropolitan areas. Almost 85% practice in metropolitan regions. These data raise the question of whether PAs are still fulfilling one of the original intentions of their creation: serving in rural and similar medically underserved communities.

Population alone cannot account for all state variations. Mississippi, for example, is ranked 31 in population and is tied with Guam for the lowest number of PAs and the

EXHIBIT 3-4

North American Distribution by Province, State, and Territory in Which Physician Assistants Practice, 2008 (N = 26,192)

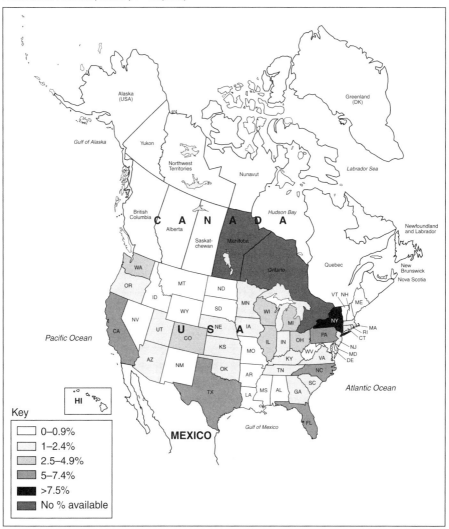

A total of 73,893 known to be eligible PAs were invited to participate in the census, accounting for 86.6% of the 85,345 individuals ever eligible as PAs.

Data from American Academy of Physician Assistants. (2008a). 2008 AAPA Physician Assistant Census Report. Alexandria, VA: Author.

highest population to PA ratio in the country. A reason for the concentration of PAs in states such as New York, Texas, and California is that they have high concentrations of PA training programs. Implicit in the location of state-supported PA programs is that many of the graduates will remain in the state. The geographic distribution of PAs in the health-care workforce is probably associated with the following:

- Market demand and salaries
- Enabling state legislation (ability to practice and prescribe)
- Location of PA training programs

EXHIBIT 3-5
Geographical Location of Physician Assistants in the United States, 2008

Respondents		Number	Percent
NONMETROPOLITAN	Nonmetropolitan with urban population more than 20,000, adjacent to metro area	1,109	4.5
	Nonmetropolitan with urban population more than 20,000, not adjacent to metro area	596	2.4
	Nonmetropolitan with urban population of 2,500 to 20,000, adjacent to metro area	926	3.7
	Nonmetropolitan, with urban population of 2,500 to 20,000, not adjacent to urban area	707	2.9
	Nonmetropolitan with urban population less than 2,500, adjacent to metro area	159	0.6
	Nonmetropolitan with urban population less than 2,500, not adjacent to metro area	247	1.0
METROPOLITAN AREAS	Metropolitan with more than 1 million population	11,942	48.1
	Metropolitan with 250,000 to 1 million population	6,151	24.8
	Metropolitan with less than 250,000 population	2,984	12.0

Data from American Academy of Physician Assistants. (2008a). 2008 AAPA Physician Assistant Census Report. Alexandria, VA: Author.

PRACTICE SETTING

Practice setting, as defined by the AAPA census, is the patient care environment in which the clinican works—the primary employer of the PA. Although concise nomenclature has not emerged for identifying where PAs practice, the AAPA Division of Research has created a classification system for analyzing data and a set of useful terms that identify where PAs are principally employed. At some point, international consensus may be necessary to create a more generic list of practice settings.

United States

For U.S. PAs, the patterns of practice settings began primarily in outpatient general practice and then began moving to hospitals and large group practices. A shift occurred in the early 1990s, revealing an increase in hospital-based practices. However, the practice settings of PAs have been relatively stable since the new century.

As of 2008, almost 55% of all PAs work in solo or group private practices. Nearly one-half (44%) of PAs work in either single specialty or multispecialty group practices. Single specialty group practice is the largest specific category of practice setting. Another fifth of PAs (19%) are in hospitals, which includes university and other hospital settings, and the remaining are in settings such as public and private ambulatory clinics, health maintenance organizations (HMOs), geriatric facilities, occupational health settings, correctional systems, and other healthcare practices and institutions (Exhibit 3-6). Over one-tenth of PAs work in emergency medicine, and another tenth work in hospital outpatient departments. This activity has been verified by large cross-sectional studies of patient visits using the National Ambulatory Medical Care Survey data (Hooker & McCaig, 2001; Lin et al, 2002; Hooker, Cipher, & Sekscenski, 2005; Hooker et al, 2008).

About 9% of the respondents to the AAPA census work for a state or federal government agency. The federal government is the largest employer of PAs, employing more than 3,000 (Hooker, 2008b). Within the federal government, the Department of Veterans Affairs employs the most PAs—more than 1,800. Uniformed services are the second largest government employer of PAs.

EXHIBIT 3-6
**Physician Assistant Principal Practice Settings,
United States, 2007**

Setting	Percent
Intensive care unit (ICU)/critical care unit (CCU) of hospital	2.2
Inpatient unit of hospital (not ICU/CCU)	10.3
Outpatient unit of hospital	7.4
Hospital emergency room	10.1
Hospital operating room	6.5
Other unit of hospital	1.5
Federally qualified rural health center	3.5
Other federally qualified health clinic (not rural)	1.9
Other community health center	1.9
Freestanding urgent care clinic	2.9
Freestanding surgical facility	0.4
Solo practice physician office	11.9
Single-specialty group practice	22.2
Multispecialty group practice	9.3
HMO facility	1.3
Nursing home or long-term care facility	0.8
University/college health facility	0.6
School-based health facility	0.4
Other outpatient facility	1.9
Correctional facility	1.0
Industrial facility	0.5
Retail outlet	0.2
Mobile health unit	0.1
Patients' homes	0.1
Other	1.3
Total	100

*Data from American Academy of Physician Assistants. (2007a). 2007
AAPA Physician Assistant Census Report. Alexandria, VA: Author.*

The distribution of PAs by practice setting tends to parallel that of physician distribution in that most PAs practice in group settings or in hospitals. Contrary to what some might suspect, there has not been any appreciable change in the number of PAs working in urgent care or surgicenters over the past 7 years (Exhibit 3-7).

In the United States, PAs practice medicine in communities ranging from the most rural to the inner city. Fifteen percent of AAPA census respondents work in counties that are not metropolitan. Approximately 9% work in inner cities (AAPA, 2008a).

Canada

Out of the approximately 170 PAs employed in Canada in 2008, roughly two-thirds are in the military providing various services around the globe (Hooker, MacDonald, & Patterson, 2003). At least 40 PAs are in Ontario working in emergency medicine, community health clinics, and hospitals (Ashton, 2007). Another growing number of PAs are in Manitoba working in hospital-based roles (Exhibit 3-8). Both provinces have PA programs. If anticipated enabling legislation is enacted across more provinces, the total number of clinically active PAs in Canada will likely double by 2012.

Great Britain

A handful of American PAs are in Scotland working primarily in outpatient clinics (Buchan, O'May, & Ball, 2007). In England, another gourp of PAs are dispersed in working in emergency medicine settings and outpatient clinics. As of 2009, there are over 120 PA graduates educated in Great Britian. Four PA programs will be graduating over 100 per year by 2010 (Ross & Parle, 2008). The majority of PAs in Great Britian are paid through some arrangement with the National Health Service (NHS).

The Netherlands

With few exceptions, all 200 PA graduates in the Netherlands are working in some hospital-based role. All are specialized in some form but may provide services in a combination of inpatient and outpatient settings (Spenkelink-Schut, Koch, & Kort, 2006). A few PAs have been employed in a general practice role.

Australia

As of 2009, 10 clinical PAs in Australia are employees of the State (Queensland primarily) and are part of demonstration utilization projects (Sweet, 2008). Other American-trained PAs are educators. A handful are in South Australia working in hospitals. Two PA programs are in development.

EXHIBIT 3-7
Physician Assistant Trends by Practice Setting

Practice Setting	2002 $N = 17,254$	2003 $N = 7,995$	2004 $N = 20,852$	2005 $N = 19,987$	2006 $N = 20,925$	2007 $N = 23,689$
Self-employed	405 (92.3%)	466 (2.6%)	553 (2.7%)	620 (3.1%)	545 (2.6%)	676 (2.9%)
Solo physician	2,188 (12.6%)	2,349 (13.1%)	2,929 (14.1%)	2,691 (13.5%)	269 (12.9%)	2,982 (12.6%)
Single specialty, physician group	5,106 (29.5%)	5,326 (29.6%)	6,251 (30.0%)	6,121 (30.6%)	6,591 (31.5%)	7,325 (31%)
Multispecialty, physician group	2,192 (12.7%)	2,440 (13.6%)	2,700 (13%)	2,453 (12.3%)	2,644 (12.6%)	3,066 (12.9%)
University hospital	1,337 (7.7%)	1,361 (7.6%)	1,517 (7.3%)	1,503 (7.5%)	1,652 (7.9%)	2,045 (8.6%)
Other hospital	2,679 (15.5%)	2,658 (14.8%)	3,083 (14.8%)	2,988 (14.9%)	3,030 (14.5%)	3,356 (14.2%)
Urgent care center	282 (1.6%)	314 (1.7%)	388 (1.9%)	366 (1.8%)	447 (2.1%)	442 (1.9%)
Surgical center	15 (0%)	19 (0.1%)	25 (0.1%)	22 (0.1%)	27 (0.1%)	19 (0.1%)
Nursing home/ long-term care	63 (0.3%)	61 (0.3%)	55 (0.3%)	47 (0.2%)	55 (0.3%)	53 (0.2%)
Hospice	NR	NR	1 (0%)	1 (0%)	2 (0%)	2 (0%)
Health Maintenance Organization	523 (3.0%)	503 (2.8%)	550 (2.6%)	457 (2.3%)	437 (2.1%)	439 (1.9%)
Community health center	1,082 (6.2%)	1,111 (6.2%)	1,227 (5.9%)	1,215 (6.1%)	1,238 (5.9%)	1,370 (5.8%)
Medical staffing organization	31 (0.1%)	36 (0.2%)	58 (0.3%)	66 (0.3%)	58 (0.3%)	78 (0.3%)
Physician practice management organization	256 (1.4%)	237 (1.3%)	309 (1.5%)	277 (1.4%)	284 (1.4%)	421 (1.8%)
Integrated health system	193 (1.1%)	213 (1.2%)	201 (1.0%)	258 (1.3%)	246 (2.6%)	342 (1.4%)
Correctional system	239 (1.3%)	226 (1.3%)	229 (1.1%)	218 (1.1%)	217 (1.0%)	207 (0.9%)
Other	660 (3.8%)	666 (3.7%)	753 (3.6%)	684 (3.4%)	751 (3.6%)	832 (3.5%)

NR, data not reported.

Data from American Academy of Physician Assistants. (2007a). 2007 AAPA Physician Assistant Census Report. Alexandria, VA: Author.

EXHIBIT 3-8
Geographic Location of Physician Assistants, Canada, 2008

Geographic Location	Number
Alberta	0
British Columbia	0
Manitoba	70
New Bruswick	0
Ontario	40
Military	100

Note: The military are dispersed throughout Canada and PAs are part of this dispersement.

Taiwan

All 1,100 or so PAs in Taiwan are working in very large hospital settings, such as emergency medicine, intensive care units, and operating theaters. In 2008 the Taiwan government refused to recognize these PAs, both formally and informally, and so the PA movement has come to an end. The nurses trained as PAs are now referred to as Practice Nurses.

Liberia

Little is known about nonphysician clinicians in Liberia who use the name "physician assistant." As the development of PAs gains a foothold in Africa, more information will emerge about these and other PAs or prototype PAs (Mullan & Frehywot, 2007).

South Africa

Three universities are developing Clinical Associates to work in locations where doctor supervision is limited.

PRACTICE CHARACTERISTICS

Medical practice is how the clinician identifies and defines himself or herself. Practice characteristics are the features of the discipline considered typical to that PA's practice and are reflected somewhat by the physician workforce, which has become increasingly specialty oriented. The American Medical Association (AMA) annually tracks more than 125 disciplines and the specialty orientation of PAs seems to parallel this activity up to a point. After a decade in which PAs were largely deployed in primary care, more recent patterns reveal a trend toward PA practice in nonprimary care specialties and being located in urban and inpatient settings (Exhibit 3-9).

Among practicing PAs, 34% work in the primary care clinical practice specialties, which are defined by the U.S. Department of Health and Human Services as the specialties of family practice, general internal medicine, and general pediatrics. This proportion is down from the 62% reported in 1980. In 2008, 25.9% of all PAs were working in family practice, 5.2% in general internal medicine, and 2.5% in general pediatrics (AAPA, 2008a). After four decades of having PAs in the U.S. healthcare system, the percentage of those working in the primary care specialties declined, and there was a corresponding increase in PAs being employed in hospital-based and specialty care practices.

Specialization began at an early stage, marked by the founding of specialty-focused educational programs in pediatrics and surgery in the late 1960s and the establishment of a surgical postgraduate program in 1972. For many years, due largely to the influence of federal funding dollars, the direction of the profession took a turn toward primary care. In the late 1970s, a majority of PAs worked in family medicine. But as the profession evolved and grew in the 1980s and 1990s, specialization increased as more PAs entered specialty practices. This trend led to the formation of more specialty and subspecialty societies within the AAPA and the emergence of more postgraduate educational programs (Asprey, 2008; Cawley, 2008a).

As the number of PAs in specialties has increased, the numbers in primary care have consequently declined. Most practicing PAs are now in medical specialties outside of primary care. According to the AAPA Physician Assistant Census Report, the percentage of those working in primary care specialties has fallen to the lowest levels recorded in the past several decades. Only one-third (33.6%) of the nation's PAs in active clinical practice work in the areas of family medicine (25.9%), general internal medicine (5.2%), or general pediatrics (2.5%); less than one-third of all new PA graduates now enter primary care fields. These statistics are in contrast to the fact that one-fifth (22.6%) of PAs work in surgery and the surgical subspecialities and 10.5% work in emergency medicine.

The decline of PAs in primary care practice parallels that of physicians whose numbers in primary care have also been falling. Fewer medical school graduates are selecting residencies in the primary care specialties, and physicians worry that primary care will be lost to other types of providers. Dwindling numbers in primary care run counter to the long-held

EXHIBIT 3-9
Percentage Specialty Distribution Trends of U.S. Physician Assistants for Selected Years

Specialty	Year (No.)								
	1974 (939)	1978 (3,416)	1981 (4,312)	1987 (10,692)	1994 (12,281)	1996 (12,701)	2000 (16,547)	2002 (16,835)	2008 (25,187)
Family practice	43.6	52.0	49.1	38.7	37.2	39.8	36.5	32.1	25.9
General internal medicine	20.0	12.0	8.9	9.5	7.7	8.3	8.8	8.4	5.2
General pediatrics	6.2	3.3	3.4	4.0	2.5	2.7	2.6	2.6	2.5
General surgery	12.1	5.5	4.6	8.8	2.8	3.1	2.7	2.5	2.5
Surgical specialties	6.8	6.2	7.7	13.8	19.1	8.3	17.4	19.2	22.6
Medical specialties	3.9	6.3	2.7	7.1	7.4	5.8	8.11	9.4	9.3
Pediatric subspecialities									1.8
Emergency medicine	1.3	4.9	4.5	6.5	8.4	7.0	9.7	10.2	10.5
Occupational medicine	1.8	2.7	3.1	4.1	3.1	3.0	3.5	3.0	2.3
Dermatology									3.6
Cardiology									3.2
Other specialty	4.3	7.1	16.0	7.5	7.0	9.5	6.5	8.4	10.4

Data from American Academy of Physician Assistants. (2008a). 2008 AAPA Physician Assistant Census Report. Alexandria, VA: Author.

traditions and priorities for PAs to serve in generalist practice and in medically underserved communities. However, it is difficult for PA educational programs to maintain an emphasis on primary care practice for PAs when the economic and market forces pull increasing numbers of graduates to specialties.

Organizationally, specialization within the PA profession has spurred the founding of specialty and subspecialty organizations, yet most specialty PAs remain closely aligned with the AAPA. The challenge is to retain these groups under the big tent of the AAPA while the many specialty groups hold their own meetings and continuing medical education programs. Developing their own certification structure seems inevitable.

A flash point for the debate related to specialization is the recent discussion of the issue of PA postgraduate program accreditation—so-called PA residencies (Knott, 2008). Specialty groups within the AAPA support the notion that PA postgraduate programs should develop a formal accreditation process. However, the AAPA as a whole has opposed the accreditation of postgraduate PA programs primarily on the basis that such a step would give status to such education and lead to circumstances in which specialty certification would be the norm and thus become a requirement for employment, practice, licensure, and reimbursement. Central to the AAPA's argument against accreditation of postgraduate programs is that such a move could limit a cherished aspect of PA practice: the capability to move into and out of different practice specialties. PA career flexibility is a major advantage for many in the PA profession, and the AAPA contends that protecting such flexibility is in the best interest of the profession. In doing so, however, the AAPA encounters the increasing forces of professional specialization that universally continue to affect modern medical practice (AAPA, 2005). In contrast, the NCCPA has decided it will begin field testing specialty examinations in 2010. The ARC-PA began certifying postgraduate programs in 2009. Debate on this topic continues largely due to the lack of good information on the topic (Hooker, 2009).

Primary care figures also differ depending on who is counting. The AAPA and some nurse practitioner (NP) organizations include women's health (obstetrics and gynecology) as a primary care discipline. Others mention that industrial and environmental (occupational) medicine, public health, military medicine, geriatrics, and corrections medicine are largely primary care disciplines that are functioning under a unique name.

Since the turn of the century, the percentage of PAs employed by hospitals has remained fairly constant, beginning with 14% in 1974. As the proportion of PAs in primary care practice declined, the rates of PAs working in acute care settings in medical and surgical specialties and subspecialties rose correspondingly (Hooker, Cipher, Cawley et al, 2008). Key factors in expanding the role of the PA and the number of PA positions in inpatient care were hospital cutbacks in physician residency programs, curtailed availability of international medical graduates (IMGs), and cost-effectiveness of inpatient roles (Cawley & Hooker, 2006).

It may be argued that trends in PA patterns have closely mirrored those of physicians. With the physician workforce becoming increasingly specialized, and with changes in physician-determined patterns in the division of medical labor, PA use has moved to some degree toward specialty areas, a process to be expected of any developing occupation. Although primary care remains the major practice thrust of the PA profession, trends emphasizing specialty practice in the PA profession continue. An intriguing, but unanswered, question is how much primary care is provided by PAs working within specialty practices?

DATA SOURCES ON PHYSICIAN ASSISTANTS

For the first two decades of the development of PAs it was difficult to obtain reliable data on their deployment. The budding AAPA had been able to retain information on many of the programs and graduates, but systematic and uniform data gathering was not standardized. Henry B. Perry was the first to systematically survey PAs (Perry, 1978b). A research council was formed to report back to the AAPA's board of directors. The council made a series of recommendations for collecting data and determining what research questions were in need of answering. Beginning in the late 1980s, the AAPA and the associated PA programs began earnestly collecting and reporting data. This process allowed for the generation of reports about cross-sectional information and trends. As the mass of PAs grew, other agencies, such as the Medical Group Management Association, state medical boards, and federal agencies began collecting information and making it available.

After more than four decades of research and careful planning, a number of important data sources for the PA profession emerged, and more are emerging in the United States and other countries. Using these data sources allows for analysis of what is occurring and trends in the behavior of PAs. Some of the more usable databases are discussed in the following paragraphs. Together, these databases provide a remarkable breadth and depth of information about the profession.

American Academy of Physician Assistants (AAPA)

One valuable information source for Americans is the AAPA set of databases. What is known about PAs, on a cross-sectional basis, is attributable in part to the AAPA's general census database. The general census is an annual survey that provides detailed and timely information on socioeconomic aspects of the PA profession. The AAPA census collects this information as part of its annual membership renewal and has been collecting this information in some form for every PA program and their graduates. Initially, this database was used to compile information on AAPA membership, but it has expanded to contain current deployment trend data on a large proportion of the PA population. The AAPA membership has waxed and waned but by January 2009 had reached 30,846, almost half of all PAs currently eligible to practice. A total of 27,568 individuals responded to the annual census survey in 2008.

Physician Assistant History Project

The History Project is an international archive of PA history and development that is underwritten in part by the AAPA. The collection of information includes documents, publications, reports, communications, memorabilia, uniforms, photographs, and ephemera. A catalog of this information is available online.

Physician Assistant Education Association (PAEA)

The *Annual Report on Physician Assistant Educational Programs* documents the data from each program. The Physician Assistant Education Association (PAEA) membership funds this report. Whereas the AAPA census database relies on individual responses from academy members, the PAEA's annual report uses data gathered from PA programs (Exhibit 3-10).

Centralized Application System for Physician Assistants (CASPA)

The Centralized Application System for Physician Assistants (CASPA) is operated by the PAEA. This national application service emerged in 2004 and has become an important Web-based application system for more than 100 PA programs. This system standardizes the application process and documents the transcripts and characteristics of the PA aspirant. As a result, educators and analysts can obtain unique perspectives on trends in applicants.

Association of Postgraduate Physician Assistant Programs (APPAP)

The Association of Postgraduate Physician Assistant Programs (APPAP) annually surveys and collects information about the activities of these programs and their residents (Wiemiller, Somers, & Adams, 2008).

National Commission on the Certification of Physician Assistants

A source of information that overlaps somewhat with the AAPA is the National Commission on Certification of Physician

EXHIBIT 3-10
Age of U.S. Physician Assistants at Graduation, 2007

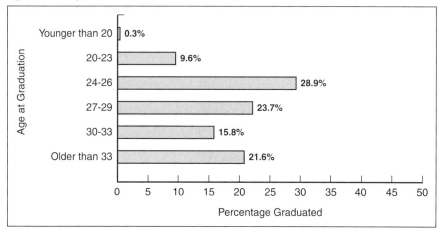

Data from Physician Assistant Education Association, 2007.

Assistants (NCCPA). The NCCPA registers all PA graduates who have sat for the Physician Assistant National Certification Examination (PANCE), NCCPA, and the National Board of Medical Examiners (NBME). It also makes available scores on the national certification and recertification examinations (Hooker, Carter, & Cawley, 2004; Arbett, Lathrop, & Hooker, 2009).

Accreditation Review Commission on Physician Assistant Education (ARC-PA)

The Accreditation Review Commission on Physician Assistant Education (ARC-PA) has a database on characteristics of developing new and existing programs. Although this database is confined to U.S. programs, its value as a source of information about new PA program trends is beginning to be explored.

State Medical and Physician Assistant Boards

All 50 states and most of the territories and the District of Columbia maintain registries and databases on PAs, where PAs practice, and their characteristics. In many states, such as Utah, Iowa, and North Carolina, annual and semiannual data on the human capital

used in healthcare services are collected (Pedersen et al, 2008). These sources provide opportunities for more detailed examination on the role and behavior of PAs.

Federal Sources

Databases within the uniform services, the Department of Veterans Affairs, and other federal agencies serve as excellent sources on the use and activites of PAs. For example, the National Practitioner Data Bank is a depository of information on litigation and misadventure regarding PA and other practitioner activity. The Bureau of Labor Statistics collects information on employment statistics by state, county, metropolitan areas, and other variables. It also projects what the demand for occupations are likely to be in 5 and 10 years. The National Centers for Health Statistics have continuous data on ambulatory care, hospital discharge data, emergency department use, and hospital outpatients.

Professional Societies

Many PA societies, such as the Society for PAs in Rheumatology (SPAR) collect information on their members and where they work (Hooker & Rangan, 2008).

Medical Groups

Information at most managed group practices, such as Kaiser Permanente and Group Health Cooperative of Puget Sound, have extensive databases on who the provider of care was for each patient encounter. Some of these large prepaid group practices record over two million visits per year.

DEMOGRAPHIC DATA

In the United States, the median age of PAs at graduation has generally declined since the 1970s. The current age at the beginning of a PA career is approximately 34 years (PAEA, 2007). Trends in the age of graduates have shifted in the span from 1984 to 2009, with a recent trend toward younger age at time of graduation than in previous years. The proportion of recent graduates in the youngest age group (younger than 24 years) has generally decreased over time with a slight increase over the previous 10 years. Conversely, the middle age group (ages 24 to 29) has increased 53% since 1994. The number of graduates in the older age group (older than 30 years) has increased 37% since 1994 (Exhibit 3-11).

The median age of all practicing PAs in the United States is 44 years (AAPA, 2007a). Since 1974, the age of practicing PAs has risen from 31 to 38 years in 1991 to 43 years in 2008 and is expected to hover at this age for the next several years (Exhibit 3-12). A trend of older PAs being replaced by younger PAs is underway at a ratio of 1:3.

The AAPA Division of Research estimates there were a total of 85,345 individuals who were ever eligible to work as a PA (primarily gradautes of a PA program) at the beginning of 2009. Of this total, there were 73,893 PAs who were technically eligible to practice who had not retired or died. At the same time, approximately 65,000 people held a valid certification from the NCCPA. Thus, about 80% of all persons ever trained as PAs are still eligible to practice (Exhibit 3-13). The AAPA membership survey reports that the mean years in clinical practice for PAs is 9.2, with a median of 9 years. A sizable proportion of those in the profession have been in clinical practice for less than 3 years (22%), and 15% have been in clinical practice less than 6 years.

The attained educational degree is the highest degree reported by AAPA census respondents. About 81% of graduates have at least a bachelor's degree (42% bachelor's degree; 39% master's degree). Most U.S. PA programs have shifted from offering a certificate or bachelor's degree to offering a master's degree. Factors contributing to this shift include the desire to remain competitive with other programs and the pressure of a competitive job market that demands at least a baccalaureate degree for professional legitimacy. The PAEA has also decided that a graduate

EXHIBIT 3-11

Percentage Trends in the Age of Physician Assistant Graduates (1984–2008)

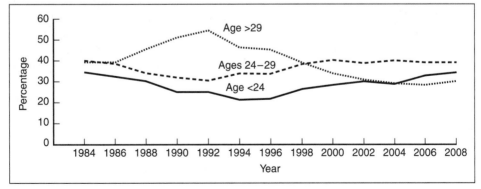

Aggregated data from Physician Assistant Education Association, 2008.

EXHIBIT 3-12

Summary Measures of Age for All U.S. Physician Assistants, 2009

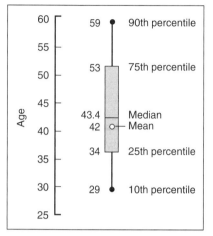

Data from American Academy of Physician Assistants. (2008a). 2008 AAPA Physician Assistant Census Report. Alexandria, VA: Author.

degree is the appropriate entry-level document for the rigor of the coursework that students attend. Additionally, more and more students already have undergraduate and graduate degrees when entering programs. More than 75% of all PA students possess at least an undergraduate degree before entering training programs, and more than 90% have a degree of some type upon graduating. The trend toward degree-granting programs and applicants with degrees already in hand is expected to continue.

Certification refers to the percentage of PAs who are nationally certified (Exhibit 3-14). Although recertification is not a requirement everywhere, most states, federal government agencies, and private employers are requiring it as a condition of employment.

The profile of the PA has changed relatively quickly, compared with that of other professions. In contrast to the three male veterans who graduated in 1967, the average PA graduate in 2008 is a woman, is approximately 44 years of age, and has a nonmilitary medical background. More than 75% have a bachelor's or a master's degree; almost 3% have a doctorate.

As the national profile of PAs changes, some predictions about what the profession will look like in 2015 can be made. First, females will likely represent two-thirds of the profession by 2015. This gender shift is seen across society in many different fields and professions (e.g., dentistry, medicine, veterinary sciences, military, and academics) Although some programs may be inclined to enroll their classes in roughly even numbers of men and women, they must draw upon the applicant pool presented. Since the mid-1980s, the PA profession has attracted more women than men and—with the exception of the military—this trend is likely to continue. Second, although the average age of PAs in the workforce has slowly increased to approximately 44 years, data from the AAPA database suggests that the aging PA is no longer remaining in the workforce into their 70s as they once did (Duryea & Hooker, 2000). Finally, the average age of entrants to PA programs is and will likely remain relatively stable (PAEA, 2007).

Although little is known about the life cycle of a PA and what the average age of retirement will be, some extrapolations can be made by examining career trends for doctors and attorneys (U.S. Department of Labor, Bureau of Labor Statistics, 2008). Based on national trends of certain professionals, it is likely that at least three-fourths of PAs will remain in their careers until the traditional retirement age between 62 and 65 years. Another relevant factor is that PAs tend to be highly satisfied with their careers, which suggests some stability of the profession (Freeborn & Hooker, 1995; Marvelle & Kraditor, 1999). Historically, physicians have had unusually long work lives, with the average 35-year-old physician practicing almost until age 70. Whether this trend holds true for PAs is not clear; however, observations made a decade ago indicate that some PAs were working beyond age 65 (Duryea & Hooker, 2000).

Gender

In 1965 the first class of PAs was all men. Women entered the third Duke University class and have been part of the PA profession

EXHIBIT 3-13

Total Number of Physician Assistants, New Physician Assistants, Accredited Physician Assistant Programs Reporting New Graduates, and Physician Assistants in Clinical Practice at Year's End, 1991–2008

	1991	1992	1993	1994	1995	1996	1997	1998	1999	2000	2001	2002	2003	2004	2005	2006	2007	2008
People ever eligible to practice as PAs*	25,131	26,668	28,310	30,214	32,384	34,917	37,720	41,346	45,188	49,223	53,595	57,803	62,171	66,563	71,216	75,260	79,706	85,345
New PAs†	1,329	1,537	1,642	1,918	2,187	2,584	2,837	3,649	3,880	4,064	4,394	4,226	4,394	4,395	4,275	4,646	4,541	4,806
New PAs as percentage of total	5.29%	5.76%	5.80%	6.35%	6.75%	7.40%	7.52%	8.83%	8.59%	8.26%	8.20%	7.31%	7.07%	6.60%	6.00%	6.17%	5.70%	5.1
PA programs with new graduates	53	55	55	58	62	71	78	93	100	115	122	124	128	131	131	131	138	142
Mean new PAs per program	25.1	27.9	29.9	33.1	35.3	36.4	36.4	39.2	38.8	35.3	36.0	34.1	34.3	33.5	32.6	35.5	32.9	34
PAs in practice at year's end‡	20,628	21,890	23,184	24,931	27,105	29,161	31,480	34,192	37,821	40,469	42,708	46,002	50,121	55,061	58,665	63,609	68,124	73,893
Percentage in clinical practice	82.1%	82.1%	81.9%	82.5%	83.7%	83.5%	83.5%	82.7%	83.7%	82.2%	79.7%	79.6%	80.6%	82.7%	82.4%	84.5%	85.5%	86.6%

*Figures represent the count of all individuals believed to be eligible to practice as PAs in each reference year. The individuals believed to have died prior to 1996 are excluded from the figures reported in 1996 and forward since year of death is not available. The individuals believed to have died in or after 1997 are excluded from the counts for each year after the year of death. Individuals for whom no graduation date is known or available are associated with the year in which they became NCCPA-certified. *Source:* AAPA Masterfile 11/1/2007.

†Figures represent the numbers of PAs believed to have graduated during each reference year from accredited PA programs reporting new graduates. Individuals for whom no graduation date is known are associated with the year in which they became NCCPA-certified. *Source:* AAPA Masterfile 11/1/2007.

‡*Source:* Estimated from 1991–1995 AAPA Membership Census surveys; 1996–2007 AAPA Physician Assistant Census surveys; and AAPA Masterfile 11/1/2007.

Data courtesy of the AAPA Research Division, 2009.

EXHIBIT 3-14
U.S. Physician Assistants, January 2009

	Percent	Number
Total U.S. PA graduates (ever graduated or ever eligible to practice as a PA)		85,345
Total employed PAs (not necessarily clinically)	85	73,893
Total currently NCCPA-certified	81.5	65,000
GENDER		
Female	59.6	
Male	40.4	
ETHNICITY		
Asian/Pacific Islander	4.8	
Black (not Hispanic)	6.1	
Hispanic/Latino origin	5.1	
Native American/Alaskan Indian	0.8	
White (not Hispanic)	83.1	
Multiethnic	0.3	
AGE		
Mean years	43.4	
Median years	42.0	
AGE DURING YEAR OF GRADUATION FROM PA SCHOOL		
Mean years	30.7	
Median years	42.0	
CURRENTLY CERTIFIED		
Yes	92.7	
No	7.3	

Data from American Academy of Physician Assistants. (2008a). 2008 AAPA Physician Assistant Census Report. Alexandria, VA: Author.

ever since. Stead (1966, 1967) conceived of the PA as being composed predominantly of men because he thought they would have a greater commitment to a career and a greater willingness to meet the demands of their work. This attitude was short lived, and by 1974 the percentage of female PAs had increased to 16% (Perry, 1977). Currently, the composition of the PA workforce is nearly 60% women and the class of 2009 is 71% women (Exhibit 3-15).

This demographic shift is not surprising. Women have been moving into formerly male-dominated professions in large numbers since 1980. For example, the percentage of female lawyers and judges rose from 4% in 1972 to 15% in 1982. Over the same period, the percentage of female accountants rose from 22% to 38% of the total. For economists, the increase has been from 12% to 25%. These changes reflect the different educational choices made by young women since the mid-1980s. In 1968, women received only 8% of all medical degrees and 4% of law degrees. The percentages were 41% and 39%, respectively, in 2001. By 2008, 51% of medical school graduates were women. For lawyers, in 2006, the number is 25% in law practice and 44% of law school graduates.

On average, women PAs are 10 years younger than males, and the average age of male PAs is rising more rapidly than women. Women are more likely than men, by a small margin, to be in family practice (39%), and more likely to be in group practices than men. Both work in towns of less than 10,000 people at about the same rate. There is a difference in the proportion of women who are not in clinical practice (17%) versus men (5%).

It is hard to determine what effect the increasing proportion of women in the PA profession will mean. If parallels are to be appropriately drawn from the literature on women physicians, it may be that female PAs emulate female physicians. However, findings on aspects of the career characteristics of women physicians may or may not apply to PAs, and there are anecdotal suggestions that women PAs may exhibit a different set of career and practice patterns than women physicians. For example, female physicians are disproportionately represented in low-paying primary care specialties, such as family practice and general pediatrics, as opposed to specialties such as orthopedics or cardiology. Women physicians spend more time with patients (Cassard et al, 1997). These practice patterns have also been said to be true of PAs, although documentation on the subject is difficult to find.

Female physicians are more likely to offer preventive services to patients (Ewing et al, 1999) and to take different pathways of communications with patients than male physicians (Seto et al, 1996). Evidence of a glass ceiling in academic medicine was present for women in the previous decade (Bernzweig et al, 1997). For the PA profession this trend

EXHIBIT 3-15
Trends in the Gender of U.S. Physician Assistant Graduates (1984–2008)

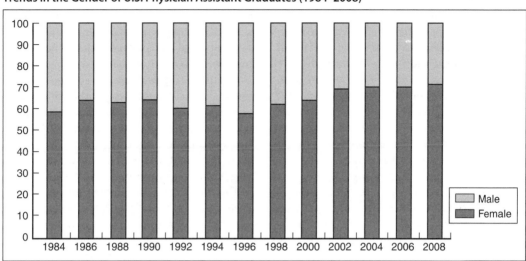

Data aggregated from the Physician Assistant Education Association.

seems to be changing. In 2006, 38% of PA education program directors were women and three of eight PAs who were deans were also female (PAEA, 2007).

For many women, the PA profession represents a preferred and attractive career choice, allowing flexibility along with a high measure of clinical responsibility. In fact, women, including those with academic records that would make them a virtual certainty to be accepted into medical school, are choosing to enter the PA profession. This tendency may be attribtuable to the fact that with a PA career women can maintain some control over their work life in a fashion that permits more lifestyle choices and family time.

Gender shifts within key professions, changing perceptions of the roles and status of physicians, and system-driven forces brought about by new requirements for institutional staffing and patient care services are redefining the division of medical labor. There is also the notion of the "deprofessionalization" of medicine—the loss of overall status in society—which is decreasing what Paul Starr calls physician sovereignty over the healthcare system (Starr, 1982). Has this trend paralleled the rising profile of the status, roles, and responsibilities of

nonphysical clinicians such as NPs, PAs, and certified nurse midwives (CNMs)? It is clear that, for many young women, the PA profession offers advantages. For some, the PA profession may be a preferable career choice vis-à-vis that of a physician, with its many demands and sacrifices. The shorter period of formal professional training, high level of clinical responsibility, increasing practice and professional autonomy, and the career flexibility options that characterize the PA profession are important factors included in the health career choices of many young women.

Because of the shift in the gender of certain historically male-dominated occupations, planning the future healthcare workforce must consider a large set of variables. Nationally, women are 11 times more likely than men to voluntarily quit a job. On average, they work 8 months in each job, whereas men work 3 years, and they are more likely to be part-time workers. Sustained work experience has an important affect on earnings, so these differences between men and women are relevant. Marriage also seems to affect women and men differently. Married men earn more than single men, but single women earn more than married women. This result may occur because historically marriage freed men of household duties and permitted more single-minded attention to jobs, but marriage has had the opposite effect for women. Women in their 30s who have worked without interruption since high school earn slightly more than men with the same background. Unmarried female faculty members at colleges and universities earn slightly more than unmarried male academics with similar credentials.

In determining whether wage differences are the result of discrimination, groups of workers are compared who are equally capable, experienced, and motivated. This comparison is not easy to make given the numerous factors that affect the current earnings of any worker. Economists, taking into account easily measured factors such as age, years of schooling, region, and hours of work, found that from one-half to three-fourths of the gross differences in earnings between men and women can be explained by these factors (Ehrenberg, Goldhaber, & Brewer, 1995). Whether the remaining differences are the result of discrimination or as yet unquantified productivity differences is and probably will continue to be a controversial issue.

Women PAs earn less than male PAs even when influencing factors such as on-call hours, years as a practicing PA, years in current practice, setting, and community size are controlled in the analysis (Carter, Emelio, & Perry, 1984; Willis et al, 1986; Oliver, 1993). Analysis by specialty also reveals that salary differences remain for family/general practice, pediatrics, obstetrics and gynecology (OB/GYN), emergency medicine, and orthopedics. However, no statistical differences emerge in the specialties of surgery, internal medicine, or occupational/industrial medicine (Willis et al, 1986). Other studies have found that female and male PAs that were hired at the same salary level did not have significant salary differences a few years later.

The reasons for salary differences are not easily explained. Shortcomings of some studies include ignoring hourly wage, productivity (patient visits per hour), and total revenues generated by the PA. Other considerations to explain the differences may relate to initial starting salaries, the ability to negotiate for raises, participation in profit sharing, strengthening of a retirement fund, and the development of partnerships when private practices are examined.

Future studies should address whether there are different expectations between women and men in specific settings and whether employers are satisfied with the job performance of both men and women. Do male PAs ask for or receive more frequent and larger raises than women? Are there changes in the way women and men are perceived in their roles and in how they are reimbursed? What experiences discourage or block female PAs from obtaining jobs with greater potential for productivity, income, and advancement? Finally, what can women do to alter discriminatory practices?

Race and Ethnicity

Racial and ethnic diversity are the cornerstones of U.S. culture, and adequate representation of all races and ethnic groups is essential to the viability of the PA profession. Without a heterogeneous mix of the U.S. population adequately representing the profession, meeting the cross-sectional needs of the U.S. population will fall short. The proportion of survey respondents from underrepresented minorities is rising within the profession (Exhibit 3-16). Groups showing the largest increases are Hispanics in the south central region and

EXHIBIT 3-16
Number and Percent of U.S. Physician Assistants by Race, 2008

	Number	Percent
Asian/Pacific Islander	3,134	4.8
Black, not Hispanic	4,016	6.1
Hispanic/Latino Origin	3,358	5.1
American Indian/Alaskan	553	0.8
White (not Hispanic)	54,259	83.1
Total	65,320	100

Data from American Academy of Physician Assistants. (2008a). 2008 AAPA Physician Assistant Census Report. Alexandria, VA: Author.

African Americans in the southeast. Trend data suggest that African Americans, Native Americans, and other distinct ethnic groups are participating more than ever before in the profession.

Organizational efforts to improve the configuration and diversity of the PA profession are ongoing. Three PA training programs actively recruit a student body of minorities (primarily African Americans). A program for Native Americans functioned for a few years in New Mexico but closed in the late 1980s. The Health Professions Educational Assistance Act and the Health Professions Scholarship Program are designed to attract minorities to the healthcare professions. Other efforts are underway, including programs to promote the sciences to minorities, an area in which they are also underrepresented.

Application to Physician Assistant School Ratios

With the advent of the centralized application for medical students and PA students, the ratio of applicants to seats has remained fairly stable since accurate counting began in 2002. That ratio is 3:1 for PA programs and 2.5:1 for allopathic/osteopathic schools (Rubeck et al, 2007).

Education

Approximately 67% of PAs received at least a bachelor's degree before enrolling in a PA program. Approximately one-half (45%) of the PAs responding received a bachelor's degree from a PA school; one-third (32.5%) received a master's level PA degree (Exhibit 3-17). Today, 62% of respondents hold bachelor's degrees,

EXHIBIT 3-17
Percent Distribution by Physician Assistant Degree Held (_N_ = 61,853)

Certificate from PA Scool	29.3
Associate from PA School	6.9
Bachelor's degree from PA School	43.1
Master's degree from PA School	35.7

Data from American Academy of Physician Assistants. (2008a). 2008 AAPA Physician Assistant Census Report. Alexandria, VA: Author.

25% hold master's degrees, and 3% hold doctorate degrees. With the change to programs granting graduate degrees, these numbers will shift to more graduates with a master's degree in the workforce.

Specialty

One remarkable aspect of the evolution of the PA profession in U.S. medicine has been its incorporation into specialty practice in addition to primary care. Although the initial mandate for PAs was to serve as primary care practitioners, more than one-half have entered specialty and subspecialty practices with equal success. Exhibit 3-18 illustrates the specialty distribution of practicing PAs in 2008.

An important group of PAs is composed of those working in general surgery and the surgical subspecialties (22%). These PAs make up more than one-fifth of the PA workforce. This group includes PAs in orthopedics (8%).

There is a good deal of overlap in the practice of PAs in specialties and those in primary care. For example, gynecology, geriatrics, corrections medicine, industrial and occupational medicine, and emergency medicine are largely composed of primary care activities but tend not be classified as primary care.

Employers

PAs are primarily employed by single specialty physician groups (30%) followed by hospitals (23.6%), multispecialty group practices (13.5%), and solo practices (12.2%). Since the year 2000, only minor shifts in the trends of practice setting have occurred, but as solo physician practices fade and changes in resident hours worked affect hospitals, a gradual shift of practices into groups and hospitals is expected. The phenomenon of self-employed PA practices is only now beginning to be recognized (Barnes & Hooker, 2001).

PRODUCTIVITY

PA _productivity_ refers to the quantity of services PAs provide to their patients. The number of patient visits to a medical office or patients

EXHIBIT 3-18
Distribution of Physician Assistants by Specialty, 2008

	Count	Percent		Count	Percent
Respondents	25,187	100	Urology	339	1.3
Addiction medicine	76	0.3	Vascular	166	0.7
Allergy	134	0.5	Bariatric	72	0.3
Anesthesiology	65	0.3	Spine	196	0.8
Dermatology	900	3.6	Other	140	0.6
Emergency medicine	2,651	10.5	General pediatrics	618	2.5
Family practice without urgent care	3,959	15.7	**PEDIATRIC SUBSPECIALTIES**		
Family practice with urgent care	2,566	10.2	Adolescent medicine	62	0.2
Genetics	12	0.0	Allergy	8	0.0
Geriatrics	162	0.6	Cardiology	25	0.1
Obstetrics/gynecology	590	2.3	Critical care	25	0.1
Occupational medicine	580	2.3	Endocrinology	14	0.1
Ophthalmology	29	0.1	Gastroenterology	32	0.1
Pain management	338	1.3	Hematology/oncology	7	0.0
Pathology	5	0.0	Infectious disease	4	0.0
Physical medical rehabilitation	168	0.7	Neonatal-perinatal	96	0.4
Psychiatry	256	1.0	Nephrology	5	0.0
Public health	40	0.2	Neurology	20	0.1
Radiation oncology	76	0.3	Pulmonology	15	0.1
Radiology	46	0.2	Rheumatology	3	0.0
Interventional radiology	216	0.9	Oncology	31	0.1
Hospital medicine	421	1.7	Other	90	0.4
General surgery	636	2.5	General internal medicine	1,303	5.2
Other	575	2.3	**INTERNAL MEDICINE SUBSPECIALTIES**		
SURGICAL SUBSPECIALTIES			Cardiology	794	3.2
Cardiovascular/cardiothoracic	775	3.1	Critical care	88	0.3
Colon and rectal	28	0.1	Endocrinology	116	0.5
Hand	53	0.2	Gastroenterology	372	1.5
Neurology	587	2.3	Hematology/oncology	46	0.2
Oncology	76	0.3	Immunology	2	0.0
Orthopedics	2,528	10.0	Infectious disease	115	0.5
Otorhinolaryngology	251	1.0	Nephrology	152	0.6
Pediatric	39	0.2	Neurology	161	0.6
Plastic	213	0.8	Pulmonology	142	0.6
Thoracic	52	0.2	Rheumatology	83	0.3
Transplant	70	0.3	Oncology	433	1.7
Trauma	120	0.5	Other	102	0.4

Data from American Academy of Physician Assistants. (2008a). 2008 AAPA Physician Assistant Census Report. Alexandria, VA: Author.

seen in the hospital are measures that capture a large proportion of overall PA use in most specialties. Time spent in practice can be measured in hours per week and patients per day. On average, PAs spend 37.6 hours per week in an outpatient setting and see 19.3 patients per day. The total number of visits per week is a unit of productivity sometimes used for comparison among organizations because routines may be accorded to specific days of the week. In 2008, the productivity of PAs was estimated to range from 53 to

99 visits per week depending on the specialty (Exhibit 3-19). These productivity figures are similar to physicians in the same specialty. The number of prescriptions per visit by the different specialty is also included in Exhibit 3-19. These findings suggest that prescribing is an important element of PA practice.

An inpatient practice is considered (although undefined in the survey) to exist when a PA makes a hospital or surgical service patient visit (commonly referred to as *making hospital rounds*). In the 2008 survey undertaken by the AAPA, 5,971 PAs responded that they worked or were employed by a hospital. The average age was 38, females were 86% of the cohort, and 52% were employed by the hospital instead of a doctor. Almost all (97%) work in an urban setting, the majority were full time (86% work greater than 32 hours a week) and 87% were salary-based. The average salary in 2008 was $89,987. Many PAs who have an outpatient practice primarily may provide some of their work in a hospital. Likewise, many

PAs working in hospitals may see only ambulatory patients.

PAs are employed by a variety of industries, agencies, and firms; however, the dominant employer is a physician or a group of physicians who provide outpatient primary care. How these employers perceive the benefit in employing a PA depends on the return they can achieve. These economic factors are discussed in detail in Chapter 11.

Patient Visits and Encounters

Because of the variety of work settings and specialty fields in which PAs practice, the types of patients they treat are varied. More than 90% of census respondents who work full time see outpatients in their primary job; the mean number of patient visits provided per week by family medicine PAs who see outpatients exclusively is 88.8 visits per week. Twenty-eight percent of respondents who work full time see inpatients in their primary

EXHIBIT 3-19
Estimated Number of Patient Visits and Medications Prescribed by Physician Assistants in 2008 and 2000

Specialty	2008		2000	
	Average No. of Visits to Each PA per Week*	*Average No. of Prescriptions per Visit†*	*Average No. of Visits to Each PA per Week**	*Average No. of Prescriptions per Visit†*
Family practice	88.8	1.5	93.7	1.3
General internal medicine	71.7	1.6	78.4	1.8
Cardiology	63.0	1.3	60.5	1.0
Other internal medicine subspecialties	59.9	1.3	59.8	1.3
Obstetrics and gynecology	69.4	0.9	64.5	1.3
Emergency medicine	84.0	1.4	93.8	1.3
General pediatrics	94.2	0.9	99.7	0.9
Pediatric subspecialty	53.0	1.3	54.2	1.2
General surgery	57.0	1.0	55.4	0.4
Cardiovascular surgery	40.7	1.2	53.1	1.4
Orthopedic surgery	67.0	0.9	78.7	0.8
Other surgical specialty	60.6	1.0	64.4	0.9
Occupational medicine	80.4	0.9	90.6	0.8
Other	65.0	1.2	77.8	1.1

*The mean number of visits per week is rounded to two decimal points; therefore, totals cannot be calculated from figures.

†Medication may be prescribed by the PA or recommended by the PA for prescribing.

Data from American Academy of Physician Assistants Marketing Research Survey, 2000, 2008; and American Academy of Physician Assistants. (2008a). 2008 Physician Assistant Census Report. Alexandria, VA: Author.

job; the mean number of patient encounters provided per week by respondents who see inpatients exclusively is 60. Eight percent of full-time PAs see nursing home patients in their primary job, and 5% of respondents see other types of patients.

Part-Time Employment

The percent of PAs who work 32 or more hours per week (considered full time in the United States) is 85.2%. Conversely, those who work less than 32 hours per week can range from one to four days per week. Characteristics of part-time PAs and their choice in trade-offs remains to be researched.

COMPENSATION

Earnings, considered either at a point in time or as a stream of revenue received over the working lifetime of an individual, strongly influences an individual's choice of occupation and is the most frequently mentioned attribute of an occupation. Although the time structure of earnings is the key determinant in measuring occupational models, the annual earnings at a point in time can give a rough idea of the relative income ranking of one occupation compared with others (Exhibits 3-20 and 3-21).

The term *compensation* includes the combination of salaries and benefits. It is the amount the employer foregos to retain the services of

EXHIBIT 3-20
Earnings for Workers in Select Occupations, May 2006

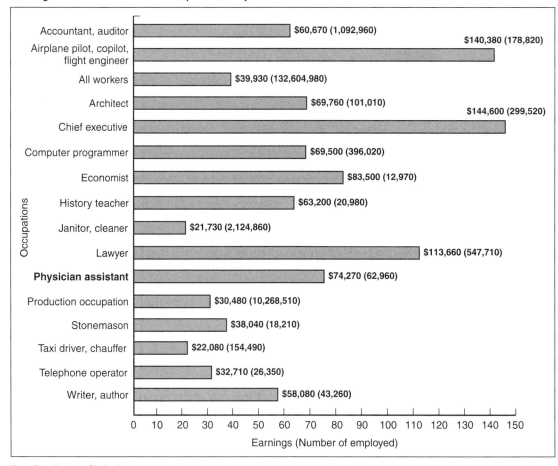

Data from Bureau of Labor Statistics, 2007.

EXHIBIT 3-21
U.S. Occupational Employment and Wages for Select Health Workers

Occupation Title	Number Employed in this Field	Median Hourly Wage	Mean Hourly Wage	Mean Annual Wage	Mean RSE
Chiropractors	25,470	$31.36	$38.97	$81,070	2.4%
Dentists, general	86,110	$63.53	$67.76	$14,950	1.7%
Optometrists	24,220	$43.77	$47.38	$98,550	1.4%
Family/general practitioners	109,400	—	$72.04	$149,850	1.0%
Pediatricians, general	28,930	$66.41	$68.00	$141,440	1.8%
Psychiatrists	24,730	—	$72.11	$149,990	4.1%
Surgeons	51,900	—	$88.53	$184,150	1.1%
Physician assistants	**62,960**	**$36.05**	**$35.71**	**$74,250**	**0.7%**
Physical therapists	156,100	$31.83	$32.72	$638,050	0.3%
Dental hygienists	166,380	$30.19	$30.01	$62,430	0.6%
Emergency medical technicians and paramedics	196,190	$13.01	$14.13	$29,390	0.7%
Licensed practical and licensed vocational nurses	720,380	$17.57	$18.05	$37,530	0.2%
Athletic trainers	15,440	—	—	$38,860	1.3%
Registered nurses	—	—	—	$52,330	
Nurse practitioners	71,300	—	—	$71,130	

RSE = Relative Statistical Estimate. The higher the number the greater the range of salary.

Data from Bureau of Labor Statistics, 2007.

the employee. Although salary is fairly easy to calculate, benefits are more nebulous. Some benefits have a definable amount, such as the cost of dental insurance for an employee and his or her family. Other benefits, such as a cellular phone or group medical liability insurance, are actually prerequisites of the job that the employer provides, and the employee is not taxed for their use. Benefits are defined in dollar amounts and usually range from 15% to 25% of the salary.

Salary

Salary is the amount of direct compensation in money that a wage earner receives. The salary range of experienced PAs is quite wide because PAs are in a wide variety of clinical settings, have many different arrangements with their employer, and have a large skill set.

Measuring the change in incomes reported by the same people for two periods provides a superior basis for examining the health of PA

income than a comparison of the incomes reported by all PAs for two periods. Understanding income change is important because it accounts for the larger constellation of static and dynamic factors that determine earnings and choice. Conversely, the change revealed by a comparison of income reported by all PAs for two distinct periods is confounded by the income-related effects of whatever differences exist between the populations of PAs represented by each period. For example, the relative proportion of recent graduates would affect the change in each period.

As a consequence, posting an average or median salary may or may not be useful to PAs interested in their market value on entry into the workforce (Exhibit 3-22). Practice specialty, years of experience, employment setting, and city size in which a PA works all have an affect on salary (Exhibits 3-23 and 3-24).

EXHIBIT 3-22
Percentile Wage Estimates for Physician Assistants, Hourly, May 2008

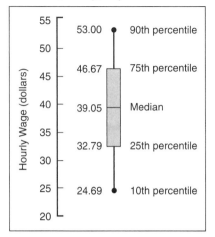

Data from Bureau of Labor Statistics, 2008.

EXHIBIT 3-23
Percentile Wage Estimates for Physician Assistants, Annual, May 2008

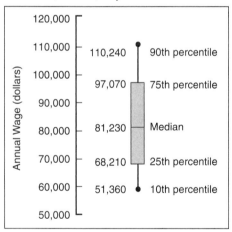

Data from Bureau of Labor Statistics, 2008.

However, the variable that influences future PA salary more than others is practice specialty. Exhibit 3-25 shows PA starting salaries for recent graduates by type of specialty. The mean starting salary in industrial and occupational medicine is approximately $80,932, versus general pediatrics in which graduates earn, on average, $70,816 per year.

Not surprisingly, PAs with more experience command higher salaries. When income distribution is viewed as a probability density, the data show a curve with the left side fatter than the right. This lopsided curve is classic for salary distributions and is predictable because income increases with experience at a fairly even pace. Eventually some peak density is attained and then decreases exponentially at higher levels of income. The ever-diminishing tail represents the very few, who for various entrepreneurial reasons, have incomes two to four times greater than their cohorts.

As the PA-physician relationship evolves on the employer-employee level, compensation arrangements negotiated by PAs will continue to undergo change. Some forms of compensation, such as overtime, are incentive bonuses directed at driving the PA to perform more work. More commonly reported compensations range from overtime pay to event-call pay to on-call pay (such as wearing a beeper or being close to home for consultation). Increasingly, PAs are being compensated with bonuses. In 2000, almost one-fifth of PAs received a bonus either because of the practice's performance or their performance. The average annual bonus earning is $9,000, although this number is a bit misleading because two-thirds earned a bonus less than $5,000 per year in additional revenue. More than 15% of the PAs report additional earnings ranging from $10,000 to more than $20,000. Other arrangements include incentive pay based on productivity, as well as partnerships and percentages of revenues (Barnes & Hooker, 2001). Eighty-two percent of respondents report receiving their base pay in the form of a salary; 17% indicated that they receive an hourly wage.

Benefits

Surveys conducted on 12,242 practicing PAs to determine the types of benefits that employers commonly offer to PAs had a 56% response rate. The distribution was reported as representative of the practicing PA population by specialty, setting, population base, and gender. Aside from the base salary information,

EXHIBIT 3-24
Practice Setting and Geographical Profiles for Physician Assistants, May 2006

Industry	Number Employed	Hourly Mean Wage ($)	Annual Mean Wage ($)
Physician offices	38,820	39.25	81,650
General medical and surgical hospitals	16,820	40.10	83,400
Outpatient care centers	6,140	41.15	85,590
Federal medical centers	2,100	37.39	77,770
University medical centers	1,960	35.50	73,830
STATES WITH THE HIGHEST CONCENTRATION OF PHYSICIAN ASSISTANTS			
Montana	580	34.07	70,860
Maine	730	40.74	84,740
South Dakota	420	38.67	80,430
North Dakota	340	36.01	74,900
Nebraska	880	38.88	80,880
TOP PAYING STATES FOR PHYSICIAN ASSISTANTS			
Alaska	290	46.99	97,715
Nevada	490	45.75	95,160
Connecticut	1,290	45.37	94,360
Washington	1,820	44.13	91,800
New Jersey	980	42.57	88,540
METROPOLITAN AREAS WITH THE HIGHEST CONCENTRATION OF PHYSICIAN ASSISTANTS			
Fayetteville, NC	280	40.05	83,300
Greenville, NC	150	38.56	80,210
Lewiston-Auburn, ME	90	40.81	84,880
Niles-Benton Harbor, MI	110	41.51	86,330
Casper, WY	70	43.70	90,890
TOP PAYING METROPOLITAN AREAS FOR PHYSICIAN ASSISTANTS			
Lake County-Kenosha County, IL-WI Metropolitan Division	140	60.99	126,850
Chattanooga, TN-GA	120	59.72	124,220
Leominster-Fitchburg-Gardner, MA	40	57.37	119,330
Ocala, FL	30	56.52	117,550
Anchorage, AK	120	55.83	116,120

Data from Bureau of Labor Statistics, 2007.

questions included areas such as insurance benefits, paid leave (vacation, continuing medical education [CME], sick time, and maternity leave), and other earnings through bonuses (Exhibit 3-26).

Exhibit 3-27 describes the findings for insurance benefits, benefits other than insurance, and the mean number of days available for various leave categories. It should be noted that the average amount of funding for CME is $1,412 per year and is available to 85% of PAs who work full time.

Additional Compensation

Respondents report receiving several different forms of compensation from their primary employer. Common forms of compensation include event-call pay (9%) and overtime pay (18%). Twenty percent of respondents report receiving an incentive based on productivity or performance. Approximately two-fifths (38%) of those who receive an incentive based on productivity and performance report that the incentive is based on revenue that the PA generates.

EXHIBIT 3-25
Mean and Median Annual Income From Primary Employer for Physician Assistants by General Specialty Practiced, 2008

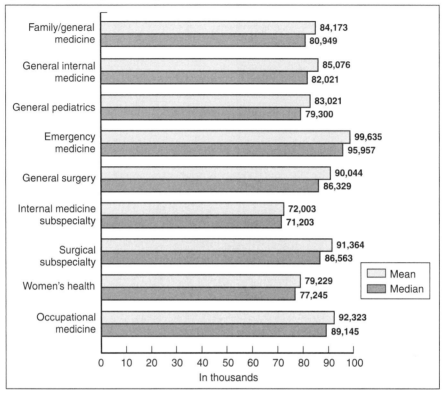

Data from American Academy of Physician Assistants, 2008.

Taking Call

More than one-third (36%) of full-time respondents report taking call for their primary employer. The mean hours on call per month for those PAs who take some call but are not always on call is 104.

CME Funding

Eighty-eight percent of respondents report having CME funds available to them from their primary employer. For those PAs who reported the amount of CME funds available to them, the mean was $1,438; the median was $1,500.

Funds for Expenses

More than 97% of respondents report having their employer pay 100% of their professional malpractice liability insurance. Approximately two-thirds of respondents also report having their employer pay their AAPA dues (64%), state license fees (70%), NCCPA certificate maintenance fees (63%), AAPA annual conference

EXHIBIT 3-26
Annual Days of Paid Vacation, Sick Leave, and Medical Education for Physician Assistants by Employer

Description	Mean	Median	Standard Deviation
Annual days of paid vacation leave (N = 14,057)	18	15	6.8
Annual days of paid sick leave (N = 9,216)	10	9	6.9
Annual days of paid medical education leave (N = 11,942)	6	5	2.3

Data from American Academy of Physician Assistants. (2007a). 2007 AAPA Physician Assistant Census Report. Alexandria, VA: Author.

EXHIBIT 3-27
Percentage of Physician Assistants Receiving Specified Fringe Benefits*

Description	Benefit Reimbursed by Employer			Benefit Not Reimbursed
	95–100 % by Employer	50–94% by Employer	1–49% by Employer	
Professional liability insurance (N = 16,595)	98	1	0	2
Individual health insurance (N = 15,325)	48	36	7	9
Family health insurance (N = 11,638)	25	36	11	29
Dental insurance (N = 14,625)	31	31	10	28
Disability insurance (N = 14,317)	44	18	8	31
Term life insurance (N = 13,597)	41	15	10	35
Pension/retirement fund (N = 15,079)	23	21	39	17
State license fees (N = 16,148)	73	2	1	24
DEA registration fees (N = 13,667)	78	1	1	20
NCCPA fees (N = 16,043)	65	2	1	33
AAPA dues (N = 15,793)	64	2	1	33
State PA chapter dues (N = 14,444)	57	2	1	41
Specialty organization dues (N = 11,571)	46	2	1	50
AAPA Annual Conference (N = 13,973)	57	8	4	30
Credentialing fees (N = 15,312)	75	2	1	21

AAPA, American Academy of Physician Assistants; DEA, Drug Enforcement Administration; NCCPA, National Commission on Certification of Physician Assistants.

*Percentages may not sum to 100 due to rounding.

Data from American Academy of Physician Assistants. (2007a). 2007 AAPA Physician Assistant Census Report. Alexandria, VA: Author.

registration fees (59%), and Drug Enforcement Administration registration fees (72%).

The benefit structure for state and federal government workers tends to be more encompassing than that for those in the private sector. For example, in the federal system, vacation time amounts to 4 weeks per year. Sick leave is generous, and health, dental, malpractice, and life insurances are automatically covered. The retirement benefits of federal, state, and sometimes municipal employment make this sector particularly attractive.

TURNOVER AND MOBILITY

PAs are fairly mobile professionals, meaning they tend to change jobs regularly. From the employer's standpoint this mobility is termed *turnover*. The standard method of determining the turnover rate is the number of PA clinical positions held divided by the total number of years in practice as a clinical PA. For all respondents to the 2002 membership census who practice full or part time, the rate is 0.47. On the whole, more than 60% of the PA profession has spent less than 3 years in their current positions (Cawley et al, 2001), and for the past few years, the percentage of PAs who have remained in the same position more than 10 years has averaged around 8% (Exhibit 3-28). Even PAs with more than 15 years of experience report that they have been with their current employer, on average, less than 3 years. This finding suggests PAs negotiate contracts frequently and are often active in the job market at advanced stages of their careers. Little is understood about this phenomenon other than the speculation that PA graduates tend to take their first job as entree to the workforce that may not be the most attractive, and then tend to look around for a way to raise their income and working conditions by switching employers.

EXHIBIT 3-28
Physician Assistant Mobility

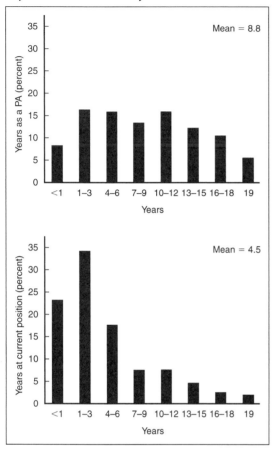

Data from American Academy of Physician Assistants.

ATTRITION

If career mobility is one side of the PA professional coin, attrition is the other. Attrition (or annulment) is the gradual and natural reduction of membership or personnel from the profession. Surveys of PAs on a nationwide basis and in selected populations confirm that about 85% of all PA graduates remain working in the U.S. labor force. This level of professional retention is higher than seen in most health professions, and may be as high as the level of physician retention. Only airplane pilots are thought to be at a higher rate of retention. Historically, at least in the early 1980s, men, former military medical corpsmen, and graduates of military PA programs had the lowest attrition rate (Perry & Redmond, 1984).

Clearly, a number of PAs drop out of the profession because of health, retirement, death, parenting responsibilities, and career burnout. Some have used their PA background and experience to branch into related fields. Still others have acquired additional formal education and used that as a stepping stone to a different career. Employment experiences and education have led many PAs into more complex and advanced roles in management, health, and academia. Some have shown the ability and interest to expand their horizons in the healthcare field by creating their own new roles and opportunities. Program alumni surveys estimate that approximately 4% of all PAs have gone on to medical, osteopathic, dental, chiropractic, or podiatric school. A considerably larger number have sought graduate education, for example, a master's degree in public health, education, business administration, or public administration. One study identified 213 PAs who had a doctorate degree other than medical (e.g., PhD, DrPH, and EdD) (Orcutt, Hildebrand, & Jones, 2006). Most of these individuals acquired their terminal degrees after graduating from a PA program. However, program directors report that applicants with doctorate degrees are also applying for PA training. In 2007, 2.4% of graduates already had a doctorate degree. Doctoral preparation is becoming an academic attainment for a career in PA education.

Employment patterns for PAs with advanced degrees are extremely varied, depending on the interests, capabilities, and personalities of the individuals. The PA credential is increasingly recognized in the healthcare field as representing a respected medical background that permits individuals to move into many types of expanded clinical and nonclinical roles. Attrition to some degree seems inevitable but does not appear to be a major problem for the PA profession. In any profession there will be a proportion of people who would be expected to explore new and expanding areas of opportunity, and the PA profession has appeared to be a reasonable springboard for these aspirations. Because a large number of PAs sought this profession after making one or more career changes, it seems only natural that they be afforded this view as well if they seek career latitude or an alternative role.

PART-TIME EMPLOYMENT

Part-time work is an integral part of the labor force in all parts of the United States and occurs in almost all careers. In the United States, *full time* means 32 or more hours per week and *part time* is typically defined as fewer than 32 hours per week. When all occupations (not just healthcare workers) are examined, women make up the bulk of part-time workers (72%) nationally. In the aggregate, they are usually married (with the husband present in the household) and are sometimes considered secondary wage earners. Although an age-participation profile is not available, most part-time PAs fall into this category as well. However, apart from the fact that only 9% of PAs practice short of full time, the distinction between full-time and part-time employment from the data presented here does not differ significantly. Part-time PAs are more likely to be in primary care (71% vs. 56%), but with the exception of the gender differences, the type of setting, ethnicity, and number of years in current position are only marginally different between full-time and part-time PAs. The fact that so few PAs are part time is seen as remarkable when compared with other healthcare professions, including nursing and medicine.

PUBLIC SERVICE: MILITARY, FEDERAL, AND STATE

Today about 11% of all PAs are employed in positions within the public sector. Among all PAs reported in the 2008 AAPA annual census, 8% are employed in the federal government, with 2% working for the state and 1% in local government agencies. The federal government is the single largest employer of all healthcare providers. Currently, about 1,150 of PAs serve in uniformed services branches on active duty.

They are distributed among the Army, the Air Force, the Navy, and the Coast Guard (Department of Homeland Security). A growing cadre are in the Department of Veterans Affairs health system, in the Department of Justice in the Bureau of Prisons (BOP) medical system, in the Indian Health Service (IHS) and other agencies in the U.S. Public Health Service. PAs are also employed in the Department of State, the Department of Health and Human Services, the U.S. Customs Service, and the Department of Defense, and serve at the White House.

The overall number of PAs employed by the Department of Veterans Affairs system in 2009 was more than 1,800. PAs are avidly recruited by agencies in the U.S. Public Health Service and the BOP, where the existing limitations in the available supply of PAs results in ongoing vacancies in medical staffing. For example, the IHS employs 98 full-time equivalent (FTE) PAs, about one-third of whom are Native Americans. The IHS and other federal agencies anticipate that medical staffing requirements for PA personnel will increase substantially. In fact, the BOP is the fastest growing federal department, and the demands for PAs and other healthcare workers are high in corrections medicine (Hooker, 2008). The distribution of PAs in the various government agencies is shown in Exhibit 3-29.

EXHIBIT 3-29
Government Employers of Physician Assistants, 2008

Employer (active duty)	Number of PAs
Army	610
Air Force	270
Navy	235
Coast Guard	42
National Guard and Reserves	410
Veterans Affairs	1,680
Bureau of Prisons	60
Public Health Service	140
Other federal government	377

Data from Hooker, R. S. (2008b). Federally employed physician assistants. Military Medicine, 173(9), 895–899.

UNDERSERVED RURAL SETTINGS

The major objective in the development of training programs for PAs was to increase the availability of health care in areas with physician shortages. These underserved areas include small communities in rural areas. The federal government defines *rural* as a county with fewer than 100,000 people and a town with fewer than 50,000 individuals. Census data classify PAs by those who live in communities with populations of fewer than 50,000 and 10,000.

About 14% of PAs are in practice in communities of fewer than 10,000 people, with an additional 14% working in communities of 10,000 to 50,000. More PAs (29%) are working in practices in communities of fewer than 50,000 than either allopathic physicians (12%) or osteopathic physicians (15%). Most rural PAs are employed in primary care practices (86%).

The reasons for the distribution of PAs in underserved communities are multifactorial, but one of the leading reasons is the federal initiative to fund programs that serve small communities. Since the late 1970s, federal statute has required that PA programs receiving grants support curricula emphasizing primary care. Programs that demonstrate successful outcomes in deploying graduates to primary care practices and medically underserved areas have promoted PA practice in rural communities. Until recently, a downward trend in the percentages of PAs practicing in small communities (less than 10,000 population) had been observed. Between 1981 and 1996, the percentage of PAs working in smaller communities declined from 27% to 14%. Major factors responsible for this decline include a changing medical market and the changing demography of the PA profession, such as the retirement of older male PAs (who are more likely than women to enter practices in underserved areas), the increasing proportion of women now entering the profession, and the increasingly strong demand and consequently higher remuneration levels offered to PAs in urban settings and hospital-based practices.

The same negative factors that discourage physicians from working in rural areas also affect PAs (e.g., large patient care load, long hours, professional and social isolation, fewer academic centers, and lower income). However, since the 1996 low of 14%, the percentages of PAs working in communities of less than 10,000 have improved. In 1992, the figure rose to 16.5% in 1993 to 18% and in 1996 to 14%. In 2002, the number remained at 14%. The effect of federal PA funding preferences on grants for PA educational programs is believed to have offset to some degree the national trend among healthcare professionals drifting away from rural practice (Exhibit 3-30) (Willis & Reid, 1990; Willis, 1993; Cawley, 2008a).

Although physicians supervise PAs, many PAs in practices in isolated rural areas function with some degree of independence. Many rural communities are dependent on a PA-staffed clinic to provide local medical care for residents (Henry & Hooker, 2007). Physicians in rural communities rely on PAs to help balance patient care duties, on-call responsibilities, and leisure time, as well as to help avoid problems of social and professional isolation. PAs are cost-effective to rural practices because their salaries are about one-third of physicians' salaries. Anecdotal reports suggest that most perform at productivity rates similar to those of physicians in these settings as well.

UNDERSERVED URBAN SETTINGS

Working with the impoverished is a part of a commitment to social services for some health professionals. For PAs and other providers who work in urban underserved areas, there is a value placed on service to humanity and a strong sense of pride in making a difference. Focus groups of primary care providers in inner city areas reveal that they thrive on the challenge of creatively dealing with their patients' complex human needs with limited healthcare resources. Factors critical to survival in an underserved urban setting include a hardy personality style, a flexible but controllable work schedule, and multidisciplinary practice teams. The camaraderie and synergy of teams generate personal support and opportunities for continuing professional development (Li, Williams, & Scammon, 1995).

EXHIBIT 3-30
Physician Assistant Specialty and Practice Settings in Underserved Areas, 2002 (%)

Practice Type	Total	High Poverty	Total HPSA*	Urban HPSA	Rural HPSA
SPECIALTY					
Primary care[†]	42.4	36.8	66.0	41.2	87.0
Medical specialty[‡]	25.4	29.8	18.9	29.2	10.2
Surgical specialty§	25.4	26.1	11.0	21.9	1.8
Obstetrician-gynecologist	4.4	4.8	3.4	6.8	0.5
Other	2.5	2.5	0.7	0.9	0.5
PRACTICE SETTING					
Group office	25.7	15.6	17.8	21.2	15.0
Clinic medical office	23.5	31.8	48.8	32.1	62.6
Private hospital	15.1	17.1	10.0	19.6	2.1
Public hospital	14.1	20.9	9.5	14.3	5.4
Solo office	12.6	7.2	11.1	7.5	14.2
Health maintenance organization	8.4	7.1	2.4	5.0	0.3
Other	0.7	0.4	0.4	0.3	0.5

*HPSA, health professional service area.

[†]Family/general practice, general internal medicine, and general pediatrics.

[‡]Allergy, dermatology, emergency medicine, geriatrics, internal medicine subspecialty, neurology, occupational medicine, pediatric subspecialty, psychiatry, and rehabilitation.

§General surgery, surgery, ophthalmology, orthopedics, and otolaryngology.

Data from American Academy of Physician Assistants. (2007a). 2007 AAPA Physician Assistant Census Report. *Alexandria, VA: Author.*

Whereas social commitment to work with the poor and transient is a strong motivator for many PAs, and many agencies exist to provide this service, very little is known about what these PAs do and how they function in their communities.

COMMUNITY AND MIGRANT HEALTH CENTERS

Shi and colleagues (1994) examined the patterns and determinants of using PAs and other nonphysician healthcare providers in rural community and migrant health centers in all U.S. geographic regions. The primary objective of the study was to compare centers that employed PAs and other nonphysician healthcare providers versus those not employing such providers. Data from the 243 responses received from rural and migrant health clinics gave findings related to the use of PAs, NPs, and CNMs. Three-quarters (77%) of respondents indicated that PA, NP, and CNM healthcare professionals were on their medical staffs. Also, 85% indicated that they were seeking to employ additional PA and NP healthcare providers. To meet anticipated demand for primary care providers, community and migrant healthcare centers would need to hire 726 physicians, 315 NPs, 218 PAs, 145 CNMs, and 169 other staff members.

A major factor in the use of PAs and other nonphysician healthcare providers in rural and migrant healthcare clinics is whether these facilities hold an affiliation with an educational program involved in the training of these providers. High proportions (77% for PAs, 67% for NPs, and 93% for CNMs) of the rural community and migrant healthcare centers surveyed nationally are involved in training activities of these healthcare professionals. Findings also suggest that the centers that actively seek to employ PAs and other nonphysician providers are more likely to establish training and employment channels with educational programs.

Working in primary care in rural community and migrant healthcare clinics, PAs, NPs, and CNMs tend to function in roles that are largely substitutive of physicians. A significant and inverse relationship exists between the number of physicians and the number of nonphysicians employed in these settings. Other factors shown to have an affect on patterns of use of nonphysician healthcare providers in these clinical settings include (1) a significant positive relationship between the number of total staff and the number of nonphysician providers employed, (2) geographic region, (3) educational program linkage, and (4) center clinical staffing policies (Shi et al, 1993).

HMO/MANAGED CARE

PAs and primary care physicians are in strong demand in HMOs and managed healthcare systems. Findings from a survey of 10 HMOs nationwide and data from several other HMO studies estimated that there are approximately 18 nonphysician healthcare providers (either PA or NP) per 100,000 HMO enrollees, with a range from 0 to 67 PAs and NPs (Weiner, 1994). A Group Health Association of America study found the mean number of full-time physicians per 100,000 enrollees to be 142.3. The number of primary care physicians was 68.7 per 100,000 enrollees. When PAs and NPs

were factored in, there was an inverse relationship (Dial et al, 1995). This observation suggests that PAs and NPs are substituting for primary care physicians in these settings in underappreciated levels (Hooker & Cawley, 1995).

Other observations from this study find PAs and NPs providing direct patient care to all categories of patients (Exhibit 3-31). NPs and CNMs tend to provide more OB/GYN care than PAs, but PAs and advance practice nurses are used extensively in primary care.

An example of the extensive integration of PAs in HMOs exists at Kaiser Permanente in Portland, Oregon. This HMO has an enrollment of more than 450,000 members, staffed by 550 FTE physicians and 150 FTE PAs and NPs within 29 clinical departments. PAs who practice in primary care areas and specialty care roles are fully integrated as members of the health provider team. The Kaiser Permanente Center for Health Research has measured longitudinally the clinical productivity, costs, and practice characteristics of both PAs and NPs in the HMO/managed care setting (Hooker, 1993).

The Southern California Kaiser Plan employs roughly 500 PAs and NPs alone. Other HMOs that employ large groups of

EXHIBIT 3-31
Clinical Responsibilities of Physician Assistants and Nurse Practitioners in HMOs*

	Percentage of HMOs	
	PAs	*NPs*
Prescriptive authority	59.5	73.3
Primary provider	70.3	68.4
Included on provider list	35.1	36.8
PROVIDE DIRECT ACCESS TO:		
Obstetrics and gynecology patients	51.5	94.7
Well adults	97.2	91.7
Chronically ill patients	91.7	91.4
Other adults	73.9	63.6
Pediatric patients	71.4	89.2
Psychiatric patients	48.4	48.4

*N = 34, NPs includes certified nurse-midwives.

Data from Dial et al. (1995). Clinical staffing in staff- and group-model HMOs. Health Affairs (Millwood) 14(2), 168–180.

PAs and NPs include Pilgrim/Harvard Community Health Plan in Boston; Health Insurance Plan of Greater New York; Group Health Association and Partners in the District of Columbia; the Mayo Clinic in Rochester, Minnesota; Group Health Cooperative of Puget Sound in Seattle; and the Family Health Plan Systems in Utah, California, and other western states. More than two-thirds of all group-model and staff-model HMOs employ PAs and/or NPs.

Performance in Managed Care Systems

Major factors receiving increased attention in managed healthcare systems relate to the clinical capabilities and cost-effectiveness of PAs in such settings. In the HMO setting, PAs and NPs have long played important roles in the clinical staffing patterns of these healthcare facilities. PAs and NPs have proven themselves capable of delivering most of the healthcare services required at physician-equivalent levels of quality of care and at lower costs than physicians (Hooker, 1993). When clinical productivity of PAs, as measured by the number of outpatient care visits per day, was compared with the patient visit rates of primary care physicians and NPs, PA clinical productivity was equal to and in some settings greater than that of the other primary care providers. In studies conducted at Kaiser Permanente Northwest, Record and colleagues (1981a, 1981b) compared the clinical performance of PAs with that of primary care physicians in a large HMO in handling episodes of four specific morbidities: strep throat, upper respiratory infection (URI), bursitis, and bronchitis. Outcome criteria included patient safety, as measured by the rate of adverse effects from antibiotics and other drugs used in patient management. Over 1 year, no differences in the rates between PAs and physicians were observed.

QUALITY OF CARE

PA utilization in medical practices has grown, partly as a result of practice efficiency and economic advantages and partly as a result of patient satisfaction with care. A number of healthcare services research studies conducted shortly after introducing a PA into practice concluded that PAs provide physician-equivalent levels of quality of patient care. Sox (1979) summarized data from more than a dozen well-conducted studies examining the clinical performance of PAs. He found that the quality of patient care delivered by PAs was at a level "indistinguishable" from that of physician care.

Patient satisfaction is a related but imperfect measure of healthcare provider quality of care and is a partial determinant of the use of healthcare personnel. High level of patient acceptance of PA services has been a consistently observed finding in many of the healthcare services research reports published after PAs were introduced into clinical practice (Office of Technology Assessment, 1986). These studies showed that the proportion of patients reporting acceptable to high levels of satisfaction with healthcare services delivered by PAs averaged between 80% and 90% among individuals not previously exposed to PA care. This figure subsequently rose more than 95% among patients surveyed after having received care from a PA (Nelson, Jacobs, & Johnson, 1974; Hooker, 1993).

Public acceptance and familiarity with PA healthcare providers have grown substantially, particularly over the last decade. Data from a report based on findings from a random sample of 687 adults surveyed by telephone in the Kentucky Health Survey indicated that 1 in 4 (25%) had received medical advice or treatment from a PA within 2 years of being surveyed. More than 90% of these subjects reported satisfaction with the care they received. Recipients of care from PAs did not differ from recipients of care from physicians with respect to income, education, insurance status, self-assessment of health status, or rural versus urban location (Mainous, Bertolino, & Harrell, 1992).

The quality of care provided by PAs was assessed in primary care clinics of the Air Force in which PAs delivered a considerable portion of primary care formerly provided by physicians. Quality of clinical care determinations were made on the basis of responses to predetermined diagnostic, therapeutic, and referral and disposition criteria. Therapeutic criteria included desirable actions on the part of the healthcare provider (e.g., prescribing the appropriate class of antibiotic for infectious otitis media at the first visit) and undesirable actions (e.g., prescribing an antibiotic for viral syndrome with gastroenteritis). On five of six such criteria, PAs performed as well as or better than physicians in identifying desirable therapeutic actions (Goldberg, 2005).

Kane, Olsen, and Castle (1978) compared the quality of clinical care performance of Medex-trained PAs to that provided by their employing and supervising physicians. Findings revealed that PAs were less likely than supervising physicians to use antibiotics in a manner judged to be inappropriate (e.g., prescribed for fevers of undetermined origin or viral URIs) and to be somewhat less likely to use systemic steroids for conditions such as contact dermatitis or asthma. These findings suggest that the patient care management decisions for these morbidities made by PAs were as good as or better than those of physicians (Kane, Gardner, et al, 1978). In another study, Wright and colleagues (1977) compared the clinical performance of several types of providers of primary care services by recording decision patterns and outcome aspects of treatment by family practice residents, faculty, and PAs in two clinics staffed by healthcare professionals in a university family practice residency program. Activities measured in the study included patient functional outcomes, patient satisfaction, and mean cost per episode of care. Findings revealed that PAs performed as well as or better than other primary care providers in delivery of services in each of the endpoint measures (Wright et al, 1977). Duttera and Harlan (1978) evaluated the appropriateness of patient care provided by PAs in 14 rural primary care settings. They concluded that PAs were clinically competent in diagnostic and therapeutic skills, as judged by performances observed in three specific practice circumstances: (1) when all patients were initially seen by the PA and then by a physician, (2) when undifferentiated patients were managed concurrently by physicians and PAs, and (3) when patients with specific problems were assigned to PAs. We conclude that quality care, based on the literature, does not seem to be an issue when PAs are the providers of care.

COMPARING PHYSICIAN ASSISTANTS WITH OTHER OCCUPATIONS

From 1987 to 2007, the income of PAs rose substantially. Thanks in part to organization of healthcare delivery, PAs have made significant gains in compensation when compared with other workers. This salary gain for PAs is substantial but is also more significant when income change is adjusted for inflation. The rising salary over this period suggests the demand for PAs continues to exceed supply.

MEDICAL LEGAL CONSIDERATIONS

PAs typically protect their medical legal risk, as well as their supervising physicians' malpractice liability risk, in one of two ways: by obtaining their own malpractice insurance (this varies by state and averages from $1,500 to $3,000 a year) or by attaching a rider to the physician's policy covering the activities of the PA. The rate of malpractice suits filed involving PAs has been quite low across a wide spectrum of practice settings and specialties (Cawley, Rohrs, & Hooker, 1998). The proportionate rate of malpractice claims for PAs versus physicians as shown from data obtained from the National Practice Data Bank is that because PA practice is associated with improved patient communication and proper documentation (two leading categories of breeches prompting malpractice lawsuits), the use of a PA can mitigate a practice's medical liability risk (Cawley, Rohrs, & Hooker, 1998; Nicholson, 2008).

BELIEFS, BEHAVIORS, AND ATTITUDES

Understanding some of the unique characteristics of PAs is important if we are to better understand the occupation. This section lists some of the health beliefs and behaviors of PAs that have been reported.

Hepatitis B Immunization

Recommendations by authorities seem to be important motivators for PA and medical students equally. At the University of Iowa College of Medicine, PA and medical students responded to recommendations to receive the hepatitis B immunization series at a higher rate than residents and staff physicians (Diekema, Ferguson, & Doebbeling, 1995).

Chemical Dependency

Impaired providers pose challenges to state medical boards that are charged with protecting their constituents' health and exposure to unhealthy conditions as well as to the professional organizations that seek to protect their legal rights. Most PAs in one study were either nondrinkers or ex-drinkers. A majority of PAs (87%) reported that they rarely or never relied on drugs or medication to affect mood or to relax. Most respondents in this study reported either occasional physical activity (47%) or regular physical activity at least three times per week (47%). It found that PAs tended to be oriented more strongly toward general health matters and prevention than toward illness or sick role-related beliefs (Glazer-Waldman, 1984).

Risks for HIV/AIDS

A 1991 national survey of PAs reported that 60% thought that treating patients with HIV placed them at risk for AIDS. About one-third thought that healthcare workers had a right to refuse care to patients with AIDS. However, more than 80% indicated they were willing to provide health care to patients with HIV and those considered to be in high-risk groups (Currey, 1992).

Thanatophobia

In caring for the terminally ill, a PA student's fear of death or dying (thanatophobia) may affect his or her ability to be an effective clinician and may influence his or her role as a patient advocate and educator. To assess the level and prediction of thanatophobia of PA students to that of medical students, an 80-item survey of both student groups was undertaken. Generally speaking, senior PA students scored significantly lower than senior medical students in thanatophobia, as well as in authoritarianism, machiavellianism, and depressed mood. For both student groups, intolerance to clinical uncertainty was a predictor of thanatophobia. PAs might be more comfortable than doctors in treating terminally ill persons and may be better suited to caring for terminally ill patients, particularly in areas such as geriatrics, hospice, and primary care in general (Chaikin, Thornby, & Merrill, 2000).

Nutrition

In a mailed survey, the nutrition knowledge and attitudes of PAs in Texas were examined. The 764 PAs (54.2%) who completed the questionnaire had a mean knowledge score of 70%. Knowledge scores were significantly related to level of education, but not to other demographic and practice variables. Most of the PA respondents supported the importance of nutrition in their clinical practices, although many PAs indicated that they were not satisfied with the amount of nutrition education in their PA programs and felt that PA programs should place a greater emphasis on nutrition education (Demory-Luce & McPherson, 1999).

Patient Education

What primary care PAs and primary care physicians do in the outpatient setting has been a focus of some research. The overlap seems to be large. In other words, what a PA does is largely similar to what a physician does in the same setting. One of the claims that PAs and NPs make is that they bring patient education to the medical office as an attribute of their training. The information to substantiate this claim is somewhat limited. Coulter, Jacobson, and Parker (2000) interviewed staff PAs and NPs from a series of HMOs. These providers stated they were more interested in preventive care than physicians. Harbert's work (1994) using a national survey of PAs in primary care suggests this finding may indeed be the case. Clearly more work is needed in this area.

Complementary and Alternative Medicine

The use of complementary and alternative medicine (CAM) is growing in the United States. Patients and their healthcare providers are increasingly accepting of CAM therapies (Jarski, 2001). A random sample of 250 PAs who were extensively surveyed found a high relationship between knowledge level of CAM and recommendations for CAM, although most believed that many CAM therapies exert a placebo effect (Houston et al, 2001) (Exhibits 3-32 and 3-33). PAs also have been shown to be more likely to incorporate clinical preventive services as advocated by the U.S. Prevention Services Task Force. PA practice is strongly preventive in orientation.

ARE PHYSICIAN ASSISTANTS PROFESSIONALS?

PAs are individuals who practice medicine, a role traditionally considered to be among the professions, yet lacking in key attributes classically considered necessary to be regarded as a true profession. There is a tendency for newly emerging occupations to aspire to professional status in part as a means to enhance prestige and societal position. Particularly in the modern U.S. healthcare sector, holding the label "professional" conveys to society and other healthcare providers the connotation of a higher position on the ladder of occupational stratification.

PAs represent a health occupation founded by medicine. PA organizations and PAs often refer to themselves as "professional" and generally assume that PAs function in practice "as professionals." The question is whether or not the American PA is a true professional. Is the American PA claim to be among the ranks of other health providers recognized as professionals valid, or does the dependent nature of PA practice and the lack of a unique body of

knowledge consign them to a lower rung in the health occupations pecking order? PAs represent a unique case study among the health occupations by virtue of their level of clinical responsibilities. Can PAs be legitimately classified as "professionals" in the delivery of health care, or are they, as some would assert, simply vassals of more powerful healthcare elite, producing wealth for their employers but not owning or controlling the means of production?

PAs have assumed a number of characteristics of professionals; they share a body of knowledge with physicians and are granted a substantial degree of work autonomy within the defined practice scope of physicians. Some would argue that PAs do not qualify as professionals as they do not possess their own body of knowledge and lack total autonomy in their work. They are also in a dependent and delegated role. Yet the standard of what constitutes a profession, even among physicians, appears to be changing. Physicians in modern medical practice are much more accountable in many respects than they were at the apparent height of their prominence as professionals in the 1960s and 1970s. PAs have made great progress in controlling their regulation and legislation, title definition and protection, rules for entry into the profession, accreditation of educational programs, and certification of graduates. Yet another consideration is that, because a wide number of health occupations now consider themselves to be professionals, the term itself has become devalued.

SUMMARY

Data on PAs indicate that they are improving the specialty and geographic maldistribution of the medical workforce in the United States. PAs are more likely to be working in primary care fields and in smaller communities and augment areas of medical need working with physicians (and are increasingly making major contributions in this area). The average age of the employed PA is 40 years and the length of employment is approximately 9 years. For students, the age is decreasing, now at 28 years.

EXHIBIT 3-32
Respondents' Perceptions of Complementary and Alternative Modalities of Treatment*

Categories of Rating (modalities rated)	No. of Respondents (%) (*N* = 245)
HIGHEST RATED THAT RESPONDENTS PERCEIVED TO EXHIBIT CONCLUSIVE EVIDENCE OF EFFECTIVENESS	
Multivitamins	50 (20)
Biofeedback	39 (16)
Antioxidants	37 (15)
Meditation	35 (14)
Chiropractic	35 (14)
Pastoral and spiritual counseling	33 (14)
HIGHEST RATED THAT RESPONDENTS PERCEIVED TO EXHIBIT A PREPONDERANCE OF EVIDENCE OF EFFECTIVENESS	
Meditation	84 (34)
Biofeedback	77 (31)
Antioxidants	61 (25)
Pastoral and spiritual counseling	58 (24)
Massage	57 (23)
Multivitamins	52 (21)
Chiropractic	52 (21)
HIGHEST RATED THAT RESPONDENTS PERCEIVED TO EXHIBIT GROWING EVIDENCE OF EFFECTIVENESS	
Massage	117 (48)
Saint John's wort	107 (44)
Garlic	103 (42)
Gingko	100 (41)
Meditation	100 (41)
Acupuncture	98 (40)
Acupressure	96 (39)
HIGHEST RATED THAT RESPONDENTS PERCEIVED TO EXHIBIT NO EVIDENCE OF EFFECTIVENESS	
Body-cleansing diets	118 (48)
Macrobiotic diets	92 (38)
Aromatherapy	87 (36)
Ergogenic aids	85 (35)
Organic food diets	84 (34)
Magnet therapy	81 (33)
Amino acids	72 (29)
Chelation therapy	72 (29)
HIGHEST RATED THAT RESPONDENTS PERCEIVED AS UNFAMILIAR	
Rolfing	148 (60)
Guided imagery	130 (53)
Coenzyme Q10	125 (51)
Reflexology	117 (48)
Chelation therapy	115 (47)
Art therapy	109 (45)
Macrobiotic diets	106 (43)

*Only the most commonly mentioned modalities in each rating category are reported here.

Data from Houston et al. (2001). How physician assistants use and perceive complementary and alternative medicine. Journal of the American Academy of Physician Assistants, 14(1), 29–30, 33–34, 39–40, 44–46 passim, 46.

EXHIBIT 3-33
Ten Most Common Complementary and Alternative Medicines Used by Physician Assistants

Modality	No. of Respondents (%) (N = 245)
Multivitamins	68 (28)
Antioxidants	54 (22)
Massage	48 (20)
Meditation	47 (19)
Pastoral and spiritual counseling	21 (9)
Aromatherapy	19 (8)
Acupuncture	18 (7)
Organic food diets	19 (8)
Acupuncture	15 (6)
Chiropractic	15 (6)

Data from Houston et al. (2001). How physician assistants use and perceive complementary and alternative medicine. Journal of the American Academy of Physician Assistants, 14(1), 29–30, 33–34, 39–40, 44–46 passim, 46.

One of the problems with the work-related rewards received by PAs appears to be that they will reach an early peak in the first several years after entry into the profession and then plateau. This issue may be a concern for individuals who enter the PA profession early in age and have career aspirations to eventually be someone other than a clinician. An older individual who has been employed for some time and then makes a career move to become a PA may see this as a major career advancement. Regardless, the PA profession is a sterling one that is attracting a wide segment of society and is blossoming globally. It is a career move for most entrants and most will remain in this career throughout their working lives. The presence of a PA in any population is a catalyst for change. How the PA profession will shape society is the next question.

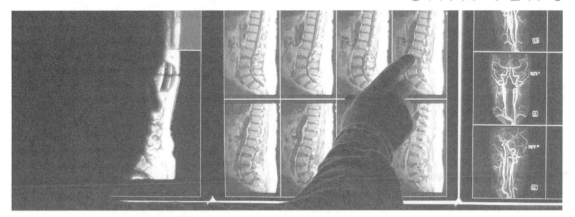

CHAPTER 4

ENTRY-LEVEL PHYSICIAN ASSISTANT EDUCATION

JAMES F. CAWLEY ■ RODERICK S. HOOKER ■ DAVID P. ASPREY

The great difficulty in education is to get experience out of ideas.

—George Santayana

ABSTRACT

Physician assistant (PA) educational programs were created in the 1960s, primarily in academic institutions preparing traditional healthcare professionals. The curricula were based on new ideas and represented a hybridization of existing medical and nursing educational models. The intent was to prepare clinicians for roles to expand medical care services. In the intervening decades, PA educational programs have become well established in academic health centers and other institutions of higher education in the United States, the Netherlands, England, Australia, and Canada. They have evolved into well-recognized and successful medical education institutions and in the process have contributed substantially to advances in healthcare delivery. Essential to the introduction of the PA was the support of the medical profession and the federal government. The medical profession encouraged legal efforts in recognition of PA practice, and the government granted financial support for the development of PA educational programs. In their development and evolution, PA programs have helped influence concepts and trends in health professions education and have pioneered methodologies in decentralized clinical education, multidisciplinary approaches, and curriculum innovation. As PA programs have evolved, they have maintained a socially responsive tradition with graduates in medically needy and rural communities to a greater degree than doctors. PA educational programs have developed a reputation of providing a practically focused and multidisciplinary approach to health professions education. These programs represent innovations in medical generalist and primary care preparation, and PA education has earned a distinct identity within medical learning.

INTRODUCTION

Shortly after World War II, medicine made a number of technological and biomedical breakthroughs and healthcare delivery changed dramatically. The development of new medical specialties and subspecialties, coupled with major growth of hospitals and hospital services, created a need for highly specialized personnel. Such change produced a fundamental restructuring of the division of medical practice labor. The country's leaders were also well aware of embarrassing inequities in the distribution of health care, and were convinced that the problem seemed to be an inadequate number of doctors.

During this time, Vietnam corpsmen and medics, battlefield tested, had no civilian role upon their return stateside. The origins of the physician assistant (PA) are indelibly linked to these paramedics, who had skills honed in trauma medicine and emergency surgical care but no comparable civilian employment opportunities. Dr. Eugene Stead and Dr. E. Harvey Estes, Jr. of Duke University and Dr. Richard Smith of the University of Washington, in founding the PA concept, tapped into this supply of ex-military corpsmen. They were able to persuade key leaders in the American Medical Association (AMA) to endorse the PA concept. Given the needs of the growing and deserving constituency and the failure of the medical establishment to come up with a solution to the shortage of physicians, it was hard to say no to the idea. Corpsmen and medics were the bridge between doctor shortages and skilled medical personnel who could ease this shortage (R. Smith, personal communication, June 2006).

The rationale for the creation of the PA profession was based on the need for a new type of clinician who would:

- compensate for the dwindling number of general practitioners by augmenting physician capabilities to deliver medical care services and help alleviate the perceived shortage of primary care physicians;
- address healthcare access problems stemming from the geographic and specialty maldistribution of physicians;
- provide an educational means by which existing healthcare personnel with broad experiences could be channeled into advanced clinical roles; and
- be a positive factor in helping to control healthcare costs and improve primary care access (Perry, 1980; Carter, Emelio, & Perry, 1984; Schafft & Cawley, 1987; Jones & Cawley, 1994).

The first PA programs began in academic medical centers and evolved with sponsorship from a wide range of educational institutions as well as clinical organizations. The Duke University program offered the initial educational model for PA training, but soon others followed. The Medex Program at the University of Washington, the 4-year program at Alderson-Broaddus College, and the Child Health Associate Program at the University of Colorado were established and fostered alternative and effective models. PA programs thereafter emerged in a variety of institutions: medical schools, universities, 4-year colleges, community colleges, and technical and vocational schools as well as in teaching hospitals, correctional systems, and the federal healthcare systems (Department of Health, Education, and Welfare, 1977). The military PA programs of the Air Force and the Navy were among the first group of health center programs beginning in 1971. Diversity in sponsoring institutions was enhanced due to the fact that PA education was not founded on an entry-level academic degree but instead was based on a competency model.

As PA programs developed, one of their hallmarks was to be educationally efficient. Early programs were structured as short versions of medical school. The diversity of sponsoring institutions resulted in various curriculum models incorporating philosophies and approaches that were innovative and on the forefront of medical education. These models were designed for the recruitment of individuals with extensive healthcare experience and intended to meet specific national, state, and community needs.

The creation of new healthcare practitioners, as well as the expansion of undergraduate medical education, significantly affected medical care delivery and education during the 1970s. This health workforce policy, developed by organized medicine and the federal government, was aimed toward the broad goals of increasing access to health care, containing costs, and improving the delivery of primary care. Economic aspects of PA education are discussed in Chapter 11.

HISTORY OF PHYSICIAN ASSISTANT EDUCATION

PA education in the new century has retained many of its historical fundamentals born in the mid-1960s, but has remained flexible enough to change with new techniques in education and science. Ideas for this type of education came from a remarkable group of academic doctors.

Leaders in Physician Assistant Education

The pioneering ideas of Stead, Estes, Smith, Myers, and Silver were major components of the larger movement to produce new types of healthcare providers. The "new health practitioner" movement—which included PAs as well as other new health professions—gained strength as dozens of training programs developed during the late 1960s and early 1970s (Exhibit 4-1).

These leaders of the "new health practitioner" movement were characterized as progressive-thinking physicians. They were respected doctors who assumed leadership positions in medical education and were capable of carrying the PA concept into academic institutions. Not only were they the founders of PA educational programs but were also champions of the PA concept to medical and regulatory organizations. All were charismatic and had a large following of admiring colleagues.

After the first PA, Medex, and Child Health Associate education programs were launched, others quickly followed. In 1970 there were 36 programs listed by the U.S. Bureau of Health Manpower Education; 10 trained personnel such as clinical technicians and emergency medical technicians, 10 were apprenticeship programs (rather than formal educational experiences), and 16 were formal educational programs training PAs, clinical nurse specialists (CNSs), nurse practitioners (NPs), or practitioners similar to NPs, termed Primex (nurses similar to Medex). These programs were considered experimental and were started primarily because federal grant support was available to support such efforts. Typically, they were 1 to 2 years in length (sometimes shorter), technically oriented, and designed to deploy providers quickly. Most of

EXHIBIT 4-1
Developers of Physician Assistant Education

Person	Description
Eugene Stead, MD	Eugene Stead is credited with founding the first formal training for PAs at Duke University in 1965. A Chairman of the Department of Medicine at Duke (and before then at Emory University) he sought to create a formal education program that would train PAs for work in any medical setting.
Richard Smith, MD, MPH	Founder of the Medex movement in 1969, Dick Smith took his concept of a person who could work alongside a doctor and launched the Medex program at the University of Washington. As a result of his efforts, eight Medex programs sprung up around the country. Smith went on to deploy the Medex model in 10 other countries, and some of those graduates still serve 40 years later.
E. Harvey Estes, Jr., MD	Harvey Estes took over the development of the Duke PA program a year after it was launched and shaped it to be a classical model of PA education—a compressed version of medical school.
Henry Silver, MD	Henry Silver was one of the most prominent pediatricians at the University of Colorado. He created a 3-year program for nurses and others to become Child Health Associates (CHAs) who would manage the majority of routine care in children.
Hu Myers, MD	Hu Myers was a general practice physician and surgeon who was professor and chairman of the Department of Medical Science and founded the PA program at Alderson-Broaddus, which started in the fall of 1968. Dr Myers' vision for a broad-based liberal arts curriculum and strong medical science studies led to the development of the nation's first baccalaureate program for the training of PAs. Dr. Myers served as medical director and an instructor for the PA program from its inception until his retirement in 1977.

these training programs created technicians (or a clinician with strong technical grounding), building on extensive nursing and/or military medical backgrounds. Although many titles were developed to describe these practitioners, including *health assistant, health associate, surgeon assistant, syniatrist, child health associate, clinical associate,* and others, two lasting models emerged: the PA and the NP.

Overlapping—and later succeeding—the initial PA founders, were other equally respected and influential medical leaders who amplified and modified the PA education model. These individuals are considered pioneers in the PA movement because they had to promote this new idea before skeptical colleagues, deans, faculty senates, and university presidents (Exhibit 4-2).

As experimenters in medical education, the focus of these leaders differed from those whose values were in traditional medical schooling, which stressed biomedical research

EXHIBIT 4-2
Influential Physician Leaders of Physician Assistant Education

Person	Description
Thomas Piemme, MD	Piemme was Professor of Medicine at the George Washington (GW) University Medical Center and a leader on multiple levels within the emerging PA concept. He worked to define the profession's educational standards and practice qualifications. Piemme founded the PA Program at GW in 1972, became president of the Association of Physician Assistant Programs (APAP) in 1974, and was the founding president of the National Commission on Certification of Physician Assistants (NCCPA). He was associated with the National Board of Medical Examiners and was central in the development of the first PA national certifying examination.
Alfred Sadler, MD	Sadler founded the Yale Physician Associate Program, which emerged from the Yale Trauma Research Project. Sadler was the first president of the Association of Physician Assistant Programs (1972) and with his twin brother, Blair, a lawyer, and Ann Bliss, a nurse, co-authored *The Physician's Assistant: Today and Tomorrow,* the first book on the PA profession. Like Piemme, Sadler was an early leader in the development of the organizations of the PA profession. He helped to found APAP and the NCCPA and was influential in advancing the PA concept within organized medicine.
John E. Ott, MD	Inheriting the creation of Henry Silver, Ott directed the Child Health Associate (CHA) Program at the University of Colorado and performed many of the early health services research studies on CHA performance. Ott succeeded Piemme as chair of the Department of Health Care Sciences at GW and served as the medical director of the GW PA Program for many years.
Malcolm Peterson, MD	At Johns Hopkins University in 1972, Peterson was appointed Dean of the School of Health Services that sponsored the Health Assistant Program, a collaboration with Essex Community College Health Associate Program.
Archie Golden, MD, MPH	Golden gained experience in designing training programs for community health workers in South America while working for Project Hope and became the director of the Hopkins/Essex Health Associate Program (which closed in 1979). This program's curriculum was designed to be different from the traditional medical model. Later, this work was described in *The Art of Teaching Primary Care,* authored by the faculty of the School of Health Services.
J. Rhodes Haverty, MD	Haverty was Dean of Allied Health at Georgia State University and a driving force in the establishment of the NCCPA.
Thomas Gallagher, MD, and Jesse Edwards, MS	Gallagher and Edwards were the founders of the PA program at the University of Nebraska.
Hal Wilson, MD	Wilson founded the PA program at the University of Kentucky and later at Wake Forest University.
Richard Rosen, MD	Chairman of Surgery at Montefiore Medical Center in the 1970s, Rosen first utilized PAs in inpatient surgical units and founded the first PA postgraduate program in 1971.
Francis Horvath, MD	Horvath, a pediatrician at St. Louis University, cofounded the PA program at that institution and was a leader in the development of the Joint Review Committee and the PA program accreditation system.
Joseph Hamburg, PhD	A Dean of Allied Health at the University of Kentucky during the 1970s, Hamburg was responsible for the institution of the PA program at that institution. An endowed chair in social research retains his name.
David Lawrence, MD, MPH, and Robert Harmon, MD	At the University of Washington, Lawrence and Harmon succeeded Dick Smith and were responsible for promulgating the Medex model of PA education.

and mechanistic approaches. PA education emerged with a philosophy of training practitioners to meet a specific societal need—increasing the supply and distribution of primary healthcare providers. Thus, there was a strong community orientation and service focus in these leaders and the programs they created. They were creative individuals who urged traditional institutions to start PA educational programs and to take a chance in a national experiment with a new type of practitioner. Often, they developed curricula from scratch or with minimal resources. Their work was mission-driven and clinically focused. Frequently, they were called upon to describe and justify the role of the PA to legislators, health regulators, and skeptical medical groups. The job could be summarized as one where the educators need to be internal as well as external ambassadors for the PA concept. In addition to being teachers in the classroom and clinic, they served many roles: administrators, counselors and advisors, curriculum designers, educational researchers, and community service providers. That they were well-respected clinicians and academics, or had valued careers in government, provided a foundation for their work.

Denis Oliver, PhD, of the University of Iowa deserves a special place in PA education. A biochemist by training, Oliver developed the Iowa PA program and instituted a number of health services research studies demonstrating the effective deployment of Iowa graduates in rural and medically underserved counties in that state. One of his legacies is the annual survey of PA education in the United States, which started in 1985. Oliver constructed a survey template that has been administered annually by the Physician Assistant Education Association (PAEA), formerly the Association of Physician Assistant Programs (APAP). The *Annual Report on Physician Assistant Educational Programs in the United States* uses a standardized questionnaire to provide longitudinal trends within PA education. It is regarded as the primary source of information on PA educational programs.

Other individuals who were not physicians but made important contributions to the development of PA education include the following:

- Suzanne Greenberg, MSW, who founded the PA program at Northeastern University in 1970 and was later a president of APAP
- Harriet Gayles, who founded the program at what was then Mercy College of Detroit
- David Lewis, who founded the PA program at the University of Florida
- Don Fisher, PhD, who founded a PA program at the University of Mississippi and became the first executive director of the American Academy of Physician Assistants (AAPA)
- David Glazer, who began his career as faculty at the Emory University PA Program and went on to head the National Commission on Certification of Physician Assistants (NCCPA) for many years

Federal Support

For three decades the federal government supported PA education through a series of small grants. PA education was included in Public Health Service (PHS) Title VII funding through the PA Grant Award Program administered by the division of primary care in the Bureau of Health Professions of the Health Services and Resources Administration (Cawley, 2008a). Periodically, there have been threats to the levels of federal funding for Title VII programs. Federal funding has been important to the growth and institutionalization of many PA educational programs in the United States (Strand & Carter, 2003) (Exhibit 4-3).

Generally speaking, medical educators viewed the PA as a quick and effective way of improving public access to primary care. Although this conceptualization of the PA as a primary care provider departed from Stead's original views, the political momentum for primary care, as well as the widespread acceptance of the concept by organized medicine and the federal government, created the climate for PAs to emerge as primary care providers and for the formalization of federal subsidization of PA education.

EXHIBIT 4-3
Three Phases of PA Federal Policy

Strand and Carter (2003) described three phases of PA-related federal policy in support of primary care training.

Phase One

- Comprehensive Health Manpower Training Act (1971) passed, which focused on developing the capacity for training primary care practitioners, including PAs, who would assume positions in primary care in rural and medically underserved areas through grants to support directly academic units.

- NIH Bureau of Health Manpower established an Office of Special Programs to coordinate physician assistant educational program funding activities. Between 1972 and 1975, this Office spent $11.7 million to train 280 Medex PAs and 376 Primex providers (Perry & Breitner, 1982).

- Health Professions Educational Assistance Act of 1976 (Public Law 94-484) was amended by the Health Services Extension Act (Public Law 95-83) to provide for grants and contracts for PA and nonphysician training programs (Cawley, 1992). Thus began a more than 35-year history of inclusion in Public Health Service Title VII funding for PA education through the Physician Assistant Training in Primary Care grant program, first based in the Division of Medicine, then the Division of Primary Care, and most recently back in the Division of Medicine in the Bureau of Health Professions of the Health Services and Resources Administration.

Phase Two

- Period is characterized by continuing priorities to recruit learners and graduates to primary care fields through funding for faculty development and additional deployment incentives.

- The Health Professions Educational Assistance Act (Public Law 94-484) sought to increase the PA supply and provide more physicians and PAs for underserved areas.

- The 1992 Health Professions Education Extension Amendment (Public Law 100-607) and 1998 Health Professions Education Partnership Act (Public Law 100-607) specified a preference for placement of a high rate of graduates in medically underserved communities, with the 1998 act providing a priority for trainees from disadvantaged or underrepresented minority backgrounds.

Phase Three (Current Stage)

- Programs have been given support to attract primary care graduates to practice in underserved regions, and to increase the number of underrepresented minorities in training programs and practice.

- During this time, the number of PA programs grew dramatically from 55 in 1990 to 115 in 2000.

The federal government's involvement in the support of PA training began with student stipends in a National Institutes of Health (NIH) grant that Duke received in 1964 and served to attract and support the students through 1968. Following the creation of the pioneering Duke University PA program, and in the vortex of a period of federal activism in the health sector—that is, the passage of the Medicare program in 1965—the federal government started promoting the training and utilization of new types of healthcare professionals, including PAs (Fox, 1996). The means to this end started with the Health Professions Education Assistance Act (PL 88-129), that was an amendment to Public Health Service Act 42 U.S.C. of 1944, and the first of its kind to address the supply of healthcare professions (Vangsnes, 2005). In addition, several federally sponsored PA programs were initiated, the first at the U.S. Public Health Service Hospital in Staten Island, New York, in 1966 and later the Federal Bureau of Prisons program in Springfield, Missouri. In 1967, the National Advisory Commission on Health Manpower recommended that the federal government give high priority to the training of new categories of health practitioners. The following year, the National Center for Health Services Research was established and charged to produce a national protocol for evaluation of health manpower innovations (National Advisory Commission on Health Manpower, 1967). This agency soon thereafter began to directly fund a number of demonstration projects supporting the training of Medex PAs and Primex NPs. Richard A. Smith, MD, founder of the Medex program, obtained federal funding through the then Bureau of Health Manpower to begin his program at the University of Washington in 1968 (Smith et al, 1971).

After 1970, the federal government became even more involved in health workforce policy. In 1972, federal support for PA education focused on start up, primary care, rural health access. Since then, funding has totaled more than $200 million (Exhibit 4-4). Title VII funding in the amount of $2.4 million was available for PA educational program support in fiscal year 2009. Congressional appropriation of PA

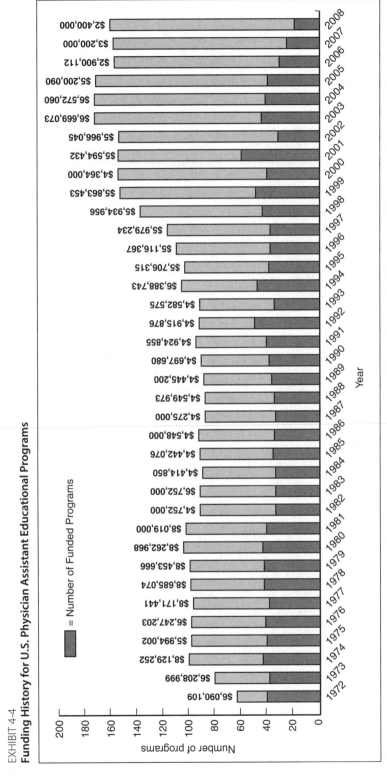

EXHIBIT 4-4
Funding History for U.S. Physician Assistant Educational Programs

The authority for these grants were Health Manpower Educational Initiative Awards, Public Health Service Contracts. The dollar amounts listed represent the total awared for that year.
Data from Cawley, J. F. (2008a). Physician assistants and Title VII support. Academic Medicine, 83, 1049–1056.

educational programs through Title VII has promoted the desired boost in PA graduate output into primary care areas (Vangsnes, 2005). Increased federal funding has supported the expansion of enrollment within existing PA programs and has provided start-up funding for more universities, academic health centers, and colleges seeking to establish new PA programs.

Federal support has provided a base for the operations and special activities characteristic of PA education, which include creative recruitment and retention strategies, primary care training approaches, and cost-effective operation. Although the expansion of PA programs and the increase in the number of available seats in these programs suggest PA education is growing in popularity, federal restrictions on grants, which specify recruitment of applicants from underrepresented areas or underrepresented minorities, also hinders program enrollment among interested PA applicants who do not fit within such criteria. Additional issues facing PA educational programs are the related forces of the loss/competition for clinical training sites, managed care, and payment for clinical student training. If there are to be increases in the enrollment capacities of PA educational programs, many programs will need to change how they do business. These include increasing efforts in the recruitment of new faculty members, strengthening minority recruitment and retention, and adding new clinical training sites and practice affiliations. All of these efforts, linked to expanded enrollments, are dependent on increased financial support from external sources.

The level of federal support for health professions educational programs is uncertain due to the future of congressional appropriations related to Title VII. At times congressional health policy leaders, whose ideological adversaries are often anxious to cut discretionary federal spending categories, have shied away from continuing health professions education program subsidies. An ongoing question for the PA profession is the status of the grant award support for PA programs under Title VII of the Public Health Service Act (Cawley, 2008a).

A long-term workforce policy goal for PA education, popular among PA educators, is to attain Medicare-linked support for graduate clinical PA education, similar to the mechanism established for physician graduate medical education (GME). The Comprehensive Health Manpower Act of 1971 (Public Law 92-157) provided the first large federal provision for PA training programs. Later, in 1977, the Health Professions Educational Assistance Act of 1976 (Public Law 94-484) provided for grants and contracts for PA and nonphysician training programs (Title VII, Section 747 of the Public Health Act). By 1981, the now defunct Congressional Office of Technology Assessment estimated that the federal government spent about $65 million to train nonphysician providers, from $1 million in fiscal year 1969 to $21 in fiscal year 1979 (Vangsnes, 2005). By 2008, almost $200 million federal dollars have been spent in support of PA education over a span of 40 years (Edwards et al, 2006; Cawley, 2008a).

For the 2009 fiscal year, a total of 18 programs were awarded federal grant support under the Title VII PA Grant Award Program, down from the 32 funded programs in fiscal year 2007. The investment in PA programs appears to have been a sound policy, and the rate of return has been higher than anticipated. Programs have been responsive to federal grant initiatives that target service in rural areas, medically underserved areas, and delivery of primary care to needy populations (Grumbach et al, 2003; Staton et al, 2007). Relative to other health professionals, the deployment record of PAs to practices in rural communities and medically underserved areas has been impressive. More than one-half of all federally funded PA programs have developed specific curricular content addressing the health and social problems of medically underserved populations. These include people living in inner cities, remote areas, correctional systems, geriatric facilities, or rehabilitation facilities.

Not only have federal funds helped PA program development, PA curriculum has been influenced by the government's policy to develop health programs and deploy PAs to underserved communities. Depending on public health issues, programs were flexible enough to include instruction in management of persons with HIV or AIDS, counseling regarding the risks of adolescent pregnancy, measures to reduce infant mortality, required schedules of pediatric immunization, domestic violence, and behavior to lower the risk of cancer and heart disease. These are skills needed in the management of health problems that occur disproportionately among medically underserved populations. To ensure that students receive adequate clinical opportunities to complement didactic instruction, many PA educational programs have links with area health education centers, rural health clinics, community/migrant health centers, and other primary healthcare agencies within their geographic region.

Accreditation

Establishment of formal accreditation standards for PA programs marked an important milestone for the PA profession. The Accreditation Review Commission on Education for the Physician Assistant, Inc. (ARC-PA) is the sole accrediting agency responsible for establishing the standards for U.S. PA education and for evaluating programs to ensure their compliance with the standards. A stand-alone agency not embedded in any professional society, the ARC-PA is unique in the American system and is an important influence in the legitimization of PA education in the state licensing process of PAs (see Appendix V).

ARC-PA was initially established by affiliated organizations of the AMA in 1971. The AMA's Council on Medical Education first wrote the standards for PA program accreditation and was the primary overseer of many allied health standards. Thus, the Subcommittee of the Council on Medical Education became the de facto accreditation body and included representatives from the American Academy of Family Physicians (AAFP), American Academy of Pediatrics (AAP), American College of Physicians (ACP), American Society of Internal Medicine (ASIM), AMA, and Association of American Medical Colleges (AAMC). A document produced by the Subcommittee Council

on Medical Education became the *Essentials of an Accredited Educational Program for the Assistant to the Primary Care Physician.* The AMA House of Delegates, with the endorsements noted and on recommendation of the Council on Medical Education, adopted these "Essentials," clearing the way for the approval of educational programs that met or exceeded these requirements.

As the quality of accreditation and the sophistication of assessing PA programs improved, the evolution of the accreditation process dictated that it become its own regulatory agency. The ARC-PA became an independent accrediting body in 2000. It reviews new applications for accreditation, periodically evaluates programs for reaccreditation, appoints site evaluators for the accreditation process, and determines accreditation status according to the *Accreditation Standards for Physician Assistant Education* (McCarty, Stuetzer, & Somers, 2001). A group of collaborating member organizations, consisting of the AAFP, AAP, AAPA, ACP, American College of Surgeons (ACS), AMA, and PAEA collectively monitors and assesses program compliance.

The *Standards* document has undergone a number of revisions (1978, 1985, 1990, 1997, 2000, 2006, and 2009 [expected]). Prior versions of the *Standards* have set the tone for all aspects of PA program operation including curriculum design and content. One of the areas of the *Standards* that has been underappreciated is the promotion of PA program curriculum creativity and innovation, particularly in institutions that have relied on traditional modes of medical education. All key aspects of program operation are addressed in the *Standards*. These areas include administration and sponsorship, personnel, financial resources, operation, curriculum, evaluation, fair practices, laboratory and library facilities, clinical affiliations, faculty qualifications, admissions processes, publications to include on websites, and record-keeping. Programs must demonstrate an ongoing self-study process and must undergo an onsite evaluation before the request for accreditation is approved.

Accredited PA programs are subject to periodic reviews and onsite evaluations;

a requirement for maintenance or retention of accreditation status. Semiannually the ARC-PA meets to consider applications for provisional and continuing accreditation. Institutions considering accreditation for a proposed or existing program must use specific guidelines in conducting a comprehensive self-analysis.

The *Standards* state the traditional philosophy of PA education while recognizing advances in medical practice. Although the opportunity for creativity and innovation in program design remains, the *Standards* reflect the realization that a commonality in the core curriculum of programs has become not only desirable, but also necessary in order to offer curricula of sufficient depth and breadth to prepare PA graduates for practice in the dynamic and competitive healthcare arena.

Although the ARC-PA does not prescribe curriculum length, preclinical and clinical content must include supervised clinical practice experiences, instruction in interpersonal and communication skills, and a number of patient-assessment and patient-management topics. Clinical education is required in a variety of settings to reflect breadth and depth of content, and includes outpatient and inpatient settings as well as emergency and long-term care facilities. This is conducted in academic teaching facility settings, and inpatient clinical rotations are usually conducted in an experiential team format consisting of PA students, medical students, and residents, led by a staff attending physician on a clinical rotation assignment basis. The required content areas

of the preclinical curriculum are anatomy, physiology, pathophysiology, pharmacology and pharmacotherapeutics, and genetic and molecular mechanisms of health and disease. In the clinical curriculum, the required areas are emergency medicine, family medicine, general internal medicine, general surgical care (including operative experiences), geriatrics, pediatrics, prenatal care, and women's health.

ARC-PA accreditation is a voluntary determination and nearly all U.S. PA programs participate in the accreditation process. Lacking ARC-PA accreditation makes one ineligible for federal grants, and their graduates risk ineligibility for national certification or state licensure.

CHARACTERISTICS OF PHYSICIAN ASSISTANT PROGRAMS

As of 2009 there are 159 PA programs in the world: 145 in the United States, 2 in Australia, 3 in Canada, 5 in the Netherlands, and 4 in the United Kingdom (Exhibit 4-5). The programs outside of the United States are situated on traditional university campuses. Three-quarters (73%) of U.S. PA programs are in university institutions, but the remaining one-quarter of U.S. PA programs are situated at 4-year colleges and community colleges. One is on a military reservation. These smaller learning institutions reflect, to some extent, the historical development of early PA programs, sometimes being viewed as technical programs or allied health programs. (A list of current PA programs is

EXHIBIT 4-5
Distribution of Physician Assistant Programs in 2009

	Australia	Canada	Netherlands	United Kingdom	United States
University-based	2	2	5	4	108
4-year college					28
Community college					7
Hospital-based but degree granted from a university					2
Military		1			1
TOTAL	2	3	5	4	146

located in Appendix II.) Additional statistics that provide an overview of today's PA programs include the following:

- Five new PA programs began in 2008.
- Over 83% of all PA programs award a master's degree.
- The most common start date was August (35%).
- In 2007–2008, the mean total budget for a PA program was $1,364,120.
- For PA students enrolled in 2007, the mean resident tuition was $48,649 and for nonresidents it was $57,280; this is for the 26-month (average) professional phase of the program.
- In 2008, there were 11,040 unique e-submitted applications to PA programs.

U.S. Physician Assistant Programs

U.S. PA programs are distributed across 44 states. Those states with the most programs are New York (19), Pennsylvania (15), California (10), Texas (8), North Carolina (6), Ohio (6), and Florida (6), reflecting somewhat the geographical concentration of the population (Exhibit 4-6).

Historically, the overall growth of U.S. PA programs has been fairly uneven (Exhibit 4-7).

Length of Programs

Early in PA education, the length of PA curriculum varied. Initially, Duke's program was 24 months and the Medex program at Northwest was 12 months. As of 2009, almost all programs are at least 24 months in duration. The mean (and median) length of PA curriculum is 27 months with a range of 16 to 36 months. Over the past two decades the average length of the U.S. curriculum increased from 24 to 27 months. Non-American PA programs are 24 months.

A few PA programs involve a 5-year master's curriculum that admits students as freshmen. Students spend 3 years studying liberal arts and preparatory sciences followed by 2 years of PA studies. Because three-quarters of PA programs are at the graduate level, these programs admit students with a baccalaureate degree and the PA coursework tends to involve experiences in research in addition to the professional curriculum.

EXHIBIT 4-6
Geographical Distribution of U.S. Physician Assistant Programs

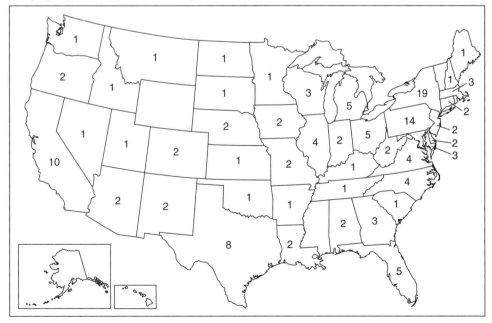

EXHIBIT 4-7
Periods of U.S. Physician Assistant Program Development

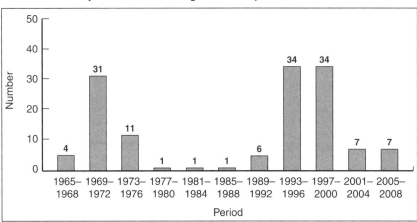

Data from *Physician Assistant Education Association. (2008a)*. Twenty-Third Annual Report on Physician Assistant Educational Programs in the United States, 2006–2007. *Alexandria, VA: Author.*

Program Personnel

There are four main types of personnel associated with PA programs: administrative, clerical, educational, and research. Within three of these types (excluding clerical) personnel can be classified as PAs or other. All but a few program directors are PAs. On average, there are 8.4 full-time equivalent (FTE) faculty members and 1.9 FTE staff. There were on average 1.6 clinical coordinators and one academic coordinator in a PA program. The mean number of faculty without any administrative role was 3.5 FTE (PAEA, 2008a). Faculty, staff, and research personnel may be PAs, doctors, scientists, or academics. They may be employed for a specific program or come from other departments within the institution.

Program Organizational Role

The hierarchy of a program within a sponsoring institution varies (Exhibit 4-8). A program may be a division (subdepartment) of a medical school department (e.g., Duke University School of Medicine, Department of Family Medicine, Division of Physician Assistant Studies), or it may be a department in a School of Medicine or Allied Health (e.g., University of Texas, Southwestern School of Allied Health, Department of Physician Assistant Studies).

Some programs are in schools of medicine within health sciences divisions or departments (e.g., The George Washington School of Medicine and Health Sciences, Health Sciences Programs Division). Two programs are schools within themselves (e.g., Pacific University School of Physician Assistant Studies). It appears that PA programs are increasingly set in academic units such as departments or divisions; in a 2008 survey, 26 of 92 responding PA programs were set in their own departments (Wright et al, 2009).

In a 2008 survey of 91 PA programs, 65% of programs were sections within departments and 29% were stand-alone departments. Three-fifths (59%) resided in private institutions; of these institutions, two-thirds (67%) were sections within departments and 26% were, themselves, departments. Approximately one-half of all programs surveyed (46%) were located in academic health centers (AHCs). The majority were embedded within a department (64%); 26% were at the departmental level. One-fifth (18%) of all PA programs reside in medical schools.

One-half of PA program directors (52%) report directly to a dean, 9% to an associate dean, 21% to a department chair, 6% to a provost (or equivalent), and 12% to "other" staff members. Between 2000 and 2008,

EXHIBIT 4-8
Examples of Physician Assistant Program Hierarchies with Sponsoring Institutions

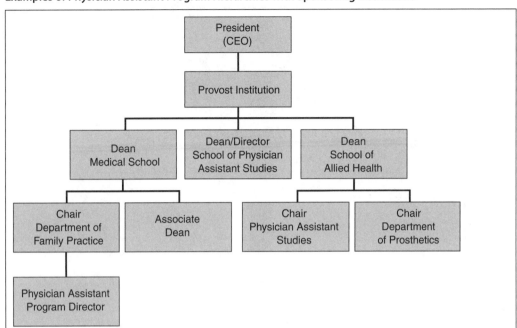

one-quarter (26%) of all programs moved up in their hierarchical arrangement within the institution and 14% anticipated change by 2010 (e.g., shifting from a section in a Department of Family Medicine to a Department of PA Studies). This substantial variation among institutions sponsoring PA programs likely reflects evolutionary development more than organizational rationale. How programs function and affect change within institutions remains to be explored.

Student Enrollment

Spread over 141 accredited programs in 2008, the average number of students in a PA program at any time (first, second, and third years combined) was 77. The mean number of students enrolled in first-year classes is 42 (range 11–195). The highest number (195) is in the Interservice Physician Assistant Program (IPAP), with more than 200 students enrolled annually (three classes each year), which is substantially larger than the next size program (110). Almost all students in U.S. programs are full time.

First-year enrollment in PA programs has increased from 24 students in 1984 to 44 in 2008 (Exhibit 4-9). The trend is increasing, and may be due to a number of factors, such as efficiency in teaching large classes, demand for employment, application demand, quality of applicants, and institutional pressure to enroll more and/or maximize tuition. The irregularity of the trend is due to new programs entering with smaller classes, pulling the mean down until they ramp up to their desired size.

Military Physician Assistant Education

Two programs run by the military are operational in 2009: the U.S. IPAP and the Canadian Forces Medical Services School (CFMSS) Physician Assistant Program. Both train PAs for combat roles, public health, occupational medicine, and humanitarian service. The CFMSS PA program, located in Borden, Ontario, graduates 16 to 20 PAs per year. Because members of the Canadian Forces Medical Services are intended to be interchangeable for all services, all PAs are trained

EXHIBIT 4-9
Trends in Physician Assistant Education Enrollment (Mean), 1984–2008

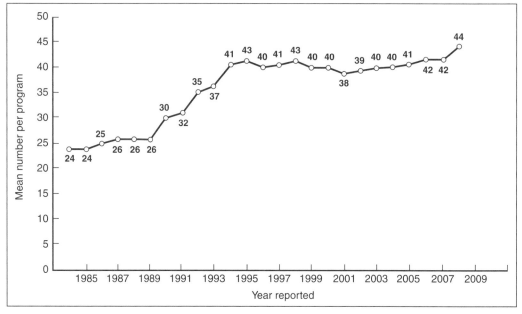

Data from Physician Assistant Education Association. (2008c). Twenty-Fourth Annual Report on Physician Assistant Educational Programs in the United States, 2007–2008. *Alexandria, VA: Author.*

for any role: be it in air, land, or sea. The CFMSS program is accredited by the Canadian Medical Association (Exhibit 4-10). The IPAP, located in San Antonio, Texas, is the world's largest PA program, and graduates more than 200 PAs per year (Exhibit 4-11). The Department of Defense (Army, Navy, and Air Force) and the U.S. Coast Guard PAs are trained at the IPAP.

EVOLUTIONARY PHASES OF PHYSICIAN ASSISTANT EDUCATION

Historically, PA education may be divided into four epochs. The first was the initial introduction in the 1960s. This phase was followed by rapid expansion that took place in the early 1970s, largely fueled by the availability of federal funding. As a result, more than 35 programs emerged between 1972 and 1975.

The second epoch was one in which the number of PA programs declined due to the Graduate Medical Education National

Advisory Committee's influence on the perception of a looming surplus of physicians by the 1990s. This trend, which existed from roughly 1980 through 1988, resulted in a decrease in the output of graduates and a depression in the applicant pool.

EXHIBIT 4-10
Canadian Medical Services School Physician Assistant Program

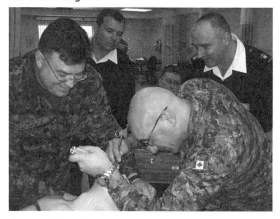

Courtesy of the authors.

EXHIBIT 4-11
U.S. Interservice Physician Assistant Program

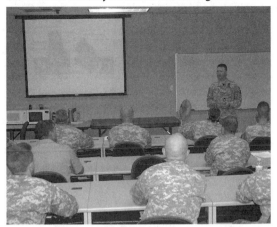

*Courtesy of Colonel William Tozier, Director, Interservice
PA Program, Ft. Sam Houston.*

The third epoch was one of significant expansion of the number of PA programs and took place in the mid and late 1990s. During this period, the number of programs virtually doubled between 1994 and 2001. Interestingly, this expansion was brought about not by the availability of federal subsidies, but by expansion taking place in the private sector of higher education. This sector of the American higher education system is likely to have viewed the rising popularity of the PA profession, the acceptance of medicine tentatively embracing PAs, and the demand for programs as an opportunity to improve revenue (Exhibit 4-12).

A fourth epoch is the growth of PA programs globally. This growth is in response to the doctor shortages; an activity similar to the early development of U.S. PA programs. Most of these efforts outside the United States tend to occur in universities with medical schools (Hooker, 2007; Ross, 2008; Simkens et al, 2009).

COMPETENCY-BASED EDUCATION

The traditional philosophy of PA education has been based on a model of demonstrating a standard level of clinical competency. Unlike most other health professions, PA education initially avoided assignment of a specific academic degree for entry-level preparation.

EXHIBIT 4-12
Physician Assistant Educational Program Growth

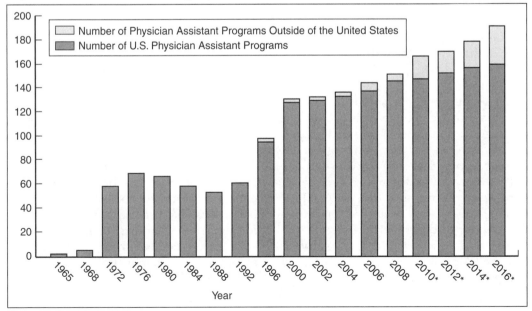

In describing this philosophy, the PAEA Graduate Education Council stated that:

> . . . proficiency in the clinical skills identified as being necessary for future competence in primary care/generalist practice would be the "gold standard" of PA educational preparation, rather than necessitating adherence to institutional requirements for a specific academic degree. (Joslin et al, 2006)

Originating from military utilization of health providers, the competency-based educational model prepared PAs to enter clinical practice based on their training and certification status. State PA practice laws and regulations were fashioned largely upon this model and typically do not refer to academic degrees with regard to PA qualification for practice. The fact that the PA clinical role is inherently tied to the physicians' practice made the need for early graduates to possess an academic degree less critical (Joslin et al, 2006).

The emphasis on competency rather than an academic degree enhanced the recruitment into PA programs of individuals from diverse ethnic, cultural, and educational backgrounds. Additionally, awarding a certificate instead of a degree tended to be an effective approach in preparing PA healthcare professionals to assume a wide range of roles in clinical practice settings and specialties (Exhibit 4-13).

Competency-based PA education appears to be effective in preparing healthcare professionals to qualify for the national certifying examination and to meet state licensing board requirements. The generalist philosophy of PA education is to produce graduates who can assume clinical practice roles in a wide range of healthcare settings and specialties. Although the competency basis of PA practice began to lose relevance in the late 1980s when programs began to award graduate degrees for PA training, the AAPA, APAP, ARC-PA, and NCCPA approved in 2005 a jointly developed document, *Competencies for the Physician Assistant Profession*, to communicate to the PA profession and the public a set of competencies that all PAs are expected to

EXHIBIT 4-13
Physician Assistant Student at George Washington University

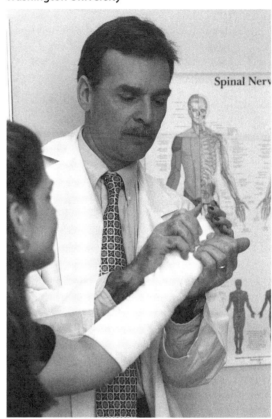

Courtesy of the authors.

acquire and maintain throughout their careers (see Appendix VII). The document outlines the kind of analysis, integration, evaluation, and information management skills that have traditionally been considered "graduate level." It is the first document of its kind to be endorsed by all of the entities representing the PA profession at a national level.

Today, the introduction of degrees (bachelor's or master's) has been a popular and enticing recruitment tool. A strong academic background has been advocated as a necessity for success in handling the intensity of a PA education—although there is little empirical evidence that demonstrates this assertion (Ballweg, 2004).

PHYSICIAN ASSISTANT CURRICULA

The philosophy of PA programs is one of a broad-based approach to primary care health professions education. This focus has resulted in curricula that provide PA students with a strong foundation in primary care and general medicine while preparing them to enter a wide range of specialized clinical areas.

Curriculum Overview

The format of the typical PA program is an intensive 26-month (range, 24 to 36 months), medically oriented curriculum that educates the student in medicine. Approximately one-half of that time (12 months) involves didactic instruction in the basic and clinical sciences, followed by a similar period of rotating clerkships and preceptorships in all major clinical disciplines (although this is increasingly blended with clinical experience in the first year and additional theoretical lectures in the second year [Ross, 2008]). Didactic courses include anatomy, physiology, microbiology, biochemistry, pathology, pharmacology, and the behavioral sciences. Instruction is also provided in the clinical sciences with coursework in history taking, physical examination, pathophysiology, clinical diagnosis, communication and interpersonal skills, epidemiology and preventive medicine, clinical procedures and surgical skills, and interpretation of laboratory test results and imaging studies. Courses in the basic medical sciences constitute a majority of the total didactic portion of PA curricula. Instruction devoted to the behavioral and social sciences averages more than 124 contact hours per program. The range of subjects includes health behavior, interpersonal communication skills, psychosocial dynamics, health promotion and disease prevention, bioethics, medical sociology, death and dying, and cross-cultural medicine (Exhibit 4-14).

During their second year, PA students obtain focused clinical training in select disciplines, typically 4 to 8 weeks long, conducted over a wide range of inpatient and outpatient care settings. Most students complete rotations

EXHIBIT 4-14

A Template of a Physician Assistant Program Curriculum

YEAR 1, DIDACTIC INSTRUCTION (COURSES)
Basic sciences
Anatomy
Physiology
Biochemistry
Medical microbiology/immunology
Pathology
Pharmacology
Clinical sciences
Clinical assessment (physical diagnosis)
Behavioral science/human behavior
Clinical medicine (cardiology, rheumatology, nephrology, hematology, pulmonary medicine, dermatology, neurology, oncology, gastroenterology, allergy/immunology, endocrinology, infectious disease, geriatrics, toxicology)
Geriatrics
Pediatrics
Clinical decision-making
Medical genetics
Clinical laboratory sciences
Surgery (otolaryngological, urological, vascular, neurological, orthopedic, thoracic, trauma, ophthalmologic)
Radiology/imaging science
Research methods/interpretation of the literature
Epidemiology and medical statistics
Preventive medicine and public health
Role of the physician assistant/Health systems and economics

YEAR 2, CLINICAL INSTRUCTION
Clinical rotations
Family medicine
Internal medicine
Surgery
Pediatrics
Obstetrics and gynecology (woman's health)
Emergency medicine
Psychiatry
Medical/surgical subspecialties (as electives)

PRECEPTORSHIP
PRIMARY CARE
SPECIALTY FIELD
GRADUATE EDUCATION/CAPSTONE PROJECT

in core medical, pediatric, surgical, and primary care clinical disciplines before moving into specialty settings. PA clinical education typically includes experiences in inpatient medicine, primary care and ambulatory medicine, surgery, pediatrics, obstetrics and gynecology, emergency medicine, and psychiatry. Clinical experiences also include elective rotations and a final preceptorship in a primary care practice setting. In serving on these clinical rotations and clerkships, PA students are instructed and mentored by practicing physicians, physician residents and house officers, graduate PAs, and various other healthcare professionals.

The basic science curriculum is usually structured to provide an in-depth understanding of structural features characterizing body tissues and organ systems, biochemical mechanisms regulating body metabolism, and nutrition. Next are the physiological controls governing body system functions, pathophysiology, and behavioral alterations causing clinical manifestations of illnesses and the management of these illnesses and injuries.

In most of the U.S. PA programs, the curriculum is based on the medical school model. A typical PA program is about 50 weeks shorter than a typical medical school program, but the primary educational objectives are similar. Both physician and PA education provide students with the theoretical knowledge and technical skills needed to perform therapeutic and diagnostic procedures accurately. Like medical schools, PA programs use a format of didactic and clinical training. However, the average PA program spans 27 months with minimal breaks, whereas the average medical school spans 48 months of instruction and breaks between school years 1 and 2.

Curriculum Topics

A few studies have dealt with the subject of what should be learned in PA programs. Golden and Cawley (1983) found that most PA programs were teaching what medical school educators had proposed—that the core of medicine is history taking and physical examination. In addition to teaching the proper approach to the patient and certain clinical skills, programs included technical skills such as urinalysis, blood analysis, electrocardiogram (ECG) interpretation, hearing and vision screening, Papanicolaou scrapings, applying and removing casts, tuberculosis skin testing, interpreting radiographs, parenteral injections, bacteriology testing, suturing, and pulmonary function testing.

Primary Care Education

Curricular innovations in health professions education that have focused on the clinical preparation of providers for primary care roles originated within now-prominent PA programs. PA programs using decentralized training approaches, such as those seen at the University of Washington Medex Northwest PA Program; the Stanford University Primary Care Associate Program; the University of California, Davis; Lock Haven University; and the University of Utah PA Program, have paved the way for other programs in their efforts to develop effective methods in placing PA graduates in medically underserved areas.

PA educators remain sensitive to changes in the healthcare environment, and program curriculum undergoes regular review and modification. Experience indicates that this flexibility results in newly employed PAs who adapt easily to many practice settings. A graduate-level educational track that aims to prepare PAs for practice in rural health care, such as the one sponsored by the Alderson-Broaddus College PA Program in Philippi, West Virginia, as well as other rural health curricula, such as those at the University of Texas-Pan American and Lock Haven University are innovative curricula that prepare primary healthcare providers for practices in areas with underserved populations.

To address areas essential to the preparation of competent primary care providers, PA programs commonly include instruction on preventive medicine, substance abuse prevention and treatment, health care for the homeless, women's health care, geriatric medicine, environmental and occupational medicine, mental health, and a practical orientation to developing skills in the delivery of clinical preventive services. Other examples of innovations of PA programs in focusing on primary care have been the long-standing inclusion of topics such as health education, epidemiology, communication skills, and biomedical ethics. These subjects have only relatively recently been regarded as important in undergraduate medical education.

Skills and Procedures

Each PA program seeks to develop within each student a strong foundation in the basic and clinical sciences of medicine. The education process may reflect a traditional medical school curriculum and even share classes with medical students, or it might introduce multidimensional assessment and decision analysis techniques that are unique to the particular PA program. Despite these variations, certain skills taught seem to be common to all programs (Cawley & Golden, 1983; Gray et al, 1995).

A comprehensive survey of Colorado PAs found that almost all of them learned 39 common procedures (Exhibit 4-15). Eight procedures (including reading chest and long-bone x-ray films, suturing, splinting, interpreting ECGs, and performing pelvic examinations, Papanicolaou smears, and urinalysis) were performed more than once per month by at least 50% of PAs in their practices. Three procedures (cardiopulmonary resuscitation, lumbar puncture, and suprapubic aspirations) were used less than once per year by more than 90% of PAs (Gray et al, 1995). The leading skills needed for any PA practice were history taking, physical diagnosis, and patient management (Cawley et al, 2001).

In examining the content of PA clinical activities, Dehn and Hooker (1999) analyzed the results of a survey of family practice PAs in Iowa and found that all respondents provided health promotion, disease prevention, health and safety education, and prescribed drugs. The procedures reported by the respondents were the same as those performed by family medicine physicians in the same state and were considerably broader than had been surmised. The size of the community in which they practiced also made a difference; the more

rural and remote the community, the more likely the PA would perform a procedure.

Telemedicine

Telemedicine refers to remote health services involving patient care interactions that are geographically disparate and enabled by telecommunications, information technology, and sensor technology. Key players involved are physicians and nonphysician clinicians,

EXHIBIT 4-15
Skills Most Frequently Learned by Physician Assistant Students

PROCEDURES
Cardiopulmonary resuscitation
Electrocardiogram (perform, interpret)
Fingerstick and heelstick
Fluorescein Wood's lamp examination
Parenteral injection (intradermal, subcutaneous, intramuscular)
Lumbar puncture
Suprapubic aspiration
Urethral catheterization
Venipuncture

LABORATORY TECHNIQUES
Agglutination test for mononucleosis (read)
Blood smear (perform, read)
Culture (streak out, read)
Gram stain (perform, read)
Sensitivity plate (read)
Stool examination for occult blood
Urinalysis (dipstick, microscopic)

PATIENT CARE
Chest radiograph (read)
Intravenous line (set up, start, monitor)
Long-bone x-ray film (read)
Papanicolaou stain (perform)
Pelvic examination
Suturing
Wound care (burns, casts, splints)

SCREENING TESTS
Articulation screen
Denver Developmental Screening Test
Hearing screen
Vision screen

Data from Gray, J. et al (1995). Do PAs use the procedures and skills they learn? Journal of the American Academy of Physician Assistants, 8, 45–51.

sick or healthy individuals, and their friends or family (Haselkorn, Coyle, & Doarn, 2007). Telemedicine is now a curricular topic addressed by some PA programs (Asprey, Zollo, & Kienzle, 2001; Goldstein, 2005).

The University of Iowa began incorporating telemedicine into its health sciences curriculum in 1999. The primary goal of the module was to teach first-year students about the value, efficacy, risks, and challenges of using telemedicine systems to diagnose and treat patients. The program focused on using various technologies to overcome issues of distance, healthcare access, and record-keeping when providing patient care rather than on computer-assisted instruction or Internet-based information resources (Exhibit 4-16). For example, a lecture on data technologies discussed how the development of the electronic medical record facilitated the practice of telemedicine with patients and clinicians in geographically disparate locations. The module was initiated with the intent of preparing PAs to utilize this technology in rural and underserved settings (Asprey, Zollo, & Kinzle, 2001).

The overall curriculum module at the University of Iowa was evaluated by the students for relevance, clarity, coordination, scope, time allotted, amount of information covered, quality of the content, class format, didactic sessions, hands-on demos, and opportunities for follow-up. One aspect of the evaluation elicited the students' subjective perceptions of their knowledge of telemedicine before and after the telemedicine class. Most of the students indicated they had minimal or no prior knowledge of telemedicine before the classes. No students had experience with telemedicine prior to the classes. After participating in the telemedicine curriculum, nearly all students reported that their knowledge of telemedicine had increased to moderate or great. Perhaps of greatest significance was the fact that nearly all respondents indicated that they were more likely or much more likely to seek out telemedicine opportunities after taking the classes.

Telemedicine has also been shown to be beneficial as an educational resource. Loera, Kuo, and Rahr (2007) used telemedicine instruments

EXHIBIT 4-16
Sample Telemedicine Curriculum Outline

SESSION 1
- Current telemedicine definitions and applications
- Reports on the viability and efficacy of telemedicine for clinical interactions
- Enabling technologies
- Challenges and obstacles to widespread telemedicine implementation
- Implications of telemedicine for rural health
- Participants and players in the telemedicine process, including reports from telemedicine users
- State and federal legislation affecting telemedicine
- Resources and pathfinders for obtaining further information about telemedicine
- Opportunities and predictions for future telemedicine development

SESSION 2
- Demonstration of how desktop videoconferencing and a high-speed Internet connection can be used to transmit patient information in real time to a distant cardiologist or neurologist for immediate consultation in an emergent situation
- Observation of a simulated teleconsultation, noting the quality of the transmission and the process involved, including asking the telemedicine physician questions, speaking to the remote-site participants, and using the telemedical peripherals and equipment such as the digital stethoscope

SESSION 3
- Presentation from a researcher whose area of interest is ethical issues in telemedicine to discuss such topics as network security, patient confidentiality, and equitable access to health care

SESSION 4
- Visit to a remote hospital in a telemedicine network to observe how teleconsultations are used and how its usefulness is perceived, including an interactive session with the academic medical center and a videoconference with an internal medicine physician to answer questions
- Session for students to ask primary care site coordinators questions in order to better understand the relative value of telemedicine to rural primary care providers and their patients

to enable faculty to teach students the skills needed to perform a history and physical examination on an elderly person. This distance mentoring study was designed as a pilot, based on limited faculty time available to determine the effectiveness of teaching students. Students essentially performed a house visit on an elderly patient without having a faculty member in attendance physically. Each student was trained on the use of the telemedicine workstation so that his or her encounter with the elderly patient could be transmitted to a faculty member at a remote location.

Students were subsequently surveyed regarding the experience of visiting an independent living facility and about the reliability and their level of comfort using telemedicine. Most students found telemedicine to be reliable, and most students gained confidence and an acceptable level of comfort using telemedicine instruments to interact with elderly volunteer residents of an independent living facility. Students improved their physical examination skills and gained confidence administering special questionnaires such as the geriatric depression scale, the Mini Mental State Examination, and the clock-drawing test.

The role of PAs in the utilization of telemedicine remains to be seen. However, the fact that PAs are distributed in many rural and underserved locations places them in a unique setting ideally situated to benefit from the utilization of this technology.

Other Components

The literature related to content of PA educational programs shows that curricula within PA programs are regularly changing and adjusted to the evolution of medical knowledge. There are few studies that present information on the entire breadth and depth of an individual curriculum. Most of the published studies relating to PA curriculum content describe specific pedagogical techniques, such as problem-based learning (Allen et al, 2003; Parkhurst & Ramsery, 2006) or expanding components, such as the use of standardized patients (Asprey, Hegmann, & Bergus, 2007; Whitman & Pedersen, 1998), service learning (Searle et al, 2003), and evidence-based medicine (DiMatteo, 2004; Keahey & Goldgar, 2004; Goldgar, 2006; Coniglio et al, 2007) as well as the inclusion of topics such as domestic violence (Phelps & Lyons, 2000), literature in medicine (Corso, 2001), women's health (Kimmos, 2005; Grant & Sullivan, 2008), geriatrics (Dieter & Fasser, 1989; Hayward et al,

2005), and cultural competency (Jacques, 2004; Parrish, 2004; Straker & LeLacheur, 2007).

Educators at the University of Texas Medical Branch at Galveston found that a majority of PA programs present instruction in health promotion and wellness. The authors also found that programs included a variety of related course topics that were usually integrated into existing courses and could be taught via telemedicine. These courses covered the fields of preventive medicine, public health, epidemiology, and health promotion/disease prevention (Perkins, Rahr, & Kurial, 2001).

In a study of nutrition education on PA programs, Sullivan (2000) conducted a national survey of PA programs. The study sought to enlist 105 programs; there was a 50% response rate ($N = 52$). She found that 94% of responding programs included nutrition education as a component of their curricula, with 20% offering nutrition as a separate course. Most responding programs (64%) included nutrition as part of their clinical medicine course.

Clinical Rotation

PA education is built on the apprentice concept—that the student learns best by doing. The clinical rotation is when the student sees patients, either in conjunction with an experienced clinician, or on his or her own with the experienced clinician assessing the student's evaluation of a patient. These clinical settings vary and can be outpatient or inpatient and in primary care offices or tertiary care centers, birth centers, or nursing homes. Although specific clinical rotations are not required for each clinical discipline, a PA program is obligated to give every student clinical experiences in family medicine, general internal medicine, pediatrics, prenatal care and women's health, general surgery, emergency medicine, psychiatry/behavioral medicine, and geriatrics.

Such clinical experiences can vary in length from a few weeks to a few months. Many programs will add components on rural health, public health, care in nursing homes, addiction medicine, and certain specialties such as orthopedics, pulmonology, forensic medicine, radiology, intensive care, urology, gastroenterology, corrections medicine, and sports medicine. Exposure to the various clinical disciplines familiarizes the student with these disciplines and offers guidance for the student to search the literature and to make appropriate referrals to specialists.

In preparation for this phase of education, regardless of when it occurs, programs must provide students with a set of skills to interview and elicit a medical history, perform a physician examination across all life spans, order and interpret diagnostic studies, and present the patient data in oral and written form.

Standardized Patients

Standardized patients (SPs) are used extensively in physician and nursing education, where they have proven to be valuable educational tools. Their benefit is mostly in developing communication skills. A survey of 96 PA programs revealed that SPs play various roles, including providing medical histories and participating in complaint-specific and organ-specific "sensitive" examinations (rectal, pelvic, etc.). Programs housed in medical schools were more likely to use professional patients. Respondents from programs not using SPs provided reasons why they were not used. Most common among these were issues related to cost, access, training, and recruitment. To a lesser extent, liability issues were also cited, as was a perceived lack of evidence that SPs add value to PA education. Details about SP compensation span a broad range of remuneration (Calhoun, Vrbin, & Grzybicki, 2008).

The Preceptorship

Traditionally, the preceptorship phase of training for PA students is the final step in the professional socialization process. (However, when this stage occurs it can vary among institutions.) During the preceptorship stage, PAs must learn the proper attitudes and techniques for managing patients with professionalism and appropriate clinical judgment—the essence of appropriate medical practice. With the science of medicine learned primarily from lectures,

books, and laboratory work, the art of relating to patients is acquired through imitative role modeling, intuition, and trial and error. Views about patients tend to change the most during this time as students gain clinical experience and expertise.

The preceptorship is an experience shared by the physician mentor and the student. This experience is not trivial because the physician may become a lasting role model in the memory of the student and shape the PA's career. The cardinal learning experiences of medicine—exploring, examining, and cutting into the human body; dealing with the fears, anger, sense of helplessness, and despair of patients; meeting urgent situations; accepting the limitations of medical science; and being confronted with death—will be experiences the physician will guide the PA through to professional self-actualization. (Exhibit 4-17).

Preceptorships do not come easily, and good preceptors are even harder to find. A PA student may have to compete with medical students from the host institution or students from other PA or NP programs for clinical slots with a preceptor. A critical issue for many PA programs is the availability of clinical training sites. With the expansion of medical student and PA student educational programs, the number of educational slots

EXHIBIT 4-17
During the Preceptorship, the Physician Guides the Student to Professional Self-Actualization

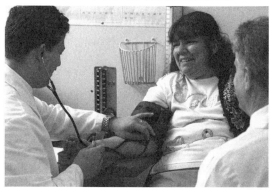

Courtesy of authors and George Washington University.

for clinical students in practices and teaching hospitals are at a premium, particularly in certain disciplines such as pediatrics and women's health. This has led some programs to begin the practice of paying precept students; in 2008, 8% (nine programs) responding to the PAEA Annual Survey reported payment to sites and/or preceptors (PAEA, 2008c). Additional factors that can impact the number of available preceptors include using one site too often (preceptor fatigue) or a facility already having clinicians with too many students (Kuttler, 2007). Higher tuition and debt burden are the reasons most often cited for not purchasing preceptorships. Outside of the United States, PA programs tend to pay preceptors for their time to work with students.

Many preceptors enjoy the intellectual and social stimulation of training students. Some see mentoring as an effective tool in recruiting new employees or the opportunity to be challenged by bright students. Others dismiss the notion of a professional obligation to train those who follow them into medicine (Kuttler, 2007). However, the pressures placed on clinicians to meet performance expectations have often been cited as a reason that some clinicians elect to discontinue as a preceptor due to the conviction that it "slows them down," thus decreasing productivity.

A survey was sent to 115 clinical preceptors of the University of New Mexico PA Program. The preceptors were asked to assess their experience as clinical teachers, interest in teaching topics, preferred delivery modes, and rewards of teaching. Their responses showed that preceptors' interests and needs varied. More importantly, it allowed the faculty opportunities to address preceptor needs and make better matches of students to preceptors at their sites (O'Callaghan, 2007).

Sometimes how students perceive a rotation and how the preceptor perceives the student may differ. A survey was conducted to examine the opinions of preceptors, PA students, and recent PA program graduates regarding the effectiveness of preceptors. Questionnaires were mailed to 100 preceptors of PA students enrolled in the Emory

PA Program and to 100 PAs graduating from the Emory PA Program in 1996 and 1997. Thirty-five current second-year and 44 current third-year Emory PA students were also surveyed. Students and graduate PAs responding to these surveys uniformly identified several qualities of effective preceptors, as did preceptors themselves. Preceptors also indicated their motivation for becoming preceptors, identified their strengths and weaknesses, and expressed interest in the Emory PA program providing faculty development. This study indicates that student evaluations of preceptors are a valuable tool in identifying qualities of an effective preceptor, as are preceptor evaluations of themselves. Findings also indicate a willingness of preceptors of PA students to participate in further training to improve clinical teaching skills (Zayas, 1999).

International Rotations

Some students undertake some of their training in other countries. Such experiences range from public health experience in the jungles of Bolivia (Pucillo, 2000) or a dermatology rotation in Brisbane, Australia. A survey of 58 programs in 1999 found that 43% would consider sending their students overseas. Several schools use medical outreach groups and missionary trips for international sites (Heinerich, 2000). A partial list of student rotation locations is shown in Exhibit 4-18.

Clinical rotations at overseas locations are popular with second year PA students. Such rotations may be challenging to arrange. Assurance of educational quality and appropriate supervision is the responsibility of the program in such instances.

Physician Assistants for Global Health (PAGH) is an official group of the AAPA. Its goal is to promote cross-cultural awareness and delivery of PA services to domestic and international healthcare professional shortage areas. PAGH has been involved with placing some students in overseas rotations. The PAEA also has a guide for international PA education programs.

EXHIBIT 4-18
Partial List of International Clinical Sites Where Physician Assistant Students Have Trained

AFRICA
Kenya
Madagascar
Tanzania
Other African countries

ASIA
India
Iran
Mariana Islands
Papua New Guinea

AUSTRALIA

EUROPE
England
Ireland
Netherlands
Scotland

NORTH AMERICA
Belize
Bermuda
Canada
Guatemala
Haiti
Honduras
Jamaica
Trinidad

SOUTH AMERICA
Bolivia
Brazil
Other South American countries

Graduate Level Education

Educators and researchers in many health profession disciplines have long wrestled with the "degree debate" regarding the appropriate entry-level credential. This process represents a natural progression in the maturation of many professions. Debates are often discomforting and require many years to achieve general consensus within the representative educational programs. For example, as early as 1958 the field of occupational therapy began deliberations as to what educational level was best suited for the profession. Nearly 30 years later, the American Occupational Therapy Association (AOTA) endorsed a gradual shift to the master's degree as the entry-level degree

for its profession. Similarly, the physical therapy profession began a transition to an entry-level master's degree over a 10-year period back in 1979, which met with continued debate. Their guidelines for educational programs, as revised in 1997, standardized the physical therapy entry-level degree at the master's level. NPs have determined that the NP education award the MSN degree, and now the doctorate of nursing practice (DNP) to be awarded to all advance practice nurses upon graduation (Brown-Benedict, 2008).

A similar pattern of evolution is being observed in the PA profession. When the first educational program was founded, the mandate for programs was to produce safe and competent clinicians and to get them into the field as soon as possible. PA education was a competency-based model, consisting of 2 or 3 years of college work with certain prescribed courses plus vocational training. Often, a certificate of completion was the only credential awarded upon completion of the educational program. As time went on and as PA educational programs evolved, sponsoring institutions, such as Alderson-Broaddus College in 1970, began to award academic degrees along with the certificate of program completion.

The first PA program to award the master's degree for entry-level training was the Child Health Associate Program at the University of Colorado. In 1975, this program was among the first of the specialty-focus PA programs. Recruits to this program tended to be individuals who did not possess a great deal of previous healthcare experience but instead were high-achieving undergraduates, heralding a trend seen among applicants to PA educational programs many years later.

As PA education evolved, individuals argued that a master's degree is consistent with the quantity and quality of intellectual work to which PA students are subjected and that the level of academic rigor in PA programs was well beyond bachelor-level work. PA students develop the power of critical reasoning, the capacity to generalize, and the ability to find and evaluate clinical information so they can practice evidence-based medicine. Using this line of reasoning, one can conclude that PA education is at a higher level than under graduate, and that a master's degree is the appropriate credential for the profession.

In 1999, a Degree Task Force surveyed accredited programs to determine how many programs planned to change the academic degree in the next 5 years (Miller et al, 2001). Of the 96 responding programs, 45 indicated they were planning to change the credential awarded, and of those 45 programs, 62% said they were planning to grant a master's degree. Considering at the time 51% of programs were already awarding a master's degree, it appeared that most PA programs intended to confer a master's degree. Additionally, the Degree Task Force recommended that all programs be required to graduate PAs with a master's degree by 2007. Although the task force did not address the question of enforcement, one could presume the likely mechanism would be through changing the accreditation standards to require programs to award the master's degree.

In 1990, only three programs (6% of all programs) awarded a master's degree; by 2008, 76% of programs awarded a master's degree. Typically, programs award the master's of physician assistant studies (MPAS), master's of health science (MHS), or master's of science (MS) degree. Some PA programs award the bachelor's degree, but also offer a master's degree option. The average program length has increased from 24 months in 1987 to 26 months in 2007 (range 12 to 31 months). Didactic curriculum has increased from 1,004.5 hours in 1991 to 1,594 hours in 2007. The increases in didactic curriculum and consequent increase in total program length are likely related to the higher degrees granted by contemporary programs. Exhibit 4-19 shows the various degrees awarded by PA educational programs.

Until recently, the ARC-PA Standards have not addressed the educational level at which PA education should be provided. In the second edition of the *Standards* (2001), the operative language was: "this version of the Standards reflects the realization that a commonality in the core curriculum of programs has become not only desirable, but also necessary in order to offer curricula of sufficient depth and breadth to prepare PA graduates for practice in a

dynamic and competitive health care arena." Additionally, the Standards are intended to "reflect a graduate level of curricular intensity." In 2005, the ARC-PA modified the third edition of the *Standards* to indicate that the establishment of new PA programs may occur only at institutions that can award a bachelor's degree or higher (Miller et al, 2001). Yet, the *Standards* do not specify any delineation of curricular content relative to the credential awarded upon successful completion of the educational program. Unlike other health professions, there is not a single type of master's degree awarded for PA education, but instead there has emerged a wide variety of master's degrees granted by sponsoring institutions.

EXHIBIT 4-19

Credentials Awarded by Physician Assistant Programs (*N* = 122)

Credential	Number
Certificate	**32**
Associate	**4**
Baccalaureate	**20**
Bachelor of Science (BS)	10
Bachelor of Science in Physician Assistant (BSPA)/ Bachelor of Science in Physician Assistant Studies (BSPAS)/Bachelor of Physician Assistant Studies (BPAS)/Bachelor of Physician Assistant (BPA)	9
Bachelor of Clinical Health Services (BCHS)	1
Master's	**107**
Master of Science (MS)	19
Master of Physician Assistant Studies (MPAS)/Master of Science in Physician Assistant Studies (MSPAS)/Master of Physician Assistant Practice (MPAP)/Master of Physician Assistant (MPA)	57
Master of Health Science (MHS)/ Master of Science in Health Science (MSHS)	9
Master of Medical Science or Master of Science in Medicine (MMS/MSM/MMSc)	12
Master of Public Health (MPH)	4
Other Master's degree	6
Other degree	**4**
Total Number of Credentials	**167**

Data from Physician Assistant Education Association. (2008c). Twenty-Fourth Annual Report on Physician Assistant Educational Programs in the United States, 2007–2008. Alexandria, VA: Author.

The Council on Graduate Medical Education (COGME) endorsed educational content that includes "principles of statistics and epidemiology, learning how to search efficiently for 'current best evidence,' knowing the relative value of different types of evidence, and knowing when and how to apply evidence to the care of an individual or patient group" (COGME, 1994). Achieving this degree of knowledge and clinical expertise requires a greater breadth and depth of graduate professional education than competency-based undergraduate models are typically able to accommodate.

In some instances institutional requirements dictate the form the master's degree is to take. In other institutions, the award of a master's degree means that such a degree comprises a set number of graduate credits and contains specific quantitatively oriented courses. Finally, the configuration of the master's degree should take a distinctly academic identity as opposed to a professional degree in which traditional institutional academic requirements may not be present (Zellmer & Hadley, 2004).

As programs converted to the master's degree, most adjusted their curricula to include additional courses in research-related subjects such as biostatistics, research methodology, and data analysis. The majority of programs made this change during the years 1998 through 2003. Converting programs were surveyed as to which course(s) were added to the curricula. Common responses were research methods in epidemiology (20%), research methods in statistics (11%), and a long list of research/quantitative courses. When converting PA programs were asked if the conversion necessitated a change in their mission and goals, 34% indicated that it did and 21% indicated that it did not. In terms of whether or not changing to the master's degree caused them to lengthen the program, 32.6% indicated that it did and 22.5% indicated that it did not.

In the early 1990s, new models of PA education developed. One of these programs combined PA education with a related graduate degree program: the PA/master's of public health (e.g., program at the George Washington University) (Benzie et al, 2003). There are now at least six PA/MPH programs. Others offered distance education master's degree programs aimed at practicing PAs (Exhibit 4-20).

Capstone Projects

An integral component of a graduate degree curriculum is a capstone project—usually some form of research involving data collection, analysis, or a library review of a subject.

EXHIBIT 4-20
Examples of Master's of Public Health/Physician Assistant Dual Degree Programs, 2008

Program	Year Founded	Applicants/ Enrollees	Admissions Criteria	Cost	Length	Curriculum Integration
Emory University	2006	21/2	Academics and experience	$46,000	38 months	10 credits
Arcadia University	2001	N/A		N/A	3 years	6 credits
Touro College	2003	500/25	Diversity	$30,000	32 months	Total program
The George Washington University	1987	150/12	Narrative	$90,000	3 years	8 credits
University of Washington	2004	551/81	Diversity/ academics	$37,000	37 months	None
Yale University	2009					

Such projects generally require the student to apply the knowledge and skills obtained in the course of their graduate work to a specific research or practical experience-oriented activity. The specific skills developed can include critical evaluation of the medical literature, an in-depth comprehension of the research process, and an awareness of potential research questions related to clinical practice (Zellmer & Hadley, 2004).

A national survey examined the content and requirements of PA program capstone projects. The sample included 43 of the existing 90 PA programs that offer a master's degree. A project usually requires a formal proposal, takes 12 months to complete, and does not always require institutional approval. The majority (84%) of programs required a capstone project for the degree. In some instances a paper was required, followed by a formal oral presentation, poster presentation, and community service. When the authors compared programs that were considered academically based or professionally based, a systematic review of the literature was the most frequently reported activity (Zellmer & Hadley, 2004).

RANKING PHYSICIAN ASSISTANT PROGRAMS

Since PA education has moved toward awarding graduate degrees, PA programs have been ranked according to opinions of faculty and graduates. *U.S. News and World Report (USN&WR)* publishes a popular list for individuals with an interest in comparing educational programs by ranking all graduate schools. The news magazine began ranking PA programs in the mid-1990s. Critics of the rankings have expressed concern regarding methodological shortcomings of the survey. For some PA educators, particularly those critical of the rankings, the survey is viewed as a popularity contest, which may or may not reflect the true quality of the programs. Academic institutions have been ranked by reputation and other attributes since 1924.

Rankings of American medical schools published annually by *USN&WR* are widely used to judge the quality of the schools and their programs. In a sharp critique of the news magazine's rankings of medical schools, McGaghie and Thompson (2002) criticized the rankings on methodological and conceptual grounds, arguing that the annual medical school evaluations fall short in both areas. The authors concluded that the annual rankings of American medical schools are ill-conceived, unscientific, and poorly conducted; they ignore medical school accreditation; judge medical school quality from a narrow, elitist perspective; and do not consider social and professional outcomes in program quality calculations. McGaghie and Thompson (2002) note that medical school rankings have no practical value as published in the news magazine and fail to meet standards of journalistic ethics. There are those in PA education who feel that these findings would apply as well to the rankings of PA programs.

Others make the point that there are many programs spanning a wide variety of disciplines that appear in the rankings of *USN&WR*, and these include graduate programs in business administration, education, and law, as well as numerous disciplines within the health professions, such as physical therapy, pharmacy, and nursing. It is also well known that a number of institutions sponsoring highly ranked PA programs promote the survey results extensively in their promotional and student recruitment materials.

There is little organizational consensus regarding the rankings. Blessing and colleagues (2001) conducted a survey of PA educators' opinions on the rankings shortly after the second survey appeared in *USN&WR*. The Blessing survey asked PA program directors to identify program characteristics that would best objectify reputations. One hundred and twenty-six program directors were mailed a 75-item survey in the fall of 2000 and 95 responded (75%). The most notable aspect of the survey results was the lack of agreement on which PA program attributes should be measured. The greatest agreement was on factors such as faculty-to-student ratio, graduation rate, student attrition rate, and PA National Certifying Examination (PANCE) scores. Agreement was nearly unanimous among responding programs that program rank should not be a component of the accreditation process (Exhibit 4-21). Despite the human need to compare and contrast, there is little agreement among PA program directors on the elements that should determine a program's ranking. Without near-unanimous support across PA programs for internally developing objectives by which to rank programs, Blessing

and colleagues concluded that this aspect of PA education is best left to outside agencies and organizations. Thus, there appears to be a distinct ambivalence among PA educators with regard to the rankings.

SATELLITE PROGRAMS

As PA programs matured and extended their missions to improve healthcare access, several programs, with federal grant support, instituted what have been termed *satellite programs*. These

EXHIBIT 4-21
Physician Assistant Program Directors Opinions on Program Ranking

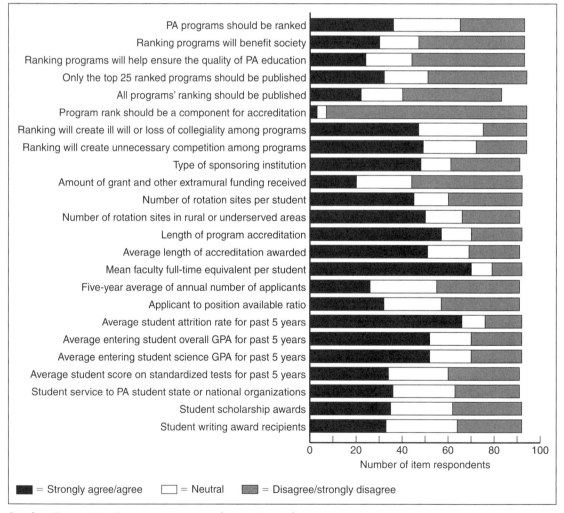

Data from Blessing, J. D. et al (2001). An investigation of potential criteria for ranking physician assistant programs. Perspective on Physician Assistant Education, 12(3), 160–166.

ventures are essentially outreach segments of existing programs designed to serve a particular region or population, or to take advantage of particular resources in an area separate from the sponsoring program. Examples of such satellite programs are the Yakima and Spokane branches of the Medex Northwest Program at the University of Washington in Seattle, the Clearfield branch of the Lock Haven University PA Program, and the University of Kentucky-Lexington/Moorhead University PA Program in eastern Kentucky. The University of Texas-Pan American PA Program in Edinburg, Texas, began as an extension of the PA Program of the University of Texas Medical Branch in Galveston and is now a separate freestanding program.

The question of the effectiveness of curriculum in satellite programs has been studied and their quality of curriculum has been shown to be equivalent to the education given in the base program. In a comparison of the satellite programs of the University of Washington Medex Northwest PA programs (Seattle, Yakima, Spokane, Washington, and formerly, Sitka, Alaska), there was little difference in grades and pass rates among graduates over a period of 5 years. Because the overall academic performances in all training sites were comparable, the authors concluded that administrative and curricular controls in the home institution could achieve parity in education across their various training sites (Ballweg & Wick, 1999).

BECOMING A PHYSICIAN ASSISTANT

The data examining why aspirants seek to become PAs are sparse. Using anecdotal sources, a list of motivators that are thought to influence individuals who apply to PA school was compiled (Exhibit 4-22). No one single motivating factor has emerged to explain why people choose a career as a PA. Some faculty believe the prime factor for young women to select a PA education over medical school is that the shortened time to achieve a professional career allows more options for family planning. However, factors that influence an

individual's decision to become a PA have been identified.

Factors Influencing the Decision to Become a Physician Assistant

Although typical students plan a career in health care during high school, the decision to become a PA commonly occurs later in life. Most students decide to become PAs after first ruling out medical school and researching the PA profession. Dissatisfaction with a previous healthcare career is a moderate motivator. After potential students learn about the profession, it may take 3 to 4 years before they begin the enrollment process. The lag time from learning about the PA profession to starting the enrollment process results from

EXHIBIT 4-22
Motivations for Applying to Physician Assistant School

1. Interest in medicine
2. Interest in health care but not in becoming a physician or nurse
3. Interest in helping people and contributing to the community
4. Financial reward, steady income, job security
5. Career in respected profession
6. Job satisfaction
7. Constant challenge of job
8. Preparation for medical school too long or too difficult or doubts about being accepted to medical school
9. Personal experience (e.g., health problem in a family, a friend, or self)
10. Influence of a family, friend, or teacher to choose a specific career
11. Faster route to practicing medicine than medical school (shorter schooling and no residency required)
12. Less costly than medical school
13. Easier to get into PA school
14. Career advancement (i.e., applicant was already in a health-related field)
15. Less responsibility than becoming a physician (less legal risk and malpractice)
16. Lifestyle issues (more time for family and friends, more recreation time, fewer work hours than a physician)

time spent meeting application requirements, applying, being accepted, and finally
enrolling. Personal contact with practicing
PAs is probably the most effective recruitment
tool for the profession.

A number of other factors influence a person's choice to become a PA (Exhibit 4-23). PAs
and other professionals continue to be the
dominant force influencing students to consider a PA career. However, the factor of "following in a parent's footsteps" has started to
emerge as an influence. Since 1985, dozens of
adult children have followed their PA parents'
careers to become PAs (a few even enrolling at
the same time). Having a family member who
is a PA or a physician or having a PA as a primary care provider is a strong influence on the
decision to become a PA.

Applications to Physician Assistant Programs

In response to forces in the healthcare professions marketplace, PA educational programs
have seen steady increases in the number of
program applicants. This is thought to be due
to factors such as:

- improved visibility of the PA profession over 40 years;
- opportunity to pursue a graduate degree;
- attractive income of PAs; and
- ability to enter medicine without pro- longed education.

The Centralized Application Service for Physician Assistants

Individuals apply to PA educational programs
through the Central Application Service for
Physician Assistants (CASPA). Established in
2001, the CASPA has improved the ability to
understand the PA applicant pool. Now in
its eight application cycle, more than three-
quarters of PA programs participated in the
service in 2008. CASPA allows a single application to be completed electronically and sent
to the PA programs of choice. Centralizing the
process enhances student choice and decreases falsifying applications. As more programs
participate, more data characterizing the PA
applicant pool emerges (Exhibit 4-24).

EXHIBIT 4-23
Summary Measures of Level of Influence on Decision to Become a Physician Assistant of New Program Enrollees, 2000*

Influence Factor	Score
American Academy of Physician Assistants (AAPA) literature	1.6
Association of Postgraduate PA Programs (APPAP) literature	1.4
PA program literature	2.0
Television program	1.2
Television public service announcement	1.1
Radio program	1.1
Radio public service announcement	1.0
Cinema	1.1
Other nonwritten media	1.3
Project Access (PAs visiting schools)	1.3
AAPA staff	1.2
APPAP staff	1.2
PA program faculty or staff	1.9
Family member	1.7
Career counselor or teacher (high school or college)	1.5
Physician who treated individual or a family member	1.8
PA who treated individual or a family member	1.8
Other PA acquaintance	2.3
Other health professional	2.2
Other factor	2.1

*The amount of influence was rated according to a 3-point scale: 1, no influence; 2, moderate influence; 3, strong influence.

Data from American Academy of Physician Assistants. (2001). Report of the Census Survey of New Physician Assistant Students, 1995–2000, Alexandria, VA: Author. Retrieved from http://www.aapa.org/research/95-00enrollees.html.

In early 2009, 115 of the 143 accredited PA
programs had elected to participate in
CASPA. Applying to programs through this
service allows applicants to complete one
online application and designate multiple programs to receive it. CASPA first verifies the
materials for authenticity. The PA profession
appears to be popular among young adults
and applications to the nation's 145 PA programs is competitive. The number of applications in 2008 was 11,040 for approximately

EXHIBIT 4-24
Centralized Application Service for Physician Assistant Applicants (CASPA) Trends, 2002–2007

Year	2002	2003	2004	2005	2006	2007
Programs participating in CASPA	68	68	80	90	93	97
Applicants	4,669	5,047	5,885	6,812	7,608	9,031
Applications	15,392	18,906	23,660	30,109	36,459	45,664
Average number of programs applied to (destination of application)	3.6	3.6	3.9	4.3	4.8	5.1

Data from CASPA. Presented at the Annual Education Forum, October 26, 2007.

5,000 entering seats. Applicants in 2008 designated an average of 5.59 schools on the CASPA application. The data from CASPA showed that there were 2.7 applicants per available seat out of the designated 3,835 seats available at programs in 2008 that are listed with CASPA (at that time, 101 programs). These proportions are similar to figures reported for medical school applicants.

Trends continue to show that more females than males apply to PA programs (ratio of about 3:1). Among CASPA applicants in 2007, 72.9% were women. The average age of students has decreased to 26.7 years in 2007. This declining trend continues, in 2005 the average age was 27.5 years and 27.8 years in 2002. States with the most applicants were Texas (9%), California (8%), New York (7%), Pennsylvania (6%), Florida (6%), and Michigan (5%).

In terms of ethnicity, in 2007, 70.8% of applicants were white, 6.4% Asian, 6.0% African American, with the remainder distributed among other ethnic groups. Applicants that matriculated into programs in 2008 presented a 3.36 science grade-point average (GPA), 3.5 nonscience GPA, and overall GPA of 3.36. The top majors who applied to PA school cited in the CASPA 2007 report were biology, psychology, health science, exercise, nursing, medical technology, premedical, and sciences. The mean number of years of prior healthcare experience was 3.60 years; 55% of the self-reported healthcare experience is direct patient care. Applicants identified health-related work experience as the leading influence in learning about the PA profession

and for choosing to apply to the PA profession. Over 50% of applicants took either the Graduate Record Examination (53.9%) and 4.2% took the Medical College Admissions Test (McDaniel, 2008).

Selection Criteria

PA programs have varying criteria for selecting qualified students. Selection measures for predicting successful completion of PA training may include the Scholastic Aptitude Test (SAT), Minnesota Multiphasic Personality Inventory (MMPI) scores, the Graduate Record Examination (GRE), transcript grade point averages, and records of length of previous healthcare experience (depending on the program). Other criteria may include a personal essay, letters of recommendation, and an interview. How these elements are weighted in a given program depends on the mission of the PA program and factors relating to institutional preference. In one study, it was determined that test results of intellectual ability and achievement are the most efficient predictors of success in training programs. Specifically, SAT scores alone predicted excellent or poor student performance in the program. The MMPI test scores and previous healthcare experience had little or no significance in predicting success or failure in the program or on the PANCE (Oakes et al, 1999).

Selection criteria may change based on institutional funding, reputation, and state resident preferences (if the program is publicly funded). Some programs have well-defined goals, such as Christian service (e.g., Trevecca Nazarene

University, Kettering College of the Medical Arts, and Union College), a strong nursing or NP background (at one time at the University of North Dakota School of Medicine; University of California, Davis), a commitment for graduates to practice in a medically underserved area, or fluency in Spanish that factor into their decisions regarding applicants.

Course Prerequisites

Because PA program curricula vary considerably in content and structure, the sponsoring institution determines which courses are required for entry to PA education. Jones and Miller (2003) conducted a national survey in which the entrance criteria of all of the then 130 existing accredited PA educational programs were examined. In looking at PA program prerequisites, they found that the courses most commonly required were chemistry (86%), followed by physiology (83%), anatomy (72%), psychology (69%), microbiology (66%), biology, (60%), and English (51%). The authors hypothesized that an applicant would face an unattainable task if they attempted to qualify for admission to all existing PA programs. Because of the wide breadth of courses required for entry into PA programs, the authors suggested that a standardized set of prerequisite courses for applicants be developed. As PA programs converted to a master's degree, prerequisites were restructured to adjust to the new curriculum (Exhibit 4-25).

Prior Healthcare Experience

Although most programs emphasize prior health-related experience as a requirement for admission, the literature demonstrating the utility of this prerequisite is almost nonexistent. There is no indication that students need prior healthcare experience in order to succeed in PA school and practice. In fact, one examination found no association between prior healthcare experience on the academic performance, graduate skill preparation, and employer perceptions of PA graduates (Kelly, 2000). However, anecdotally, students with extensive healthcare experience are perceived as "easier" to teach by some faculty. This preference on the part of PA programs is a

reflection of the early models of PA education, which tended to be based on students possessing extensive prior healthcare experience. (Recall that throughout the 1960s and 1970s former military corpsmen and medics were viewed as the most suitable PA students.)

The requirements and acceptable definitions of "experience" vary by program. CASPA categorizes experience into "direct patient care" and "health-related" experience. Some programs require a definitive number of hours of direct patient care experience. Some schools do not recognize volunteer hours as sufficient, whereas

EXHIBIT 4-25

Prerequisites for Physician Assistant Entry to Master's Level Program

Prerequisite	Percent of Programs for Which Course Is Required	Average Semester Hours Required
Basic or inorganic chemistry	86	6.9
Physiology	77	3.7
Anatomy	74	3.7
Microbiology	70	3.7
Biology	63	7.1
Organic chemistry	52	5.0
Psychology	51	4.2
Statistics	43	3.0
Math/algebra	37	3.3
English	30	5.0
Social science	24	6.1
Biochemistry	21	3.7
Medical terminology	16	2.4
Humanities courses	16	7.6
Sociology	11	3.2
Genetics	7	3.4
Writing composition	7	3.8
Human growth/development	6	3.0
Physics	6	4.0
Art	4	3.0
U.S. History	4	4.8
Pathophysiology	3	4.8

Data from Dehn, R. (2007). 2006 national survey of PA program admission prerequisites. Journal of Physician Assistant Education, 18(1), 45–47.

other schools "strongly recommend" or simply do not require any healthcare experience at all.

Because there remains a great diversity in the type and duration of prior healthcare experience required by schools and recommended by practicing PAs, prospective students often are forced to ask themselves (and admissions committees): "Does experience really matter?" As admissions committees try to look at the "total package" in each applicant, it becomes difficult to justify how much prior healthcare experience is necessary to enter a PA program. Furthermore, because schools vary on what they consider appropriate experience, a prospective student may find himself or herself eligible for some programs but not others. Individuals accepted to PA programs in 2007–2008 had a mean undergraduate GPA of 3.4 and a mean science GPA of 3.4. The median number of prior healthcare experience expressed in total hours worked was 2,139.

A 2008 annual survey by the PAEA reported that 75% of new students responding had previously worked in a healthcare field, regardless of patient contact, with 11% having worked in health care for more than 9 years (PAEA, 2008a). In the 2007 AAPA new student survey, 31% of new student respondents had never worked in a healthcare field with direct patient-contact experience. When that number is compared with the percentage of students who reported any healthcare experience in 2007, a significant number of students start PA school with no direct patient contact experience. In previous years, students reported higher rates of patient contact experience. The number of students reporting no direct patient experience in 2003, 2002, and 2001 was 28%, 19%, and 17%, respectively. Whether this trend is a temporary fluctuation in numbers or an indication of a changing population in PA students remains to be seen.

Despite the lack of evidence correlating previous healthcare experience with success in PA education and the profession, some still feel it is important to mandate healthcare experience in new applicants. It is not unreasonable to assume that some experience in health care would help a student learn more in the limited amount of time they have as a PA student. Students with a background in health care know some of the language and culture of medicine and may have less difficulty deciphering classes and lectures. Another strong argument for the experience requirement is that it brings with it a degree of exposure to the "real world," which usually involves holding a job and possessing the sense of responsibility that comes with it (Dehn, 2002). Finally, some believe that students who enter a PA program with significant clinical experience may find it easier to get through the clinical phase of the program.

However, prerequisites that are too diverse from program to program or prerequisites that are difficult to fulfill, such as 3 to 4 years of hands-on healthcare experience, may be detrimental for the profession because such restrictions would limit potentially successful individuals from pursuing the career. Ultimately, as the profession grows, more work is needed in determining the influence and effects of previous healthcare experience on matriculating and graduating students because many inexperienced but compassionate and motivated first-career individuals make good PAs.

Of those starting PA school with experience, the average student enters school with about 3.5 years of experience (Exhibit 4-26). In 2007, new PA students reported an average of 32 months experience, down from an average of 56 months in 1992. These statistics do not differentiate between direct patient contact experience and "other" experience. Therefore, the average 32 months of experience reported by new students may be in healthcare positions requiring fairly different skill sets and experiences than those required for PAs.

Many applicants come from decidedly clinical settings, such as former emergency medical services, nursing, medical assisting, or medical laboratories. In fact, nurses, including NPs and licensed practical nurses, made up almost one-fifth of the 2002 student body. Paramedics accounted for 20% of the 2001 entry-level student body and have ranged from 10% to 15% between 1990 and 2001. Some applicants come from other branches of the medical field, such as psychology, pharmacy, or allied health disciplines (Exhibit 4-27).

Factors Influencing the Decision to Enroll in a Program

Among those accepted in a PA program, the most common factors that influenced the decision to become a PA were primarily the desire for "health-related work" and the encouragement of a "PA acquaintance" or some "other health professional." These factors account for one-half of all reasons for choosing a PA career and have important implications for recruiting additional PAs.

Once an applicant has selected or has been selected by a PA program, two of the most influential reasons for almost one-half of all decisions to enroll in a particular program are "PA program location" and "program reputation." The reputation factor is interesting because there is no consensus among applicants regarding which programs have high reputations. Once a student has selected a program or has graduated from that program, there is an inherent belief among individuals

that he or she made the correct educational institution decision.

STUDENT DEMOGRAPHIC

Demographic patterns observed among PA students for the first decade of the profession showed clear male predominance. As a result of a steady increase in the proportion of women in the PA profession since 1985, women now comprise more than 64% of all practicing PAs and an even larger percentage of PA students. An estimated 5,600 first-year students enrolled in 141 programs in 2008, and most of these students were female.

In 2008, there were approximately 5,700 available first-year PA student seats with an expected 5,300 new graduates. The average first-year enrollment was 44 students per program. Among PA students enrolled in 2008, 22% were members of racial and ethnic minorities, 72% were women, and 63% were single. Furthermore, 11% had been in the military at one time, and 76% possessed at least a bachelor's degree. The mean age of students

EXHIBIT 4-26
Trends in Healthcare Experience of Physician Assistant Enrollees, 1993–2005

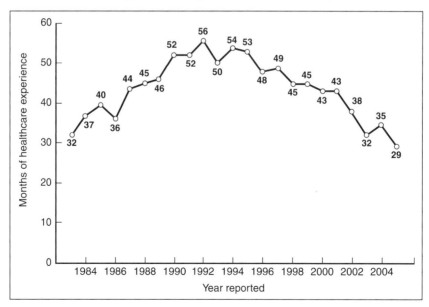

Data from Physician Assistant Education Association, 2005, Authors

at the time of enrollment in 2008 was 27 years, down from the 36-year figure observed in 1992 (Exhibit 4-28).

The mean age distribution of students for the first-year class in 2007 is shown in Exhibit 4-29. More than one-fourth of the students

EXHIBIT 4-27
Field of Prior Healthcare Occupations of Physician Assistant Program Enrollees, 2001

Healthcare Field	No.	%*
Athletic trainer	222	5
Case manager	66	2
Chiropractor	18	0
Dental assistant	68	2
Emergency room technician	396	10
Emergency medical technician/ paramedic	803	20
Healthcare administration	82	2
Health educator	222	5
Health services researcher	69	2
Home health aide	243	6
Medic/medical corpsman (military)	202	5
Medical assistant	695	17
Medical lab technician	247	6
Medical reception/records	229	6
Medical technician	155	4
Nurse practitioner	1	0
Nurse, licensed practical	82	2
Nurse, registered	208	5
Nurse, other	273	7
Nutritionist/dietitian	64	2
Operating room/ surgical technician	154	4
Occupational therapist	34	1
Optometrist	5	0
Pharmacist	44	1
Phlebotomist	420	10
Physical therapist	143	4
Physician (MD/DO)	48	1
Podiatrist	5	0
Radiology technician	114	3
Respiratory technician	90	2
Social worker	55	1
Other	1187	29

*Respondents were permitted to indicate multiple fields, so the sum of all fields exceeds 100%.

Data from the American Academy of Physician Assistants. (2001). 2001 survey of new enrollees in physician assistant programs. Retrieved July 31, 2008, from http://www.aapa.org/research/enrollees01/index.html.

EXHIBIT 4-28
Characteristics of Physician Assistant Students by Year Entering Education

	1995	2000	2007
Respondents			4,893
Average age	30.4	28.6	26.4
Women (%)	61	65	72
Non-white/non-Caucasian (%)	22	19	22
Married/single/other (%)	43/54/3	35/63/2	29/68/2
Ever in military* (%)	12	11	8
Bachelor's degree or higher (%)	61	73	81
ORIGINS OF RESIDENCE OF NEW PA STUDENTS			
Inner city	—	15	15
Urban	—	35	37
Suburban	—	62	63
Rural	—	42	40
Indian reservation	—	1	1
Other	—	2	2
NEW PA STUDENTS			
No. of students†	—	40	40
Knew a PA before applying	79	90	90
College grade point average (mean)	3.41	3.44	3.43
Average no. of programs applied to	2.4	2.4	1.2
No. of programs accepted to	1.2	1.4	1.6
Worked in a healthcare field (%)	85	86	73

*Active duty, Reserves/National Guard/Veteran.
†Full time and part time.

Data from American Academy of Physician Assistants. (2007). Regional Report of the 2006 Student Census Survey. Alexandria, VA: Author.

enrolled in the first-year class were older than age 30; more than one-half were between the ages of 20 and 26, and 2% were younger than age 20.

By 2008, the average size of the entering PA class was 44 students, 72% of whom were women. The senior class averaged 40 students per program with 9% of the maximum capacity of the class unfilled (due largely to attrition from the program). Using the mean values of the responding programs, the total enrollment (all classes) across 141 programs was estimated

EXHIBIT 4-29
Enrollees by Age Distribution, 2007

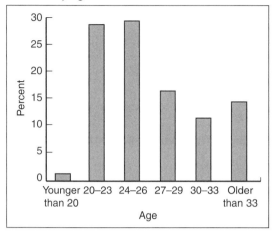

Data from Physician Assistant Education Association, 2007, Authors.

to be 10,267. The estimated first-year enrollment was 5,306 students with less than 2% enrolled as part-time students. The Eastern region had the largest number of students enrolled (46.5/program). Programs in the Midwestern region had the fewest number of students enrolled (36.4/program). The typical entering student was described as a white/non-Hispanic female, 27 years of age, with a grade point average of 3.4 and 29 months of healthcare experience prior to admission. The proportion of minority students enrolled in the first-year class has increased from 13.8% in 1983–1984 to 22.8% in 2008 (PAEA, 2008a).

Diversity of Student Population

The expansion of ethnic and racial minorities in PA educational programs since 1970 reflects social progress in shaping the healthcare professions to look more like the population at large. Percentages of minorities enrolled in PA educational programs from 1983 through 2001 averaged 18.3% per enrolled class; that is, the number of minority students doubled from a mean of four students per program in 1983 to more than nine per program in 2008.

Two of the accredited PA educational programs, the Howard University PA Program and the PA Program at the University of Maryland, Eastern Shore, are set within a historically and predominantly black college or university. Programs at Drew University and Harlem Hospital/City University of New York enroll higher numbers of individuals who are racial or ethnic minorities than other programs.

Amid trends for students to come from smaller towns and have more academic preparation, student backgrounds are more diverse than ever before. Most students possessed substantial previous healthcare experience—a mean of 43 months in the class beginning in 2001 (PAEA, 2007). About 10% of all individuals admitted to PA educational programs held a graduate degree (master's or doctoral degree) in 2007; 18 individuals were unlicensed graduates of international medical schools.

Attrition

Attrition from PA programs is typically low. In 2008, the mean percentage of enrolled students who were decelerated was 2.7% and the mean percentage withdrawn or dismissed was 2.6% (PAEA, 2008a). Overall, attrition among PA students is disproportionate for racial and ethnic minority individuals (Carter, 2000; Whitman, 2000). The overall attrition rate for PA students was 4.2% in 2008; the percentage withdrawn was 7.3% and decelerated was 5.1% among non-whites (PAEA, 2008a). Underrepresented racial and ethnic minority persons, in particular African American women, were more likely than nonminority individuals either to be lost to attrition or to be assigned to decelerated tracks in PA programs (Whitman, 2000).

International Medical Graduates

International medical graduates (IMGs) are doctors who have been to medical school outside of the United States. Some IMGs are U.S. citizens who were simply not educated in the United States, whereas others are not U.S. citizens. Historically, the relationship between IMGs and PAs has had its share of controversy in regards to IMGs attempting to become PAs. Concern arose over IMGs attempting to obtain advanced placement in

PA programs and shortcut their way through the codified steps to PA licensure. Additional controversy resulted when some states funded "fast-track" to recruit IMGs into PA programs. In fact, IMGs constitute between 23% and 28% of physicians in the United States, the United Kingdom, Canada, and Australia. Low-income countries supply between 40% and 75% of these IMGs (Mullan, 2005).

Despite such controversy, IMGs have a presence in PA education, including in programs outside of the United States. Canada, in its effort to build its PA profession, is recruiting IMGs for PA education (Magnus, 2007). Additionally, Medex Northwest, the University of Washington's PA Program, has trained 30 IMGs since 1980. The success of this venture is in contrast to other PA programs, some of who do not accept IMGs. One reason for its success is that Medex prides itself on a rigorous selection process that includes three group interviews for each candidate as well as writing samples, student interactions, and orientation content. More than 50 IMG candidates for Medex Northwest were screened. Reasons for not selecting a candidate included language issues, incomplete knowledge of the PA role, interviewer concerns about potential dissatisfaction with the PA role, and/or general communication concerns.

The academic performance of Medex IMGs created few issues during the didactic phase of the Medex program. These students tended to be "average" students academically. Some IMGs had communication difficulties or role socialization and transition concerns; some had issues regarding a lack of assertiveness and discomfort dealing with crisis. The Medex clinical training model, however, includes close monitoring of student performance and frequent clinical site visits. This ongoing evaluation allows faculty observation of the IMGs and how they adapt as PA students. The IMGs—many of whom had been working as translators or lower level health workers in the United States—generally made an easy transition to the clinical phase of training. Most expressed gratitude to be back in significant clinical roles. All graduated "on time" and none were required to repeat any clinical rotations.

All Medex IMG PAs have passed the national PANCE on the first try. Ballweg and colleagues believe that IMGs not eligible for medical licensure in the United States and Canada may be an overlooked applicant pool for PA education and deployment. Application screening may be the best criteria for successful matriculation (Ballweg, 2008). Other PA programs that have had a long and positive experience in training IMGs to become PAs include the Essex/Towson University PA program in Baltimore.

Predicting Success as a Physician Assistant Graduate

Without a definition regarding what constitutes an "effective PA," educators have turned to the only quantifiable indicator: the PANCE. Researchers have studied predictors of success in education programs to validate and improve admission requirements and course curricula. Oakes and colleagues (1999) examined the predictive value of the PANCE among a small sample of 88 PA students and found little to predict in terms of demographics. McDowell, Clemens, and Frosch (1999) examined the PANCE scores of 38 programs in the early 1990s and found master's-prepared PAs had higher average percent pass rates on the PANCE and higher average core scores than bachelor's-level program graduates. Programs with long accreditation status were found to perform significantly better on the clinical skills portion of the PANCE than those with less-established accreditation. Similarly, Asprey and colleagues (2004) found that master's-prepared PA graduates performed better on the PANCE examination than non-master's-prepared graduates.

Hooker, Cipher, and Hess (2002) examined 18,000 test takers and found that master's-prepared graduates did slightly better on the PANCE than bachelor's-level graduates. Program characteristics, such as tuition, length of program, public versus private, medical school affiliation, and region of the country made no difference in PANCE scores. Neither did the size of class, age, or gender of the student. The authors concluded that in this sample there was very little quantitative difference to predict who will pass and who will fail the PANCE in relation to an academic degree.

FACULTY

A mixture of healthcare professionals and professional educators are used within PA education programs. These educators include physicians and PAs (both master's- and doctoral-level instructors) with backgrounds in the basic medical sciences, the behavioral and social sciences, and various other disciplines. In 2008, approximately 450 PAs and 300 non-PAs were employed in U.S. PA programs nationwide.

The professional faculty of a PA program typically consists of a full-time program director (usually a PA who holds a master's or doctorate degree), a medical director (usually a physician serving part time), and an average of 4.3 FTE personnel serving in various PA faculty instructional roles (Exhibit 4-30). The total number of employees per program ranges from 3 to 13, with an average of one employee for every 7.7 students enrolled. This ratio has been stable since the mid-1990s (Whitman, 2000).

In 2008, the average annual income for PA academicians was $79,685 (as compared with the average annual income of $86,204 for practicing PAs). Whereas females fill the majority of PA program faculty positions, males hold the majority (60%) of program leadership positions, such as the role of program director. In addition, male PA faculty members earn on average around $8,000 per annum more than female faculty members (PAEA, 2008a).

Like other relative newcomers in health professions education, PA educational programs have experienced difficulty in identifying, recruiting, and retaining qualified faculty members. The combination of an increasing number of applicants and a growing demand for PA services has resulted in an "academic hourglass" effect. There is a bottleneck in processing PA students because there are not enough programs to train them. This is further complicated by an existing shortage of qualified educators.

Advancement and Tenure

Traditional criteria for promotion and tenure tend to present difficulties for PA faculty because faculty members are responsible for the academic administration of programs. Typically, administrative accomplishment is a minimal consideration in promotion and tenure decisions that usually reflect a "publish or perish" academic attitude. On the other hand, PA program faculty, given a finite timeframe and limited faculty resources, tend to believe that the successful implementation of academic programs and production of competent graduates takes precedence over research and publications. Alternative definitions of scholarship have been developed by higher

EXHIBIT 4-30
Typical Physician Assistant Program Faculty Roles and Salaries Based on 40 Students per Year, 2008

Title	Rank	Full-Time Equivalent (FTE)	Annual FTE Salary ($)	Budget Salary	Salary Range ($)
Program Director	Professor	1.0	101,246	101,246	70,120–187,000
Academic Coordinator	Associate Professor	1.0	87,000	87,000	NA
Clinical Coordinator/Instructor	Assistant Professor	2.8	75,820	212,296	NA
Associate/Assistant Director	Associate Professor	1.0	80,000	80,000	NA
Medical Director	Associate Professor	0.3	135,000	40,500	4,500–300,000
Office Manager		1.0	40,680	40,680	NA
Secretary/Receptionist		1.4	36,000	50,400	NA
TOTAL		8.5		612,122	

education and need to be used by institutions to broaden their criteria for consideration in faculty promotion and tenure decisions affecting health professions faculty (Boyer, 1990; Nora et al, 2000; Beattie, 2000).

Trends of PA program faculty in tenure-track positions or holding tenure over the past 5 years are shown in Exhibit 4-31. Despite the growth of PA educational programs and student numbers during this timeframe, the percentages of faculty either in tenure-accruing positions or tenured has declined. Nationally, about one-third of all college and university faculty members are tenured. In PA education, the mean jumped from approximately 5% early in the century to 10% tenure by 2008.

Less than 3% of all PA faculty members had earned the rank of professor. Around 10% earned the rank of associate professor, whereas 87% were classified as either assistant professors or instructors (Exhibit 4-32). The composition of PA faculty remains largely at the junior level in most sponsoring institutions. In 2008, only one-quarter of PA faculty members were in tenure-stream positions and 6.5% held tenure. Among the senior ranks, less than 15% held the rank of associate professor and 2% held the rank of professor.

The proportion of PA faculty in the senior ranks (associate professor or professor) and those in relatively secure types of positions (tenure and long-term [3 to 5 year] contracts) is lower than comparable programs in disciplines such as nursing and physical therapy. Although PA education in America is a relatively young enterprise, it seems that more faculty members should have risen into the higher academic ranks and attained tenured status. One reason for why these percentages are so low is that PA education has evolved on

EXHIBIT 4-32

Academic Rank of U.S. Physician Assistant Faculty, 2002–2006

Academic Rank	2002 (N = 403)		2006 (N = 455)	
	No.	%	No.	%
Full professor	8	2.0	11	2.4
Associate professor	41	10.2	55	12.1
Assistant professor	208	51.6	265	58.2
Instructor/lecture	146	36.2	124	27.3
Tenure track				24.8
Hold tenure				3.7

Data compiled from Physician Assistant Education Association's Annual Reports of PA Educational Programs in the United States, 2002–2006.

the competency-based educational model and has avoided dependence on academic degrees to define its identity. Faculty in many institutions has been hired primarily as teachers and administrators and often has not been required to publish as readily as their peers in other departments. Whereas this trend has been a positive one in many instances, it may not be the model for the future, particularly if PA education hopes to become more permanently established in academe.

Some programs are debating the pros and cons of tenure and considering whether alternatives exist. This debate is especially a concern for institutions with new PA programs. An advantage of establishing tenure is that it provides a sense of a major achievement in the life of an academic and reflects a high level of recognition by one's peers and the institution, suggesting that one has advanced in the field by dint of his or her scholarly contributions. Tenure also provides a level of permanence within the institution for the faculty member

EXHIBIT 4-31

Percentage of Faculty in Physician Assistant Educational Programs Tenured or in Tenure Track Positions, 2003–2007

	2003 (N = 421)	2004 (N = 461)	2005 (N = 535)	2006 (N = 484)	2007 (N = 476)
Tenure	32 (7.3%)	24 (5.3%)	23 (4.3%)	18 (3.7%)	25 (5.3%)
Tenure track	117 (26.6%)	102 (22.3%)	143 (26.7%)	120 (24.8%)	112 (23.5%)

Data compiled from Physician Assistant Education Association's Annual Reports of PA Educational Programs in the United States, 2003–2008.

and his or her discipline; that is, the faculty member's position is something that cannot easily be done away with if political winds shift and deans get antsy about admission numbers or other factors. For example, if applications to programs decrease or if demand for graduates diminishes, PA programs and their faculty would be placed into a more risky environment in the competitive world of academe. Faced with falling enrollment, some institutions may waiver in their commitment to PA program sponsorship and, unless faculty have the protection of tenure and seniority, it could be too easy for such institutions to cut faculty or eliminate programs.

The major disadvantage of establishing a traditional tenure-granting system in the minds of most people is the burden on faculty in terms of scholarly productivity. PA faculty tend to be stretched thin in terms of teaching workload and tend not to have the doctoral preparation that gives them the tools to conduct original research and/or similar forms of scholarship. Most PA faculty come from a background as a clinician and may not have sufficient background preparation to successfully meet the traditional requirements for tenure (excellence in at least two of the three key areas—teaching, scholarship, and professional service—and to do so in 6 or so years).

One alternative to traditional tenure is the semi-tenure system introduced by some institutions. Semi-tenure is essentially a modernized version of tenure in which the institution provides long-term contracts (3 to 5 years). This approach gives deans an opportunity to cancel contract renewals to make way for more productive newcomers.

Attrition

Attrition is the reduction of a workforce due to members leaving an agency or institution. According to annual surveys conducted by the PAEA, faculty attrition rates in PA programs have averaged roughly 11% per program per year over the past 10 years, and 12% for the 2006–2007 academic year (Exhibit 4-33). Over the 20-year period examined by the PAEA, respondents reported that 1,387 personnel left their positions. The overall 20-year mean is 69.3 personnel departing per year; an average of 0.9 persons departing/program per annum.

In the 2003–2004 academic year the three predominant reasons for personnel leaving their academic positions were (1) career advancement, (2) return to clinical practice, and (3) geographic relocation, representing 22%, 18%, and 16% of the exiting personnel, respectively. Job dissatisfaction and salary dissatisfaction accounted for less than 5% of the reasons. Other reasons were retirement (7%), returning to school (4%), and family obligations (3%). A fairly large category (17%) was "other," which reportedly included such factors as resignation and military service. Of some interest is that most program personnel did not report salary dissatisfaction as a reason for leaving in 2003 (Reed, 2006).

EXHIBIT 4-33
Program Personnel Turnover, 1986–2005

Academic Year	Total Number Departing	Mean/ Program
1986–1987	13	0.3
1987–1988	16	0.3
1988–1989	30	0.6
1989–1990	45	0.9
1990–1991	58	1.2
1991–1992	45	0.8
1992–1993	42	0.8
1993–1994	53	0.9
1994–1995	65	0.9
1995–1996	57	0.7
1996–1997	92	1.0
1997–1998	83	0.9
1998–1999	74	0.7
1999–2000	101	1.1
2000–2001	105	1.1
2001–2002	92	0.9
2002–2003	108	1.0
2003–2004	92	0.8
2004–2005	112	1.1
2005–2006	103	1.5
20-year mean	69.3	0.9

Data from Physician Assistant Education Association, 2007, Authors.

Faculty Evolution

The directors and faculty of early PA programs were typically physicians. As programs evolved, more PAs, as well as a wide variety of professional educators and other healthcare professionals, were employed in PA educational programs. In the 1980s, because more PAs were trained and became interested in entering faculty positions, the number of PAs assuming positions as program directors increased, as did the number of PAs in various faculty roles. This new wave of PA faculty was typified by individuals who were trained as clinicians and who held clinical positions for some time prior to entering education. These educators were part of the pioneering spirit of that generation of PAs, commonly being the first PAs to work in a particular town, county, hospital, or practice. According to one observer "they were creative, determined people with an overwhelming sense of ownership of the PA profession . . . who brought these values and energies to PA education" (Hammond, 2003). As a result, PA education changed in a number of ways. For example, because these educators were more clinically oriented, their teaching styles tended to reflect this orientation and tended to bring a student-centered focus to PA education.

Program Directors

The role of the PA program director has expanded dramatically in scope and qualifications over the past two decades. Program directors administer academic units with an annual budget averaging $986,987, teach and evaluate an average of 44 students per program per year, and supervise an average of 10.1 faculty and 2.5 administrative staff. Once a position that was open to and held by various types of healthcare professionals, PA program directors should now be certified PAs or physicians; others may still assume the role but institutions must provide the ARC-PA with justification for such appointments.

In comparing the 2008 with the 2004 PAEA annual survey data, the proportion of program directors credentialed as PAs remained static (88%), salaries increased by 6%, and the number of months spent in the position decreased from 81 to 77 months. The majority of program (94%) and medical (92%) directors were classified as faculty and were on a tenure track. Less than one-fifth were tenured. Fourteen percent of the program directors had doctoral-level degrees (typically the PhD or EdD). Since 1984 there has been a 159% increase in mean salary for program directors.

The role of the PA program director has evolved and become more complex. Directors are essentially academic unit administrators who are responsible for setting and maintaining the mission and goals of the program, supervising and evaluating the faculty, selecting qualified students, supervising administrative staff, attaining and maintaining compliance with accreditation criteria, managing the budget, relating to senior institutional administration, and promoting the program and the PA profession within and external to the institution.

Medical Directors

The role of the PA program medical director has consolidated over the years. Once a central member of the program faculty, medical directors now usually serve on a part-time basis (0.2 to 0.5 FTE). A survey found that 50% of medical directors have a time commitment of less than 15%, and one-sixth have a time commitment of more than 50%; 100% participated in curriculum planning and committee function, most notably the admissions committee; 100% participate in direct student instruction. Rarely do medical directors mentor students or faculty or participate in or guide research projects (Green, 2000).

GRADUATES

One of the useful ways of examining outcomes of the PA education process over time is to note changes and trends. The *Annual Report on Physician Assistant Education* conducted by the PAEA describes the graduating cohort and contains the reported level of employment as well as unemployment (defined as the number of graduates still looking for a job as a PA at the time of the survey). Because each survey is performed at the same time of year, this measurement is useful in tracking year-to-year changes.

Employment

In the decade covered by the sixth through the 24th annual reports, unemployment in PA graduating classes averaged 4.0%. The lowest rate of 2.3% was reported for the graduating class of 2006, and the highest was for the class of 1992 at 5% (Exhibit 4-34). Anecdotally, it is widely known that the demand for newly-minted PAs is strong with far more jobs available to graduating PA students than can be filled.

Starting Salary

The average starting salary for new graduates increased from $31,352 in 1989 to $68,757 in 2001 to $74,353 in 2008. An increase occurred every year from 1989 to 2002, and the average annual increase was 7.6% over the past decade. The highest annual increase was from 1989 to 1990 (14.4%), and the smallest from 1997 to 1998 (1.2%).

Exhibit 4-35 shows the estimated starting salary of recent graduates in 2006 by region. The overall average was $68,886, an increase of 5.0% from the 2005 average of $65,595. Mean salaries were above $65,000 for graduates from programs located in all but the Eastern region. Data from the 24th annual survey where programs provided data on graduate starting salary shows that the mean was $74,154 with a range of $63,000 to $95,000 per year (PAEA, 2008c).

Minority Graduates

The graduation of minority PAs has been one of the distinguishing characteristics of PA programs from other healthcare occupations in the United States. The graduation rate of

EXHIBIT 4-34
Employment of Recent Graduates in Primary and Nonprimary Care Medicine, 1985–2006

Academic Year	Primary Care		Nonprimary Care		Total (N)
	N	%	N	%	
1985–1986	399	59.9	278	41.1	677
1986–1987	404	55.6	322	444	726
1987–1988	418	56.4	323	43.6	741
1988–1989	422	52.2	387	47.8	809
1989–1990	398	48.2	427	51.8	825
1990–1991	508	58.1	367	41.9	875
1991–1992	511	53.5	444	46.5	955
1992–1993	674	55.7	537	44.3	1,211
1993–1994	826	58.0	597	42.0	1,423
1994–1995	852	55.5	684	44.5	1,536
1995–1996	817	52.2	702	44.8	1,566
1996–1997	970	62.3	588	37.7	1,558
1997–1998	1046	56.9	792	43.1	1,838
1998–1999	1113	54.5	928	45.5	2,041
1999–2000	1176	53.7	1,015	46.3	2,191
2000–2001	1143	53.9	977	46.1	2,120
2001–2002	1014	46.5	1,166	53.5	2,180
2002–2003	964	49.0	1,003	51.0	1,967
2003–2004	623	33.7	1,228	66.3	1,851
2004–2005	837	38.3	1,346	61.7	2,183
2005–2006	660	35.2	1,214	64.8	1,874
2006–2007	604	37.5	1,008	62.5	1,612
22-year mean	745	51.3	737	48.6	1,483

Data from American Academy of Physician Assistants, 2008, Authors.

EXHIBIT 4-35
Program Directors' Reports of Starting Salaries for Physician Assistant Graduates by Region

Consortia Region	N	Mean	Median	Change From 2005
Northeastern	13	$70,519	$71,452	5.9%
Eastern	5	$63,633	$64,000	6.4%
Southeastern	8	$70,638	$72,700	6.0%
Midwestern	10	$66,620	$66,000	2.0%
Heartland	6	$72,500	$71,000	6.5%
Western	12	$68,219	$68,000	3.4%
TOTAL	54	$68,886	$69,150	5.0%

Data from Physician Assistant Education Association. (2008c). Twenty-Fourth Annual Report on Physician Assistant Educational Programs in the United States, 2007–2008. Alexandria, VA: Author.

EXHIBIT 4-36
Percent of Minority Graduates by Year, 1984–2007

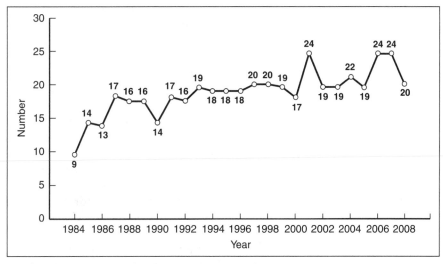

Data from Physician Assistant Education Association, 2008, Authors.

minority students has increased from 9% in 1984 to 24% in 2007 (Exhibit 4-36). The average for the past two decades has been 21%. In 2007, 4.7% of graduates were African American, 6.5% were Hispanic, 7.8% were Asian, and 8.1% were identified as "other."

Research and Physician Assistant Education

In spite of 40 years of experience, the literature about the education of PAs is limited (Lane & Jones, 2009). Following is a list of research areas in need of attention.

■ **Case reports:** Writing about the development of a program from its initial conception and development to the first class can provide insight into policy development and educational start-up costs. Case reports can show how a program is structured in an institution and the organizational roles for each educator.

■ **Role delineation:** What is the role of the educator in a PA educational setting? What percent of PA educators work clinically? Are there lines of demarcation between the academic coordinator and the clinical coordinator? Does size of program matter in the educational load of a PA academic? Are increasing numbers of PA faculty attaining doctoral degrees?

- **Organizational arrangements:** What are the lines of influence and organization for a PA program in a host institution? What is the optimal academic unit (school, department, division, program) for a PA program within an educational institution? Does the degree of separation from the president of the university to the PA director have any influence on how the program functions?

- **Breadth of knowledge:** How many diagnoses should a PA know by the time he or she graduates? What measures do PA programs apply to ensure that graduates are attaining minimal levels of competence?

- **Comparing programs:** What can a student expect that distinguishes a PA program in a university from a community college? What distinguishes a public versus a private university or a school of allied health versus a medical school?

- **Quality of care:** How do programs know that the students they are graduating are prepared to deliver adequate quality of care ?

- **Outcomes:** What does PA education produce that predicts outcomes of care?

- **Retention:** What are the social and economic factors that contribute retention or attrition of PA faculty? Is the turnover of PA program directors excessive?

- **Education:** What are the education strategies that can contribute to successful deployment of PAs to rural settings?

- **Global comparisons:** How does PA education differ by country?

SUMMARY

PA education entered its fifth decade in 2006. It was created by several visionaries in U.S. academic medicine and then grew and developed through the coordinated efforts of organized medicine, educational institutions, and federal support. During this process of maturation, education transitioned from a set of vaguely structured, disparate, fledgling efforts to well-established, progressive, and flourishing academic programs. While most PA programs are anchored in academic health centers and other health-related institutions of higher learning across the country, the movement contains a wide diversity of types of educational institutions. Overall, PA development has been characterized as a great experiment in medical education. In its short history it lays claim to a string of medical curricular innovations and provider deployment success. Nowhere is this more apparent than in primary care. PA educational programs have developed a well-respected system of accreditation and have been a prominent and long-term fixture in federal legislative primary care training initiatives.

Two of the most dominant trends in PA education are the marked expansion of the numbers of programs since the 1990s, as well as graduates' recent resolution of the issue of the academic credential awarded on completion of PA studies. Yet despite these achievements and the significant recognition of the PA profession evident in U.S. medical education, there remain a number of challenges facing programs and sponsoring institutions. The constantly changing forces in the U.S. healthcare delivery system and in educational institutions have brought some of these challenges.

The growth and acceptance of the PA concept and education domestically and globally in the last several decades has been nothing short of amazing. For the most part, these U.S. programs are relatively homogenized in that they all meet the proscribed *Standards* for accreditation but at the same time retain their original values, innovations, and unique characteristics. Finally, these programs have been shown to be socially responsive and to do a better job of meeting workforce demands than many other health profession programs.

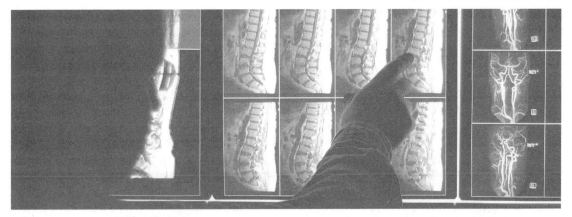

CHAPTER 5

POSTGRADUATE PHYSICIAN ASSISTANT EDUCATION PROGRAMS

DAVID P. ASPREY ▪ JAMES F. CAWLEY ▪ RODERICK S. HOOKER

Experience teaches only the teachable.
                                        —Aldous Huxley

ABSTRACT

Postgraduate residency education for physician assistants (PAs) developed in response to a perceived need for instruction beyond the entry-level programs, increased specialty training, and labor shortages in hospitals. Trainees of postgraduate programs perform medical tasks at a level comparable to a physician resident and may provide some economic benefit to the healthcare system. However, postgraduate residency training programs face substantial challenges. These include lack of documented value, standardized curricula, or chronicled outcomes through research. On the other hand legitimacy of postgraduate education is a voluntary accreditation process. Generally, PA residents report substantial gains in their knowledge and skills during their training, including improvements in their abilities to establish a diagnosis; to recognize disease and pathology; to think critically; and to develop a differential diagnosis. Educators, policymakers, employers, and members of the profession have relatively little systematic information which to formulate

opinions and make judgments about the value of PA postgraduate education programs, but these programs are established and expected to grow.

INTRODUCTION

The physician assistant (PA) has educational requirements that begin immediately upon graduation from the entry-level program. Such education ranges from formal courses of concentration to on-the-job training. For most it is a lifelong learning process. Postgraduate education, commonly referred to as PA residency programs, is an advanced training process available to some PAs and has steadily grown since the new millennium. It is an additional period of training in a formal setting with a concentration in a medical or surgical discipline.

Postgraduate education for PAs has been in existence since 1971 (Rosen, 1986). Such programs developed in response to a perceived need for education beyond the entry level and increased specialty training (Anonymous,

2000; Jameson, 2000). Such programs also developed in response to perceived needs for standardization of education beyond the entry level (Stanhope, 1991; Timmer, 1991). Graduates of postgraduate education programs are skilled clinicians capable of performing medical tasks at a level comparable to a physician resident at the same time providing some economic benefit to the healthcare system (Reynolds & Bricker, 2007).

Although PA residency programs have been in existence for more than three decades, they have yet to establish themselves as an essential component of the profession. However, increased autonomy and specialization have resulted in a need for practical, postgraduate specialty education. The numbers of PAs seeking formal postgraduate training prior to entering the specialty of their choice, or transferring from one specialty to another is slowly increasing. If the PA profession follows the pattern of physicians and several other healthcare professions, postgraduate residency education may become an expectation for practitioners.

HISTORY OF POSTGRADUATE PROGRAMS

The first PA postgraduate program was developed in the surgery department at Montefiore Hospital in New York (in affiliation with the Albert Einstein School of Medicine) in 1971, just 6 years after the first PA program opened. At the time, Dr. Richard Rosen, a surgeon, was concerned that the large size of the surgical residency-training program was compounding the already apparent overproduction of surgeons. He believed that PAs could provide the same type of patient care as physician surgical house staff, thereby limiting the need for future surgeons in what was becoming an overcrowded field. The notion that PAs could augment house staff was quite different from the existing mainstream philosophy of how PAs were to be utilized. Rosen recruited PAs to work on inpatient units, first in surgery and later expanding into other departments. He thought that PAs ought to be used in settings where there were many physicians (e.g., in hospitals) and was convinced that PAs should be allowed to provide care that does not have to be given solely by a physician (Rosen, 1986).

This unique utilization of PAs led to other postgraduate residency programs. The Norwalk Hospital, affiliated with the Yale University School of Medicine program, began in 1976. A 12-month training experience was instituted, consisting of a 4-month didactic training session in the fundamentals of surgical anatomy and physiology, followed by 8 months of clinical rotations through surgical wards at Norwalk. By 1980 there were six postgraduate residency programs.

As of 2009, 16 clinical disciplines, representing primarily subspecialty areas of medicine, are represented among postgraduate programs (Exhibit 5-1). Most are located within larger teaching hospitals or clinics throughout the United States (Exhibit 5-2).

Association of Postgraduate Physician Assistant Programs

In May 1988, a group of postgraduate PA residency programs met at the American Academy of Physician Assistants (AAPA)

EXHIBIT 5-1
Types of Specialty Training Offered by Postgraduate Physician Assistant Programs, 2008

- Cardiothoracic surgery
- Critical care
- Dermatology
- Emergency medicine
- Hospitalist
- Neonatology
- Neurosurgery
- Obstetrics and gynecology
- Oncology
- Orthopedics surgery
- Psychiatry
- Rheumatology
- Sleep medicine
- Surgery
- Trauma/Critical care
- Urology

EXHIBIT 5-2
U.S. Postgraduate Residency Programs for Physician Assistants

Specialty	Location
CARDIOTHORACIC SURGERY	
The Methodist DeBakey Heart Center	Houston, Texas
St. Joseph Mercy Hospital Cardiothoracic Surgery Program	Grand Rapids, Michigan
CRITICAL CARE	
The Johns Hopkins Hospital Postgraduate Physician Assistant Critical Care Residency Program	Baltimore, Maryland
The University of Massachusetts Memorial Medical Center Physician Assistant Residency Program in Critical Care	Worcester, Massachusetts
Oregon Health and Sciences University	Portland, Oregon
DERMATOLOGY	
University of Texas Southwestern's Dermatology Physician Assistant Training Program	Dallas, Texas
EMERGENCY MEDICINE	
Albert Einstein Medical Center Physician Assistant Emergency Medicine Residency	Philadelphia, Pennsylvania
Johns Hopkins Bayview Medical Center Emergency Medicine Residency	Baltimore, Maryland
University of Iowa Emergency Medicine Physician Assistant Residency Program	Iowa City, Iowa
University of Texas Health Sciences Center San Antonio	San Antonio, Texas
U.S. Army Medical Department Emergency Medicine Physician Assistant Programs	Tacoma, Washington San Antonio, Texas
Wright Patterson Emergency Medicine Physician Assistant Fellowship	Wright-Patterson Air Force Base, Ohio
HOSPITALIST	
Alderson-Broaddus College	Philippi, West Virginia
Mayo Clinic Arizona Postgraduate PA Fellowship in Hospital Internal Medicine	Phoenix, Arizona
NEONATOLOGY	
University of Kentucky PA Residency in Neonatology	Lexington, Kentucky
NEUROSURGERY	
Geisinger Medical Center Advanced Practice Postgraduate Neuroscience Residency	Danville, Pennsylvania
University of Arizona—Tucson, Neurosurgery PA Residency	Tucson, Arizona
OBSTETRICS AND GYNECOLOGY	
Riverside-Arrowhead Regional Medical Center	Colton, California
ONCOLOGY	
M.D. Anderson Cancer Center—The University of Texas	Houston, Texas
ORTHOPEDIC SURGERY	
Arrowhead Regional Medical Center	Colton, California
Illinois Bone and Joint Institute	North Chicago, Illinois
Watuga Orthopaedics	Johnson City, Tennessee
PSYCHIATRY	
Cherokee Mental Health Institute	Cherokee, Iowa
Regions Hospital Psychiatry Fellowship for Physician Assistants and Nurse Practitioners	St. Paul, Minnesota
RHEUMATOLOGY	
University of Texas Southwestern/Dallas VA Medical Center	Dallas, Texas
SLEEP MEDICINE	
Neurology and Neuroradiology Residency Program	Bethlehem, Pennsylvania

Continued

EXHIBIT 5-2
U.S. Postgraduate Residency Programs for Physician Assistants—cont'd

Specialty	Location
SURGERY	
Alderson-Broaddus College	Philippi, West Virginia
Arrowhead Regional Medical Center—General Surgery Physician Assistant Residency	Colton, California
Bassett Healthcare	Cooperstown, New York
Duke University Medical Center	Durham, North Carolina
Geisinger Medical Center Physician Assistant Surgical Residency Program	Danville, PA
Grand Rapids PA Surgical Residency	Grand Rapids, Michigan
The Johns Hopkins Hospital Postgraduate Surgical Residency for Physician Assistants	Baltimore, Maryland
Montefiore Medical Center—University Hospital for Albert Einstein College of Medicine	Bronx, New York
The Hospital of Central Connecticut PA Residency in General Surgery	New Britain, Connecticut
Norwalk Hospital/Yale University School of Medicine (General)	New Britain, Connecticut
Mayo Clinic Arizona Postgraduate Physician Assistant Fellowship in Otolaryngology/Head and Neck Surgery	Phoenix, Arizona
Medical College of Wisconsin Post Graduate Physician Assistant Training Program	Milwaukee, Wisconsin
WakeMed Health and Hospitals Physician Assistant Residency in Trauma, Critical Care, and General Surgery	Raleigh, North Carolina
University of Texas Southwestern/Parkland Health and Hospital System Physician Assistant Residency Program in Surgery	Dallas, Texas
TRAUMA/CRITICAL CARE	
Bridgeport Hospital PA Trauma, Surgical Critical Care, and Burn Fellowship	Bridgeport, Connecticut
Pacific University Rural Trauma and Hospital Care	Hillsboro, Oregon
St. Luke's Hospital Trauma and Surgical Critical Care	Bethlehem, Pennsylvania
WakeMed Health and Hospitals Physician Assistant Residency in Trauma, Critical Care, and General Surgery	Raleigh, North Carolina
UROLOGY	
Northwest Metropolitan Urology Associates	Park Ridge, Illinois

Source: Association of Postgraduate Physician Assistant Programs.

annual meeting to formalize a national, postgraduate PA program organization. Bylaws were drafted and approved by the eight founding programs listed in Exhibit 5-3. Subsequently, the Association of Postgraduate Physician Assistant Programs (APPAP) was formed to further specialty education of PAs through advanced training.

The stated goals of the APPAP include:

- assisting in the development and organization of postgraduate educational curricula and programs for PAs;
- assisting in defining the role of the PA (with emphasis on the specialties);

- assisting in the development of evaluation methodologies for postgraduate educational curricula and programs;
- providing information about postgraduate educational curricula and programs to individual PAs, training at the entry level, other medical and healthcare disciplines, and the public.

All members of APPAP are formal postgraduate programs that offer structured curricula, including didactic and clinical components, to educate those eligible for certification by the National Commission on the Certification of Physician Assistants (NCCPA)

EXHIBIT 5-3
Founding Association of Postgraduate Physician Assistant Programs

- LAC+USC Emergency Medicine Physician Assistant Residency
- LAC+USC Physician Assistant Neonatology Residency Program
- Montefiore Postgraduate Residency in Surgery and Masters in Health Sciences
- Montefiore Residency in Gynecology for Physician Assistants and Optional Masters in Health Sciences
- Norwalk Hospital/Yale University Pediatric Physician Assistant Postgraduate Training Program
- Norwalk Hospital/Yale University School of Medicine PA Surgical Residency Program
- Sinai Hospital Postgraduate Physician Assistant Surgical Residency
- USC Physician Assistant Fellowship in Geriatric Medicine

or NCCPA-certified PAs for a defined period of time (usually 12 months) in a medical specialty. As of 2009, 16 areas of specialization are available at 45 postgraduate APPAP member programs. A number of programs are established in institutions that also conduct a physician residency program of the same specialty. APPAP member programs follow several models of training with varying titles including fellowships, master's degree programs, and residencies. All APPAP member programs award a certificate or degree.

APPAP maintains formal relationships with the AAPA, the Physician Assistant Education Association (PAEA), and the Accreditation Review Commission for Physician Assistants (ARC-PA) and works on mutual goals to further PA education. In the early years of the organization, there was no formal office location; rather the organization was maintained by the officers who served as the contacts for individuals, institutions, and organizations in need of information. In 2007, APPAP contracted with PAEA to provide administrative services to their organization. In 2008, the first programs were formally accredited by the ARC-PA.

TYPES OF RESIDENCY PROGRAMS

Asprey and Helms (1999) described postgraduate residency programs in the late 1990s and classified the programs into two types: the internship model and the academic model. The internship model involves a modest, practically oriented, didactic curriculum combined with intensive clinical rotations and educational experience. These programs tend to lead to a certificate of completion.

Academic model programs combine a highly structured and formalized didactic education (through courses taken for graduate credits) with clinical rotations, and lead to a master's degree or credit toward a master's degree upon completion. Programs following the academic model focus on skill development in clinical and nonclinical areas. Included in the curriculum are courses in advanced clinical areas/ clinical training, research methodology, interpretation of the biomedical literature, computer medicine, clinical prevention, health systems management, health policy, clinical decision sciences, and medical ethics. A research paper is sometimes required as the capstone project. Tracks for clinical, research, PA education, or health administration can be developed. Curriculum emphasizes preparation in those areas that students believe are important in expanding their professional potentials and advancement in the healthcare system.

The prototype academic model of PA postgraduate education is the master of medical science (MMS) PA program sponsored by St. Francis University in Loretto, Pennsylvania. In operation since 1993, this program uses multiple clinical and nonclinical disciplines in its 33-credit curriculum. In 1995, Alderson-Broaddus College began a postgraduate master's degree programs (emergency medicine and rural health).

In 2009, approximately 95% of the postgraduate programs awarded a certificate of completion as their credential (as compared to 82% in 1992 [Asprey & Helms, 1999]). The remaining programs awarded a master's degree. In some instances this master's degree was offered through a distance learning program, such as those at the University of Nebraska, George Washington University, the Arizona School of Health Science, and Nova Southeastern University. The declining percentage of academic model programs may be a result of the rapidly increasing number of entry-level programs that offered a master's degree coupled with the expanding number of master's completion programs for PAs who did not receive a master's degree from their entry-level PA program.

In 1999, the mean length of residency programs in existence at the time was 14 months with a range of 12 to 22 months. The average length of a PA residency program is now 12.5 months with a range from 6 to 20 months.

Despite some growth in PA residency training programs, only a small percentage of PAs have completed them. Thus, on-the-job training remains the primary means by which PAs gain the necessary knowledge and skills needed for specialty practice. Almost all PAs (98%) have entered clinical practice roles in specialty and subspecialty areas having acquired their preparation through on-the-job experiences learning from physician employers within their practice or institution.

Curriculum

Curriculum content varies based upon the credential granted upon completion of the residency (Exhibit 5-4). All residencies have a didactic component that may either occur at the beginning of the residency or is incorporated throughout the residency. The didactic element may involve formal courses or a series of lectures, conferences, grand rounds, etc. Regardless of the type of residency, the majority of the curriculum content is completed using elements of an internship model of education.

EXHIBIT 5-4
Physician Assistant Postgraduate Program Curriculum Topics

Research methods/biostatistics/epidemiology
Advanced pharmacology
Family medicine/primary care/clinical issues
Emergency medicine/clinical training experiences
Healthcare systems management
Clinical ethics/clinical decision-making
PA professional issues/PA studies/health services research
Healthcare policy/health policy analysis
Interpretation of biomedical research information
Computer applications in medicine
Medical/scientific writing/biomedical communication

The 17 programs studied in 1999 had a separate didactic curriculum component that involved classroom instruction, and formal lecture series, as part of the residency training experience. The mean number of didactic curriculum hours for all programs (as reported by residency directors) was 299 hours. For the 14 internship model programs, the mean was 249 hours of didactic instruction. The three academic programs reported a mean of 532 hours (Asprey & Helms, 1999). Exhibit 5-5 summarizes the differences identified between the two types of programs. Exhibit 5-6 shows a summary of resident activities from the perspective of program directors.

PA residents (as opposed to residency program directors) estimated the total number of hours of formal didactic curriculum included in their program to be 370 hours. Those attending an academic model residency program estimated spending an average of 414 hours in didactic curriculum. Residents attending internship model programs estimated spending 350 hours. The cohort as a whole was asked to estimate the average number of clinical hours related to patient care spent per week in their residency program. Those enrolled in academic model programs estimated spending approximately 44 hours weekly (SD = 6.5, range = 36–60) in patient care. Internship model program residents spend approximately 72 hours (SD = 28.1, range = 28–150) in clinical care per week on average. This represents an average difference of 28 additional hours per week spent in clinical care for residents enrolled in internship model programs.

Furthermore, PA postgraduate trainees were asked to estimate the average number of hours per week spent in educationally related activities related to patient care (reading texts, journals, studying). PAs in academic model programs estimated that on average they spent nearly 8 additional hours per week (average = 16 hours, SD = 14.5, range = 4–60) on educational activities when compared to the internship model residents (average = 8.4 hours, SD = 4, range = 2–20). The number of hours spent participating in research-related activities and research-related education during their program was approximately 186 additional hours of research-related education on average.

EXHIBIT 5-5
Residency Director Estimates of Total Hours of Didactic Curriculum

	Internship Programs (N = 13)	Academic Programs (N = 3)	All Programs (N = 16)
Average hours	249 hours	532 hours	299 hours
Standard deviation	187 hours	234 hours	218 hours
Range	645 (5–650) hours	445 (350–795) hours	790 (5–795) hours

Data from Asprey, D., & Helms, L. (1999). A description of physician assistant post-graduate residency training: The director's perspective. Perspectives on Physician Assistant Education, 10(3), 124–131. Reprinted with permission of the Physician Assistant Education Association.

EXHIBIT 5-6
Summary of All Resident Activities (Average Hours/Week)

Resident Educational Activity	Hours/Week	% of Total
Patient care	61.4	75.6
Educational activities related to patient care	10.7	13.2
Didactic education	7.4	9.1
Research-related educational activities	1.7	2.1
TOTAL	81.2	100

Postgraduate programs typically expose trainees to interdisciplinary roles such as PA students (74%), physician residents (63%), and medical students (54%). The least common team members included dentists (17%), nurse practitioners (17%), pharmacists (7%), physical therapists and nursing students.

Supervision

Various health professionals are responsible for supervising PA residents during their clinical work in the residency program. Most PA residents were typically supervised by staff physicians (96%) and staff PAs (56%). Other supervisors included physician residents (39%), PA residency staff (33%), and other healthcare professionals (7%) (Asprey & Helms, 2000).

Evaluation

Evaluation of the resident's performance during their residency program has also been investigated. Written and verbal evaluations of the resident's performance are the most common methods (61% and 50%, respectively,

$N = 46$). Other methods included written evaluations from PA residency staff (35%), written clinical examinations (35%), other forms of evaluation (4%), and practical clinical examination (2%) (Asprey & Helms, 2000).

Educators

Program directors of five programs estimated the percentage of teaching in the program by the faculty's position. Attending physicians were the most common faculty member to teach in the programs (46%) followed by PA house staff or residents (24%), others (17%), and resident physicians (13%).

Rheumatology Fellowship

One institution's experience in training PAs in rheumatology was quantified by logging the number of patients seen, diagnoses treated, procedures performed, and didactic courses attended. Four PA fellows over 4 years were tracked at the Department of Veterans Affairs Medical Center in Dallas, Texas. Each PA trainee had a similar profile of patients and was assigned similar clinical experiences. On average, each PA saw 476 outpatients and 56 inpatients over the 12-month period of their fellowship. Rheumatoid arthritis was the disorder seen most, followed by spondyloarthritis, other forms of connective tissue disorders, and autoimmune diseases. Seminars in immunology, clinical rheumatology, and internal medicine augmented regular clinical training (Exhibit 5-7).

While such a fellowship is intense it tends to remain true to the tradition of apprenticeship where the preceptor instructs the novice in how to approach the patient and uses the tools available for diagnosing and treating.

EXHIBIT 5-7
Summary of Rheumatology Physician Assistant Fellowship Activity, 2004–2009

	2005	2006	2007	2008	Average
Number of ambulatory patients	505	486	470	444	476
Number of inpatients	54	48	59	71	58
Number of injections	41	79	51	36	52

Data from Hooker, R. S. (2009). An Analysis of a Rheumatology Physician Assistant Fellowship. Unpublished report.

In annual surveys, the trainees and faculty viewed this particular fellowship as valuable. Administrators for Veterans Affairs viewed this as a source of additional labor providing needed access to rheumatology services. Whether the patient benefits from the exposure of a trainee was not assessed. The validity of a PA rheumatology fellowship such as this awaits validation by other agencies and in different settings.

ADMISSION TO A POSTGRADUATE PHYSICIAN ASSISTANT PROGRAM

Residency programs have varying prerequisites when selecting candidates who are appropriate for their program. All programs require an individual to be a graduate of an accredited PA program. Other prerequisites may include current NCCPA certification or eligibility. Exhibit 5-8 presents a summary of

EXHIBIT 5-8
Summary of Residency Program Prerequisites (*N* = 16)

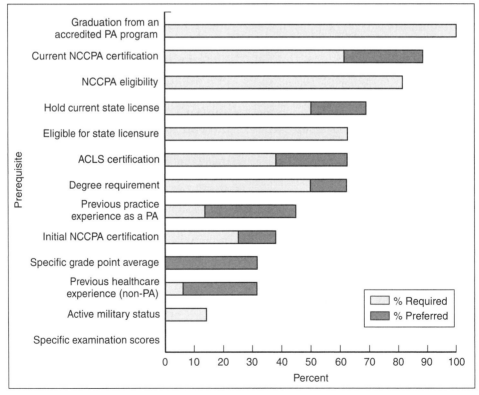

Data from Asprey, D., & Helms, L. (1999). A description of physician assistant post-graduate residency training: The director's perspective. Perspectives on Physician Assistant Education, 10(3), 124–131.

EXHIBIT 5-9
Physician Assistant Residency Program Admission Factors

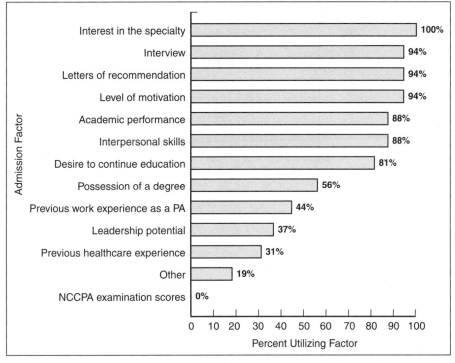

Data from Asprey, D., & Helms, L. (1999). A description of physician assistant post-graduate residency training: The director's perspective. Perspectives on Physician Assistant Education, 10(3), 124–131.

program expectations in terms of required or preferred prerequisites (Asprey & Helms, 1999). Exhibit 5-9 shows factors reported by program directors that influence admission to a postgraduate program.

Number of Applicants

The competition for admission to residency programs varies widely. Programs may experience applicant to enrollee ratios in excess of 10:1 (Asprey & Helms, 1999). Class sizes vary up to 18. Exhibit 5-10 displays the average number of applications received per residency program between 1971 and 1998. A maximum of 93 applications per year was reached in 1978 with a 28-year average of 30 applications per residency program. The average number of applications received was at or above the 28-year average from 1977 through 1990. These admission data have not been reported for the years after 1998.

PA POSTGRADUATE PROGRAM AWARENESS AND SELECTION

Studies have found that the majority (89%) of entry-level PA students are aware of the existence of postgraduate residency programs (Fishfader, Henning, & Knott, 2002). Residents become aware of such programs through a number of sources, including entry-level PA programs (the most common source), friends and colleagues, and advertisements (Asprey & Helms, 1999).

Factors influencing an individual's decision to attend a PA residency include the ability to compete for a job in a particular specialty, interest in clinical knowledge and skills prior to working as a PA, and improved future earning potential (Exhibit 5-11). Several factors influence a prospective resident's decision to attend a specific program (Exhibit 5-12). Program reputation and curriculum were the most commonly

EXHIBIT 5-10
Average Number of Applications per Year

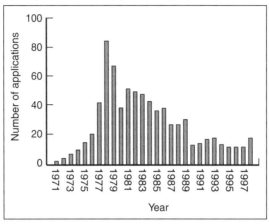

Data from Asprey, D., & Helms, L. (1999). A description of physician
assistant post-graduate residency training: The director's
perspective. Perspectives on Physician Assistant Education, 10(3),
124–131. Reprinted with permission of the Physician Assistant
Education Association.

EXHIBIT 5-11
Items Influencing the Decision to Attend a Residency

Item	Frequency of Selection (N = 46)	Percent	Rank Order
Increased ability to compete for a job in a particular specialty	41	89	1
Interest in additional clinical knowledge and skills prior to going into practice as a PA	39	85	2
Improved future earning potential	37	80	3
Current level of competency in this specialty area	34	74	4
Provides flexibility to change specialty area practiced	28	61	5
Obtaining an advanced degree	28	61	5
Other	4	9	7

Data from Asprey, D., & Helms, L. (2000). A description of physician assistant post-graduate residency training: The resident's perspective.
Perspectives on Physician Assistant Education, 11(2), 79–86. Reprinted with permission of the Physician Assistant Education Association.

reported items. Salary stipend, the benefits package, and other were the only categories identified by less than 50% of residents.

PROGRAM FINANCIAL RESOURCES

Approximately one-half of postgraduate PA programs (56%) reported a single funding source; 38% relied on two sources. A specific line item budget was the most commonly reported funding source (Exhibit 5-13). Direct and indirect billing for the resident's services were infrequently cited. The mean annual budget for the residency programs was $300,437 (SD = $237,872, range = $76,000–$793,809). The average budget of the eight internship model programs that provided total annual budget data was $375,488 (SD = $239,000, range = $90,000–$793,800) (Asprey & Helms, 1999).

EXHIBIT 5-12
Items Influencing Resident Decision to Attend Their Residency

Item	Frequency of Selection (N = 46)	Percent	Rank Order
Program reputation	36	78.3	1
Didactic component of curriculum	36	78.3	1
Practical clinical education component	31	67.4	3
Geographic location	30	65.2	4
Recommendation from colleague or friend	26	56.5	5
Degree or degree option offered	25	54.3	6
Recommendation from PA program faculty member	24	52.2	7
Impression obtained during application/interview process	24	52.2	7
Salary stipend	20	43.5	9
Benefits package	15	32.6	10
Other	9	19.6	11

*Data from Asprey, D., & Helms, L. (2000). A description of physician assistant post-graduate residency training: The resident's perspective.
Perspectives on Physician Assistant Education, 11(2), 79–86. Reprinted with permission of the Physician Assistant Education Association.*

EXHIBIT 5-13
Physician Assistant Residency Program Financial Resources

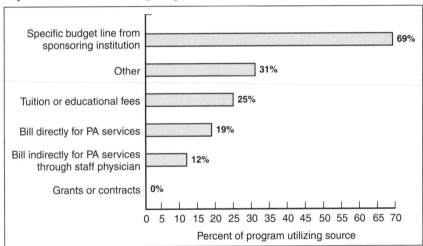

*Data from Asprey, D., & Helms, L. (1999). A description of physician assistant post-graduate residency
training: The director's perspective. Perspectives on Physician Assistant Education, 10(3), 124–131.*

PROFILE OF POSTGRADUATE PA PROGRAM RESIDENTS

The 1996 AAPA census data indicated of the 13,256 respondents, 708 or 5% of the PAs report having attended a PA postgraduate residency program. Exhibit 5-14 identifies the specialty of the residency attended by the 708 PAs who completed the AAPA 1996 Census.

The only study of demographic characteristics of enrolled residents was in 1999. Gender was evenly divided. Residents were predominantly white (86%) with African American (14%) comprising the rest. The mean age was 34 years. Thirty-seven (82%) of the residents (N = 45) reported an average of 57 months (SD = 58.7, range 6–240) of healthcare experience prior to their entry-level PA training.

However, many PA residents enter the residency without having worked as a PA; two-thirds (61%) of respondents had no practice experience compared with 39% of the residents who reported having practiced as a PA prior to entering residency. Residents with PA experience had an average of 51 months (SD = 60.7, range = 1–209) in practice. Of those with prior experience, nearly two-thirds of the respondents were practicing the specialty of family medicine immediately prior to entering the residency program (Exhibit 5-15).

EXHIBIT 5-14
Physician Assistant Postgraduate Residency Attendees (N = 708)

Specialty of Residency Attended	Total	% of Total
Anesthesiology	3	0.4%
Emergency medicine	158	22.3%
Geriatrics	9	1.3%
Gynecology	15	2.1%
Neonatology	16	2.3%
Occupational health	26	3.7%
Pediatrics	27	3.8%
Rural primary care	22	3.1%
Surgery	325	45.9%
Other	107	15.1%
TOTAL	708	100%

Data from American Academy of Physician Assistants. (1996). 1996 AAPA Census Report. Alexandria, VA: Author.

EXHIBIT 5-15
Specialty Practiced as a Physician Assistant Prior to Residency

Specialty Prior to Residency	N	Percent of Total Respondents
Family practice	9	64
Emergency medicine	2	14
Internal medicine	1	7
Internal medicine specialty	1	7
Occupational health	1	7
TOTAL	14	99.9*

*Due to rounding off of individual percentages the total is less than 100%.

Data from Asprey, D., & Helms, L. (1999). A description of physician assistant post-graduate residency training: The director's perspective. Perspectives on Physician Assistant Education, 10(3), 124–131.

Compensation

Residents typically work long hours for modest pay, but benefits must be factored into the total compensation (Exhibit 5-16).

Perceptions

Residents' perceptions of their training reveal that they are generally satisfied with their education and experienced significant improvement in their knowledge and clinical skills (Exhibits 5-17 and 5-18). In decreasing order of frequency, the clinical activities in which the residents identified increased knowledge with the greatest frequency were ability to establish a diagnosis (98%), ability to recognize disease and pathology (96%), critical thinking skills (96%), and ability to develop a differential diagnosis (96%). Clinical activities that were most commonly identified as unchanged included research skills (52%), history taking and interviewing skills (30%), physical

EXHIBIT 5-16
Benefits Provided by Internship Residency Programs, 1999

Benefit	Percent of Residencies That Provide Benefit		
	Fully	Partial	Total
Malpractice insurance	100	0	100
Vacation days	100	0	100
Health insurance	83	8	91
Life insurance	75	0	75
Continuing medical education (CME) days of paid leave	50	17	67
Allowance for meals or meals provided	42	25	67
Dental insurance	67	0	67
CME funds	25	17	42
Housing allowance	8	25	33
Transportation allowance	17	0	17
Retirement funding	8	0	8
Other	NA	NA	67

Data from Asprey, D., & Helms, L. (1999). A description of physician assistant post-graduate residency training: The director's perspective. Perspectives on Physician Assistant Education, 10(3), 124–131. Reprinted with permission of the Physician Assistant Education Association.

EXHIBIT 5-17
**Residents' Perceptions of Change in Knowledge
of Clinical Activities (*N* = 44)**

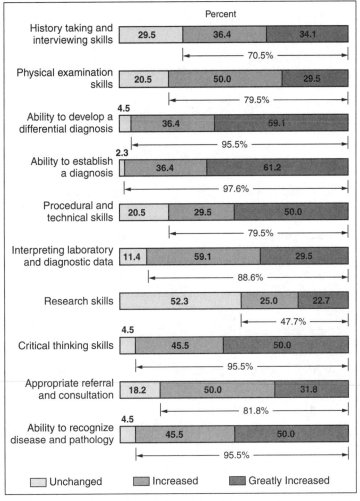

Data from Asprey, D., & Helms, L. (2000). A description of physician assistant post-graduate residency training: The resident's perspective. Perspectives on Physician Assistant Education, 11(2), 79–86.

examination skills (21%), and procedural skills (21%). The clinical skills for which residents identified the greatest growth were the ability to develop a differential diagnosis (100%), ability to recognize disease and pathology (100%), critical thinking skills (98%), and ability to establish a diagnosis (96%). The clinical skills that residents most commonly identified as unchanged included research skills (54%), history taking and interviewing skills (22%), and physical examination skills (20%).

All residents reported satisfaction in their summary evaluation of their residency training experience and substantial satisfaction in the areas of degree of responsibility and didactic and clinical education (Exhibit 5-19). Residents were least satisfied with the salary and benefits packages. When asked if they would recommend their residency program to other PAs interested in their specialty, 33 (72%) answered "definitely" and 13 (28%), "probably" (Asprey & Helms, 2000).

EXHIBIT 5-18
Residents' Perceptions of Change in Their Clinical Skills (*N* = 46)

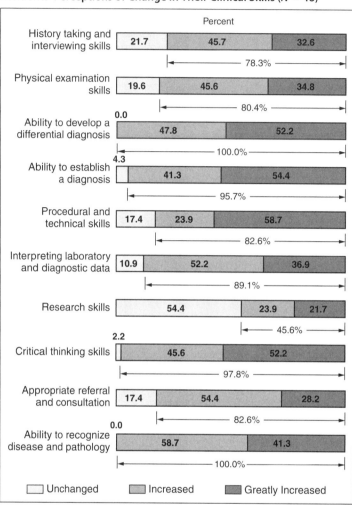

Data from Asprey, D., & Helms, L. (2000). A description of physician assistant post-graduate residency training: The resident's perspective. Perspectives on Physician Assistant Education, 11(2), 79–86.

EMPLOYMENT OPPORTUNITIES

Although little objective data are published comparing the number of employment opportunities and salaries of PAs who have gone through a residency program with those PAs who do not have postgraduate training, there is anecdotal information and a general belief that the residency-prepared PA has a competitive edge when applying for PA positions and that they command additional salary.

In 1987, Keith and Doerr surveyed graduates of the Montefiore Medical Center Surgical Residency Program. Between 1971 and 1977, 43 PAs entered the 12-month internship and 27 (63%) graduated. Between 1978 and 1985, 102 PAs entered the 15-month PA internship; 86 (85%) of these PAs completed their education. The overall completion rate of the 145 trainees of the program was 78% and 86% of respondents remained employed as PAs. In addition, it was noted that of the 110 respondents, 86 (78%) were employed by

EXHIBIT 5-19
Summary of Residents' Satisfaction Levels

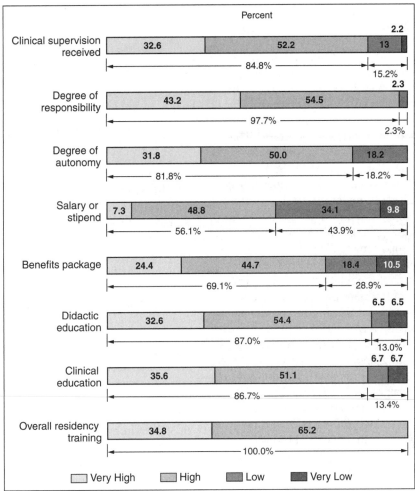

Data from Asprey, D., & Helms, L. (2000). A description of physician assistant post-graduate residency training: The resident's perspective. Perspectives on Physician Assistant Education, 11(2), 79–86.

institutions and 24 (22%) were employed by physicians in private practice. Postgraduate residency graduates earned significantly higher pay than PAs practicing in the same specialty without completing a postgraduate residency program. The average salary was 21% greater than the national average salary of PAs at the time. Of those surveyed, 72% indicated satisfaction with the preparation they received, 20% believed they were overprepared, and 8% felt inadequately prepared for the positions they held.

Some data reveal that the salary edge of a PA resident may be canceled out when the amount of hours worked are factored into the equation. In 2007, salaries of PAs who graduated from a surgery residency and the salaries of non-residency-trained PAs practicing in the same specialty had shifted somewhat. On average, the residency-trained PA earned a 15% higher salary than the PA without residency training. However, on average, residency graduates reported working 16% more hours than the average of all surgical PAs. When the salaries are adjusted for hours worked, the compensation per hours worked is nearly identical (Brenneman, Hemminger, & Dehn, 2007).

ACCREDITATION

In an attempt to accomplish the goal of PA residency accreditation, APPAP met with several organizations, including the AAPA and ARC-PA, to discuss the feasibility of developing a collaborative mechanism for PA residency program accreditation. APPAP took an initial step by developing its own set of "program essentials" that are intended to identify the desirable elements of a PA residency program. These essentials were developed and approved in 1991 by APPAP's member programs. Although compliance with these essentials is voluntary for PA programs and is not reviewed by any external entity, programs must agree to adhere to the essentials if they are to be APPAP members.

Several groups have called for establishing standards for the PA postgraduate education process because of the relative lack of information on PA postgraduate programs. PA educators, policymakers, employers, and members of the profession still have relatively little systematic information on which to formulate opinions or make judgments about the value of the PA postgraduate programs. A clear, long-term outcome of postgraduate education should be undertaken and compared with outcomes of PAs who were trained on the job. To date, PA postgraduate programs have not objectively documented their value, standardized their curricula, legitimized their educational processes and outcomes through research, or implemented an accreditation or certification process for postgraduate education (Cawley & Jones, 1997; Hooker 2009).

Historically, the topic of accreditation of postgraduate programs is one dating to the 1980s (Exhibit 5-20). A survey of residency directors in 1999 found that directors supported seeking accreditation of PA residency programs. Specifically, 88% indicated that residency programs should seek to implement an accreditation process. APPAP deliberated the merits of accrediting PA postgraduate programs and ARC-PA provided an accreditation process for the postgraduate programs. The standards governing the postgraduate programs can be found at the ARC-PA website at http://www.arc-pa.org. Exhibit 5-21 outlines the initial process that has been adopted and implemented by the ARC-PA for postgraduate PA programs.

CHALLENGES FOR PHYSICIAN ASSISTANT RESIDENCY PROGRAMS

Directors of residency programs perceive several challenges including clinical curriculum, recruitment and retention of residents, and program evaluation. The most significant challenges are shown in Exhibit 5-22. (Note that this study occurred prior to the establishment of the current accreditation system.)

Standardization of the postgraduate residency education process is also an ongoing concern for programs. Another substantial challenge is the fact that programs have not objectively documented their value, standardized their curricula, or chronicled their outcomes through research. Perhaps the greatest step forward in adding legitimacy to their educational processes is the recent implementation of an accreditation process for postgraduate education.

In a survey of 712 orthopedic PAs in 2008, 52% approved a recommendation for advanced clinical training (12 months) before entering orthopedics. However, of those who disapproved, a strong preference was expressed for a model of "on the job" training in specialty medicine and surgery (H. D. Larson, personal communication, May 2009).

Research and Physician Assistant Education

The literature about the education and deployment of postgraduate-trained PAs is incomplete. Following is a brief review of areas in need of attention.

- **Case reports:** Writing about individual programs or a group of programs within a specialty can show how a program is structured in an institution and the organization of roles for each educator so that new programs can be constructed.

EXHIBIT 5-20
Clinical Postgraduate PA Program Accreditation History

Date	Activity
February, 1980	The Joint Review Committee (JRC) was first approached to review the issue of accrediting postgraduate PA programs.
February, 1981	An ad hoc committee was appointed and reported its findings. The JRC determined that it was inappropriate to review postgraduate PA programs at that time.
March, 1985	The JRC revisited the issue of reconsidering the advisability of expanding the scope of its review to include postgraduate PA programs. No decision was made. Later the JRC was replaced by the Accreditation Review Commission for Physician Assistants (ARC-PA).
September, 1992	The ARC-PA entertained a presentation from representatives of the Association of Postgraduate Physician Assistant Programs (APPAP). Over the ensuing months additional information was garnered.
March, 1994	The JRC declined to be involved in accrediting of postgraduate programs but offered technical assistance regarding the development of separate standards.
March, 1999	The ARC-PA received a request from the APPAP president to reconsider accrediting its member programs. A workgroup was appointed.
September, 1999	Workgroup reported issues identified and requested a meeting of the ARC-PA and APPAP to further explore the issue.
May, 2000	Meeting of APPAP representatives and ARC-PA.
March, 2001	Issue further discussed at ARC-PA meeting. ARC-PA invites APPAP, AAPA, and APAP to join in a task force.
October–December, 2002	Task force members surveyed regarding issues related to accrediting postgraduate PA programs.
March, 2003	ARC-PA decided that if there is to be an accreditation process, the ARC-PA should administer the process.
May, 2003	Task force meets in New Orleans, Louisiana, to discuss possible standards.
October, 2003	Task force meets in Scottsdale, Arizona.
June, 2004	Task force meets in Las Vegas, Nevada. APPAP formally asks ARC-PA to develop an accreditation process with cost estimates.
November, 2004	Task force meets in Nashville, Tennessee. Task force discusses working draft of accreditation process, policies, time line, costs, and standards.
May, 2005	AAPA House of Delegates passes policy statement in opposition to accreditation of postgraduate programs. APPAP passes motion reaffirming its desire to have ARC-PA proceed in developing an accreditation process. Task force has final meeting in Orlando, Florida.
September, 2005	ARC-PA appoints committee to continue study of accreditation of post entry-level PA programs.
February, 2006	ARC-PA appoints committee to continue study of accreditation of post entry-level PA programs.
March, 2006	ARC-PA votes to begin providing accreditation services for clinical postgraduate PA programs.
March, 2007	ARC-PA approves accreditation standards for clinical postgraduate PA programs.
March, 2008	ARC-PA accredits first two clinical postgraduate PA programs.

Source: Accreditation Review Commission on Education for the Physician Assistant. (2009). Clinical postgraduate PA program accreditation history. *Retrieved September 2, 2009, from http://www.arc-pa.org/Post_Grad/post_gradhx.htm.*

■ **Role delineation:** What does a graduate from a postgraduate PA program do? Is there some way to distinguish a postgraduate-trained PA and a PA trained on the job in the same specialty?

■ **Organizational arrangements:** What are the lines of influence and organization for a PA program in a host institution? Does the degree of separation from the president of the university to the PA director have any influence on how the program functions?

■ **Economics:** What are the opportunity costs of a formally trained surgical PA versus a

EXHIBIT 5-21
ARC-PA Postgraduate Residency Accreditation Process

The clinical postgraduate PA program accreditation process conducted by the Accreditation Review Commission for Physician Assistants (ARC-PA) is a voluntary one entered into by institutions and programs that sponsor a structured educational experience. To be eligible to apply for accreditation, programs must be operational with at least one enrolled PA resident at the time of application.

SELF-ASSESSMENT

A requirement of accreditation is ongoing self-assessment of the clinical postgraduate program to review the quality and effectiveness of its educational practices and policies. During this process, the clinical postgraduate program identifies strengths as well as problems, develops plans for corrective intervention, and evaluates the effects of the interventions. Ongoing self-assessment provides the means by which clinical postgraduate PA programs can envision, attain, and maintain quality education. The accreditation application includes questions that address issues related to a well-conceived self-assessment process. The applicant must identify the physician specialty organization or other specialty organization the institution plans to use to review its curriculum content and required clinical experiences. The ARC-PA must pre-approve the organization from which review of their curriculum will be solicited.

SITE VISITS

Site visits are required for initial accreditation and are scheduled after clearing the administrative review of the application. The purpose of the site visit is to allow the site visit team to verify, validate, and clarify the information supplied by the program in its application. The site visit team also reviews the nature and manner in which the program's objectives are being pursued, and the manner in which the program's self-identified concerns and problems are being addressed.

Within a specified period of time after the site visit, programs are invited, but not required, to respond to any of the observations contained in the site visit summary in order to eliminate errors of fact or challenge perceived ambiguities and misperceptions. The response is not to be used to provide new information regarding changes made since the visit or plans for changes in response to the observations contained in the report.

DURATION OF ACCREDITATION

Accreditation for clinical postgraduate PA programs is time limited. Initial accreditation is limited to 3 years. If the program chooses to continue its accreditation, it must complete a continuing application and will be eligible for 3 additional years of accreditation. There is no site visit associated with the second review. (However, a site visit may be scheduled if the review of documents submitted indicates that a visit is needed to verify, validate, or clarify information.)

After a 6-year period of accreditation, another site visit will be a required component of the accreditation process for any clinical postgraduate PA program wanting to continue its accreditation.

ANNUAL REPORTS

All accredited clinical postgraduate PA programs are required to submit an annual report.

Source: Accreditation Review Commission on Education for the Physician Assistant. http://www.arc-pa.org.

EXHIBIT 5-22
Greatest Challenges to the Future of Residency Programs

Challenge	N
Funding needs	8
Accreditation of the residency programs	5
Recognition of PA residencies by PA profession	4
Other	4
Sustaining education in managed care environments	3
Demonstrating/documenting the quality and value of residency education	3
Recruitment of residents	2
Market demand for residency graduates	2
Perceived threat of PA residents to physicians	2
TOTAL	33

Data from Asprey, D., & Helms, L. (1999). A description of physician assistant post-graduate residency training: The director's perspective. Perspectives on Physician Assistant Education, 10(3), 124–131. Reprinted with permission of the Physician Assistant Education Association.

postgraduate-trained PA versus an on-the-job trained PA? Do these differences in cost of education have any predictive value on the role the PA selects?

■ **Breadth of knowledge:** Does the matriculate of a postgraduate PA program exhibit a different degree of knowledge than the informally trained PA?

■ **Program closures:** Why have one-third of PA programs failed?

■ **Procedures:** What are the procedures that a PA resident learns prior to graduation?

■ **Patient satisfaction:** Do patients have any different perceptions of PAs in training in a fellowship versus doctors in training in a fellowship?

■ **Retention:** Do PAs in a residency remain in their specialty for their career?

■ **Education:** What is the optimal balance between didactic learning and clinical experience?

SUMMARY

Postgraduate education for PAs has been slow to develop for a number of reasons. For many PAs, prolonging their ability to work in the medical setting they were trained for is less attractive than seeking employment. For others, the idea of specialization may offset some concerns about their ability to function or their desire to be specialized for various reasons. Additionally, the programs themselves have struggled to mature and stabilize due to their previous lack of an accreditation mechanism and the tenuous nature of PA residency program funding. The programs are small in enrollment, and the stipend pays about half of what they can earn in a non-trainee setting. However, as of 2009, over 42 programs exist and over 500 PAs have been trained in some formal way for a specialty role. The postgraduate programs are surviving for the most part, and some are thriving. If the profession follows the pattern of physicians (and several other healthcare professions), postgraduate residency education may become an expected element for practitioners' education. For many settings, postgraduate programs provide a steady workforce in times of scarcity, but funding continues to be a challenge for PA programs.

Educators, policymakers, employers, and members of the profession still have relatively little systematic information on which to formulate opinions and make judgments regarding the value of PA postgraduate residency education programs. The PA profession may benefit from a more active interest in this form of education and working with the residency programs to develop more systematically its postgraduate education system to serve the interests of a broad array of stakeholders. Better record-keeping and careful evaluation both of programs and outcomes both of programs and outcomes for graduates would be an important starting point.

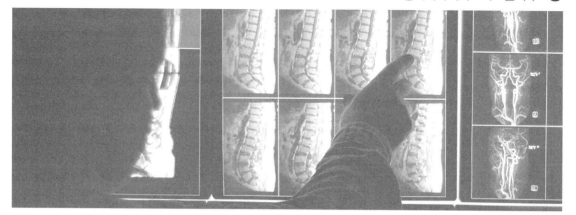

CHAPTER 6

PHYSICIAN ASSISTANTS
IN PRIMARY CARE

RODERICK S. HOOKER ■ JAMES F. CAWLEY ■ DAVID P. ASPREY

ABSTRACT

Primary care is a central component of western healthcare systems and is the focus of services that most patients enter and return to for continuity of care. Traditionally, primary care includes diagnosis, prevention, therapeutic services, health education, counseling, minor surgery, and longitudinal care from birth to death. That physician assistants (PAs) are central to primary care is not surprising given their genesis and development in many countries. This chapter includes the disciplines of general/family medicine, general pediatrics, internal medicine, and women's health. Together these disciplines make up nearly 40% of American PA roles, and a larger segment in other countries. Because primary care is undergoing change at the same time as PAs are experiencing worldwide growth, this chapter identifies primary care not only in North America, but globally.

INTRODUCTION

The entry point for most people into the healthcare system is primary care. Not surprisingly, primary care–oriented disorders make up the vast majority of all medical conditions seen by healthcare providers. Starfield (1994) pointed out that countries whose health systems are oriented toward primary care achieve better health levels, higher satisfaction with health services among their populations, and lower expenditures in the overall delivery of health care.

A substantial amount of research documents that physician assistants (PAs) are ideally suited and well qualified to deliver primary care services. PAs are trained to diagnose and treat most general medical conditions, and a substantial proportion of clinical PAs work in the primary care disciplines. In terms of medical specialties, primary care is defined as family medicine, general internal medicine, general pediatrics, and sometimes obstetrics and gynecology (commonly referred to as *women's health*). To most clinicians, the term *primary care* is synonymous with ambulatory care because less than 0.5% of all conditions seen in primary care result in hospitalization. In many countries, general medicine serves as the entry point to the health system (although not necessarily in the United States). Countries with well-established primary care systems have physicans serving as "gatekeepers," meaning that patients do not visit specialists, nor are they admitted to hospitals without being referred by primary care doctors. To some, "gatekeeping" represents a negative element of healthcare delivery systems because patients may be denied needed care. The practice, however, is associated with the avoidance of unnecessary procedures and overtreatment, thus facilitating the appropriate distribution and utilization of limited resources (Franks et al, 1992). In the United States, people can access some specialists directly (e.g., dermatology), which many believe leads to increased cost and fragmentation of services.

The major focus of medical education for PAs, doctors, and most nurse practitioner (NP) programs is primary care. Curricula for the would-be primary care clinician are organized so that the graduate can manage most medical conditions in a typical community with a normal population distribution. In many instances, primary care forms the foundation on which other areas of medicine rest. The student entering medicine learns the principles and practice of general medicine. These principles are often incorporated within other specialties, and in turn, specialties develop principles that are adopted in primary care. To understand this crucial role, which PAs have increasingly helped to define, we first define *primary care.*

Primary Care Defined

Primary care is the provision of integrated, accessible healthcare services by clinicians who are responsible for meeting most personal healthcare needs, developing sustained partnerships with patients, and practicing in the context of family and community. Definitions of primary care typically focus on the type or level of health services such as preventive, diagnostic, and therapeutic sevices; health education and counseling; and minor surgery, although it is possible for specialists to provide primary care. For example, a cardiologist who offers advanced specialized care for myocardial

conditions will also provide health education and preventive counseling.

The most commonly accepted definition of primary care is medical care services that are characterized by the following attributes:

- First-contact care
- Longitudinality
- Coordination
- Comprehensiveness (Starfield, 1993)

Primary care is distinguished from two other classifications of healthcare delivery: secondary and teritary care. *Secondary care* is usually thought of as short-term service delivery, infrequent consultation from a specialist, or surgical or other advanced interventions that primary care clinicians are not equipped to provide (Shi & Singh, 2008). This type of care includes hospitalization, routine surgery, specialty consultation, and rehabilitation. *Tertiary care* is regarded as the provision of care for complex conditions and usually involves an institution with advanced technology and specialty and subspecialty services (Hooker, 2008c). Examples include organ transplants, burn centers, cardiothoracic surgery centers, and advanced trauma centers.

The World Health Organization (WHO) Meeting on Primary Care, Family Medicine/General Practice in Barcelona, Spain, in 2002 proposed a definition of *primary care:* "Primary care refers to a span or an assembly of first-contact healthcare services directly accessible to the public."

Primary care (as opposed to primary *health* care) has gained increased attention since the new century and raises several questions. For example, how does it fit into the healthcare delivery system? Is it the same as primary health care? What strategies should be used to link primary care with other levels of care? What are the implications of developments in technology for primary care functions and professionals? These are some of the issues many countries in the WHO European Region are facing when trying to develop primary care as part of the overall healthcare system.

The participants of the 2002 WHO conference in Barcelona concluded that primary care is part of the provision of healthcare services and has to be looked at in the context of the overall services, not in isolation. In light of the confusion about commonly used terms— notably *primary healthcare, primary care, primary medical care, general practice,* and *family medicine*—the consensus was that a clear distinction between *primary health care* (as presented in the Declaration of Alma-Ata in 1978) and *primary care* (which refers to local level healthcare services) was necessary. More work in this area will emerge before the end of this decade.

Evolution of Physician Assistants as Primary Care Specialists

The initial purpose of the creation of PAs was not specifically to become primary care providers, but to support and augment the general services of the physician, regardless of specialty. The fundamental role of the PA as a clinician was initially described as one designed to examine and gather clinical information on the patient.

For more than three decades, federal government policies and state legislation have encouraged the use of PAs and encouraged their utilization in primary care. Due to the federal grant award program for PA educational programs, many PA training programs emphasized primary care as the centerpiece of their curriculum. Strong incentives were offered to programs that graduated large numbers of primary care PAs or deployed them into practices with primary care physicians. The result has been an impressive production of healthcare services in the United States. Hooker and McCaig (2001) analyzed primary care physician office encounter data from the National Ambulatory Medical Care Surveys. There were remarkably few differences in the types of patients, diagnoses made, and treatment rendered by the three providers, with the exception that the mean age of patients seen by physicians was slightly greater than that for PAs or NPs. On the other hand, NPs provided counseling and education during a higher proportion of visits than PAs or physicians. These factors aside, this study suggests that PAs and NPs are providing primary care in a manner that is similar to physician care.

In the U.S. healthcare system, it is estimated that there were approximately 1.2 billion outpatient visits in 2006 (combination of federal and nonfederal medical sites, urgent and nonurgent). Approximately 60% were broadly defined as "primary care" (internal medicine, family practice, pediatrics, and obstetrics and women's health). Primary care is provided in a wide variety of clinical settings. Using the aforementioned study, which consolidated 5 years of national ambulatory data, the estimate was that the productivity and distribution of PAs and NPs conservatively accounted for 11% (and perhaps as much as 15%) of all U.S. ambulatory visits in 2005 (Burt & McCaig, 2007).

How did a national system evolve where one in 8 or 9 visits is attributable to a PA or NP? This has been a slow evolutionary process. As the concept matured, the role of the PA transformed from merely assisting the primary care physician to one of close interdependence with the physician employer. This evolution was not strategically planned, yet this outcome was the inevitable product of delegation and expansion of duties that occurs in almost any apprenticeship and assistantship.

In the beginning, the role of the PA was conceived to be one in which the PA would initially see the patient and then present the major findings to the physician. Together they would complete the patient visit. Usually, the doctor would be the one to decide on the final diagnosis and treatment and then delegate aspects of a further diagnostic or treatment plan. The PA performed the diagnostic or treatment plan based on the PA's level of experience and skill, as well as the degree of trust between the PA and the physician. Something of a hand-off from doctor to PA would occur. A further evolution of the PA role, now commonplace, is that the PA sees the patient often without having the physician present for any part of the visit. With experience and trust, particularly in which the patient's problems are routine and typically straightforward, the physician-PA relationship develops. This is the point at which the physician may delegate a good portion of diagnostic and treatment responsibilities without the physician seeing or reviewing each patient. This process is referred to as "negotiated performance autonomy" and is the cornerstone of the PA movement (Schneller, 1978).

In some instances, patients will preferentially request the PA. With time, as the supervising doctor's confidence becomes reinforced by the skill and performance of the PA, the PA may be delegated more advanced work tasks (Schneller & Simon, 1977). As the PA assumes more responsibility for the management of patients, he or she begins to work longitudinally with chronic diseases such as hypertension and diabetes. Evolution is not static and the desire to learn well or even excel tends to move the PA into more challenging roles without jeapordizing patient safety.

In the new millenium, the PA in a practice may manage most of the common primary care disorders and may have as much experience with these conditions as associated physicians in the same setting. In some instances, a recently trained physician who is more familiar with hospital care than ambulatory care may employ a more experienced outpatient-based PA as a complement to the practice. In these cases, there are clearly trade-offs as to who can do what task best. As the PA profession and PA educational programs evolve, there will likely be an increasing emphasis on independent evaluation and management of common primary care disorders by the PA. Such complementary roles strengthen the team concept in healthcare delivery.

Primary Care Ecology

Human medical ecology may be defined as the study of relationships between people and the medical care system. One of the most famous and revealing studies of primary care was conducted by Kerr White and colleagues, titled "The Ecology of Medical Care" (White, Williams, & Greenberg, 1961). They drew a portrait of people, illness, and medical care that assumed a typical population of 1,000 citizens in an average month. The results were drawn from 1,000 noninstitutionalized adults; 750 were symptomatic for some illness each month, 250 received care from doctors in the office setting, 9 were hospitalized, 5 were referred to a specialist, and no more than 1 was admitted to a tertiary medical center or hospital. The authors were trying to make the point that health policies in the United States tended to overemphasize hospital-based care and that the common problems that people had most of the time were relegated to the underfunded, underappreciated system of primary care.

Forty years later, the study was replicated with expanded and updated data (Green, 2001). The results were remarkably similar. In an average month, again using 1,000 men, women, and children in the United States, about 800 were symptomatic, 327 considered seeking medical care, 217 visited a doctor, 65 visited a provider of complementary and alternative medicine, 21 visited a hospital outpatient clinic, 14 received care in their home, 8 were hospitalized, and no more than 1 was hospitalized in an academic medical center. These findings indicate the relative occurrence and severity of health problems in the U.S. population and the choices that persons make regarding the medical care system. The 2001 findings reaffirm the portrait of a health system that has a well-funded, high-technology tertiary health component that serves only a fraction of the ill population that needs a more extensive and better supported system of primary care (Green, 2001).

Federal Policy and Primary Care

The intent of U.S. federal health policy was (and continues to be) to utilize PAs in primary care. Early conceptualization of PAs was that they would work with generalists or specialists in augmenting physician services. Evidence to date shows that this policy device is accomplishing its goals. PAs are helping to ease the maldistribution of physicians by delivering primary care to many areas in which access is difficult and physicians are not likely to practice.

Some of the early PA programs, such as the Medex program and the PA program at Alderson-Broaddus College, focused on supporting the generalist physician in rural areas, whereas other programs prepared PAs for broader roles. At the other end of the spectrum were programs whose mission included training PAs to meet the needs of specialist physicians and hospitals. However, in 1973, federal incentives were established to provide training in primary care, and that policy has shaped many PA programs.

The deployment of PAs in primary care continues to be a sound policy to many observers. In the 1970s, most PAs were employed in some type of primary care practice or ambulatory setting and seemed to be fulfilling the ideals of their creators (Lawrence, 1978; Steinwachs et al, 1986). Some of the early studies of PAs in communities in which they served demonstrated improvement in the health status of patients beyond what was present before their arrival. Other benefits of PA utilization appeared because studies suggested healthcare costs were less expensive and the financial viability of the clinics improved (Greenfield et al, 1978; Hooker, 2000).

In 1978, the Institute of Medicine (IOM) issued a major report on primary care. This report recommended that PAs and NPs be given important roles in delivering primary care. The IOM study was wide sweeping and included recommendations on a number of important issues, such as PA prescriptive practices, third-party reimbursement, and enabling legislation (Peterson, 1980). These recommendations were endorsed by the American College of Physicians (ACP) and were reiterated in many healthcare policy reports over the next few years (Burnett, 1980; Record, 1981a).

By the early 1980s, the differences in roles between PAs and physicians in primary care became less distinct. Both seemed to be providing similar services in many settings such as rural practices, health maintenance organizations (HMOs), and public health clinics (Nelson, 1982; Repicky, Mendenhall, & Neville, 1982; Hooker, 1986; Steinwachs et al, 1986). Based on these observations, the following healthcare policy question arose: What is the appropriate balance of the primary care workforce between family practice physicians, PAs, and NPs? Subsequent studies all examined the use of and the contributions that PAs and NPs make in primary care practices. One idea emanating from these studies is the estimate of primary care staffing that PAs can provide. Compared with the physician service in question, PA/NP staffing ratios ranged from 20% in pediatric services to 50% in adult services (Hooker, 2000; Johnson, Hooker, & Freeborn, 1988; Salmon & Stein, 1986; Steinwachs et al, 1986; Synowiez, 1986). In the aggregate these researchers believed that PAs could be substituted for a physician in a practice for at least 50% of services.

Many PAs and health workforce researchers have wondered how much of the clinical primary care function a PA can assume. Record et al (1981) examined a representative population of patients managed by physicians and PAs in primary care in a large HMO. Using a number of conservative assumptions, she determined that PAs could manage at least 83% of all primary care encounters. Follow-up investigations by Hooker (1986) and Hooker and Freeborn (1991) found that, based on diagnoses rendered, there was a 90% overlap in types of patients managed by physicians and PAs in the departments of internal medicine and family practice.

Additional evidence showed that PAs could assume a wide variety of medical care services that had been the traditional domain of primary care physicians. By the 1990s, there was compelling evidence not only that PAs could expand the delivery of primary care services going unfilled by physicians, but that national policies should be promulgated to promote this trend (Osterweis & Garfinkel, 1993; Schroeder, 1992). This concept was never more clearly expressed than in President Bill Clinton's attempt to reform health care and improve primary care delivery in the mid-1990s (Health Security Act of 1993). The intent of this legislation was to expand the role of primary care PAs, NPs, and certified nurse-midwives (CNMs).

Primary care was the underlying pinning for the development of the PA profession, although it was not stated at the time of inception. A focus on primary care was in large part responsible for the profession's development and remains a major theme of PA education.

In 2008, approximately one-third of PAs in practice are in the federally designated primary care specialties of internal medicine, general and family medicine, and general pediatrics. Some argue that many primary care services are provided by PAs who are working in certain specialty areas such as occupational medicine, geriatrics, correctional medicine, military medicine, and public health. If the percentages of PAs in clinical practice working in emergency medicine (10.1%), women's health care (2.5%), industrial medicine and occupational medicine (3.6%), and geriatrics (1%) are included, the percentage of PAs engaged to some degree in primary care clinical activities approaches over 50% (Exhibit 6-1). Finally, what is lacking is our understanding of the extent of services in these specialities that would be considered primary care.

The characteristics of patients, the reason for a medical office visit, the most frequently reported principal diagnoses, and the medications prescribed in primary care are featured in Exhibits 6-2, 6-3, 6-4, and 6-5, respectively. These data are drawn from a national study on the content of ambulatory visits undertaken in 2006. Because of the high volume and frequency of these diagnoses seen in primary care, the PA is tutored and apprenticed in managing these and more complex cases.

PAs are commonly used in roles as primary care providers by a wide variety of healthcare organizations and in various settings, including:

- multispecialty group practices expanding primary care service delivery;
- managed care organizations expanding primary care capacities;
- private rural systems of care delivery and small community hospitals seeking to extend ambulatory care and primary care services;
- public health clinic settings, community and migrant health centers, and rural health clinics (RHCs);
- clinical settings in which they may provide clinical preventive services and wellness and preventive care (i.e., private clinics);

EXHIBIT 6-1
Distribution of Practicing Physician Assistants by Specialty

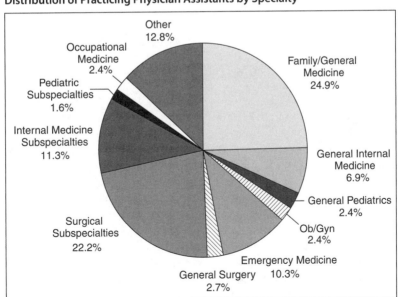

Data from American Academy of Physician Assistants. (2007a). 2007 AAPA Physician Assistant Census Report. Alexandria, VA: Author.

EXHIBIT 6-2
Number and Percentage of U.S. Office Visits by Patient Age and Sex, 2006*

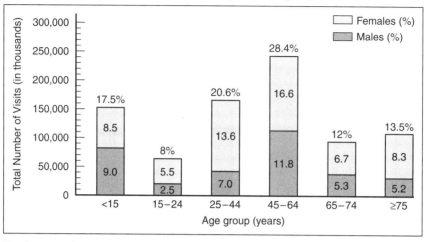

*Based on a reason for visit classification for ambulatory care.

Data from Cherry, D. K., et al. (2008). National ambulatory medical care survey: 2006 summary, National Health Statistics Report, *no. 3, Hyattsville, MD: National Center for Health Statistics.*

EXHIBIT 6-3
Distribution of Medical Office Visits by the Most Common Principal Reasons for Visit, United States, 2006*

Most Common Principal Reason for Visit	Percentage
General medical examination	7.4
Progress visit, not otherwise specified	5.7
Cough	3.0
Postoperative visit	2.6
Routine prenatal examination	2.4
Medication, other and unspecified kinds	2.1
Stomach pain, cramps, and spasms	1.8
Knee symptoms	1.7
Symptoms referable to throat	1.5
Back symptoms	1.5
Well-baby examinations	1.5
Vision dysfunctions	1.4
Earache or ear infection	1.3
Fever	1.3
Hypertension	1.3
Headache, pain in the head	1.1
Skin rash	1.1
Nasal congestion	1.0
All other reasons	58.8

Data from Hing, E., Cherry, D. K., & Woodwell, D. A. (2006). National ambulatory medical care survey: 2004 summary. Advance Data From Vital and Health Statistics, *no. 374, Hyattsville, MD: National Center for Health Statistics.*

EXHIBIT 6-4
Number and Distribution of Office Visits by the Most Common Principal Diagnosis Groups, United States, 2006

Most Common Diagnosis	Percentage
Routine infant or child health check	4.4
Essential hypertension	4.0
Acute upper respiratory infections, excluding pharyngitis	3.4
Arthropathies and related disorders	3.1
Diabetes mellitus	2.6
Spinal disorders	2.6
Specific procedures and aftercare	2.5
Malignant neoplasms	2.3
Normal pregnancy	2.2
Rheumatism, excluding back	1.8
Gynecological examination	1.7
Follow-up examination	1.5
General medical examination	1.5
Heart disease, excluding ischemic	1.5
Otitis media and eustachian tube disorders	1.5
Chronic sinusitis	1.4
Allergic rhinitis	1.3
Asthma	1.2

Data from Hing, E., Cherry, D. K., & Woodwell, D. A. (2006). National ambulatory medical care survey: 2004 summary. Advance Data From Vital and Health Statistics, *no. 374, Hyattsville, MD: National Center for Health Statistics.*

EXHIBIT 6-5
Number and Percentage Distribution of Drug Mentions by Therapeutic Drug Categories, United States, 2006

Therapeutic Class	Number of Occurrences (in thousands)	Percentage Distribution
Analgesics	209,936	11.1
Antihyperlipidemic agents	101,640	5.4
Antidepressants	85,331	4.5
Antidiabetic agents	68,742	3.6
Anxiolytics, sedatives, and hypnotics	66,968	3.5
Beta-adrenergic blocking agents	63,428	3.3
Antiplatelet agents	62,430	3.3
Bronchodilators	60,170	3.2
Diuretics	54,571	2.9
Dermatological agents	53,135	2.8
Anticonvulsants	49,800	2.6
Antihistamines	45,181	2.4
Ophthalmic preparations	40,197	2.1
Sex hormones	36,777	1.9
Calcium channel blocking agents	36,529	1.9
Adrenal corticosteroids	36,276	1.9
Vitamins and minerals	33,634	1.8
Thyroid drugs	33,340	1.8

Data from Hing, E., Cherry, D. K., & Woodwell, D. A. (2006). National ambulatory medical care survey: 2004 summary. Advance Data From Vital and Health Statistics, no. 374, Hyattsville, MD: National Center for Health Statistics.

- geriatric facilities and occupational and worksite health settings;
- correctional health systems;
- university and college student health facilities; and
- residency programs.

Physician Assistants as Primary Care Providers: Making the Case

Clearly, PAs have established themselves as a vital part of the U.S. primary care workforce and will be central for other countries as their numbers expand. Essential to any discussion of healthcare system policy is the question of workforce supply, distribution, and use. The imbalance of specialist physicians, the growth of managed care, and the issues affecting various types of healthcare personnel take on greater importance in a changing market-driven environment. All of this has spurred a critical reexamination of the roles, accountability, cost-effectiveness, and social responsibility of healthcare professionals in various nations, which is why the WHO revisited the definition of primary care in 2002.

Yet the role, scope of practice, and range of service of PAs is clearly not homogeneous. A number of interacting influences in the healthcare workforce explain why the practices of PAs differ so much. One reason is that the demand for PA services is related to external factors such as state licensing and regulation policy, which affect both the scope of practice and the prescribing authority. Primary care PAs working in states where legislation enables wide latitude with regard to physician supervisory requirements may be used more effectively (Wing et al, 2004). Another influence are market forces that shape the demand for PAs to assume different roles than those for which one was originally trained (Hooker, 1992). These differences are fading as legislation becomes more standardized.

Effectiveness of primary care delivery depends, at least in part, on using the correct mix of healthcare personnel. Starfield (1993) showed that this mix maximizes the clinical capabilities of healthcare professionals. In primary care practice, it is neither necessary nor particularly efficient for each patient to be seen by a physician. Because PAs are, by definition, physician-supervised clinicians, the very nature of their clinical role is to work with doctors in collaborative interdisciplinary settings.

A number of physician and nonphysician healthcare professional groups have laid claim to the title of primary care (such as obstetricians and NPs, asserting that they should be included as primary care providers). Attempts to answer the question of which types of physicians should be defined as primary care providers have prompted systematic analyses of the competencies of various physician specialists to provide the range of medical and preventive care services required (Mullan, Rivo, & Politzer, 1993). The conclusion was that only the disciplines of general or family practice, internal medicine, and general pediatrics fulfilled all of the criteria to be considered primary care disciplines.

Using these same criteria, the competency of PAs to provide primary care was assessed by Hooker and Cawley (1997). A matrix identified educational preparation, clinical practice, and professional certification measures of competency in the provision of primary care. Four national data sources were used as indicators of PA clinical practice performance and competency in primary care: educational preparation, national certification examination content, profession-defined role delineation, and actual data on use. The data overwhelmingly indicated that PAs are educated well enough to function as primary care providers and are successfully performing a large portion of tasks typically required in primary care.

COMMUNITY-ORIENTED PRIMARY CARE

Community-oriented primary care (COPC) is an advanced approach to primary care practice—one designed to better serve the health needs of populations (Mullan & Epstein, 2002). Since PA educational philosophy is related to primary care, it is useful to understand the concept of COPC's relevance to the PA profession.

Population health tends to improve when a community approach assumes the responsibility of care beyond the individual level (Kark, 1981). A COPC approach meets the demand for curative care and at the same time considers the total population and its health needs:

> [The COPC model] is a way of practicing medicine and nursing or of providing primary care, which is focused on care of the individual who is well or sick, or at risk for illness or diseases, while also focusing on promoting the health of the community as a whole, or any of its subgroups. (Kark & Kark, 1983)

The COPC model has been further defined as "a continuous process by which primary care is provided to a defined population on the basis of its health needs by the planned integration of public health with primary care practice"

(Gofin & Cawley, 2004). This COPC approach in health services delivery is one in which providers take responsibility for the health of all members of the community, whether or not they seek care. COPC is considered a practical approach to rationalize, organize, and systematize the existing resources through health interventions directed to prioritize health problems. The impact of COPC in different countries and health systems is considered relevant in the practice and teaching of family medicine as well as in healthcare reform movements addressing the future of general practice in the United Kingdom (Koperski & Rodnick, 1999).

The COPC Approach

The main elements in the development and application of the COPC model are:

- **Determination of a Defined Population**—the assessment of the population served, which may be a community, a neighborhood, a school, a working place, a clinic, or the people registered with a practitioner. In all of these cases, essential demographic information of all members of the population is critical. This information will enable access to the total population for critical intervention.
- **Assessment**—the assessment of the health needs of the community; findings will be used for priority setting and intervention planning.
- **Community Health Programs**—integration of health interventions that address all stages of the natural history of disease (incorporating promotion, prevention, treatment, and rehabilitation functions) and a comprehensive focus addressing all the physical, mental, and social determinants of health.
- **Accessibility**—to the services, taking into consideration economic, fiscal, and cultural barriers.
- **Multidisciplinary Health Team**—a team composed of different disciplines according to the specific health needs of the community and the available human resources. Together with the clinical skills needed to provide high quality health care, epidemiological and

sociobehavioral skills are needed to respond to the community health needs while performing the activities required by the COPC approach.

- **Outreach Approach**—"working outside the clinical walls" to enable the team to assess directly the physical and social determinants of health at the microenvironment level.
- **Community Involvement**—requiring, promoting, and facilitating community participation in healthcare activities as a means for active involvement (individually and collectively) in the improvement of health. Important determinants of health, such as behavior, attitudes, and beliefs, are closely related to individual decisions in their social environment. Therefore, the involvement of members of the community can enhance the positive effects of the community-oriented health interventions. If health services are not able to meet all the needs of the population, then a COPC program should include an inter-sector coordination with other services serving the population (Gofin & Cawley, 2004).

There are at least three educational programs that provide orientation in COPC to PA students: The University of Utah, the University of Texas Southwest, and the George Washington University.

DELINEATION OF THE ROLE OF THE PHYSICIAN ASSISTANT

PAs are aware of the need to communicate what goes on in clinical practice with the designers of educational programs and certification examinations. As a maturing profession, it requires diligent self-evaluation to balance its origins with the expanding levels of authority and responsibility it is evolving toward. This self-evaluation is accomplished by role delineation studies. Through serial role delineation analysis, the PA profession became codified and set into a structured framework of rules and regulations to convince those early innovators that taking an assistant into the physician's practice would be safe and convenient and would not threaten patient confidence.

Role delineation research is a fundamental way in which information about the professional activity of an occupation is gathered and analyzed (Cawley et al, 2001). In this case, the following nine general clusters of activities are common to PA practice across specialty lines:

- Gathering data
- Seeing common problems and diseases
- Conducting laboratory and diagnostic studies
- Performing management activities
- Performing surgical procedures
- Managing emergency situations
- Conducting health promotion and disease prevention activities
- Prescribing medications
- Using interpersonal skills

Role Delineation for the New Century

In 1998, the National Commission on Certification of Physician Assistants (NCCPA) conducted a detailed study of the knowledge, skills, and abilities important for safe and effective PA practice. The purpose of the NCCPA's Practice Analysis was to update and revalidate the content blueprints for NCCPA certifying and recertifying examinations. Results of the study revealed:

- the tasks and essential knowledge and skills that are representative of the actual clinical practice roles of PAs;
- differences in the practices of entry-level PAs and seasoned professionals; and
- the tasks, knowledge, skills, and abilities that are specific to PA practice in primary care and in specialty areas.

This work continues the efforts of the National Board of Medical Examiners, which conducted early role delineation studies in the beginning of the 1970s and by the American Academy of Physician Assistants (AAPA) in 1979 and 1985.

In 2004, an NCCPA's study was undertaken on a sample of 5,236 practicing PAs and examined their professional roles and functions. It also examined the frequency of specific medical activities and determined the required knowledge and skills deemed most important to PA clinical practice. The distribution of responses (47%) by demographic variables and by clinical specialty and setting indicates that survey respondents reflect the same profile observed in other national surveys of PAs. Two-thirds (66%) of survey respondents were in practice as a PA for more than 6 years, 21% practiced between 3 and 6 years, and 13% practiced up to 2 years. More than one-fourth (28%) worked in three or more specialty areas (Arbett, Lathrop, & Hooker, 2009).

Results identified the following domains of knowledge as most important for PAs:

- Subjective data gathering
- Assessment
- Objective data gathering
- Formulation and implementation of plans
- Clinical intervention procedures
- Health promotion and disease prevention
- Ancillary professional responsibilities

Overall, survey responses identified few differences in the tasks performed by PAs based on the length of time practicing in the profession. Response patterns differing across specialties were noted, particularly in the areas of cardiovascular and thoracic surgery, general surgery, and orthopedic surgery. The knowledge and skill areas rated most highly by practicing PAs were the following:

- Skill in identifying pertinent physical findings
- Knowledge of signs and symptoms of medical conditions
- Skill in recognizing conditions that constitute medical emergencies
- Skill in performing physical examinations
- Skill in conducting a patient interview (Exhibit 6-6)
- Knowledge of conditions that constitute medical emergencies
- Skill in associating current complaints with presenting history and identifying pertinent factors
- Knowledge of physical examination directed to a specific condition
- Knowledge of physical examination techniques
- Skill in effective communication

EXHIBIT 6-6
Conducting a Patient Interview

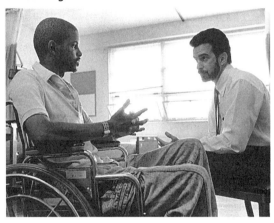

Courtesy of the American Academy of Physician Assistants.

Results of the NCCPA study reveal that PAs engage in and highly value those tasks essential for clinical practice. Ratings were consistently high in terms of frequency and importance of the daily functions of PA clinicians—history-taking and physical diagnosis. The expected knowledge areas required for practice are consistent with competencies identified in previous surveys. PAs also value diagnostic acumen and judgment and knowledge in developing an effective management plan. The consistency and high ratings of these findings suggest that there is a central core of medical knowledge, tasks, and skills valued that is performed often and consistently by practicing PAs. This core of knowledge and skills appears to apply to virtually all specialties and settings.

This information reveals a picture of PAs as professionals who have a great deal in common with physicians. The tasks are in terms of obtaining subjective and objective patient data; reviewing and interpreting diagnostic tests; formulating diagnoses; establishing or implementing treatment plans; prescribing certain medications; and providing patient education, counseling, and follow-up care. PAs also engage in many specialized practice activities. There are wide individual differences in the specific clinical interventions and procedures performed by PAs in different practice settings. Although they perform procedures in widely varied practice domains, it is clear that all PAs do not perform procedures in all areas. However, PAs rated the knowledge and skills required for clinical procedures and interventions as important (except for knowledge of advanced surgical equipment). This finding may reflect PA willingness to be trained in and to perform whatever procedures are appropriate and required by the particular physician or practice setting (Cawley et al, 2001; Arbett, Lathrop, & Hooker, 2009).

United Kingdom: The Competence and Curriculum Framework for the Physician Assistant

In 2005, the United Kingdom's National Health Service (NHS) published *The Competence and Curriculum Framework for the Medical Care Practitioner.* The report used the term "medical care practitioner" as a working title for the profession equivalent to the PA in the United States. A definitive decision on the title was made by the regulator (Department of Health, National Practitioner Programme). "Physician assistant" was the title most advocated and is now official.

This document sets the standards for the education, training, and assessments of PAs in the United Kingdom and, possibly, in all of Europe, by outlining the knowledge, skills, and core competencies expected at the point of qualification. For many, establishing these standards is seen as an opportunity to improve and develop the skill mix in primary care (with carryover to secondary care) while recognizing the unique skills and knowledge of other healthcare professionals.

Because the new PA in the United Kingdom is skilled in all the primary care roles and will maintain professional competence, an assessment as to how these factors translate into waiting times and patient satisfaction will be undertaken periodically. This document may find uses in other countries as they try to align their citizens' healthcare needs with the providers available to deliver some of those needs.

Clinical Practice Guidelines and Protocols

At one point, protocols were developed in an attempt to standardize the performance of the PA and to ensure physicians and patients that medical treatment provided by this new healthcare practitioner would be adequate. These protocols began with the patient's presenting complaint and continued step-by-step through the questions that should be asked, the tests that should be run, and the medications that should be prescribed. There cannot be a protocol for every situation, but dozens were written by PA educators and physicians and were used extensively in training and practice. With time, these protocols have been replaced by clinical practice guidelines.

Clinical practice guidelines have become the standard for many medical providers as managed care and corporate interests transform the U.S. healthcare system. Along with guidelines come corporate mandates for efficient use of resources, assessment of provider productivity, and measurement of clinical outcomes. The courts tend to expect providers to justify their medical decisions in terms of published clinical guidelines.

Guidelines for providing optimal medical care are not a new idea. The experiences of individual physicians and opinions of professors in medical schools, medical textbooks, clinical journals, and clinical trials have guided the practice of medicine for most of the 20th century. The medical community has traditionally standardized medical care to some degree to provide the best care possible, efficiently use resources, satisfy patients, and withstand third-party scrutiny. The increased level of standardization in today's clinical practice guidelines, however, is relatively new. When predicated on sound medical and scientific data, these guidelines can lessen provider variability in treatment and diagnosis. Evidence-based medicine and standardization improves measurement of resources used and assessment of benefits obtained. These guidelines can be particularly effective when applied to high-prevalence, high-cost diseases or conditions.

Clinical practice guidelines come from many sources, including professional medical societies, health-related associations, and governmental authorities. In the U.S. healthcare system, among the most prominent organizations that promulgate clinical practice guidelines is the Practice Guidelines Partnership (PGP), composed of 13 national medical specialties societies, the American Medical Association, the Agency for Healthcare Research and Quality (AHRQ), the American Hospital Association (AHA), the Joint Commission, and the Center for Medicare and Medicaid Services (CMS). For access to evidenced-based clinical practice guidelines, visit the National Guideline Clearinghouse website at http://www.guideline.gov.

As for PAs in practice, it is neither desirable nor common for them to practice strictly according to written practice protocols. Practice management systems can serve as an initial "security blanket" in the PA's clinical practice until the supervising doctor's confidence is sufficient to allow the PA to develop competent clinical skills and judgment. As the physician becomes comfortable with the PA's performance, there appears to be less concern with the external supports that inform the PA of correct procedures. Consequently, the PA develops a necessary sense of clinical judgment and critical thinking, particularly in regards to knowing when the patient needs to be referred to the physician.

PRIMARY CARE PROVIDERS

This section identifies the core primary care disciplines. It also defines the role of the primary care PA and evaluates how much more there is to discover about this discipline.

Family Medicine

Family medicine (historically referred to as *general medicine*) is the trunk from which all aspects of medicine grow. It is the discipline that deals with the general medical needs of the individual and his or her family, from pregnancy and children through adolescents to adults, and on into geriatics. The family medicine doctor treats acute and chronic illnesses and provides preventive care and

health education for all ages and both sexes. She or he has spent 2 to 3 years in postgraduate training learning all aspects of general medicine as it affects the individual, the famiy, and the community as a whole. Educated in health, fitness, and all aspects of medicine, including obstetrics, gynecology, and pediatrics, the family practitioner is the source of continuity of care for the community. The rural practitioner is more likely to be a family doctor than any other discipline in medicine.

The titles *family practitioner* and *family physician* have become widespread in Canada, the United States, and many other countries (see following text). The term *general practitioner (GP)* is common in the United Kingdom along with most other Commonwealth countries, where the word *physician* is largely reserved for certain other types of medical specialists, notably internal medicine.

Many GPs do minor procedures in their offices, such as repairing lacerations and removing skin lesions. Historically, they carried out major surgery, such as tonsillectomies, hernia repairs, and appendectomies. In the more rural parts of many countries, this style of medical practice continues. However, throughout much of the world in the past few decades the number and type of medical specialists has increased, whereas the number of family physicians or GPs has steadily decreased. These changes may have many causes, including long working hours, the relative isolation of a solo general practice, and the lower pay compared with that of most specialists.

The development of a formal family medicine doctor to replace the GP occurred almost at the same time as the development of the PA profession in the United States. Outside of the United States, how the family practitioner or GP is viewed differs depending on the country.

United States

In the United States, the family medicine doctor (also known as a family physician), has completed a 3-year family medicine residency in addition to undergraduate and doctoral studies, and is eligible for the board certification now required by most hospitals and health plans. The scope of practice of family doctors typically includes general medicine, general pediatrics, and sometimes, obstetrics and outpatient gynecology. Most family physicians practice in solo or small-group private practices or as hospital employees in practices of similar sizes owned by hospitals.

Canada

In Canada, all medical students go on to a specialty, and family medicine accounts for almost 40% of the residency positions for graduating students. Following 4 years in medical school, a resident (postgraduate doctor) will spend 2 to 3 years in an accredited family medicine program. At the end of this period, residents are eligible to be examined for certification in the College of Family Physicians of Canada. Many hospitals and health regions now require this certification.

There is little private family medicine practice in Canada. Most family practitioners are remunerated through their provincial government health plans. Various payment mechanisms include fee-for-service, salaried positions, and alternate payment plans. As standard office practice has become less financially viable in recent years, many family practitioners now pursue areas of special interest. However, in rural areas, the majority of family practitioners still provide a broad, well-rounded scope of practice.

Australia

General practice in Australia has undergone many changes in education requirements since the 1990s. The basic medical degree in Australia is the twin Bachelor of Medicine and Bachelor of Surgery (MB BS or MBBS) degree, which has traditionally been attained after completing a 6-year course. Since the mid-1990s, 4-year postgraduate courses have become more common. After graduating, a 1- or 2-year internship (dependent on state) is required for registration before specialist training begins. For general practice training, the doctor applies to enter the 3-year Australian General Practice Training Program, a combination of coursework and apprenticeship-type training, leading to the awarding of the Fellowship of the Royal Australian College of General Practitioners (FRACGP). Since 1996, this qualification or its equivalent has been required in order for the GP to access rebates from Medicare, Australia's universal health insurance system. Without access to Medicare, most GPs cannot effectively work in private practice in Australia. Most GPs work under a fee-for-service arrangement, although a portion of income is increasingly derived from government payments for participation in chronic disease management programs. There are shortages of GPs in rural areas and, increasingly, in outer metropolitan areas of large cities. Such shortages have led to the utilization of internationally (overseas) trained doctors.

United Kingdom

In the United Kingdom, doctors wishing to become GPs take at least 4 years of training after medical school, which usually involves an undergraduate course of 5 to 6 years or a graduate course of 4 to 6 years, leading to the degrees of Bachelor of Medicine and Bachelor of Surgery (MB BS or MB ChB). GPs then serve as the portal of entry for patients into the NHS.

Up until 2005, those wishing to become a GP had to do a minimum of the following postgraduate training:

- 1 year as a pre-registration house officer (formerly called a houseman), in which the trainee would usually spend 6 months on a general surgical ward and 6 months on a general medical ward in a hospital
- 2 years as a senior house officer commonly on a General Practice Vocational Training Scheme (GP-VTS), in which the trainee would normally complete four 6-month jobs in hospital specialties such as obstetrics and gynecology, pediatrics, geriatric medicine, accident and emergency, or psychiatry
- 1 year as a general practice registrar

This process has changed under the Modernising Medical Careers program, a major reform of postgraduate medical education that is designed to improve patient care by delivering a contemporary and clear career structure for doctors. Doctors graduating from 2005 onwards have to do a minimum of

5 years postgraduate training, which involves the following:

- 2 years of foundation training, in which the trainee does a rotation around six 4-month jobs or eight 3-month jobs; these rotations include at least 3 months in general medicine and 3 months in general surgery, but will also include jobs in other areas
- 2 years on a GP-VTS, in which the trainee completes four 6-month jobs in hospital specialties such as obstetrics and gynecology, pediatrics, geriatric medicine, accident and emergency care, or psychiatry
- 1 year as a general practice registrar

At the end of the 1-year registrar post, the doctor must pass an examination in order to be allowed to practice independently as a GP. This summative assessment consists of a 2-hour video of consultations with patients, an audit cycle completed during the registrar year, a multiple-choice questionnaire, and a standardized assessment of competencies by a trainer.

Membership to the Royal College of General Practitioners is optional and can be awarded by examination or by systematic assessment of an existing practitioner. After passing the examination or assessment, the doctor is awarded the specialist qualification of Member of the Royal College of General Practitioners (MRCGP). GPs are not required to hold the MRCGP, but it is considered desirable. In addition, many hold qualifications such as the Diploma in Child Health of the Royal College of Paediatrics and Child Health (DCH), the Diploma of the Royal College of Obstetricians and Gynaecologists (DRCOG), or the Diploma in Geriatric Medicine of the Royal College of Physicians (DGH). Some GPs also hold the Member of the Royal College of Physicians (MRCP) or other specialist qualification, but they generally only do so if they had a hospital career or a career in another specialty before training in general practice. The career grades of the GP and other specialties have undergone significant change to allow for a more focused GP practitioner and to allow the Medical Modernization Act of the United Kingdom to meet changes in the European Union (Exhibit 6-7).

GPs in the United Kingdom can work under many arrangements. Although the main career aim is to become a principal or partner in a GP practice, many become salaried or nonprincipal GPs, work in hospitals in GP-led acute care units, or perform locum work. Whichever of these roles they fill, the vast majority of GPs receive most of their income from the NHS. Principals and partners in GP arrangements are self-employed, but they have contractual arrangements with the NHS, which give them considerable predictability of income.

The MB ChB medical degree is generally considered equivalent to the North American MD medical degree. Doctors educated in the

EXHIBIT 6-7
Medical Career Grades in the United Kingdom's National Health System

Year	Old System		New System (Modernizing Medical Careers)	
1	Pre-registration House Officer for 1 year		Foundation House Officer for 2 years	
2 3	Senior House Officer for a minimum of 2 years, although often more		Specialty Registrar (StR) in a hospital specialty for 6 years	Specialty Registrar (StR) in general practice for 3 years
4 5 6–8 9	Specialist Registrar for 4 to 6 years	General Practitioner; total time in training = 4 years	Consultant; total time in training = 8 years	General Practitioner; total time in training = 5 years
Optional	Training may be extended by pursuing medical research (2 to 3 years), usually with clinical duties		Training may be extended by obtaining an Academic Clinical Fellowship for research	

United States, Canada, Ireland, and Great Britain have more ability to move between the countries than those educated in other national systems.

Netherlands

General practice in the Netherlands is considered fairly advanced and consists of 3 years of specialization after completion of internships. The *huisarts* (literally: "home doctor") administers all first-line care and makes required referrals. Many have a specialist interest, such as palliative care. Only a few PAs in the Netherlands are involved in general practice (Simkens et al, 2009).

Role

The role of the family medicine PA is to provide primary care (entry-level care and longitudinal care) for a defined population in any geographical setting. All U.S. and Commonwealth PAs are trained in the generalist model of acute and chronic illnesses and provide preventive care and health education for all ages and both sexes. Skilled in preventive care, the PA is experienced with more than 40 immunizations. Knowledgeable about chronic care, the PA in family medicine is skilled in managing a host of conditions, such as diabetes, hypertension, heart failure, early-stage renal insufficiency, dementia, osteoarthritis, and select gastric and endocrine conditions. The PA in family practice is also able to switch from family counseling to acute care management, which includes suturing, and treating pneumonia, acute cardiac symptoms, fractures, tendinitis, and minor injuries. For many PAs, the change of pace that family medicine brings is what keeps them in the PA role. Finally, it is the foundation of family medicine—the core and extended family and its passage through birth, aging, middle age, family planning, and wellness—that provides its own rewards.

History

More PAs identify their practice specialty as family medicine than any other. In 2008, approximately one-fourth of PAs who responded to the AAPA Census identified family medicine or general practice as the specialty they practiced for their primary employer. No studies have been done to identify all of the specific activities of PAs in family medicine; however, the work by Dehn and Hooker in 1999 detailing the daily activities of family medicine PAs in rural Iowa is profiled in Chapter 9. The eclectic and humanitarian orientation of family medicine is also epitomized in the book *Kernal in the Pod*: "I have finally found a place to rest, where the pod of peas is big enough for a kernal or two" (Jones, 2002). The largest contingent of PAs in rural practice identify their role as oriented to family practice.

PAs enjoy strong support from family physicians, as evidenced by statements by the American Academy of Family Practice (AAFP) affirming PAs' capabilities in delivering primary care services. Several postgraduate training programs are available for PAs in family practice, providing an additional year of clinical education in this specialty.

The efficacy of PAs in diagnosing patients was supported by Goldstein's examination of whether primary care providers, especially PAs, could recognize, diagnose, treat, or triage rare gastrointestinal disorders. Concern about whether primary care providers in general (and PAs in particular) could diagnose, treat, or triage anorectal disorders as a proxy for other referrals was retrospectively examined. Charts of the first 100 consecutive consultations for anorectal complaints were analyzed for accuracy of diagnosis and appropriateness of care. Correct diagnoses were made by 45 of 85 primary care physicians (53%), 6 of 15 PAs (40%), and 8 of 15 general surgeons (53%). A delay in diagnosis or appropriate treatment occurred in 25 patients (25%), resulting in adverse outcomes in 15 patients. Of these patients, five complications were caused by delayed diagnosis, and 10 patients had symptoms that persisted from 5 months to 14 years (mean, 4.5 years). Seven unnecessary referrals to a gastroenterologist resulted in three unnecessary colonoscopies. Of the 19 patients evaluated by a general surgeon, 4 had inadequate or inappropriate operations, 5 were untreated because of misdiagnosis, 3 were correctly diagnosed but untreated, 3 had inappropriate follow-up, 1 was referred to a gastroenterologist, and 2 were advised to have appropriate treatment. The authors concluded that primary care PAs and doctors correctly diagnosed anorectal disorders in 51% of cases and referred patients promptly 75% of the time. Of the 25% with delay, 60% experienced a complication of persistent symptoms. Fifteen of 19 patients seen by a general surgeon (79%) were inappropriately managed (Goldstein, 1996).

Profile

A survey undertaken by the AAPA (Exhibit 6-8) in which 6,525 PAs in family medicine responded found that the average age was 43, females were 64% of the cohort, and 23% worked in a single specialty physician group practice. Most respondents (70%) worked in an urban setting. The majority (82%) worked full time (at least 32 hours per week) and 78% were salary-based. The average salary in 2008 was $84,173 (AAPA, 2008a).

Professional Society

The Association of Family Practice Physician Assistants (AFPPA) is the organization that represents PAs in family practice. Its mission is:

> to foster the educational and professional interests of Family Practice Physician Assistants by promoting clinical and academic excellence and providing a forum for assembling and distributing information important to our profession. Pursuant to this

EXHIBIT 6-8
Family/General Medicine Physician Assistants, 2008

Number of respondents to the survey	6,525
Age (mean years)	43
Number (percent) female	4,145 (64%)
Solo practice physician's office	16%
Single specialty physician group practice	23%
Multispecialty physician group practice	16%
Hospital based	8%
Years in current position	11
Percent in urban practices	70%
Percent who work more than 32 hours per week	82%
Percent who precept PA students	34%
Percent who are salary-based	78%
Mean salary	$84,173

Data from American Academy of Physician Assistants. (2008a). 2008 AAPA Physician Assistant Census Report. Alexandria, VA: Author.

mission, the association seeks to provide a base for mentoring and/or precepting future PAs, promotes relevant CME resources, and disseminates employment information. Additionally, the AFPPA provides information relevant to the Family Practice discipline and/or a list of subject matter experts to all interested parties. (AFPPA, n.d.)

The AFPPA claims to be the "largest and fastest growing specialty organization of the AAPA" and invites PAs practicing in family practice, internal medicine, emergency medicine, pediatrics, obstetrics and gynecology, occupational medicine, or a related area, to join.

Internal Medicine

Internal medicine is another component of the main trunk of medicine that deals with the general medical needs of the individual adult, from adolescence through geriatrics. The specialists of internal medicine are referred to as *internists* and spend at least 3 years of postgraduate training learning how to prevent, diagnose, and treat diseases of the internal organs that affect adults. Internal medicine includes 13 subspecialities of medicine, such as rheumatology, endocrinology, nephrology, cardiology, infectious disease, and gastroenterology. The term "internal medicine" comes from the German term *innere medizin*, a discipline popularized in Germany in the late 1800s in which physicians combined the science of the laboratory with the care of patients. Internists are more likely to be basic scientists than the other primary care disciplines.

In the United States, the general internist practices medicine from a primary care perspective, but they can treat and manage many ailments and are usually the most adept at treating a broad range of diseases affecting adults. In other countries, the internist is a specialist who accepts referrals for consultation, but may not follow patients longitudinally. Outside of the United States the internist is usually not a primary care provider.

Role

Internal medicine PAs in the United States tend to work closely with general internists, often in medical groups, and follow patients longitudinally for illness and diseases that may need more attention. Examples of such diseases include progressive pulmonary diseases, renal insufficiency, type I diabetes mellitus, labile hypertension, and common maladies. PAs in internal medicine often have to solve puzzling diagnostic problems and handle severe chronic illnesses and situations in which several different illnesses may be present at the same time. They also bring to patients an understanding of wellness (disease prevention and the promotion of health), substance abuse and mental health, as well as effective treatment of common problems of the eyes, ears, skin, nervous system, and reproductive organs. Because internists commonly have patients hospitalized, some PAs share the role of checking up on the progress of the patient with the internist and report the findings back to the internist.

History

In 2008, approximately 5% of all PAs in clinical practice identified general internal medicine as the specialty they work in for their primary employer. Internal medicine physician groups, as expressed in published statements of the ACP, support the role of PAs working in general internal medicine. Like internists, PAs in internal medicine have practices skewed toward geriatrics. Among internists, the hospitalist movement has become increasingly popular, driven in part by a desire by physicians to better control the circumstances of their work. It would be a mistake to believe that physicians as we know them are going to fade from the healthcare delivery scene, yet it is clear that their roles in the division of medical labor are changing (Cawley, 2000).

Profile

In a survey undertaken by the AAPA, 1,303 PAs in general internal medicine responded (Exhibit 6-9). The average age was 43, females were 70% of the cohort, and 21% worked in a single specialty physician group practice. Almost all (84%) work in an urban setting. The majority (82%) were full time (worked at least 32 hours per week) and 84% were salary-based. The average salary in 2008 was $85,076 (AAPA, 2008a).

EXHIBIT 6-9
General Internal Medicine Physician Assistants, 2008

Number of respondents to the survey	1,303
Age (mean years)	43
Number (percent) female	904 (70%)
Solo practice physician's office	20%
Single specialty physician group practice	21%
Multispecialty physician group practice	21%
Hospital based	20%
Years in current position	10
Percent in urban practices	84%
Percent who work more than 32 hours per week	83%
Precept PA students	33%
Percent who are salary-based	86%
Mean salary	$85,076

Data from American Academy of Physician Assistants. (2008a). 2008 AAPA Physician Assistant Census Report. Alexandria, VA: Author.

Professional Society

There is no organization that specifically represents PAs who work in general internal medicine.

Pediatrics

Pediatrics is the branch of medicine that deals with the medical care of infants, children, and adolescents. The upper age limit ranges from age 14 to 18, depending on the country (or institutional inclination), although a new area of pediatrics specialization is adolescent medicine, which can include youth up to age 21. The pediatrician may be more holistic than the internist as a result of having a depth of knowledge about premature birth, family dynamics, death and dying, growth milestones, mental health disorders, genetics, behavioral disorders, preventive medicine, reproduction, and injury.

Role

In pediatrics the responsibility of the PA is more likely to be team-based than most other specialties. Collectively, the pediatrician, PA, nurse, and social worker have many lines of communication to work with, and these individuals tend to perform roles that commonly overlap. In addition, each team member tends to be knowledge rich; understands parental needs, family dynamics, and school-based learning; and remains alert to the idiosyncrocies of dysmorphology. Much of the role of the pediatric PA, which includes measuring milestones of growth and intellectual achievement, is routine. However, while recognizing deviations from normal in terms of testing and responses, the PA also serves as a resource and a comfort to parents.

Although the role of the PA in pediatrics was initially to assist the physician in the provision of primary care for well children and those with acute illnesses, subspecialty areas such as neonatalology have developed over the past 40 years. PAs have been used more extensively in hospital departments of surgery, in which they may obtain initial histories and perform physical examinations and minor surgical procedures under physician supervision.

For PAs on the pediatric inpatient units, roles continue to expand in response to new technology and pediatric provider shortages. PAs who are used in such positions require additional supervised education beyond that required for certification. The additional supervised education tends to be the responsibility of the pediatric unit director and may include orientation to hospital and departmental policies and protocols and direct teaching of clinical skills needed for the specific unit. Hospital-based PAs work under the supervision of an attending physician, and the patient's primary physician must always remain available to answer questions and provide backup to the PA. Decisions regarding the need for admission, management plans, and appropriateness for discharge are typically made with the involvement of the attending physician (American Academy of Pediatrics, Committee on Hospital Care, 1999).

History

Pediatrics is considered one of the three or four specialties that make up primary care. Many PAs specialize in pediatrics with formal and on-the-job training. One entry-level PA program specializes in pediatrics and two postgraduate programs are in neonatology. The number of PAs who practice general pediatrics

or a pediatric subspecialty has been steadily increasing from approximately 1,300 PAs in 1997 to approximately 3,000 PAs in 2008. There were more than 11.5 million patient visits to PAs in general and subspecialty pediatrics in 2006 (Burt & McCaig, 2007). In addition, PAs in various other specialties see pediatric patients. Considering that PAs in family medicine and emergency medicine see large numbers of children and adolescents, more than 40% of practicing PAs routinely treat pediatric patients (Cornell, 2007). The range of pediatric PA practices mirrors that of pediatricians. Most work in general pediatric settings, whereas a smaller number choose subspecialties of pediatric care. Of all pediatric PAs, two-thirds practice with general pediatricians and one-third work with pediatric subspecialists.

Most PAs working with pediatricians are graduates of programs that offer a broad general medical education that includes pediatrics. The one entry-level PA program that offers a special focus in pediatrics is the University of Colorado School of Medicine's Child Health Associate/PA (CHA/PA) program. Although this is a primary care PA program, it specializes in the care of infants, children, and adolescents. Students originally fulfilled a 3-year curriculum, with in-depth didactic course work serving as a foundation for a 12-month internship in the third year. Through required rotations in general pediatrics, newborn nursery, adolescent medicine, family medicine, inpatient pediatric medicine, and service in underserved or rural areas, PA students in the CHA/PA program gain generalist medical training with a special pediatric emphasis. This program has since been reduced to 24 months.

Pediatric PAs are specialized as well. They are used on pediatric bone marrow transplant units (Trigg, 1990) and work with the homeless, uninsured, poor, and underserved (Rada-Sidinger & Connor, 1992). Some are members of social service child protection units (Gray & Fryer, 1991) and work with inpatients to address the problems associated with resident overwork and educational needs of hospital services (Giardino, Giardino, & Burns, 1994).

Although most PAs go immediately from PA school to medical practice, opportunities also exist for postgraduate training in pediatrics and other specialty fields. The University of Kentucky has a neonatology fellowship for PAs and NPs.

PAs working in the pediatric inpatient setting typically fit one of two models. Either they are employed outside the hospital and have privileges to provide inpatient care or they are employed as medical staff on the pediatric or neonatal unit. Because pediatric PAs draw on the generalist and the specialist aspects of their medical training, they can effectively handle routine pediatric issues and can address a wide range of acute problems. Common responsibilities for PAs in the pediatric hospital setting include taking patient histories and performing physical examinations, working with physicians in diagnosing and treating illnesses ranging from common infections to more complex congenital diseases, attending to premature babies, and assisting in surgery. PAs in pediatric hospital practice tend to act as stabilizers within the intense and transient pediatric setting, providing continuity of care to the young patients who need it most. A 1999 report by the American Academy of Pediatrics on the role of PAs and NPs in the care of hospitalized children concluded that they "have a meaningful role in the management of hospitalized children. Having already demonstrated their ability to perform in supervised intensive care settings, they should be effective in the general inpatient unit and can play a valuable role in the care of hospitalized children by contributing specialized skills that improve the quality of patient care" (American Academy of Pediatrics, Committee on Hospital Care, 1999).

Patient satisfaction tends to increase when PAs are on staff for several reasons. PAs facilitate patient flow, shorten waiting periods, and ease staff scheduling. By handling routine pediatric questions and concerns, PAs help patients and parents understand their illnesses and treatment options. A PA on the team can help with patient education and follow-up, which improves compliance.

The role of PAs in child care has a rich history. Much of this history derived from the

CHA program developed by Henry K. Silver, MD, and Loretta Ford, RN, in the 1960s at the University of Colorado.

In the 1970s, Fine, Silver, and others, conducted numerous studies examining the roles and capabilities of the pediatric PA in general and the CHA in particular. They found that CHAs provided a wide range of diagnostic, preventive, and therapeutic services in pediatrics. CHAs and pediatric PAs demonstrated knowledge and skill to care for more than 90% of patients seen in a pediatric practice (Fine & Silver, 1973; Silver, 1973a; Silver, 1973b; Silver & Ott, 1973; Fine, 1977a; Fine, 1977b; Fine & Scriven, 1977). When compared with pediatric residents and medical students, CHA students demonstrated a comparable level of factual knowledge in the pertinent basic sciences and clinical pediatrics (Fine & Machotka, 1973; Machotka et al, 1973; Ott et al, 1974). Patient acceptance and the quality of care associated with pediatric PAs and CHAs are high (Wallen et al, 1982) (Exhibit 6-10).

One study of CHA care reported favorable marks by all mothers surveyed. Almost all (90%) indicated a desire to have their children cared for by a CHA (Dungy, 1974; Dungy, 1975). In spite of the research that demonstrates that pediatric PAs and NPs are widely accepted by the parents of patients and can perform well when compared with physicians, many physicians at the time were still slow to

EXHIBIT 6-10
Clinical Assessment

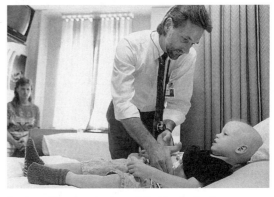

Courtesy of American Academy of Physician Assistants.

accept them as additions to their pediatric staff (Dungy & Silver, 1977; Silver et al, 1981).

As of 2008, there does not appear to be an increase in the number of pediatricians being trained. To confront the challenges of providing quality healthcare services to more children with more diverse and difficult problems, pediatricians will increasingly rely on PAs and NPs to perform certain tasks. This trend may give rise to more collaborative teams of pediatricians, PAs, and NPs, and more involvement of nurses. Shifting of pediatric services to family medicine is expected to continue.

Profile

In a survey undertaken by the AAPA, 1069 PAs in pediatrics responded (Exhibit 6-11). The average age was 40. Females were 80% of the cohort, and 36% worked in a single specialty physician group practice. Almost all (89%) worked in an urban setting. The majority (78%) were full time (worked at least 32 hours per week) and 86% were salary-based. The average salary in 2008 was $83,021 (AAPA, 2008a).

Professional Society

The Society for Physician Assistants in Pediatrics (SPAP) is a nonprofit specialty organization of the AAPA. Founded by and consisting of PAs, PA residents, and PA

EXHIBIT 6-11
Pediatric Physician Assistants, 2008

Number of respondents to the survey	1,069
Age (mean years)	40
Number (percent) female	854 (80%)
Solo practice physician's office	14%
Single specialty physician group practice	36%
Hospital based	27%
Years in current position	9
Percent in urban practices	89%
Percent who work more than 32 hours a week	78%
Precept PA students	53%
Percent who are salary-based	86%
Mean salary	$83,021

Data from American Academy of Physician Assistants. (2008a). 2008 AAPA Physician Assistant Census Report. Alexandria, VA: Author.

students, the SPAP welcomes affiliates and associate individuals who share a common interest in pediatric medicine. SPAP supports members in promoting high standards in the delivery of pediatric health care and provides the opportunity to network with other PAs and individuals interested in the well being of children. The mission of SPAP is to improve the health care of children by supporting the physician-PA teams who provide cost-effective, quality care to pediatric patients and by promoting a network for communication and education between providers dedicated to the well being of children.

Women's Health

Women's health (obstetrics and gynecology) is the specialty dealing with health of the female reproductive system (uterus, vagina, and ovaries), with obstetrics being the surgical specialty that deals with the care of a woman and her offspring during pregnancy, childbirth, and the puerperium. Midwifery is equivalent to a nonsurgical specialty of this discipline. Most family practitioners are trained in obstetrics and gynecology.

Women's health is a term not universally adopted, but it derives from the growing body of research about unique characteristics of women, their hormones, and their reproductive, social, and psychological issues. The term is used here to reflect the contemporary use in North America. Some researchers, advance practice nurses, and policy analysts include obstetrics and gynecology as part of primary care because the definitions for primary care are broad enough to fit this specialty.

Role

PAs in women's health tend to practice in outpatient settings, provide care regarding routine health matters, and evaluate for complaints. The role of a PA in women's health includes taking a history, performing a physical examination with emphasis on the reproductive organs, screening for breast disease, screening for cancer and sexually transmitted diseases, and providing family planning and birth control measures and advice.

Obstetric and gynecological care provided by PAs includes comprehensive annual reproductive organ examinations. They evaluate and manage common gynecologic conditions, such as vaginal infections, sexually transmitted diseases, and menopausal issues. They provide prenatal, intrapartum, and postpartum care. Many PAs are included on teams that evaluate and treat infertility. PAs also provide patient education and counseling on contraception, breast self-examination, lactation, and other topics.

PAs perform many obstetric and gynecological procedures, including but not limited to ultrasound, colposcopy, cryotherapy, intrauterine device insertion and removal, insemination, endometrial and vulvar biopsies, and loop excision electrocoagulation. In addition, many women's health PAs who work in ambulatory practices have hospital privileges to first assist in surgeries such as hysterectomies and cesarean deliveries.

History

PAs have practiced in teams with physicians for more than 40 years, providing a broad range of obstetric and gynecological and primary care services to women in outpatient and inpatient settings. In 2002, nearly 1,200 PAs practiced exclusively in the field of women's health. Thousands of other PAs across the spectrum of medical and surgical specialties provide primary and specialty care to women. Studies have shown that these PAs provide cost-effective, physician-quality medical care with high levels of productivity and patient acceptance. PAs' general medical education allows them to provide the primary care services many obstetricians and gynecologists seek to offer their patients in this era of proliferating managed care. Many PAs work in practices in which women would be likely to receive their primary medical care.

With the growth of managed care plans, many obstetricians and gynecologists are providing more primary care. PAs are ideally suited to provide not only treatment of ambulatory gynecologic problems, but also primary care for women. Because they are educated as generalists, PAs are well prepared to handle conditions such as respiratory infections, headaches, mild hypertension, diabetes, and urinary tract infections, as well as to provide health promotion, disease prevention, and screening for women in all stages of life.

Use of PAs in obstetric practices also can be an effective way to keep patient appointments on track when deliveries would otherwise disrupt the physician's schedule. PAs commonly share night and weekend call for deliveries, particularly in rural practices in which there may be a scarcity of doctors to serve the community.

In a 1994 study specific to obstetric and gynecological practices, the Collaborative Practice Advisory Group of the American College of Obstetricians and Gynecologists surveyed 3,257 patients in 10 practice settings to ascertain their satisfaction level with care provided in practices that used physicians and PAs, NPs, CNMs, or clinical nurse specialists. Patients felt these team practices provided quicker appointments (80.6%), more time with their provider (82.2%), and more health information (86%). "Few differences were evident in their perceptions of the care provided by physicians and nonphysicians." Patients perceived nonphysicians as being less rushed and spending more time with them than physicians. However, they perceived physicians as providing more complete information (Hankins et al, 1996).

Goldman and colleagues (2004) compared complication rates after surgical abortions performed by PAs with rates after abortions performed by physicians. A 2-year prospective cohort study of women undergoing surgically induced abortion was conducted. Ninety-one percent of eligible women (1,363) were enrolled. The total complication rates were 22.0 per 1,000 procedures (95% confidence interval [CI] = 11.9, 39.2) performed by PAs and 23.3 per 1,000 procedures (95% CI = 14.5, 36.8) performed by physicians ($P = 0.88$). The most common complication that occurred during PA-performed procedures was incomplete abortion; during physician-performed procedures the most common complication was infection not requiring hospitalization. A history of pelvic inflammatory disease was associated with an increased risk of total complications (odds ratio = 2.1; 95% CI = 1.1, 4.1). The authors concluded that surgical abortion services provided by experienced PAs were comparable in safety and efficacy to those provided by physicians.

Profile

In a survey undertaken by the AAPA, 590 PAs in women's health responded (Exhibit 6-12). The average age was 39. Females were 97% of the cohort, and 38% worked in a single specialty physician group practice. Almost all (91%) worked in an urban setting. The majority (72%) were full time (worked at least 32 hours per week) and 76% were salary-based. The average salary in 2008 was $79,229 (AAPA, 2008a).

Professional Society

The Association of Physician Assistants in Obstetrics and Gynecology (APAOG) is a support organization whose mission is to improve the health care of women. They support physician-PA teams who provide cost-effective, quality care to female patients and promote a network of communication and education between providers dedicated to

women's health. As stated on their website, the purpose of APAOG is:

- to promote clinical and academic excellence for members of APAOG, and to enhance quality medical care to patients;
- to provide the general membership of the AAPA with a forum for informal assembly regarding the issues that relate to PAs practicing in the field of obstetrics and gynecology; and
- to facilitate mutual assistance and support of physician assistants, health professionals, and health services by organizing and disseminating healthcare information through forums, panels, and other similar programs concerning the delivery and quality of healthcare services within women's health.

HEALTH MAINTENANCE ORGANIZATIONS

HMOs are prepaid group practices that provide capitated care for a large group of patients. Because of the economic structure of HMOs and their need to seize innovative, cost-containing measures, PAs were quickly adopted. The HMO experience with non-physician providers sharing and offsetting traditional physician responsibilities dates from the 1950s, when optometrists were employed to assume the role of refraction from ophthalmologists, nurse anesthetists were used to assist anesthesiologists, and psychiatrists shifted mental health patients to psychologists. It was not surprising that when PAs came along, HMOs embraced them.

Background of HMOs

Although HMOs have existed in the United States in some form since the first capitated plan was set up in Elk City, Oklahoma in 1929, it has only been since the early 1970s that substantial numbers of U.S. citizens have had access to this alternative to traditional fee-for-service health care. Sidney Garfield, a physician hired by the industrialist Henry Kaiser in the 1930s, started the first prepaid

EXHIBIT 6-12
Obstetrics and Gynecology (Women's Health) Physician Assistants, 2008

Number of respondents to the survey	590
Age (mean years)	39
Number (percent) female	563 (97%)
Solo practice physician's office	17%
Single specialty physician group practice	35%
Hospital based	17%
Years in current position	10
Percent in urban practices	91%
Percent who work more than 32 hours a week	72%
Precept PA students	45%
Percent who are salary-based	76%
Mean salary	$79,229

Data from American Academy of Physician Assistants. (2008a). 2008 AAPA Physician Assistant Census Report. Alexandria, VA: Author.

group practice. Kaiser wanted to provide care to workers who were building aqueducts in the California desert to reach southern California communities. When World War II broke out, Dr. Garfield was recruited to provide the same type of worker health benefit to the Kaiser shipbuilders in Walnut Creek, California. A similar program was incorporated in the Kaiser shipyards of Vancouver, Washington (near Portland), under Dr. Ernest Saward. In 1945, with the cessation of the war and the release of workers to other jobs, the two Kaiser plans opened enrollment to the public.

In 1970, there were 39 prepaid group practices operating in the United States. At this time, most of the legal and political battles against this managed care option had been fought, yet few U.S. citizens had access to this kind of plan. The Health Maintenance Act of 1973 is generally credited for being the impetus for an explosion of HMO growth. As a result, by 1985 there were 323 HMOs, and by 2000 there were more than 700. The number of preferred provider organizations today is almost double this amount (more than 1,200) and growing. Beginning in the new century more than 100 million U.S. citizens are in some form of managed care plan.

As HMOs have developed, several variations on their basic structure have evolved. The primary organizational type is the staff model, which is composed of salaried employees and providers and a group of beneficiaries whose health care is provided by the HMO. An example is Group Health Cooperative of Puget Sound. Similar in structure is the group model, which is organized by a prepaid population of patients, but the physicians are in a separate structure, usually as shareholders, which contract with the parent structure. Kaiser Permanente is the prototypical group model HMO. A third model, the network model, has characteristics of both of the other types.

Physician Assistants in HMOs

The first HMO to hire a formally trained PA was Kaiser Permanente, based in Portland, Oregon. In 1970, a Duke graduate PA was employed by the Department of Internal Medicine. The medical director at the time wrote that this strategy was not only to assist in staffing, but also to gain experience for future staffing needs. To the medical staff, PAs seemed like a natural fit for primary care (Lairson, Record, & James, 1974). This organization had experience with nurse-midwives, psychologists, and nurse anesthetists and believed that PAs and NPs could be useful adjuncts to the primary care physician staff. Within a decade, 10 departments had incorporated a PA or an NP, and 35 years from their first hire, more than 220 PAs and NPs work alongside 600 physicians to serve more than 500,000 Kaiser Permanente members. Other Kaiser Permanente regions have similar staffing arrangements, and other classical model HMOs have followed suit. The fact that a few HMOs still do not employ PAs is more of an anomaly rather than the norm in an era that stresses team approach and organizational efficiency in healthcare delivery.

In some HMOs the nonphysician providers are organized as a separate department, such as the Department of Physician Assistants at the LaGuardia Medical Group in Queens, New York (Goldberg, 1983), or the Department of Physician Extenders at Geisinger Medical Center in Pennsylvania (Regan & Harbert, 1991), or as affiliated staff at Group Health Cooperative of Puget Sound. In others, they are incorporated within the departments that employ them and are considered representative members of that department (Hooker, 1993; Jacobson, Parker, & Coulter, 1998; Coulter, 2000). In one HMO, PAs are shareholders in the medical group that contracts services with the health plan.

Various organizational theories have been postulated as to why HMOs employ PAs and NPs. The most reasonable explanation is that HMOs and other types of managed care systems have strong incentives to contain personnel costs, and their structure and size provide the opportunity to capitalize on the economy of scale and division of labor that the use of PAs and NPs can offer.

Early in the 1970s, most employers realized that PAs and NPs could meet the majority of primary care needs. Harvard Community Health Plan examined its providers' and patients' views on the role of NPs and PAs in its Internal Medicine Department. The analysis suggested that 28% of visits required the attention of a physician, though physicians actually provided 66% of visits. The authors concluded that it may be possible to increase the use of NPs and PAs if the health plan can educate members, particularly younger women, about the role of NPs and PAs so as to encourage their preferentially selecting these practitioners for their routine care (Frampton & Wall, 1994).

Based on a 1994 survey of medium-sized plans (45,000 to 100,000 enrollees) and large plans (more than 100,000) by the Group Health Association of America (GHAA), a surprisingly high number of PAs and NPs were used in a representative number of group and staff model HMOs (Dial et al, 1995). In Exhibit 6-13 the median number of physicians ranges from 119 to 123 per 100,000 enrollees. In addition, the PA and NP ratios range from 10.6 to 15 per 100,000 enrollees. The PA/NP staffing ratios of about 30 per 100,000 must be taken into consideration when physician ratios are extrapolated as national requirements (Weiner, 1994).

Studies also have revealed that NPs and PAs perform at rates of clinical productivity in a manner in which the quality of care provided is maintained at levels that are "indistinguishable" from those of physicians. PAs practice orientation tends to place an emphasis on interpersonal skills, patient education, and preventive care (Institute of Medicine, 1978).

Other studies showed that a PA or an NP can provide approximately 81% to 91% of the medical care in a primary care setting in an HMO (Record, 1981b; Hooker, 1993; Frampton & Wall, 1994; Hummel & Pirzada, 1994). Steinwachs and colleagues (1986) demonstrated that in one HMO, PAs and NPs tended to manage more acute diseases than chronic diseases. A study a decade later, however, showed that patients managed by PAs and physicians in adult primary care settings had a 90% overlap of diagnoses (Hooker, 1986; Hooker & Freeborn, 1991).

Because PAs are cost-effective in the delivery of primary care services, two of the largest employers of PAs—the federal government and HMOs—have incorporated PAs and similar healthcare providers in clinical staffing. Managed care health delivery systems using PAs and similar providers gain certain economic advantages by using a team approach. HMOs are ideally suited to employ PAs and NPs because of the nature of preventive care, by stressing health education and disease prevention, and by carefully integrating primary care and specialty care.

EXHIBIT 6-13

Full-Time Equivalent Provider per 100,000 Enrollees in Group/Staff Model Health Maintenance Organizations

Providers	No. of Enrollees	
	45,000–100,000 (12 plans)	More than 100,000 (16 plans)
Total physicians	118.7	122.6
Primary care physicians	68.8	59.1
Specialty care physicians	49.9	63.5
Physician assistants	10.6	11.2
Nurse practitioners	15.0	14.6
Other advanced practice nurses	6.3	2.3

Data from Dial, T. H., et al. (1995). Clinical staffing in staff- and group-model HMOs. Health Affairs (Millwood) 14(2), 168–180.

ISSUES AND NEW ROLES OF PHYSICIAN ASSISTANTS IN PRIMARY CARE

House Calls

Although the era of house calls by physicians may be remembered by a diminishing number of people in the United States, they still occur, but in different forms. In Las Vegas, for example, a group of two physicians, six PAs, and one NP use vans to visit patients. Two-thirds of the patients are seniors, and most of the visits are scheduled. Many of the patients are established with the group and prefer the ambulatory service coming to them instead of having to journey to the medical office. Most services are reimbursed by Medicare (Swann, 2000).

Referrals to Specialists

Referring is an important activity in primary care, but is poorly understood. The referral may help bring an episode of care to a conclusion, such as a referral to an ear surgeon to place tubes in the tympanic membrane for chronic recurrent otitis media. It can also represent an alternative to treatment, such as a referral to physical therapy for acute shoulder tendinitis when the patient declines a shoulder injection. However, not all insurance carriers want their providers to liberally refer, and not all specialists openly welcome referrals from PAs.

To begin understanding referrals by PAs, Enns, Muma, and Lary (2000) surveyed 500 primary care PAs across the United States about their referral practices and perceived barriers to referrals (Exhibit 6-14). They found that 71% of respondents identified barriers to referral of patients to specialists and 86% were satisfied with their level of autonomy in making referrals. The most frequently identified barrier (38%) was the patient's insurance company. This is not an unexpected finding, considering the managed care environment in which medicine is practiced in the United States. In addition, the longer the PA was in practice the fewer barriers were perceived by the PA. The high degree of autonomy expressed by the surveyed PAs may reflect the level of confidence that

EXHIBIT 6-14
Weekly Patient Referrals by Physician Assistants to a Specialist and to the Supervising Physician

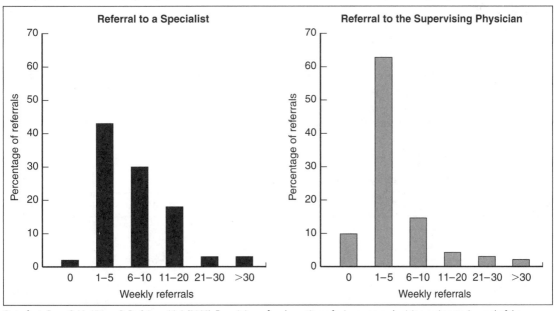

Data from Enns, S. M., Muma R. D., & Lary, M. J. (2000). Examining referral practices of primary care physician assistants. Journal of the American Academy of Physician Assistants, 13*(5), 81–82, 84, 86, 118.*

supervising physicians have in the PA's ability to make appropriate decisions regarding referrals.

Clearly the interactions between specialist physicians and primary care providers can result in improved patient outcomes. Subspecialists and primary care physicians have complementary roles to play in this form of chronic disease management. One examination found that the outcome of postmyocardial infarction care was better for patients for whom both primary care physicians and subspecialists provided care than for patients seen by specialists alone or primary physicians alone (Ayanian et al, 2002). Whether or not interaction between primary care PAs and specialty physicians would result in similar beneficial outcomes is not known and requires further investigation.

A CRISIS IN PRIMARY CARE?

Near the end of the 20th century, many medical leaders considered primary care to be in crisis. The American College of Physicians stated in 2006 that "primary care, the backbone of the nation's health care system, is at grave risk of collapse" (American College of Physicians, 2006).

The reason for this crisis, in part, is the ever-dwindling number and percent of doctors selecting general internal medicine, general pediatrics, and family medicine as careers. Like NP and PA education, family practice residency training capacity expanded significantly in the later part of the 20th century.

Positions in family practice residency programs increased 34%, from 2,393 in 1990 to 3,206 in 2000 (Exhibit 6-15). However, since that time, the trend in primary care has steadily decreased. The number of newly garduating medical students choosing primary care residency positions has declined significantly. Fewer young physicians are choosing residency training that leads to careers in primary care (Goodman, 2008; Phillips et al, 2009).

The 2007 national "fill rate" for family medicine residency programs was 2,313 positions filled out of 2,621 positions offered (88%). This finding represents an increase in the percentage of family medicine residency positions filled through the National Residency Matching Program (NRMP) over 2006. Included in this category are family medicine-psychiatry and internal medicine-family medicine programs. Compared with 2006, 106 fewer family medicine positions (3.8%) were offered in 2007, and 5 fewer positions (0.2%) were filled in 2007 compared with 2006 (2,313 [88.2%] vs. 2,318 [85.0%]) (American Academy of Family Physicians, 2007).

Fewer U.S. medical school graduates are filling family medicine training slots. In 2007, for the 10th consecutive year, a smaller percentage of U.S. seniors participating and matching through the NRMP matched into family medicine in comparison with the previous year, although this trend started to slow in 2002.

Anecdotes about primary care physicians leaving practice are plentiful, although we lack documentation that the rate of exodus is increasing. A field is in trouble when the number of practitioners is getting smaller while the demand for services remains strong (Sox, 2003).

EXHIBIT 6-15
Trends in Family Medicine Residency Positions, Selected Years

	1995	1998	2000	2004	2007
Family practice residency positions offered	2,941	3,293	3,206	2,884	2,621
Family practice residency positions filled	2,563	2,814	2,603	2,273	2,313
Percent filled	87.1%	85.5%	81.2%	78.8%	88.2%
U.S. medical school graduates	2,081	2,179	1,833	1,198	1,107
Percent with U.S. medical school graduates	70.8%	66.2%	57.2%	41.5%	42.2%

Data from American Academy of Family Physicians. (2007a). National Residency Matching Program. Retrieved March 8, 2008, from http://www.aafp.org/online/en/home/residents/match.html.

There are multiple interacting reasons for physician disaffection with primary care practice (Moore & Showstack, 2003). Income is a major reason for the declining attractiveness of careers in primary care. Primary care physicians earn less than specialists, even though they work longer hours than physicians in some better-paid specialties. Increased workload is another issue raised by primary care physicians. These physicians are working harder to meet their payroll and maintain their income despite lower payment rates. Modern physicians want more time with family and seek a more circumscribed professional and personal life. Physician groups have reorganized practice to respond to these needs, but it is hard to overcome the perception of the primary physician who is always on call. Satisfaction with practice is falling as the complexity of the primary care physician's work day increases. Whereas the length of the primary care office encounter increased slightly between 1989 and 1998, physicians also indicate that increasing administrative requirements and the needs of sicker patients leave less time for effective patient communication (Mechanic, 2001).

Because of the pressing need for primary care clinicians and the potential for increasing access while containing labor costs, the role of the primary care PA is generally believed to be secure for the near term. Health policies determining the future of the healthcare workforce are dictating that PAs and other nonphysician providers need to be part of the labor force mix.

Other experts agree that forces in medicine spell a confluence of factors that represents "disaster" for the future of primary care, noting that patients are increasingly dissatisfied with their care and with the difficulty of gaining timely access to a primary care physician. Primary care physicians, in turn, are unhappy with their jobs, as they face a seemingly insurmountable task. The quality of care is uneven, reimbursement is inadequate, and fewer U.S. medical students are choosing to enter the field (Bodenheimer, 2006).

The majority of patients prefer to seek initial care from a primary care physician rather than a specialist (Grumbach et al, 1999a). Primary care physicians are expressing frustration that

the knowledge and skills they are expected to master exceed the limits of human capability, making it impossible to provide the best care to every patient (Østbye et al, 2005). The scope of primary care extends from uncomplicated upper respiratory and urinary tract infections to the longitudinal care of elderly patients with diabetes, coronary heart disease, arthritis, and depression, who may also have limited proficiency in English.

Reimbursement based primarily on the quantity of services delivered, rather than on quality, forces primary care physicians onto a treadmill, devaluing their professional work life. The short, rushed visits with overfilled agendas that cause patient dissatisfaction simultaneously breed frustration among physicians. The suggested solution to remedy the declining status of primary care among physicians is to create greater financial incentives. Given modern trends to cut rather than increase physician reimbursement rates, however, such a solution seems improbable.

Thus, it appears that physicians are likely to continue to avoid primary care and that the 70% to 30% imbalance in physician specialty distribution will only worsen. If doctors are abandoning primary care, and if PAs are following a similar path, who will provide primary care services for the population? Advanced practice nurses have declared themselves to be fully capable of stepping into this practice area and have taken steps to secure this niche (Mundinger, 2004).

Research and Primary Care

The literature about the deployment of PAs in primary care is limited. We offer a brief review of areas in need of attention.

- **Case reports:** Writing about PAs in primary care provides a PA in training an idea of what a primary care PA does and what a typical day is like.

- **Role delineation:** Role delineation studies are needed every 5 years or so to identify the skill sets and activities of PAs. These studies need to be undertaken for all types of primary care PAs, including those in urban and rural settings, in large multispecialty clinics, and solo practices. The Physician Assistant National Recertification Exam (PANRE) and PANCE are developed by these role delineation studies.

- **Organizational arrangements:** How do large multispecialty groups arrange the care of a defined population and utilize PAs? What are the trade-offs organizations make in employing PAs and NPs? What are the overlaps in care by doctors, PAs, and NPs in the same setting?

- **Economics:** What is the ratio of compensation to revenue of various types of primary care PAs? Is there an ideal ratio of primary care PA to doctor for a given size population? What is the substitution ratio of PAs to doctors?

- **Breadth of knowledge:** How does a primary care PA obtain his or her knowledge set once in practice? Does the acquisition of knowledge have different trajectories depending on age, gender, and experience?

- **Career selection:** Do PAs in primary care have different expectations and aspirations than those in specialty practices?

- **Procedures:** What are the procedures that a PA in primary care needs to know?

- **Patient satisfaction:** How do patients of primary care PAs perceive the quality of care received?

- **Retention:** What are the factors that contribute to retention or attrition of PAs in primary care?

- **Education:** What are the links between training in primary care and patient outcomes?

SUMMARY

PAs have displayed an impressive track record in primary care. This has been accomplished through role delineation studies guiding the education process, and physicians who are willing to apprentice assistants in their offices and places of practice. For decades PAs have shown themselves to be safe and capable providers of primary care services. Despite the success of the PA, it remains a challenge for practices to attract enough of these providers to rural and other needy areas. Where there were once clear barriers to their full practice effectiveness, there is now the recognition by state boards, insurance carriers, and physician groups of the vital roles that PAs play in the delivery of primary care health services.

The PA profession has determined that primary care should remain the cornerstone for PA education. A report published by the AAPA states that the PA profession should remain rooted in its primary care foundation, with an emphasis on lifelong learning. Although PAs do work in specialty areas, the generalist basis of their education remains critically important to their future. Lifelong learning is an important component of PA education. The healthcare system is rapidly changing; a commitment to continuous lifelong learning is a way for PAs to enhance the value they bring to physician practices as well as the health system at large (Benjamin et al, 1999).

By the end of 2008 there were at least 110,000 NPs who held an NP license and close to 71,000 PAs certified to work in clinical practice. These providers, along with family physicians, general internists, and general pediatricians, comprise the U.S. primary care workforce, yet there remains little planning or coordination among the professions in terms of meeting health system and societal needs for primary care services. Family physicians, NPs, and PAs have complementary and interdependent functions that are important to primary care. PAs always work with physicians, as do most NPs. Despite this functional interdependence, since 1990 there has been tremendous growth in the production capacity of all three professions without joint workforce planning. The AAFP's Robert Graham Center for Policy Studies in Family Practice and Primary Care identified the issue of the uncoordinated growth of the U.S. primary care workforce noting that family physicians, NPs, and PAs are distinctly different in their clinical training, yet they function interdependently. Together, they represent a significant portion of the primary care workforce.

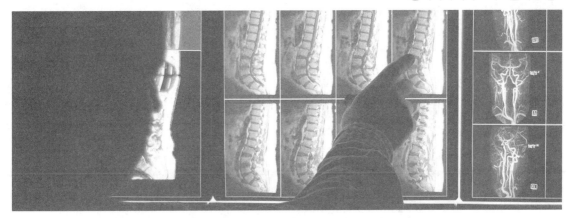

CHAPTER 7

PHYSICIAN ASSISTANT SPECIALIZATION: NONPRIMARY CARE

RODERICK S. HOOKER ■ JAMES F. CAWLEY ■ DAVID P. ASPREY

Specialization is a feature of every complex organization, be it social or natural, a school system, garden, book, or mammalian body.
—*Catharine R. Stimpson, U.S. scholar and educator, 1992*

ABSTRACT

Although the primary care role of the physician assistant (PA) is the root of the profession and remains the basis of PA education, the profession has undergone increased specialization since the mid-1990s, primarily as a result of economic pressures. One of the major rationales for the development of the PA profession was to augment the supply of medically trained providers in those specialties in greatest need of assistance. The diversity of employment settings is an indication of the maturity of the profession. These areas of specialty mix represent the significant employment opportunities and offer expanded roles for PAs.

Specialty pathways involve PA residencies, master's degrees in clinical and nonclinical disciplines, and entry into other fields through experience and formal training. Many PAs enjoy membership status in physician specialty societies or professional specialties of their own making. Narrowly focused medical and surgical roles will remain an important component of the PA profession.

INTRODUCTION

The profession of medicine is broadly divided into two disciplines: medicine and surgery. Like tree branches, these disciplines then divide into numerous specialties and subspecialties. This chapter follows a similar format. The trunk is the basis of specialities and the main branches are surgery and medicine. Smaller branches describe the different surgical and medical specialities.

From the earliest days of physician assistant (PA) development, the medical profession recognized their value and employed them in a diverse number of disciplines. Although approximately 40% of all PAs are in primary care, almost one-quarter of PAs are involved in a surgical practice (general surgery, orthopedics, cardiovascular surgery, or some other surgical activity). Another quarter have roles in medical disciplines such as cardiology, nephrology, oncology, rheumatology, hematology, pulmonology, and gastroenterology. Smaller branches produce the disciplines of radiology (diagnostic and interventional), pathology, and psychiatry. Postgraduate programs have sprung up to accommodate PAs who wish to have additional training in various areas of medical care.

The wave of specialization that has swept over the medical profession over the past 50 years is exerting its effects on the PA profession. Specialization, seemingly an inexorable phenomenon, has influenced the practice of medicine in profound ways, from the demise of the American general practitioner to the rise of a Byzantine world of specialty and subspecialty societies, examination processes, certification systems, and credentialing arrangements.

Some would observe that it was only a matter of time before specialization would transform the PA profession just as it has that of physicians. In 1972, Ann A. Bliss wrote that "immediately upon graduation, the physician's assistant (*sic*) is in considerable danger of being swallowed whole by the whale that is our present entrepreneurial subspecialty medical practice system. The likely co-option of the newly-minted physician's assistant by subspecialty medicine is one of the most serious issues confronting the PA" (Sadler, Sadler, & Bliss, 1972). Although Bliss believed that this "danger" would occur much sooner than it has, it appears that the time of reckoning with specialization has finally arrived.

The raison d'être of the PA profession was to provide basic medical services to populations that were underserved or that did not receive any care. Although this is fully recounted in the history of the profession (see Chapter 2), the original intention of Eugene Stead, Richard Smith, and Harvey Estes in creating the profession is not fully appreciated. They envisioned these new practitioners as assistants to doctors in a very general and literal sense; they did not confine the activities of PAs to working only with primary care physicians (Hooker, 2009). Estes intended that PAs would provide a wide number of services

for physicians in all types of medical practice (Estes, 1993). The original Duke curriculum, for example, not only provided training in performing and interpreting electrocardiograms, but also gave instructions on how the machine could be repaired if broken. In many ways, the development of specialities occurred with the first PA class at Duke as students were taught barometric pressure medicine. Thus, the original design of the Medex and Duke programs was that the PA would perform medical tasks—some involving diagnosis and therapeutic management and some involving technical and routine procedures. This training relieved the busy doctor and allowed him or her more time for continuing professional education, dealing with complex patient illnesses, and seeing more patients (Estes, 1968b). Both models trained PAs as all-purpose generalist assistants to doctors. This concept became markedly altered as the PA movement gained momentum in the early 1970s.

Another movement in specialization that took place in the late 1960s was a surge of new programs to train nonphysician providers in certain specialty areas of medicine. It was a time of experimentation. Some of these programs included the orthopedic assistant and the urological physician's assistant, which were 2-year programs designed to train personnel to work directly for specialists. Another experiment was the 4-month "health assistants" training program sponsored by Project Hope in Laredo, Texas. The only requirement was that the student be 18 years of age and be interested in health care. Of the 11 students who entered the first class, 8 lacked high school equivalence but were able to earn their general equivalency diploma certificate upon completion of the program (Sadler, Sadler, & Bliss, 1972). Other programs of various training missions and duration were developed in gastroenterology, allergy, dermatology, and radiology. None survived past 1975, with the exception of the surgical assistant, the pathologists' assistant, and the child health associate programs. In a health profession that was once comprised of mostly generalist clinicians and that for several decades was roughly evenly balanced between primary care providers and specialists, the trend has now gradually shifted to the majority of U.S. PAs working in specialties. This trend brings with it good and bad aspects for the PA profession. It is worth exploring a few of the implications of these trends as they affect PAs.

In an historic sense, specialization in medicine would appear to be an inexorable phenomenon. Medical specialization emerged in the 19th century as a result of expanding medical knowledge and the notion that patients could be best managed through grouping patients, providers, and diseases into specific categories. Specialization was influenced by factors such as disease prevalence, advances in medical knowledge, and the use of technology, and it became well established throughout the 20th century as more and more groups of physicians formed specialty societies and formal certification processes.

Among the first of these specializations was ophthalmology, which emerged in 1916. Later, between 1974 and 1992, 28 new specialties and subspecialties came to be recognized by the Accreditation Council for Graduate Medical Education (ACGME). Today, ACGME recognizes 26 physician specialties and 84 subspecialties. Specialization is a compelling force in medicine and medical practice, and it is not at all surprising that the PA profession has been influenced by this movement.

Within the PA profession, specialty mix began at an early stage, marked by the founding of specialty-focused educational programs in pediatrics and surgery in the late 1960s and the establishment of a surgical postgraduate program in 1972. For many years, largely due to the influence of federal funding dollars, the direction of the profession took a marked turn toward primary care, and in the late 1970s a majority of PAs worked in family medicine. But as the profession evolved and grew in the 1980s and 1990s, specialization increased as increasing numbers of PAs entered specialty practices. This, in turn, led to the formation of an increasing number of specific specialty and subspecialty societies within the American

Academy of Physician Assistants (AAPA) and increasing numbers of postgraduate educational programs.

These trends have continued, and as the number of PAs in specialties has increased, the numbers in primary care have consequently declined. A majority of practicing PAs are now in specialties. According to the 2008 AAPA Physician Assistant Census Report, the percentage of PAs working in primary care specialties fell to the lowest levels recorded in the past several decades. Only 37% of the nation's 73,500-plus PAs in active clinical practice work in the areas of family medicine (24%), general internal medicine (7%), obstetrics and gynecology (2%), or general pediatrics (2%); less than a third of all new PA graduates now enter primary care fields. This trend is in contrast to the fact one-quarter (25%) of PAs work in surgery and the surgical subspecialties and more than 10% work in emergency medicine (AAPA, 2008a).

FACTORS INFLUENCING PHYSICIAN ASSISTANT SPECIALIZATION

The decline in interest of PAs in primary care practice parallels that of physicians, whose numbers in primary care also have been falling. Fewer medical school graduates are selecting residencies in the primary care specialties, and physicians worry aloud that in the future primary care will be lost to other types of providers.

For the PA profession, the decline in the numbers in primary care runs counter to long-held traditions and priorities for PAs to serve in generalist practice and in medically underserved communities. It is difficult for PA educational programs to maintain an emphasis on primary care practice for PAs when the economic and market forces pull increasing numbers of graduates to specialties.

Organizationally, specialization within the PA profession has, as would be expected, spurred the founding of a number of specialty and subspecialty organizations, most of which are still closely aligned with the AAPA. The challenge is to retain these groups under the big tent of the AAPA because many of these specialty groups hold their own meetings and continuing medical education programs, and they may even develop their own certification structure.

Because PAs are employed by physicians and emulate physician behavior in many ways, it is not surprising that they would move into specialty practices. Most of the trends observed among physicians are also seen in PA specialization, including the trend to work in a nonprimary care role and the increase in wages that specialization brings (Exhibit 7-1).

As the profession evolved, PAs were attracted to many roles in medicine. Today, the profession is composed of a broad array of primary care and nonprimary care PAs. Why this occurred has only been theorized. Hooker (1992) hypothesized that PAs probably respond to the same forces that shape physician specialty choices: the training process, the specialty that fits the lifestyle and geographic preferences of the physician, and market forces (Exhibit 7-2). Genova (1995) examined the influence of market forces on PA practice settings in Maine and concluded that (at least there) the market was weaker for primary care PAs than for the services of specialty care PAs. Cawley and colleagues (2000), examining new graduate employment, showed that the specialty distribution of new graduates closely resembles that of the entire profession and the

market has the same influence on new graduates as experienced PAs. Finally, the 2007 AAPA Census Report suggests that the earnings of PAs in many specialties tends to track more or less with the earnings of doctors in various specialites (Morgan & Hooker, 2009).

In approaching the issue of specialization, we divide this chapter on nonprimary care PAs into surgical and nonsurgical specialties. As noted, PAs who participate in surgery or work in the surgical specialties represent a significant component of PA practice. Their history begins shortly after the formal PA was created. The remainder of the chapter is devoted to many of the nonsurgical disciplines. Information for this chapter is from public reports, published studies, or conversations with PAs in these roles.

Physician Assistants in Specialties and Subspecialties

Exhibit 7-3 is a list of some of the clinical practice specialties and subspecialties in which PAs are used. The list is far from complete.

Increasing demand for and use of PAs in specialized roles tends to fluctuate as the result of many factors (supply and demand being the leading factor). However, the presence of PAs in medical subspecialty areas has expanded considerably since 1980. Specialty practice areas expected to remain strong for PAs in nonprimary care roles include

EXHIBIT 7-1
Physician Assistants, Specialty Groups: Trends, by Percent, 1997–2008

Specialty	1997	1998	1999	2000	2001	2002	2003	2004	2005	2006	2007	2008
Family/general medicine	38.4	39.6	38.0	36.5	34.5	32.1	30.9	29.5	28.4	26.5	23.8	25.9
General internal medicine	8.9	8.5	9.2	8.8	8.5	8.4	7.8	7.8	7.6	7.1	6.4	5.2
Emergency medicine	9.8	9.5	9.9	9.7	10.1	10.2	10.0	9.9	9.7	9.7	11.5	10.5
General pediatrics	2.7	2.9	2.8	2.6	2.6	2.6	2.7	2.5	2.5	2.5	2.2	2.5
General surgery	3.1	2.8	2.8	2.7	2.5	2.5	2.6	2.8	2.8	2.7	3.0	2.5
Internal medicine subspecialties	6.2	6.4	6.9	8.1	8.6	9.4	9.5	9.8	10.3	11.1	10.0	7.2
Pediatric subspecialties	1.5	1.3	1.4	1.5	1.4	1.5	1.3	1.5	1.5	1.5	1.4	1.8
Surgical subspecialties	15.7	16.3	16.8	17.4	18.4	19.2	20.4	21.1	21.9	22.2	22.2	22.6
Obstetrics and gynecology	2.7	2.7	2.4	2.7	2.5	2.7	2.8	2.6	2.4	2.3	2.1	2.3
Occupational medicine	3.3	3.4	3.4	3.5	3.6	3.0	2.7	2.4	2.4	2.4	2.4	3.6
Other	7.9	6.6	6.4	6.5	7.4	8.4	9.3	10.2	10.5	11.6	12.8	10.4

Data from American Academy of Physician Assistants, AAPA Census Reports 1997–2008.

EXHIBIT 7-2
The Effect of the Education Process on Physician Assistant Specialty and Location

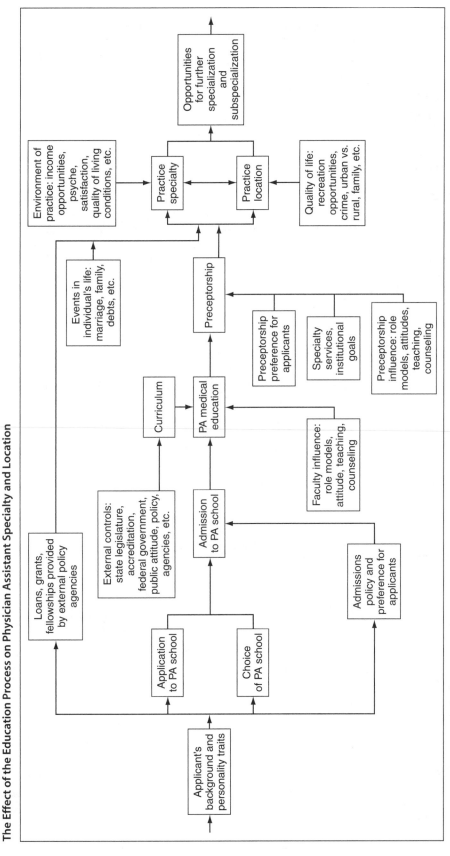

Data from Hooker, R. S. (1992). Employment specialization in the PA profession. Journal of the American Academy of Physician Assistants, 5(8), 695–704.

EXHIBIT 7-3
Partial Listing of Nonprimary Care Areas Employing Physician Assistants

Allergy	Neonatology
Anesthesiology	Neurosurgery
Cardiothoracic surgery	Obstetrics and gynecology
Clinical research	Occupational health
Critical care units	Oncology (including pediatric oncology)
Dermatology	Ophthalmology
Emergency medicine	Organ procurement and transplantation
Forensic medicine and pathology	Orthopedics and sports medicine
Gastroenterology and endoscopy	Otorhinolaryngology (head and neck surgery)
Gerontology	Physical medicine and rehabilitation
Hematology	Plastic surgery and burn care
Infectious disease and immune deficiency	Public health
Interventional radiology	Rheumatology
Invasive cardiology	Substance abuse
Mental health and psychiatry	Urology
Preventive medicine	

emergency medicine, cardiovascular surgery, orthopedic surgery, dermatology, and a large number of internal medicine subspecialties.

Another factor at work is the demand for medical labor at a time when medical education is expanding. The trend of using PAs—sometimes as replacements for residents—raises several policy issues in healthcare workforce planning. When the resident work week was restricted to 80 hours, a significant effect on the use of PAs in hospital settings was observed with the number of PAs being employed. The most immediate effect was that between the years 2000 and 2006 the number of hospital-based PAs increased by nearly one-third (Cawley & Hooker, 2006).

Other reasons for PAs shifting into specialty roles include an unfilled niche for a provider in a particular specialty or a physician specifically inviting and directing the PA into this specialty. The result of program growth has been because there is demand for PAs. This growth is illustrated in a brief encapsulation of the PA phenomenon in the United States (Exhibit 7-4).

Factors Influencing Specialty Choice

What factors influence or lead PAs to choose a particular specialty or practice? In 2008, the level of debt of newly graduating PAs must be

a strong determinant of specialty choice, just as it is for graduating medical students. Beyond this factor, why PAs choose a particular specialty is only partially known. Clearly,

EXHIBIT 7-4
Growth of Select Physician Assistant Specialities

Specialty	1997	2001	2007
Total PAs	31,480	42,708	63,609
Family/general medicine	12,088	14,734	16,858
General internal medicine	2,802	3,630	4,516
Emergency medicine	3,085	4,314	6,170
General pediatrics	850	1,110	1,590
General surgery	976	1,068	1,717
Internal medicine subspecialties	1,952	3,673	7,061
Pediatric subspecialties	472	598	954
Surgical subspecialties	4,942	7,858	14,212
Obstetrics and gynecology	850	1,068	1,527
Occupational medicine	1,039	1,537	1,527
Other	2,487	3,160	7,506

Data from American Academy of Physician Assistants, 2006 survey, reported in 2007.

employment opportunities play a significant role, but studies show that differences between primary care and nonprimary care PAs do exist. For PAs in nonprimary care roles the most influential factors determining specialty choice are technical orientation and income (or employment). These factors seem to differ from PAs in primary care, who identify prevention, academic environment, debt/scholarship, intellectual content, and peer influence as influencing factors (Singer & Hooker, 1996) (Exhibit 7-5).

SURGICAL PHYSICIAN ASSISTANTS

It seems that early in the development of PAs, doctors' attitudes about surgical PAs were positive (Legler, 1983). With cost-containment, surgical residencies going unfilled, advancements

in surgical techniques, and increasing acceptance of PAs and surgical assistants, the field of surgery for PAs is likely to continue to grow because of the growing shortage of surgeons (Exhibit 7-6).

Meeting the educational needs and requirements of surgical residents has been a challenge for postgraduate program directors. Balancing resident training while achieving optimal patient care requires collaborative measures. In one large community teaching hospital, a group of PAs and nurse practitioners (NPs) were employed to improve continuity of care and to augment the surgical teaching service by giving resident surgeons the flexibility to participate in classroom, operative, and clinical educational experiences. The PAs and NPs were integrated into the surgical program by creating a supportive environment in which the administrative

EXHIBIT 7-5

Mean Scores for Factors Influencing Specialty Choice of Physician Assistants Who Choose or Did Not Choose Primary Care in Their First Practice Year

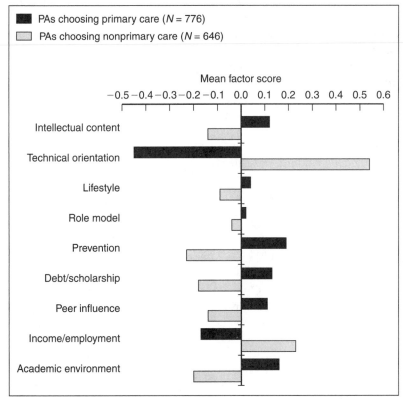

Data from Singer, A. M., & Hooker, R. S. (1996). Determinants of specialty choice of physician assistants. Academic Medicine: Journal of the Association of American Medical Colleges, 71(8), 917–919.

EXHIBIT 7-6
Physician Assistant in Surgery

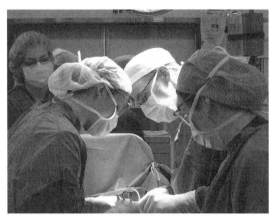

Courtesy of Linda Kortora, American Association of Surgical PAs.

leadership stated approval of the use of PAs and NPs, developing positive relationships, decreasing resistance, and rewarding those who demonstrated acceptance of the PA and NP team members. Technically, the PAs and NPs functioned at the level of a junior resident physician and participated in the teaching process. Instituting the program required providing financial justification to administration and flexibility in meeting diverse needs of the stakeholders. As a result, the surgical resident was freed from service activities and instead capitalized on learning activities that ranged from surgeries to conferences. The authors concluded that the integration of PAs and NPs was a positive force in enhancing resident education (Reines et al, 2006).

Other studies were along a similar line of observation but with some qualification. Resnick and colleagues (2006) examined the results of the introduction of PAs and NPs into service teams with residents. A total of one to three PAs and/or NPs were hired for each of four surgical teams at a large hospital. Overall, 63% of residents believed that lines of communication between surgery team members were clear, and 58% of residents and 71% of PAs and NPs believed that attending faculty, residents, and PAs or NPs worked together effectively. A total of 91% of residents believed that the addition of PAs and NPs to the teams was positive overall, and 80% of the PAs and NPs were satisfied with their positions (Resnick et al, 2006).

The distribution of PAs in surgery continues to grow, with orthopedics being the leading specialty, followed by cardiothoracic surgery (Exhibit 7-7). For many observers this growth seems characteristic of the market forces because of the scarcity of surgeons. Because the occupational projections for doctors, PAs, and NPs is not growing faster than demand, this shifting into better paying careers for PAs is likely to continue (Morgan & Hooker, 2009).

Cardiovascular and Thoracic Surgery

Cardiovascular surgery and thoracic surgery are separate surgical specialties but are frequently grouped together as cardiothoracic surgery (primarily in the United States). Cardiovascular surgery generally refers to surgery of the heart and great vessels, and thoracic surgery generally refers to surgery of the chest other than the heart.

Role

The role of PAs in cardiovascular and thoracic surgery ranges from first assisting in surgery to providing preoperative and postoperative care in the hospital and seeing patients in the medical office. Responsibilities include performing a complete pulmonary and circulatory examination, explaining the surgical procedure to the patient and family members, and answering their questions. PAs may insert and remove vascular lines and monitoring devices, such as Swan-Ganz catheters and arterial lines; insert

EXHIBIT 7-7
Distribution of Surgical Physician Assistants, 2007

Surgical Specialty	% of Total PA Population	% of Surgical PA Population	Total Number
Orthopedics	10.6	43	6,900
Cardiovascular and thoracic surgery	3.2	13	2,100
General surgery	2.7	11	1,750
Neurosurgery	2.5	10	1,625
All other surgical subspecialties*	5.8	23	3,800

*For example: oncology, otorhinolaryngology, pediatrics, plastic surgery, transplant, trauma, urology, vascular surgery, and bariatric surgery.

Data from American Academy of Physician Assistants, 2006 survey, reported in 2007.

and remove wound drains; and regulate the metabolic needs of the patient. Procedures include heart or lung transplantation, liver transplantation, and routine heart procedures. Technical skills involve placing and monitoring intra-aortic balloon pumps, right and left ventricular assist devices, cardiopulmonary support systems, and extracorporeal membrane oxygenators. At least 10% of PAs specializing in cardiovascular and thoracic surgery are also certified clinical perfusionists, and may operate heart-lung machines. Another important task of the cardiovascular and thoracic surgery PA is harvesting the saphenous veins for coronary artery bypass grafting (Chaffee, 1988).

PAs have been working alongside vascular surgeons since the first Duke class was enrolled in 1965 (Cooper & Willig, 1971; Rothwell, 1993). From 1970 to 1974, a program at the Oregon Health Sciences University in Portland trained approximately 15 PAs in cardiovascular surgery and other disciplines.

Postoperatively, cardiothoracic PAs manage the patient in the intensive care unit (ICU) and the hospital wards, and watch for early postsurgical complications. Providing optimal patient care includes managing the patient's surgical condition as well as other disease processes the patient may have, such as hypertension and diabetes. Other roles include overseeing cardiac rehabilitation, teaching about diet, and discharging the patient. The PAs' involvement with the patients continues in the form of answering telephone calls regarding their concerns after returning home and seeing them in the office for postoperative visits (Gray, 1997).

History
Only a few studies have examined the safety of cardiothoracic PAs. In one 3-year retrospective examination of 1,226 central venous cannulations in 732 patients undertaken by PAs in a vascular surgery section of Geisinger Medical Center, seven patients experienced a pneumothorax as a complication. Six of the seven procedures were performed by different PAs. Although statistics were not included for physicians, the less than 1% incident of pneumothorax for this procedure is considered low compared with the 4% overall major complication rate of surgical house officers, anesthesiologists, and other house officers (Marsters, 2000).

At Yale University the number of PAs in cardiothoracic surgery increased from 2 (in 1973) to 23 (in 2003). PA employment expanded from one to five hospitals, and the service expanded from 300 to 4,000 cases per year. In spite of this expansion, the PA role of taking histories, performing physical examinations, harvesting veins, inserting invasive cathethers and chest tubes, assisting in surgery, closing the chest, providing optimal ICU management, and providing nighttime in-house call changed very little. The authors conclude that the addition of PAs has allowed this university service to resolve many staffing problems and improve the safety and efficiency of the surgical teams without increasing the number of residents (Marsters, 2000).

A survey of cardiovascular and vascular PAs in 2000 found that the average surgical practice had three to six (average five) PAs and five to six (average five) surgeons. Sixty-seven percent of the 572 PA respondents were based in private practice, 16% in universities, 7% in hospitals, 3% in health maintenance organizations (HMOs), 3% in clinics, and 2% in the military. In the practices that employed a PA, other providers were employed as well: registered nurses (RNs) (52%), NPs (26%), resident physicians (20%), RN first assistants (RNFAs) (15%), and nonsurgeon physicians (10%). Those most often involved in preoperative care and evaluation consultations were PAs (71%), followed by NPs (15%), RNs (13%), nonsurgeon physicians (7%), certified surgical technicians CSTs (5%), and RNFAs (4%). Other settings in which PAs were used included postoperative ICU care, postoperative care on the ward, and outpatient care (Lee et al, 2000).

Profile

In a survey undertaken by the AAPA, 775 PAs in cardiothoracic surgery responded (Exhibit 7-8). The average age was 40. Females were 49% of the cohort, and 24% worked in a single specialty physician group practice. Almost all (95%) worked in an urban setting. The majority (94%) worked full time (greater than or equal to 32 hours per week) and 89% were salary-based. The average salary was $110,468 and all received bonuses and overtime (AAPA, 2008a).

Professional Society

The Association of Physician Assistants in Cardiovascular Surgery (APACVS) includes PAs who participate in the surgical treatment of cardiovascular disease that encompasses three specialty areas: general thoracic surgery, surgery for congenital heart disease, and surgery for acquired heart disease. The APACVS began in 1981 as an educational organization and represents the professional interests of the CVPA. The primary objectives are to promote the clinical and academic excellence of its members, and enhance the quality of medical care to their patients. Today, the APACVS is the educational, scientific, and political subspecialty organization representative of surgical PAs practicing in the field of cardiovascular and thoracic surgery. With over 700 members, the APACVS

EXHIBIT 7-8
Cardiovascular or Cardiothoracic Physician Assistants, 2008

Total respondents	775
Age (mean years)	40
Females	375 (49%)
Solo physician practitioner	13 (2%)
Single specialty physician group practice	187 (24%)
Multispecialty physician group practice	94 (12%)
Hospital	423 (55%)
Years in clinical practice	11
Work in urban setting	95%
Precept PA students	48%
Percent who work more than 32 hours per week	94%
Mean income	$110,468

Data from American Academy of Physician Assistants. (2008a). 2008 AAPA Physician Assistant Census Report. Alexandria, VA: Author.

is recognized and endorsed by the Society of Thoracic Surgeons and the American Association for Thoracic Surgeons. Their website is http://www.apacvs.org/. The American Academy of Surgical Physician Assistants maintains a website that opens its membership to CVPAs: https://www.aaspa.com/cts.asp.

General Surgery

General surgery focuses on surgical treatment of abdominal organs such as the intestines (including esophagus, stomach, colon, liver, gallbladder, and bile ducts), the thyroid gland (depending on the availability of head and neck surgery specialists), hernias, and sometimes, the breast.

Role

PAs in general surgery assist in the operating room and provide preoperative and postoperative care to patients as members of surgical teams in hospital or outpatient settings. General surgery PAs may be the first assistant in the operating room, surgically opening access to the patient. They may close the patient's wound and then follow the patient into the surgical ICU or recovery area, where they may write the orders for a patient's immediate care and accompany the doctor on rounds. Perioperative PAs may dictate the operative report, insert and remove monitoring devices, and regulate the pharmaceutical needs of the patient (Stahlfield, Robinson, & Burton, 2008). Other roles include placing and removing temporary pacemakers; applying and removing casts, sutures, and skin clips; and relieving the surgeon of many routine matters. Some PAs in general surgery work exclusively in pediatrics; others in gastrointestinal (GI) diseases. Some serve as permanently employed staff working closely with the chief resident in surgery to maintain continuity of care for residents (Todd et al, 2004). Their ability to reduce the workload of surgeons in training (residents) has been significant during the period the 80-hour work week was initiated in the United States (Gordon, 2006; Reines et al, 2006; Stahlfield, Robinson, & Burton, 2008).

In some instances general surgery PAs are employed by surgeons to be outpatient specialists. They work almost entirely in the office seeing preoperative and postoperative patients. The roles may include undertaking physical examinations; processing necessary insurance forms; communicating with the family, hospital, and surgical center; and changing dressings. Some of these PAs may provide an element of primary care in maintaining continuity of care.

History
The history of the PA in general surgery runs parallel to the history of the PA. Almost from the beginning of the Duke PA program, surgery and surgical experience were part of the curriculum. Because of cost containment, surgical residencies going unfilled, and advancements in surgical technique, the acceptance of surgical PAs and surgeons' assistants came easily.

Profile
In a survey undertaken by the AAPA, 636 PAs in surgery responded (Exhibit 7-9). The average age was 39. Females were 69% of the cohort, and one-half (52%) were employed by a hospital. Most (89%) worked in a large urban setting. The majority worked (89%) full time

(at least 32 hours per week). At least 77% were salary-based, but all received bonuses and overtime. The average salary in 2008 was $90,904 (AAPA, 2008a).

Professional Society
The American Association of Surgical Physician Assistants (AASPA) was originally established as the American Association of Surgeon Assistants by a group of surgical PAs in 1972 in spite of opposition from some primary care PAs that the PA profession, in the aggregate, would be fragmented. Surgical PAs, on the other hand, countered that they are fundamentally PAs and as such represent the diversifying interest of PAs. Presently, the AASPA maintains an active relationship with the AAPA as well as the American College of Surgeons (ACS). Their website is http://www.aaspa.com/.

Hospitalist
See Chapter 8 on the role of hospitalist PAs.

Neurosurgery
Neurosurgery is the surgical discipline focused on treating the central and peripheral nervous system and spinal column diseases amenable to mechanical intervention.

EXHIBIT 7-9
Surgical (General) Physician Assistants, 2008

Total survey respondents	636
Age (mean years)	39
Female	431 (69%)
Solo physician practice	31 (5%)
Single specialty physician group practice	87 (14%)
Multispecialty physician group practice	111 (18%)
Hospital	329 (52%)
Years in clinical practice	9
Work in urban setting	89%
Precept PA students	49%
Work more than 32 hours per week	89%
Mean income	$90,094

Data from American Academy of Physician Assistants. (2008a). 2008 AAPA Physician Assistant Census Report. Alexandria, VA: Author.

Role

The role of PAs in neurosurgery ranges from first assisting in surgery to providing preoperative and postoperative care and handling patients' medical office visits. Responsibilities also include performing a complete physical and neurological examination, explaining the surgical procedure to the patient and family members, and answering their questions (Sonntag, Steiner, & Stein, 1977). PAs in neurosurgery may insert and remove lines and monitoring devices, insert and remove drains, and regulate the medical needs of the patient (Andrews, 1999). Procedures include brain or peripheral nerve surgery, spinal cord surgery, and routine neurological procedures. Neurosurgical PAs sometimes perform certain procedures, such as carpal tunnel releases, on their own. They are involved in developing treatment plans for neurosurgical conditions within the scope of practice and in conjunction with the neurosurgeon as well as implementing therapeutic interventions for specific conditions when appropriate.

The neurosurgical PA commonly closes deep and superficial wounds and assists with all neurosurgical procedures including craniotomies, spinal procedures, fine instrumentation of nerves, and microscopic procedures. Neurosurgical PAs conduct hospital rounds of all patients, including those in ICUs, on a daily basis. Daily tasks may include writing orders and progress notes, performing admission histories and physical examinations, and ordering appropriate laboratory and imaging studies, such as magnetic resonance imaging (MRI), myelograms, and bone scans, as needed or indicated. Neurosurgical PAs also perform appropriate laboratory and diagnostic studies, such as lumbar punctures, ventriculostomies, and myelograms, and may place tong traction or halo fixation devices on the cranium. For the most part, neurosurgical PAs evaluate and clarify clinical conditions, formulate and implement a treatment and therapeutic plan for hospitalized patients, write discharge plans, and dictate discharge summaries (Odom, 1975).

Office duties for neurosurgical PAs include seeing new office patients and completing a thorough history and physical examination that is oriented for neurosurgical conditions. They present patients to the attending neurosurgeons, help formulate a treatment plan, order appropriate radiographic studies, and perform office procedures such as local blocks. Other roles include evaluating postoperative patients, handling routine follow-up visits, and being available to see those patients that require same-day office visits. They return phone calls from patients, handle prescription refills, review radiographic and laboratory reports for abnormalities, and review imaging studies with the attending neurosurgeon. Neurosurgical PAs also evaluate, screen, and counsel patients on health maintenance, and promote use of community resources.

Obtaining the necessary skills and expertise to be of value to a neurosurgical team requires time and training. A new graduate or someone without any neurosurgical experience works approximately 1 year to obtain the confidence in handling the day-to-day office and hospital routine.

History

Neurosurgery is a labor-intensive surgical subspecialty. It is not surprising that neurosurgical PAs have a role in this discipline. This surgical specialty tends to be in a high pay range for PAs, particularly when they first assist in lieu of another surgeon. In the late 1970s, a study indicated that the PA functions in an intern-equivalent capacity in neurosurgery. This study suggests that patient care and patient acceptance were improved overall (Sonntag, Steiner, & Stein, 1977).

Profile

In a survey undertaken by the AAPA, 587 PAs in neurosurgery responded (Exhibit 7-10). The average age was 39, females were 56% of the cohort, and 37% were employed by a hospital. Almost all (96%) worked in an urban setting. The majority (95%) worked full time (at least 32 hours per week) and 92% were salary-based. The average salary in 2008 was $98,024 (AAPA, 2008a).

EXHIBIT 7-10
Neurosurgery Physician Assistants, 2008

Total survey respondents	587
Age (mean years)	39
Female	325 (56%)
Single specialty physician group practice	193 (33%)
Multispecialty physician group practice	81 (14%)
Hospital	90 (37%)
Other practice	220 (16%)
Years in clinical practice	8
Work in urban setting	95%
Precept PA students	32%
Work more than 32 hours per week	95%
Mean income	$98,024

Data from American Academy of Physician Assistants. (2008a). 2008 AAPA Physician Assistant Census Report. Alexandria, VA: Author.

Professional Society

The AASPA includes neurosurgical PAs. Their website is http://www.aaspa.com/ns.asp.

Orthopedic Surgery

Orthopedic (also spelled orthopaedics) surgery is concerned with acute, chronic, traumatic, and overuse injuries and other disorders of the musculoskeletal system. Orthopedic surgeons manage most musculoskeletal ailments, including trauma, congenital deformities, and the effects of arthritis. The discipline uses surgical and nonsurgical interventions.

Role

The role of the formally trained orthopedic PA (graduate of an accredited PA program and eligible for certification by the National Commission on the Certification of Physician Assistants [NCCPA]) is varied. PAs who practice in orthopedics are licensed healthcare professionals who practice medicine and provide surgical services within the scope of practice of their supervising physician. They also exercise autonomy in diagnosing and treating bone and joint diseases and injuries.

In hospitals, some PAs work primarily in surgery as first assistant in joint reconstruction (Gordon, 2006). They may write preoperative and postoperative orders and may close deep and superficial wounds when assisting with surgical procedures (including joint reconstructions, joint prostheses, spinal procedures and instrumentations, and microscopic procedures). They conduct hospital rounds of all patients, including ICUs, on a daily basis. Tasks include writing orders and progress notes; performing all admission history and physicals; and ordering appropriate laboratory and radiographic tests such as MRIs, myelograms, and bone scans as needed or indicated (Larson et al, 2009). PAs also perform appropriate laboratory and diagnostic studies, such as joint aspirations and injections and placement of traction devices. All PAs in orthopedics evaluate and clarify clinical conditions, formulate and implement a treatment and therapeutic plan for hospitalized patients, write discharge planning, and dictate discharge summaries. NCCPA-certified PAs in orthopedics provide a host of roles that closely juxtapose the orthopedic surgeon. They provide pre-admission physical examinations, write admitting orders, first assist in surgery, and conduct fracture clinics (Samsot & Heinlein, 1996).

Another group of orthopedic PAs may be primarily in the outpatient setting, evaluating acute bone and joint injuries, stabilizing bone fractures, removing hardware and sutures, and placing patients in rehabilitation programs (inpatient or outpatient). A third group may move between the two roles (surgical and outpatient) as the surgeon or surgical group may need them.

History

There is a great deal of confusion about PAs who work in orthopedic settings, technicians who call themselves orthopedic PAs (OPAs), and the different organizations of PAs who specialize in orthopedic medicine. Formally trained PAs who work in an orthopedic setting differ from another group of technicians trained to assist the orthopedic surgeon. Both groups have *orthopedic* in the title, and each may refer to themselves as *OPAs*. To add to this confusion, there is the American Society of Orthopedic Physician Assistants (ASOPAs), OPAs, and the Physician Assistants in Orthopedic Surgery (PAOS).

The history of OPAs begins with technician assistants to the orthopedic surgeon. They have been present at least since 1954 in some capacity, whether to assist applying a cast or to hold a retractor, and many developed expertise while in the military. It is unclear when the first formal orthopedic technical program started; however, the American Medical Association (AMA) House of Delegates first adopted minimum educational standards for OPA education in 1969 upon a recommendation from the American Academy of Orthopedic Surgeons (AAOS). Eight OPA programs had been accredited by 1973. This involvement proved somewhat controversial, and 1 year later the AAOS announced its intent to withdraw sponsorship from the accreditation program. After substantial consultation with the AAOS, the AMA Committee on Medical Education (CME) announced a moratorium on the accreditation of any additional orthopedic programs and informed accredited programs that accreditation would be discontinued upon graduation of the classes that would be matriculating in the fall of 1974. It is important to note that the AMA, without the involvement of the medical specialty society, does not sponsor accreditation efforts in allied health education or societies and the related allied health organizations most closely associated with the occupation.

None of the eight OPA programs accredited by the AMA CME remain in existence. The one at Kirkwood Community College in Cedar Rapids, Iowa, graduated its last class in 1988. The AMA Committee on Allied Health Education and Accreditation never accredited any OPA programs as PA programs.

The orthopedic assistant programs were confined to training technical orthopedic tasks without the substantial background in the basic medical sciences that the primary care PA programs stressed. The educational qualifications of the two groups—OPAs and PAs—differ substantially. Orthopedic assistants were trained as technologists in an 18-month course at a junior college, which was more closely related to other technical programs, such as respiratory therapy, surgical technology, and medical or dental assisting. Anywhere from 500 to 1,000 graduates are estimated to have matriculated from these eight programs, along with some similar programs in the Air Force.

Graduates of the orthopedic assistant program are not eligible to sit for the Physician Assistant National Certification Examination (PANCE), which is administered by the NCCPA. The National Board for Certification of Orthopedic Physician Assistants (NBCOPA) handles an examination for certifying OPAs. This examination is not equivalent to the NCCPA's examination, and the organizations are not affiliated in any way (Kappes, 1992).

Although both PAs and OPAs work for orthopedists, Minnesota is the only state with a law regulating OPAs. In 1978, Michigan included a grandfather title protection for "orthopedic physician's assistants," but OPAs remain an unlicensed occupation in that state. OPAs were also given a finite period to register in Minnesota when regulation of PAs became effective in 1986. In Iowa, home of the Kirkwood Community College program, the 1988 Physician Assistant Practice Act explicitly states that "orthopedic physician's assistant technologists" are not required to qualify as PAs.

Formed in 1971, the ASOPA represents approximately 400 practicing OPAs. Medicare does not cover services provided by OPAs.

PAOS, the latest special interest group for formally trained PAs, was formed in 1992 at the annual AAPA Conference in Nashville, Tennessee. This seems to be the most active organization. It reports working with the Southern Orthopedic Association to develop a membership category for PAs.

Broughton's study (1996) examining the range of tasks and the dynamics of practice of orthopedics by PAs helps illustrate the degree of service these PAs perform (Exhibit 7-11). From a survey of 440 PAs in orthopedic practice, all perform history and physical examinations and prescribe medications. Most interpret x-rays, apply casts, suture wounds, assist in surgery, and reduce fractures. Postgraduate-trained PAs seem to have higher levels of responsibility than NCCPA-certified PAs or OPAs (Broughton, 1996).

EXHIBIT 7-11
Tasks Performed by Physician Assistants in Orthopedic Surgery

Task	Percent
History taking	99.0
Physical examination	99.0
Interpretation of x-ray studies	94.2
Cast application	94.5
Wound suturing	93.8
Assistance in surgery	92.9
Joint aspiration/injection	80.8
Brace application	76.0
K-wire removal	73.4
Wound incision and drainage	67.5
Fracture reduction	57.1
Dislocation reduction	54.5
Hardware removal	50.3
Compartment pressure measurements	31.2
Administer regional anesthesia	22.1
Tendon repair	22.1
Percutaneous pinning of fractures	21.4

Data from Broughton, B. (1996). A delineative study of physician assistants in orthopaedic surgery: Tasks, professional relationships, and satisfaction (doctoral dissertation, Columbia Pacific University, California).

Profile

In a survey undertaken by the AAPA, 2,528 PAs in orthopedic surgery responded (Exhibit 7-12). The average age was 39, females were 46% of the cohort, and 20% were employed by a hospital. Almost all (88%) worked in an urban setting. The majority (93%) worked full time (at least 32 hours per week) and 92% were salary-based. The average salary in 2008 was $94,916 (AAPA, 2008a).

Professional Society

PAOS is an organization created by and for PAs who are NCCPA-certified and work in orthopedics. This is an official specialty organization of the AAPA and has an official liaison with the AAOS. The official website for PAOS is http://paos.org/.

Otorhinolaryngology (Head and Neck Surgery)

Otorhinolaryngology is the specialty in the diagnosis and treatment of ear, nose, throat, and

EXHIBIT 7-12
Physician Assistants in Orthopedic Surgery, 2008

Total survey respondents	2,528
Age (mean years)	39
Female	1145 (46%)
Single specialty physician group practice	1,133 (45%)
Multispecialty physician group practice	476 (19%)
Hospital	498 (20%)
Other practice	392 (18%)
Years in clinical practice	8
Work in urban setting	88
Precept PA students	39%
Work more than 32 hours per week	93%
Mean income	$94,916

Data from American Academy of Physician Assistants. (2008a). 2008 AAPA Physician Assistant Census Report. Alexandria, VA: Author.

head and neck disorders. The full name of the specialty is otolaryngology-head and neck surgery. Practitioners are called otolaryngologists-head and neck surgeons, or sometimes otorhinolaryngologists. A commonly used term for this speciality, although somewhat out of favor, is ENT (ear, nose, and throat).

Role

Some otorhinolayrngology-head and neck surgery PAs are primarily surgically oriented and others are exclusively outpatient oriented. A few straddle surgery and inpatient and outpatient services. Otorhinolayrngology-head and neck surgery PAs are involved in diagnostic tests and procedures such as fine-needle aspiration biopsies, tympanostomy tube insertion, and sinus irrigations (Lewit et al, 1980). Many PAs in this specialty assist in facial reconstruction surgery, oncology surgery, and staging surgery. They also coordinate admissions, dictate discharge summaries, and provide follow-up care.

Office procedures may include cleaning ear canals and mastoid cavities, performing electrocautery for the control of epistaxis, inserting nasal packing, and providing immediate postoperative care of patients in the inpatient and outpatient setting (Poppen, 1996). They may also perform rhinopharyngolaryngoscopy, videostroboscopy, and vocal/voice recordings. Survey results from the Society of Physician

Assistants in Otorhinolaryngology/Head and Neck Surgery (SPAO-HNS) (2003) provide greater detail of office procedures completed by PAs in this specialty.

History

PAs have been employed in relatively small numbers in the orhinolaryngology specialty. According to AAPA census data, only 52 (0.5%) of PAs were employed in this specialty in 1996. By 2001, the number had risen to 104 (0.6%) and in 2008 it was 251 (0.9%). This steady increase over several years suggests that PAs are fufilling an important role within the specialty.

Profile

In a survey undertaken by the AAPA, 251 PAs in otorhinolaryngology responded (Exhibit 7-13). The average age was 39, females were 63% of the cohort, and 39% worked in a single specialty physician group practice. Most (89%) worked in an urban setting. The majority (85%) worked full time (at least 32 hours per week) and 91% were salary-based. The average salary in 2008 was $86,856 (AAPA, 2008a).

Professional Society

The SPAO-HNS was founded in Kansas City during the American Academy of Otorhinolayrngology-Head and Neck Surgery's annual meeting in 1991. The Society was developed to enhance the professional growth development of PAs who work in the field of ear, nose, and throat diseases. The organization was formed to provide an opportunity to meet and interact with PAs who share a common interest and to obtain continuing medical education specific to their field. At least 75 PAs belong to this organization, which has a liaison with the American Academy of Otorhinolaryngology-Head and Neck Surgery. Their website is http://www.entpa.org/.

Plastic and Reconstructive Surgery

Plastic surgery is a specialty that uses a number of surgical and nonsurgical techniques to change the appearance and restore the function of a person's body. Procedures involve cosmetic enhancements (also referred to as *cosmetic surgery*), functionally reconstructive operations, or both.

Role

PAs in plastic and reconstructive surgery work in a variety of settings that encompass cosmetic surgery, burn management, and reconstruction of congenital and trauma-related injuries. Because many plastic surgeons practice in office-based operating rooms and "surgicenters," PAs must be able to first assist on all cases, provide suture skills equal to that of the surgeon, and be knowledgeable of anatomy and the latest surgical techniques (Lennox, 2008). Perioperatively, PAs in plastic and reconstructive surgery must perform physical examinations and discharge planning, oversee rehabilitation, communicate with various members of the surgical team, and be knowledgeable about surgical supplies and prostheses. In the clinic setting the PA may see postoperative patients. They may order routine laboratory tests, dictate discharge summaries, monitor patients, and change dressings (Gittins, 1996).

Because the plastic surgery PA works in all settings from the office to the emergency department (ED), she or he must be knowledgeable about reimbursement issues and patient insurance plans, have the ability to

EXHIBIT 7-13
Otorhinolarongology—Head and Neck Surgery Physician Assistants, 2008

Total survey respondents	251
Age (mean years)	39
Female	156 (63%)
Solo physician practitioner	53 (21%)
Single specialty physician group practice	97 (39%)
Multispecialty physician group practice	43 (17%)
Hospital	46 (18%)
Other practice	12 (5%)
Years in clinical practice	10
Work in urban setting	89%
Precept PA students	29%
Work more than 32 hours per week	85%
Mean income	$86,856

Data from American Academy of Physician Assistants. (2008a). 2008 AAPA Physician Assistant Census Report. Alexandria, VA: Author.

communicate with insurance companies in writing, and perform consultations in the surgeon's absence. PAs in plastic and reconstructive surgery receive formal surgical assistant or postgraduate training, or on-the-job training.

History

The plastic surgeon has used and continues to use the PA in a variety of ways. In fact, reconstructive microsurgery has relied on trained PAs in this area to reduce operating time since the 1970s (Toth, Pickrell, & Thompson, 1978; Gould & Gould, 1984). Sigurdson (2007) theorized that the introduction of a reconstruction surgical PA in a Canadian practice could improve productivity by 37%.

Profile

In a survey undertaken by the AAPA, 213 PAs in plastic surgery responded (Exhibit 7-14). The average age was 38, females were 84% of the cohort, and 32% were employed by a hospital. Essentially all (97%) worked in an urban setting. The majority (86%) worked full time (at least 32 hours per week) and 90% were salary-based. The average salary in 2008 was $92,633 (AAPA, 2008a).

EXHIBIT 7-14
Plastic (Reconstructive) Surgery Physician Assistants, 2008

Total survey respondents	213
Age (mean years)	38
Female	177 (84%)
Solo physician practitioner	67 (32%)
Single specialty physician group practice	31 (15%)
Multispecialty physician group practice	24 (11%)
Hospital	68 (32%)
Other practice	23 (10%)
Years in clinical practice	8
Work in urban setting	97%
Precept PA students	31%
Work more than 32 hours per week	86%
Mean income	$92,633

Data from American Academy of Physician Assistants. (2008a). 2008 AAPA Physician Assistant Census Report. Alexandria, VA: Author.

Professional Society

The AASPA includes plastic and reconstructive PAs. Their website is http://www.aaspa.com/prs.asp.

Trauma Surgery

Trauma surgeons are general surgeons who have concentrated their practice on the care of injured and critically ill patients. In the United States, trauma surgeons generally work in large urban hospitals specifically designated as trauma centers by the ACS (Martin, 2007).

Role

PAs working in trauma surgery tend to be in large hospital settings that are prepared for massive trauma-related injuries. These PAs must be current in advanced cardiac and advanced trauma life support and skilled in managing cardiac and respiratory emergencies. They must be able to first assist on all cases, provide advanced skills, be knowledgeable of anatomy, and remain current on the latest surgical techniques. Perioperatively, PAs in trauma surgery perform physical examinations and discharge planning, oversee rehabilitation, communicate with various members of the surgical team, and are knowledgeable about surgical supplies and prostheses (Nyberg et al, 2007).

Because the trauma surgery PA interfaces with the ED, the PA must be able to quickly assess a patient's needs in the surgeon's absence. For example, the PA may be the first member of the trauma team to evaluate the injured victim and institute immediate therapy. A trauma PA may also assist in the operating room, with postoperative management, and following the patient through the critical care portion of recovery. This PA will often attend to the patient closely on the hospital surgical ward. In most trauma centers, patient follow-up occurs in the trauma surgery clinic, where the PA may provide continuity of care not usually possible with surgical residents. The trauma surgery PA may make rounds with the attending surgeon and reports on pertinent issues regarding patient care. Other responsibilities include dealing with patient calls after hospital discharge and answering general follow-up questions. These responsibilities may include triaging patients to the ED or to the trauma clinic (Christmas et al, 2005).

PAs in trauma surgery obtain their skills through formal training (e.g., surgical assistant or postgraduate training) or on-the-job training (Wiemiller, 2008; Salyer, 2008). Most PAs in trauma surgery have a minimum of 2 years of general and emergency medicine experience.

History

The history of PAs in trauma surgery is rooted in military medical experience that found that PAs in advance trauma support were capable of working closely with trauma surgeons. At first they were involved with ordering and interpreting appropriate laboratory and diagnostic studies, collating information, requesting and following up on recommendations of consultants, and assessing fluid and electrolyte balance. Other skills taken up included managing and removing tubes and drains, formulating differential diagnoses, and confirming or refuting the treatment options according to the physical examination findings and other data obtained. Increasingly, PAs in trauma surgery were involved in identifying and prioritizing surgical, medical, and psychosocial problems and assisting the trauma surgeon.

One study was undertaken to assess the quality of patient care during transition from a resident-assisted to a PA-assisted trauma program (without residents). The study was controlled for other factors such as support services available. A retrospective analysis of patient care during two 6-month segments was carried out: one during a resident-assisted program at a level II trauma center in 1998, the other at a PA-dedicated trauma program in 1999. Regression analysis indicated the only statistically significant outcome was decreased length of stay (LOS) when patients were transferred directly from emergency center (EC) to floor in 1999. The mean LOS was 2.54 ± 4.65 compared with 3.4 ± 5.81, and no statistical difference in other assessments was noted. Focused analysis in 2002 showed 100% participation of PAs during the trauma alert compared with 51% by residents. Substitution of residents with PAs had no impact on patient mortality; however, LOS (from EC to floor), was statistically reduced by 1 day. The authors believe that trauma programs can benefit with collaboration of residents and PAs in patient care (Oswanski, Sharma, & Shekhar, 2004).

The timely treatment of patients with head injuries is affected by the availability and commitment of neurosurgeons. To test whether PAs permit more efficient neurosurgical coverage, a study on intracranial pressure (ICP) monitoring, one of the most frequently used neurosurgical procedures, was performed. The purpose of the study was to examine the placement of ICP monitors by PAs. Medical records and trauma registry data for a level I trauma center were reviewed from December 1993 to June 1997. Patients who had ICP monitors placed were included. Patient data recorded were age, mechanism of injury, injury type, ICP monitor placement and length of placement, complications related to the ICP monitor, and outcomes.

In the study, 210 patients had 215 monitors placed. ICP monitors were placed by neurosurgeons (105), PAs (97), and general surgery residents (13) and remained in place a mean of 4 days. No major complications attributable to ICP monitor placement occurred; 19 minor complications (malfunction, dislodgment) were noted. Eleven monitors placed by neurosurgeons (10%), seven placed by PAs (7%), and one placed by a resident (8%) had complications. The authors concluded that ICP monitor placement by PAs is safe and their use may aid neurosurgeons in providing prompt monitoring of patients with head injuries (Kaups, Parks, & Morris, 1998).

Oswanski and colleagues (2004) compared the quality of care during off-hours between trauma residents to PA-assisted trauma management. When the PA was involved with the care, the length of stay decreased by 1 day when compared to the resident. Substitution of residents with PAs had no impact on patient mortality.

EXHIBIT 7-15
Trauma Surgery Physician Assistants, 2008

Total survey respondents	120
Age (mean years)	37
Female	67 (57%)
Single specialty physician group practice	8 (7%)
Multispecialty physician group practice	7 (6%)
Hospital	99 (83%)
Years in clinical practice	7
Work in urban setting	97%
Precept PA students	66%
Work more than 32 hours per week	95%
Mean income	$91,417

Data from American Academy of Physician Assistants. (2008a). 2008 AAPA Physician Assistant Census Report. Alexandria, VA: Author.

The contemporary trauma surgery PA is expected to be able to manage patients undergoing a broad range of procedures including orthopedic, ENT, urology, and vascular. The PA must also know when appropriate consultation is warranted and speak with that service.

Profile
In a survey undertaken by the AAPA, 120 PAs in trauma surgery responded (Exhibit 7-15). The average age was 37, females were 57% of the cohort, and 83% were employed by a hospital. Almost all (97%) worked in an urban setting (usually a tertiary medical center) in facilities with staffing for casualties and high-end technological equipment. The majority (95%) worked full time (at least 32 hours per week) and 81% were salary-based. The average salary in 2008 was $91,417 (AAPA, 2008a).

Professional Society
The AASPA includes trauma surgery PAs. Their website is http://www.aaspa.com/ts.asp.

MEDICAL SPECIALTIES

Medical specialities are the nonprimary care disciplines that physicians and PAs pursue. Some of the medical specialities listed are surgically based, but the PA tends to function outside the operating theater.

Addiction Medicine (Alcohol and Drug Abuse)

Addiction medicine, also known as *substance abuse medicine* or *addictionology*, is a medical specialty that deals with the treatment of chemical dependency. The specialty commonly crosses over into other areas because various aspects of addiction fall within the fields of public health, psychiatry, and internal medicine (among others). Incorporated within the specialty are the processes of detoxification, rehabilitation, harm reduction, abstinence-based treatment, individual and group therapies, oversight of halfway houses, treatment of withdrawal-related symptoms, acute intervention, and long-term therapies designed to reduce likelihood of relapse (Ball et al, 1986). Some specialists also provide treatment for disease states commonly associated with substance abuse, such as hepatitis, tuberculosis, and HIV infection.

Role
A growing number of PAs provide alcohol and drug abuse management from the clinical side. Their roles include admitting and discharging patients from detoxification units and providing medical management of substance abuse patients in outpatient settings (Rosenblum et al, 2002). About one-third of PAs in addiction medicine work in a hospital setting, and 15% work for the Department of Veterans Affairs (AAPA, 2008a).

History
Early in the development of PA education, psychiatry and psychosocial medicine were introduced as critical areas of learning. The issues of alcoholism and drug addiction became part of the curriculum. These topics were emphasized more in programs for PAs preparing for inner-city work than in programs geared toward rural deployment (Alexander, 2006). Eventually, the standards for PA education included some aspect of substance abuse. As of the new century, substance abuse and chemical dependency is taught in almost all PA programs (Judd & Hooker, 2001) (Exhibit 7-16).

EXHIBIT 7-16
Number of Hours of Physician Assistant Education Instruction on Substance Abuse

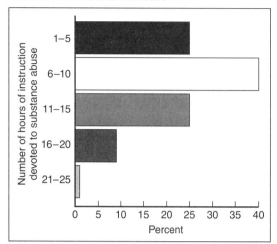

Data from Judd, C. R., & Hooker, R. S. (2001). Physician assistant education in substance abuse. Perspectives on Physician Assistant Education, 12(3), 172–176.

Profile

In a survey undertaken by the AAPA, 76 PAs in addiction medicine responded (Exhibit 7-17). The average age was 51, females were 59% of the cohort, and 37% were employed by a hospital. Most (88%) worked in an urban setting. The majority (72%) worked full time (at least 32 hours per week) and 80% were salary-based. The average salary in 2008 was $84,627 (AAPA, 2008a).

Allergy and Immunology Medicine

Immunology is the study of all aspects of the immune system including allergies. This discipline deals with the physiological functioning of the immune system in states of health and disease; malfunctions of the immune system in immunologic disorders (autoimmune diseases, hypersensitivities, immune deficiency, allograft rejection); and the physical, chemical, and physiological characteristics of the components of the immune system in vitro, in situ, and in vivo. Allergy is the application of immunology to diagnose the allergic responses to environmental stimuli

EXHIBIT 7-17
Addiction Medicine Physician Assistants, 2008

Total survey respondents	76
Age (mean years)	51
Female	45 (59%)
Employed in a hospital	20 (37%)
Years in clinical practice	17
Work in urban setting	88%
Precept PA students	21%
Work more than 32 hours per week	72%
Mean income	$84,627

Data from American Academy of Physician Assistants. (2008a). 2008 AAPA Physician Assistant Census Report. Alexandria, VA: Author.

and determine their treatments. Allergists tend to be internists or pediatricians, although many family medicine physicians perform allergy testing and treatment. Allergy and immunology are combined because a large overlap exists between the two disciplines and many doctors are trained in both areas of medicine. Some doctors are trained in allergy, immunology, and rheumatology.

Role

Historically, allergy and immunology have not been areas widely occupied by PAs, although more than 130 PAs identify these areas as their primary areas of practice in the AAPA annual survey (AAPA, 2008a). Based on the patient's history and accompanying physical examination findings, the PA typically orders a range of tests for allergens and lung functions via bronchodilators and spirometry and develops a preliminary diagnosis and treatment plan. On a typical day, an allergy and immunology PA sees acute and chronic conditions. Sinus conditions tend to make up a large part of the patient load. In some settings, the PA may administer allergy densensitization injections, manage atopic dermatitis and chronic coughs, and treat acute asthma attacks. Patients may be children or adults with allergies or immunologic disorders such as immunoglobulin G subclass deficiency. Some allergy and immunology PAs serve as researchers in clinical trials.

History

In 1969, a program was developed at the University of California, San Diego, to prepare PAs as advanced skill technicians in allergy. This program trained PAs to prepare, administer, and evaluate allergens for those with suspected allergic conditions. At the time, this was a labor-intensive activity that required technical skill to prepare the allergens and perform pulmonary function testing (Perlman, 1976). Because manufacturers now prepare almost all allergens, nurses skilled in allergy have largely supplanted the role of the technical PA in allergy (Johnstone, 1977).

However, to understand the value a PA brings to an allergy and immunology practice a study on satisfaction and quality of care survey was undertaken in 2002. This telephone survey queried 23 PAs, 21 doctors, and 54 patients from asthma practices employing PAs and 21 physicians and 55 patients from practices who did not employ PAs (Exhibit 7-18). The survey found patient satisfaction was higher in terms of level of care provided, responsiveness to questions, phone calls, patient education, and time spent waiting to see a provider in practices that employed a PA compared with those who did not employ a PA (Thomas, McNellis, & Ortiz, 2003).

The survey inquired about the motivations for hiring a PA. Almost three-quarters of employing doctors said they were specifically looking for a PA to alleviate the burden on the doctor and to increase the ability to see more patients. Five physicians reported that the involvement of PAs increased the ability to see new and old patients. Four physicians and three PAs mentioned an increase in the following activities:

- Developing emergency plans for asthma patients
- Ordering and interpreting indicated diagnostic tests
- Designing and implementing treatment plans
- Obtaining patient histories and performing physical examinations
- Providing on-call coverage
- Establishing a diagnosis
- Providing patient education

An increase in patient satisfaction as well as patient volume were mentioned as the top two benefits a PA provides to an allergy clinic (Exhibit 7-19). In addition, an increase in patient education, a reduction in appointment wait time, and the ability to spend more time with the physician or PA were mentioned by respondents as the top benefits provided to the patients by a PA (Exhibit 7-20).

Profile

In a survey undertaken by the AAPA, 134 PAs in allergy and immunology responded (Exhibit 7-21). The average age was 39 and females were 77% of the cohort. Almost all (97%) worked in an urban setting. The majority (73%) worked full time (at least 32 hours per week) and 80% were salary-based. The average salary in 2008 was $81,557 (AAPA, 2008a).

Anesthesiology

Anesthesia is the medical science of blocking the feeling of pain and other sensations. This process allows patients to undergo surgery and other procedures without the distress and pain they would otherwise experience. *Anesthesiologist* is the North American term for the doctor who administers anesthesia.

EXHIBIT 7-18
Allergy Clinics With and Without Physician Assistants: Characteristics

	Interviews
ALLERGY CLINICS STAFFED BY PAS	
PAs	23
Physicians	21
Patients of PAs	54
ALLERGY CLINICS WITHOUT PAS	
Physicians	21
Patients	55

Data from Thomas, G. P., McNellis, R. J., & Ortiz G. R. (2003). Physician assistants enhance quality of care in asthma patients. Journal of Allergy and Clinical Immunology, *111(2), S71–440.*

EXHIBIT 7-19

Benefits of a Physician Assistant to the Allergy Clinic as Perceived by Each Provider (7-point Likert scale)

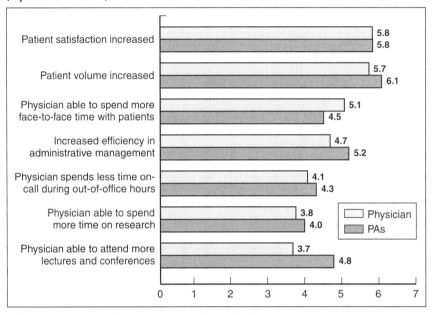

Data from Thomas, G. P., McNellis, R. J., & Ortiz G. R. (2003). Physician assistants enhance quality of care in asthma patients. Journal of Allergy and Clinical Immunology, 111(2), S71–440.

EXHIBIT 7-20

The Patient's Views: Benefits of a Physician Assistant to the Allergy Clinic as Perceived by the Patient (7-point Likert scale)

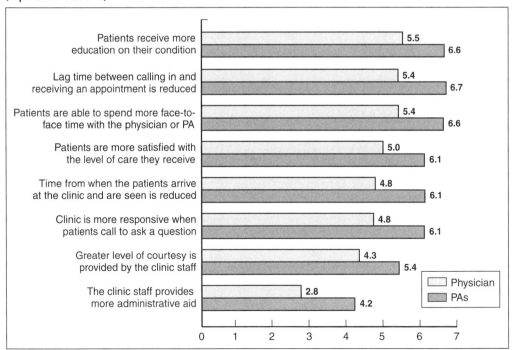

Data from Thomas, G. P., McNellis, R. J., & Ortiz G. R. (2003). Physician assistants enhance quality of care in asthma patients. Journal of Allergy and Clinical Immunology, 111(2), S71–440.

EXHIBIT 7-21
Allergy and Immunology Physician Assistants, 2008

Total survey respondents	134
Age (mean years)	39
Female	103 (77%)
Single specialty physician group practice	62 (46%)
Multispecialty physician group practice	17 (13%)
Years in clinical practice	8
Work in urban setting	97%
Precept PA students	20%
Work more than 32 hours per week	73%
Mean income	$81,557

Data from American Academy of Physician Assistants. (2008a). 2008 AAPA Physician Assistant Census Report. Alexandria, VA: Author.

Anesthetist is the British Commonwealth term that is more commonly used around the world.

Role

The PA who works in anesthesiology must be distinguished from another separately trained healthcare provider, the anesthesiology assistant (AA). The AA functions under the direction of a licensed and qualified anesthesiologist, principally in academic medical centers. There are five educational programs training AAs in 2008. The AA assists the anesthesiologist in collecting preoperative data, such as taking an appropriate health history and performing physical examinations. Preoperative tasks include the insertion of intravenous and arterial lines, central venous pressure monitors, and special catheters. In surgery, AAs monitor anesthesia, support airway management and drug administration for induction and maintenance of anesthesia, and may administer supportive therapy, such as intravenous fluids and vasodilators. In the recovery area, they perform tasks relating to the ICU or pain clinic. In most instances, a designated anesthesiologist is within the hospital and immediately available to the operating room (Exhibit 7-22). AAs are trained in general, epidural, spinal, and peripheral anesthetic nerve blockade. They may be involved in a pain management program that involves chronic pain assessment, injections, and narcotic management.

EXHIBIT 7-22
Activites of an Anesthesiologist Assistant

- Establishing noninvasive and invasive routine monitoring modalities as delegated by the responsible anesthesiologist.
- Performing or assisting in diagnostic laboratory and related studies as appropriate, such as drawing arterial and venous blood samples
- Assisting in the application and interpretation of advanced monitoring techniques such as pulmonary artery catheterization, electroencephalographic spectral analysis, echocardiography, and evoked potentials
- Assisting in inducing and maintaining and altering anesthesia levels, administering adjunctive treatment, and providing continuity of anesthetic care into and during the postoperative recovery period
- Assisting in the use of advanced life support techniques such as high-frequency ventilation and intra-arterial cardiovascular assist devices
- Assisting in making postanesthesia patient rounds by recording patient progress notes, compiling and recording case summaries, and transcribing standing and specific orders
- Performing evaluation and treatment procedures essential to responding to life-threatening situations, such as cardiopulmonary resuscitation, on the basis of established protocols (basic life support, advanced cardiac life support, and pediatric advanced life support)
- Assisting in the performance of duties in intensive care units, pain clinics, and other settings, as appropriate
- Training and supervising personnel in the calibration, troubleshooting, and use of patient monitors
- Performing delegated administrative duties in an anesthesiology practice or anesthesiology department, such as managing personnel, supplies and devices
- Assisting in the clinical instruction of others

AAs also provide technical support according to established protocols. This support includes first-level maintenance of anesthesia equipment; skilled operation of special monitors, including echocardiograms, electroencephalograms, special analyzers, evoked-potential apparatuses, autotransfusion devices, mass spectrometers, and intra-aortic balloon pumps; the operation and maintenance of bedside electronic computer-based monitors; supervised laboratory functions associated with anesthesia and operating room care; and cardiopulmonary resuscitation.

AAs are likely to be employed by hospitals with at least 200 beds and with staffs of 15 or more anesthesiologists, nurse anesthetists, and AAs. Within these settings a team approach to anesthesia service is used. In facilities for open-heart surgery a graduate medical residency training program for anesthesiologists is typically in place and will invove the AA in teaching.

The specific job descriptions and duties of AAs may differ according to geographic area and local practice. State law or board of medicine regulations or guidelines may further define the job descriptions. AAs practice under the direction of a qualified anesthesiologist. The American Society of Anesthesiologists' statement on the Recommended Scope of Practice of Nurse Anesthetists and Anesthesiologist Assistants may be found at http://www.asahq.org/Washington/09Scope.pdf. AAs are not certified by the NCCPA and their training programs are distinct from ARC-PA-accredited PA educational programs. One PA working in anesthesia has completed the equivalent of a 3-year physician residency in anesthesiology and functions on a level similar to physicians at an academic health center.

History

In the 1960s, three anesthesiologists, Joachim S. Gravenstein, John E. Steinhaus, and Perry P. Volpitto, were concerned with the shortage of anesthesiologists in the country. After studying the educational pathway for anesthesiologists and certified registered nurse anesthetists (CRNAs), they created a new educational paradigm for a "midlevel" anesthesia practitioner that included a pre-med background. This person would perform the same job as the CRNA but would be readily able to go on to medical school if appropriate. As a new professional, the AA had the potential to alleviate the shortage of anesthesiologists. The concept became reality in 1969 when the first AA training program began accepting students at Emory University in Atlanta, Georgia, followed shortly thereafter by a second program at Case Western Reserve University in Cleveland, Ohio. By 1975, the ASA was supportive of this emerging occupation.

In 1976, the ASA petitioned the AMA CME to recognize the AA as an emerging health profession. The council's recognition followed in 1978. An ad hoc committee within the ASA worked collaboratively with the AMA's Department of Allied Health Education and Accreditation on the development of educational standards. Because of differences in opinion about the level of the credential and about the need for graduates in this field, in 1981 the ASA withdrew its collaboration with the AMA in the development of accreditation standards and in the accreditation of educational programs.

By 1982, the Association of Anesthesiologist's Assistants Training Programs (AAATP) was created and incorporated. The following year, the AAATP and the American Academy of Anesthesia Associates (AAAA) petitioned the AMA CME to recognize them as collaborative sponsors for the program designed to educate AAs. In 1984, the AMA CME reinstated its recognition of the AA profession. *Essentials* for the education and training of AAs were adopted in 1987 by the CME, the AAATP, and the AAAA.

As of 2008 there are three accredited AA educational programs—those at Emory and Case Western Reserve and a consortium between South University and Mercer School of Medicine, Savannah, Georgia, which accepted its first class in 2004. In 2008, the AAPA estimated that approximately 65 people were formally trained PAs working as anesthesiologists.

AAs have sought recognition as PAs, using as justification the premise that the term *physician assistant* includes all assistants to physicians. For many years AAs have been recognized as "type B" PAs in Georgia; this designation reaches back to a recommendation by the National Academy of Sciences in 1970 that PAs be classified as types A, B, and C by degree of specialization and level of judgment involved in practice. That designation scheme is defunct. Another battle is between the AAs and CRNAs. The lines are drawn between CRNAs who are seeking independence and AAs who are maintaining their physician-dependent role.

EXHIBIT 7-23
Anesthesiology Physician Assistants, 2008

Total survey respondents	65
Age (mean years)	42
Female	42 (66%)
Single specialty physician group practice	13 (20%)
University hospital	28 (43%)
Years in clinical practice	11
Work in urban setting	95%
Work more than 32 hours per week	95%
Mean income	$93,370

Data from American Academy of Physician Assistants. (2008a). 2008 AAPA Physician Assistant Census Report. Alexandria, VA: Author.

Profile

In a survey undertaken by the AAPA, 65 PAs in anesthesiology responded (Exhibit 7-23). The average age was 42, and females were 65% of the cohort. All PAs in anesthesiology are hospital-based; 20% worked in a single specialty physician group practice and 43% were employed by a university hospital. Almost all (95%) worked in an urban setting. The majority (95%) worked full time (at least 32 hours per week) and 90% were salary-based. The average salary in 2008 was $93,370 (AAPA, 2008a).

Cardiology

Cardiology is the study and management of patients with myocardial, circulatory, and valve diseases. Interventional cardiology deals specifically with the catheter-based treatment of structural heart diseases. A large number of procedures can be performed on the heart by catheterization. This approach most commonly involves inserting a sheath into the femoral artery (or other large peripheral vessel) and cannulating the heart under x-ray visualization (most commonly fluoroscopy).

Role

The cardiology PA is one member of an organ-specific team that provides comprehensive and quality patient care. A cardiology team may include cardiologists, PAs, NPs, pharmacists, nutritionists, physical therapists, behavioral

medicine specialists, technologists, and others (Dracup et al, 1994). The PA role in cardiology involves ambulatory care, hospital admission and discharge evaluations, early myocardial infarction management, treadmill and stress testing, and other procedures (Mayes, 1991).

DeMots and colleauges (1987) evaluated the feasibility of PAs performing coronary arteriography. The complication rate and facility in performing the procedure were compared with those of cardiology fellows. The procedure and fluoroscopy times were similar and, more importantly, the mortality rate was zero. The rate of complications was very low when compared with published standards (DeMots et al, 1987). Additional experience with this same model and two additional PAs included an evaluation of more than 1,000 patients, with no mortality and low complication rates (Dracup et al, 1994). Other specialized roles for cardiology PAs are emerging as technology becomes increasingly invasive and demands on cardiologists stretch their capacity (Krasuski et al, 2003).

The work of one PA in a large cardiology practice demonstrates the range and versatility of cardiology PAs. On a typical day, this PA takes complete histories and physicals of new patients. She or he explores in depth the details of each patient's cardiovascular health and general habits. The PA presents the essentials of the patient history to the cardiologist, who directs patient care from that point forward. Consulting with the physician throughout the process, the PA conducts key tests, including stress tests, nuclear stress tests, and tilt table tests. She or he consults in the hospital, revisits patients after being discharged from myocardial infarctions and blood pressure medication titration. The PA explains cardiology procedures to patients, performs site checks after placement of catheters or pacemakers, and monitors chest pains that do not require evaluation by the ED.

In the hospital, a cardiologist reviews the PA's notes on the tests, adding a note to the interpretation and electronically signing the reports (O'Rourke, 1987). Typically, the cardiologist will call the referring physician with "positive" stress results. The PA's inpatient responsibilities include seeing non-ICU patients. She or he writes orders and progress notes, sees patient consults, and dictates the consultations. The hospital bylaws where she or he works require that a cardiologist see the patient at some point during the day.

By seeing patients, writing notes and orders, and dealing with laboratory results and imaging studies in advance, the PA enhances continuity of care, and the cardiologist gains time and ease of case management. Patients and their families appreciate having their questions and concerns addressed by the PA. Back at the office, the PA sees patients for follow-up visits. She or he performs postprocedure site checks, titrates blood pressure, coordinates medications, and promotes recovery through discussion of diet, exercise, and lifestyle issues (Hormann et al, 2004).

Using a prospective database of patients undergoing cardiac catheterization, a cardiology team compared the outcomes of procedures performed by supervised PAs with those performed by supervised cardiology fellows-in-training. Outcome measures included procedural length, fluoroscopy use, volume of contrast media, and complications including myocardial infarction, stroke, arrhythmia requiring defibrillation or pacemaker placement, pulmonary edema requiring intubation, and vascular complications. Class 3 and 4 congestive heart failure was more common in patients who underwent procedures by fellows compared with those undergoing procedures by PAs ($P = 0.001$). PA cases tended to be slightly faster ($P = 0.05$) with less fluoroscopic time ($P < 0.001$). The incidence of major complications within 24 hours of the procedure was similar between the two groups (0.54% in PA cases and 0.58% in fellow cases). The authors conclude that under the supervision of experienced attending cardiologists, trained PAs can perform diagnostic cardiac catheterization, including coronary angiography, with complication rates similar to those of cardiology fellows-in-training (Krasuski et al, 2003).

Profile

In a survey undertaken by the AAPA, 794 PAs in cardiology (adult and pediatrics) responded (Exhibit 7-24). The average age

EXHIBIT 7-24
Cardiology Physician Assistants, 2008

Total survey respondents	794
Age (mean years)	39
Female	521 (66%)
Solo physician practitioner	51 (6%)
Single specialty physician group practice	409 (52%)
Multispecialty physician group practice	117 (15%)
Hospital	175 (22%)
See inpatients	87%
Years in clinical practice	9
Work in urban setting	94%
Precept PA students	38%
Work more than 32 hours per week	89%
Mean income	$87,812

Data from American Academy of Physician Assistants. (2008a). 2008 AAPA Physician Assistant Census Report. Alexandria, VA: Author.

was 39, females were 66% of the cohort, and 52% worked in a single specialty physician group practice. Almost (94%) worked in an urban setting. The majority (89%) worked full time (at least 32 hours per week) and 93% were salary-based. The average salary in 2008 was $87,812 (AAPA, 2008a).

Professional Society

A website for PAs in cardiology is maintained by the AAPA at http://www.aapa.org/gandp/cardiology.html.

Correctional Medicine

Correctional medicine is the medical management of individuals who are incarcerated. It is a broad-based general medical service that incorporates general medical care (almost exclusively adult care), geriatric medicine, public health, occupational medicine, hospice, rehabilitation, and minor trauma.

Role

The role of the PA in correctional medicine spans a number of medical specialties. With a number of safeguards in place, correctional medicine PAs may hold sick call in the morning, see scheduled patients throughout the day, and perform some minor procedures. In some instances they communicate with medical and surgical specialists and follow through with recommendations for treatment.

History

Each county and state, like most large cities, has a jail or prison system—many with opportunities for PAs. The Department of Justice recruits PAs to staff the Federal Correctional System, better known as the Federal Bureau of Prisons, either as civil service employees or public health service officers. The mission statement of correctional institutions is the same as other heathcare systems: to provide essential health care for inmates consistent with acceptable community standards.

The Federal Bureau of Prisons was established in 1930 to maintain secure, safe, and humane correctional institutions. By 1974, the Bureau had created its own PA program at the Federal Medical Center in Springfield, Missouri. The design of the program was similar to that of today: 1 year of academic study and 1 year of clinical work. In 1976, the Bureau employed the first trained PAs. The Springfield program operated until 1978 and then discontinued, partly as a result of an inability to provide satisfactory obstetrics and gynecology and pediatric rotations, and in large measure because it was not cost-effective.

In 1978, between one-half and two-thirds of the Bureau's medical technical assistants were given the job title PA within the Bureau after they passed a written and oral examination. Several graduates of that program went on to pass the PANCE (Vause, Beeler, & Miller-Blanks, 1997). The balance of medical technical assistants is made up of personnel who qualify under the U.S. Office of Personnel Management standards for PAs (and not always technically a formally trained graduate from an accredited program who is certified by the NCCPA [Vause, Beeler, & Miller-Blanks, 1997]). When the Bureau of Prisons discusses its use of PAs a large number do not fit the criteria of NCCPA-certified PAs.

Although commonly listed as a specialty (as it is here), in reality correctional medicine is a primary care discipline that is practiced under extenuating circumstances and involves challenging behavior, ethical considerations, and certain legal constraints (Jarmul & Chavez, 1991, 602–603; Smith, 1996, 103–104). PAs often work independently and deliver a number of primary care and specialty services depending on the size of the institution (Freeman, 1981). As of 2007, there were 106 federal prisons and many PAs were working within the federal prison system. Anecdotal information suggests that this role of medicine offers a great deal of satisfaction for PAs (Brutsche, 1975; Brutsche, 1986). In the mid-1990s, a federal correctional institution in Georgia with 1,750 inmates divided healthcare responsibilities among 10 full-time PAs, 2 physicians, 3 administrators, a nurse, and numerous ancillary staff (Smith, 1996). As demonstrated in another study, the employment of a PA in a Baltimore, Maryland, city jail resulted in a decrease in use of prisoner sick call and an increase in duration of encounters. Improvement in prescribing pattern and categories of prisoner complaints was observed as well (Freeman & Rose, 1981).

A national survey of doctors, PAs, and nurses working in federal prison systems identified many personal and professional issues involved in regulated environments. The findings identified that provider attitudes affected prisoner sick roles and illness behavior. The author identifed that psychological rewards were ample and monetary rewards adequate for retention. However the nature of the institution influences the rules, regulations, concerns, and policies of the prison bureaucratic administrators and managers (Griffiths, 1986).

Profile

For new and experienced PAs, opportunities abound in the Bureau of Prisons. The great diversity of the inmates provides a challenging clinical experience, and the types of settings are uniquely different (Exhibit 7-25). There are probably no greater opportunities to examine healthcare staffing while holding a vast number of variables constant than to practice medicine in this, the quintessential managed-care setting. Prisons allow the PA to follow through with their patients longitudinally while monitoring compliance (Cornell, 2000a).

EXHIBIT 7-25
Correctional Medicine Sites Where Physician Assistants are Employed

- Central Office
- Community Corrections Management Office
- Correctional Institution
- Detention Center
- Federal Correctional Complex
- Federal Correctional Institution
- Federal Detention Center
- Federal Medical Center
- Federal Prison Camp
- Federal Transfer Center
- Medical Center for Federal Prisoners
- Metropolitan Correctional Center
- Metropolitan Detention Center
- Regional Office
- U.S. Penitentiary

Source: Federal Bureau of Prisons. Available at http://www.bop.gov/locations/locationmap.jsp.

There are two paths that healthcare professionals can take with the Bureau of Prisons: Federal Civil Service or the U.S. Public Health Service Commissioned Corps (PHS). Each path has its own pay structure, benefits, and career progression.

Although the United States has a large incarcerated population, there are but two aspects that are important to note about the types of facilities used. First, is the difference between a prison and a correctional facility or jail. Prisons are usually located outside of a major city, preferably in remote regions of the state. They provide housing for inmates who have been convicted and sentenced to serve for a period of 12 months of more. Jails, on the other hand, are usually located within close proximity of city limits and tend to have access to major trauma centers and hospitals of the respective city.

With respect to the healthcare systems, inmates of jails have access to a number of healthcare services, including but not limited to a normal sick call, ongoing treatment for a chronic illness, or a limited facility for prenatal care. In addition, because the locations of the jails are close to major trauma centers and hospitals, emergency care can be attended to at any given time if such services are not immediately available within the jail facility.

Inmates of prisons, however, are faced with a totally different set of healthcare facilities, primarily because of their remote locations and, more often than not, because of the limited number of healthcare providers assigned to the respective prison. Therefore, the prison system is where PAs are most needed and called for, simply because the available senior physicians alone cannot handle all of the health needs of the prison inmates. According to one estimate, PAs perform more than 80% of the tasks of the senior physician in the prison setting. These tasks may include conducting physical examinations, treating illnesses, diagnosing patients, ordering and interpreting tests results, and sometimes, assisting in surgery. In some settings the medical officer (doctor or PA) may be involved in stabilizing psychiatric illnesses.

One consideration of correctional medicine concerns legal proceedings. Some inmates may feel that the healthcare professional assigned to them is there to collect evidence against them. However, collecting evidence is considered a conflict of interest for the PA working in a prison setting. The responsibility of the PA is to help the inmate with their medical needs and requirements. In most instances, the ethics of correctional medicine are separated from the state or facility's legal or judicial system.

Professional Society
The American Correctional Health Services Association's (ACHSA's) mission is to be the voice of the correctional healthcare profession and serve as an effective forum for communication addressing current issues and needs confronting correctional health care. The ACHSA provides support, skill development, and education programs for healthcare personnel, organizations, and decision-makers involved in correctional health care, resulting in increased professionalism and a sense of community for correctional healthcare personnel and positive changes in health for detained and incarcerated individuals. Their website is http://www.achsa.org.

Critical Care Medicine

Critical care specialists treat patients in the ICU and critical care unit (CCU). Critical care covers all aspects of acute and emergency care for the critically ill or injured patient. The discipline includes chest physicians, surgeons, pediatricians, pharmacists and pharmacologists, anesthesiologists, critical care nurses, and other healthcare professionals. Practitioners in critical care may deal with new technologies that require advanced knowledge of physiology.

Role

The critical care PA is a hospital-based role assigned to oversee medical and surgical patients in the ICU. They are skilled in pulmonology/respirology, cardiology, nephrology, endocrinology, and neurology, and work as members of the critical care team.

History

Critical care evolved from an historical recognition that the needs of patients with acute, life-threatening illness or injury could be better treated if they were grouped into specific areas of the hospital. Nurses have long recognized that very sick patients receive more attention if they are located near the nursing station. A time line of critical care medicine is provided in Exhibit 7-26.

A study supporting the value of PAs in critical care followed two PAs who were assigned to the ICU at the Veterans Health Administration Medical Center in Allen Park, Michigan after 3 months of rigorous training.

EXHIBIT 7-26
Timeline of Critical Care Development in Hospitals

- In 1854, Florence Nightingale wrote about the advantages of establishing a separate area of the hospital for patients recovering from surgery.
- Intensive care began in the United States when a three-bed unit for postoperative neurosurgical patients at the Johns Hopkins Hospital in Baltimore opened in 1920.
- In 1927, the first hospital premature infant care center was established at the Sarah Morris Hospital in Chicago.
- During World War II, shock wards were established to resuscitate and care for soldiers injured in battle or undergoing surgery.
- The nursing shortage, which followed World War II, forced the grouping of postoperative patients in recovery rooms to ensure attentive care. The obvious benefits in improved patient care resulted in the spread of recovery rooms to nearly every hospital by 1960.
- Between 1947 and 1948, the polio epidemic raged through Europe and the United States, resulting in a breakthrough in the treatment of patients dying from respiratory paralysis. In Denmark, manual ventilation was accomplished through a tube placed in the trachea of polio patients. Patients with respiratory paralysis or suffering from acute circulatory failure required intensive nursing care.
- During the 1950s, the development of mechanical ventilation led to the organization of respiratory intensive care units (ICUs) in many European and American hospitals. The care and monitoring of mechanically ventilated patients proved to be more efficient when patients were grouped in a single location. General ICUs for very sick patients, including postoperative patients, were developed for similar reasons.
- In 1958, approximately 25% of community hospitals with more than 300 beds reported having an ICU. By the late 1960s, most U.S. hospitals had at least one ICU.
- In 1970, 29 physicians with a major interest in the care of the critically ill and injured met in Los Angeles, California, to discuss the formation of an organization committed to meeting the needs of critical care patients: the Society of Critical Care Medicine (SCCM).
- In 1986, the American Board of Medical Specialties approved a certification of special competence in critical care for the four primary boards: anesthesiology, internal medicine, pediatrics, and surgery.
- Between 1990 and the present, critical care significantly reduced in-hospital time as well as costs incurred by patients with diseases such as cerebrovascular insufficiency and lung tumors.
- The development of new and complicated surgical procedures, such as transplantation of the liver, lung, small intestine, and pancreas, created a new and important role for critical care following transplantation.
- Widespread utilization of noninvasive patient monitoring has further reduced the cost and medical or nursing complications associated with care of critically ill and injured patients.
- Widespread utilization of pharmacological therapy for critical care patients with specific organ system failure reduced time spent in both critical care units and in the healthcare facility.
- In 2007, more than 4,000 ICUs were operational across the United States.

Their performance, as well as the operation of the ICU, was evaluated over a 2-year period and then compared with the 2 preceding years—when house officers operated the ICU. There were no changes in occupancy, mortality, or the rate of complications. Instead, there seemed to be evidence for more careful evaluation of patients before admission and discharge, manifesting as slightly fewer admissions and slightly longer durations of hospitalization. The authors concluded there is a role for PAs in providing health care in critical care settings (Dubaybo, Samson, & Carlson, 1991). Experience in other hospitals has demonstrated to be similar (Grabenkort & Ramsay, 1991).

Another comparative study involving 5 PAs, 11 NPs, and 41 resident physicians in two critical care units found similar roles (Rudy et al, 1998). The tasks and activities performed by these three types of providers were similar and the outcomes of patients tended by these three providers were the same. Resident physicians tended to treat older and sicker patients and worked longer hours than PAs and NPs.

The role of the intensive care specialist sometimes involves performing a number of procedures. The activities and procedures listed in Exhibit 7-27 are those recorded over a 14-month period (Rudy et al, 1998).

In one hospital in Rhode Island, a rapid response team (RRT) led by PAs was assessed on the rates of in-hospital cardiac arrests, total and unplannned ICU admissions, and hospital mortality. There were 344 RRT calls during the study period. In the 5 months before the RRT system began, there were an average of 7.6 cardiac arrests per 1,000 discharges per month. In the subsequent 13 months, that figure decreased to 3.0 cardiac arrests per 1,000 discharges per month. Overall, the hospital mortality the year before the RRT system was 2.8% and decreased to 2.4% by the end

EXHIBIT 7-27

Activities and Procedures of Critical Care Physician Assistants, Nurse Practitioners, and Physicians in Training (Residents/House Officers)

- Formally present and discuss patient with staff, nursing, and others
- Provide hands-on treatment
- Serve as preceptor or instructor
- Chart, dictate, compute, and write orders
- Discuss care and interact with patient, family, and others
- Perform formal consultation
- Perform hands-on assessment
- Arrange, obtain, or review laboratory test results
- Review chart notes or records
- Transfer patient on or off unit, or discharge
- Conference or lecture
- Perform administrative or research duties

INVASIVE PROCEDURES PERFORMED BY CRITICAL CARE PAs AND NPs
- Venipuncture
- Arterial or venous cutdowns
- Percutaneous placement of arterial catheters
- Placement of pulmonary artery catheters
- Placement of central venous catheters

- Placement of pigtail catheter
- Placement of chest tube
- Oral or nasal endotracheal intubation
- Paracentesis
- Thoracentesis
- Arthrocentesis
- Lumbar puncture
- Insertion of drains
- Bone marrow aspiration
- Liver and other biopsy
- Wound closure (superficial and deep)
- Wound débridement
- Placement or removal of nasogastric or feeding tube
- Insertion or removal of nasal packing
- Removal of superficial foreign body
- Placement of transcutaneous pacemaker
- Application of plaster casts

Data from Rudy, E. B. et al. (1998). Care activities and outcomes of patients cared for by acute care nurse practitioners, physician assistants, and resident physicians: A comparison. *American Journal of Critical Care, 7*(4), 267–281.

of the RRT year. The percentage of ICU admissions that were unplanned decreased from 45% to 29%. Linear regression analysis of key outcome variables showed strong associations with the implementation of the RRT system, as did analysis of variables over time (Exhibit 7-28). PAs successfully managed emergency airway situations without assistance in the majority of cases (Dacey et al, 2007).

A systematic review on the role of the PA and NP in acute and critical care settings revealed 31 research studies focused on the role and impact of these practitioners in the care of acute and critically ill patients. Most studies used retrospective or prospective study designs and nonprobability sampling techniques. Only two randomized control trials were identified. The majority examined the impact of care on patient care management (N = 17), six focused on comparisons of care with physician care, five examined the impact of models of care including multidisciplinary and outcomes management models, and three assessed involvement and impact on reinforcement of practice guidelines, education, research, and quality improvement.

The authors concluded that further research that explores the impact of PAs and NPs in the ICU setting on patient outcomes, including financial aspects of care is needed. In addition, information on successful multidisciplinary models of care is needed to promote optimal use of these providers in acute and critical care settings (Kleinpell, Ely, & Grabenkort, 2008).

Profile

In a survey undertaken by the AAPA, 88 PAs in critical care medicine responded (Exhibit 7-29). The average age was 39, females were 55% of the cohort, and 77% were employed by a hospital. All (100%) worked in an urban setting. The majority (91%) worked full time (at least 32 hours per week) and 67% were salary-based. The average salary in 2008 was $96,984 (AAPA, 2008a).

Professional Society

The Society of Critical Care Medicine has a special section for PA members. Their website is http://www.sccm.org/Membership/Specialty_Sections/Physician_Assistant/Pages/default.aspx.

EXHIBIT 7-28
Cardiac Arrests per 1,000 Discharges Versus Rapid Response Team Calls (May 2004–October 2005)

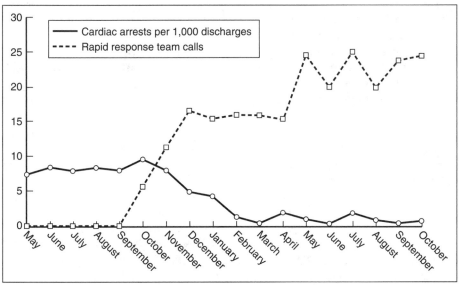

Data from Dacey, M.J., et al. (2007). The effect of a rapid response team on major clinical outcome measures in a community hospital. Critical Care Medicine, 35(9), *2076–2082.*

EXHIBIT 7-29
Critical Care Physician Assistants, 2008

Total survey respondents	88
Age (mean years)	39
Female	47 (55%)
Multispecialty physician group practice	6 (10%)
Hospital	67 (77%)
Years in clinical practice	8
Work in urban setting	100%
Precept PA students	56%
Work more than 32 hours per week	91%
Mean income	$96,984

*Data from American Academy of Physician Assistants. (2008a). 2008
AAPA Physician Assistant Census Report. Alexandria, VA: Author.*

Dermatology

Dermatologists specialize in the diagnosis and treatment of diseases and tumors of the skin and its appendages. There are medical and surgical sides to this specialty. Dermatologic surgeons practice skin cancer surgery (including Mohs' micrographic surgery), laser surgery, cryosurgery, photodynamic therapy, and cosmetic procedures using botulinum toxin, soft tissue fillers, sclerotherapy, and liposuction. Dermatopathologists interpret tissue under the microscope (histopathology). Pediatric dermatologists specialize in the diagnosis and treatment of skin disease in children. Immunodermatologists specialize in the diagnosis and management of skin diseases driven by an altered immune system, including bullous diseases such as pemphigus. In addition, a wide range of congenital syndromes are managed by dermatologists.

Role

The role of the dermatology PA is to assess the skin complaint of the patient, biopsy the lesion (if necessary), and provide treatment. These tasks are usually done under the direction and delegation of a dermatologist, although some group practices of internists have employed PAs to function as first contact for patients with dermatological complaints. PAs in dermatology may medically treat common skin conditions such as acne. Some PAs with advanced skills may transpose surgical flaps,

remove scars and tattoos, and assist in hair transplants. A profile of a dermatology PA in a private clinic demonstrates that the patients seen range from children to 80 year olds, and the diagnoses span many conditions from adolescent skin disorders to suspicious nevi (Steiner, 2008).

History

In the late 1960s, a technical PA program developed briefly at the University of Chicago Pritzker School of Medicine in the Dermatology Department under the direction of Dr. Stanford I. Lamberg, a noted dermatologist. This was a 12-month program that graduated a certified PA in dermatology. The requirements were a high school diploma plus 3 years of healthcare experience, such as being an RN or a medical corpsman (Sadler, 1972).

Interest in expanding the role of the primary care PA into dermatology has been present for more than three decades (Krasner et al, 1977; Katterjohn, 1982). In one descriptive study, the PA was found to be a useful addition in relieving some of the burden of patient care, but neither patient flow nor income was favorably affected (Laur et al, 1981). In another dermatology practice, PAs specialized in removal of suspicious moles, acne scars, port-wine stains, and other birthmarks. Lasers were used for hair removal, tattoo removal, and the treatment of hemangiomas (Samsot, 1998). The economics of managed care and current emphasis on cost reduction continue to make PAs attractive to dermatologists (Baker, 2000; Monroe, 2001).

An analysis of the 1996 and 1997 National Ambulatory Medical Care Survey (NAMCS) data found that the dermatologic conditions evaluated by PAs accounted for 14% of all primary care visits. Dermatologic symptoms were the primary reason for a visit to all physicians 11% of the time. The NAMCS identified that approximately 2.5% of all patient visits involved a PA as the provider of care (Clark et al, 2000).

In 2008, there were more than 900 formally trained PAs who identified their clinical practice as dermatology (AAPA, 2008a). The majority worked in private dermatologists' offices and reported seeing or billing for an average of 28 patients a day (Clark et al, 2000). The procedures are listed in Exhibit 7-30. Currently, postgraduate programs in dermatology are at the University of Texas Southwestern Medical Center in Dallas and at Kirksville College of Osteopathic Medicine. These programs provide 12-month fellowships and a stipend for PAs interested in dermatology.

The American Academy of Dermatology's 2007 practice profile survey analyzed patterns of PA and NP use. Of 3,965 surveys mailed, responses were obtained from 1,243 dermatologists (31% response rate). Overall, 325 responding dermatologists (29.6%) reported using PAs, NPs, or both in their practices in 2007, a 43% increase from the proportion in 2002 (20.7%). PAs were more prevalent than NPs (23% vs. 10%). By the year 2010, 36.2% of respondents plan to hire these nonphysician providers. Younger cohorts of dermatologists were significantly more likely to use PAs and NPs as were those in group and academic practices. Respondents seeking to hire additional dermatologists and those with surgical or cosmetically focused practices were much more likely to use PA or NPs. Respondents reported supervising their nonphysician clinicians on-site 93% of the time, but 31% were off-site 10% of the time or more. Most dermatologists allowed their PA and NP colleagues to see new patients and established patients experiencing new problems. A minority of these patients were formally presented to a physician. PAs and NPs spent the majority of their time seeing medical dermatology patients, even if their supervising dermatologist was primarily engaged in surgical or cosmetic dermatology.

The authors concluded that in the setting of persistently long patient wait times and difficulty recruiting new physician staff, dermatologists have turned to PAs and NPs to help meet patient demand for care. In the aggregate, PAs and NPs are primarily caring for new and established medical dermatology patients under indirect supervision. In the absence of explicit consensus or policy as to how the field should ensure future access to care for patients with skin disease, growth in the use of nonphysician clinicians has continued, with significant variation in use and supervision patterns (Resneck & Kimball, 2008).

Concern about a perceived liability has been raised by authors from time to time (Nestor, 2005). This concern appears to be more theoretical than actual, and the number of PAs and NPs in dermatology continues to rise (Anonymous, 2004). However, if the role of PAs in dermatology expands into cosmetic surgery, this liability may be more real than theoretical (White & Geronemus, 2002).

EXHIBIT 7-30
Procedures Frequently Performed by Physician Assistants in Dermatology

- Cryotherapy of benign lesions
- Intralesional injections
- Laser surgery
- Incisional and excisional biopsies
- Wound closure of flaps and grafts
- Phototherapy
- Patch testing
- Hair transplantations
- Sclerotherapy
- Mohs' surgery
- Chemical peels

Data from Clark, A. R., et al. (2000). The emerging role of physician assistants in the delivery of dermatological health care. *Dermatologic Clinics, 18*(2), 297–302.

Profile

In a survey undertaken by the AAPA, 900 PAs in dermatology responded (Exhibit 7-31). The average age was 38, females were 79% of the cohort, and 42% worked in a single specialty physician group practice. Almost all (94%) worked in an urban setting. The majority (81%) worked full time (at least 32 hours per week) and 84% were salary-based. The average salary in 2007 was $104,474 (AAPA, 2008a).

EXHIBIT 7-31
Dermatology Physician Assistants, 2008

Total survey respondents	900
Age (mean years)	38
Female	703 (79%)
Solo physician practitioner	367 (41%)
Single specialty physician group practice	372 (42%)
Multispecialty physician group practice	74 (8%)
Hospital	40 (4%)
Minor surgical procedures	94%
Years in clinical practice	8
Work in urban setting	94%
Precept PA students	34%
Work more than 32 hours per week	81%
Mean income	$104,474

Data from American Academy of Physician Assistants. (2008a). 2008 AAPA Physician Assistant Census Report. Alexandria, VA: Author.

Professional Society

The Society of Dermatology Physician Assistants (SDPA) was founded in 1994 and is composed of members who have a medical interest in the management of dermatological conditions. The organization has over 1,200 members. Their website is http://www.dermpa.org.

The *Journal of Dermatology for Physician Assistants (JDPA)*, the official journal of the SDPA, premiered in 2007. More information about the journal can be found at http://jdpa.org/index.html.

Emergency Medicine

Emergency medicine focuses on diagnosis and treatment of acute illnesses and injuries that require immediate medical attention. Although they usually do not provide long-term or continuous care, emergency medicine physicians and nurses provide care with the aim of improving long-term patient outcomes. Emergency medicine provided within an ED must be distinguished from care provided in urgent care centers. Urgent care centers are commonly staffed by providers who may or may not be formally trained in emergency medicine. These providers offer primary care treatment to patients who desire or require

immediate care but they do not reach the acuity required for providing care in an ED.

Emergency medicine encompasses a large amount of general medicine but involves virtually all fields of the surgical subspecialties. Physicians are tasked with seeing a large number of patients, treating their illnesses, and arranging for disposition (admitting them to the hospital or releasing them after treatment as necessary). The emergency physician requires a broad field of knowledge and advanced procedural skills, which are commonly used in interventions such as surgical procedures, trauma resuscitation, advanced cardiac life support, and advanced airway management. Emergency physicians ideally have the skills of many specialists—the ability to manage a difficult airway (anesthesia), to suture a complex laceration (plastic surgery), to reduce (set) a fractured bone or dislocated joint (orthopedics), to treat a myocardial infarction (internist/cardiologist), to work up a pregnant patient with vaginal bleeding (obstetrics and gynecology), and stem epistaxsis (ENT) (Camargo et al, 2008).

Role

The PA in emergency medicine tends to be highly skilled in advanced cardiac life support, advanced trauma life support, toxicology, orthopedics, trauma, and neurology. An emergency medicine PA may be the provider directing a code for a cardiac arrest or assisting in a polytrauma stabilization. Most PAs in emergency medicine work as a team, although a few may be the only provider in a small rural hospital (with immediate backup by a doctor).

History

Shortly after the first few PA classes had graduated, they were occupying roles in hospitals, and before long they were in the EDs. PAs were used to manage the less acute patients, such as in a fast-track/urgency care clinic, and other times they were seeing undifferentiated acute medical and trauma patients. At first glance this employment seemed a natural fit because many had developed trauma expertise in the military and some had wartime experience that honed their skills further.

Others had worked as trauma nurses and technicians.

There is much consensus that the education process seems to prepare the interested PA for ED services (Gentile, 1976; Friedman, 1978). In 2006, approximately 9% of PAs reported that they were employed in an emergency medical setting.

A few studies have described the range of services a PA provides in an ED setting. In a small rural community hospital, a PA competently managed 62% of all presenting conditions (Maxfield et al, 1975). In an urban setting, PA roles were quite diverse and helped bridge complex cultural gaps in medical surgical services (Goldfrank, Corso, & Squillacote, 1980). Despite the limited studies regarding the full range of services that can be provided by an emergency PA or NP, most believe the range of services is similar to that of physicians. Regarding the concentration of both types of practitioners in some EDs, results of a 1993 survey of 111 Veterans Affairs (VA) medical centers showed that a mean of 1.9 full-time equivalent (FTE) PAs were employed in 37 EDs and a mean of 2.1 FTE NPs were employed in 29 EDs (Young, 1993).

Hooker and McCaig (1996) analyzed the results of the National Ambulatory Hospital Medical Care Survey that began in 1992. Combining PAs and NPs for statistical purposes, they found that PAs and NPs managed 3.5 million (4%) of the approximately 90 million nonfederal ED visits in the United States. They concluded that there are few differences in the type of patient seen at PA and NP visits compared with physician visits when gender, reason for visit, diagnosis, and medications prescribed are compared (Hooker & McCaig, 1996). In another study, Arnopolin and Smithline (2000) compared patient encounters between PAs and physicians and reached a conclusion that the distribution of diagnostic groups between PAs and physicians was similar. Some differences that emerged were the time for patients and the total charges (Exhibit 7-32). Overall, visits were 8 minutes longer and total charges were $8 less when a PA treated a patient. Patients who had headache, otitis, respiratory

infection, asthma, a GI or genitourinary disorder, cellulitis, laceration, or a musculoskeletal disorder had a longer visit when seen by a PA. The difference in visit time ranged from 5 minutes to 32 minutes longer than a visit with a physician (Arnopolin & Smithline, 2000). Innovative programs that utilize PAs in EDs have included laceration management. In one example, the PA was on call to manage all lacerations that presented to an ED. In one study, results indicated improved care and outcome, decreased cost, and satisfied patients (Katz et al, 1994).

Five postgraduate programs are available to train the PA in emergency medicine. Active programs include Alderson-Broaddus in West Virginia and Montefiore Hospital in New York. The University of Southern California in Los Angeles was the first with such a program, but it closed in 1995. The Army implemented a postgraduate program to train Army PAs in emergency medicine in 1992. These military programs are located at Brooke Army Medical Center in Texas and Madigan Army Medical Center in Washington State (Herrera et al, 1994). In 2007, the Brooke Army program was expanded to 18 months and a research component was introduced. Also, the Army program now awards a doctorate of science (DSc) in emergency medicine through Baylor University in Waco, Texas (Salyer, 2008).

Patient satisfaction with PAs in the ED seems to be as high as that for physicians. A 1999 study of patients who were seen in a fast-track ED were surveyed about their experience with the PA who took care of them. A total of 111 survey results were analyzed. The mean response was 93 (on a scale of 0 to 100). This demonstrates a high degree of satisfaction with ED PAs. Only 12% of the patients said they would be willing to wait longer to be seen by a physician (Counselman, Graffeo, & Hill, 2000).

Cutbacks in residency programs of surgical specialties have necessitated substitutions for traditional trauma providers. Miller and colleagues (1998) examined the use of PAs in a large trauma center in Flint, Michigan. Over the 3 years spanning 1994 through 1996, the use of a team of trauma surgeons and PAs was

EXHIBIT 7-32
Comparison of Emergency Department Patient Encounters

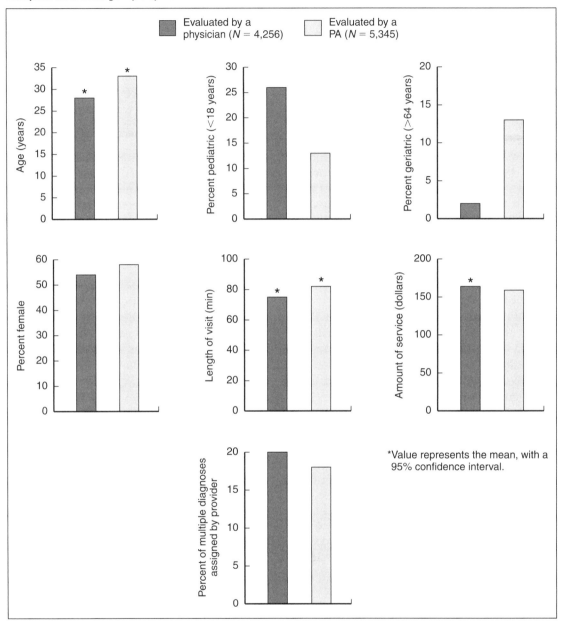

Data from Arnopolin, S. L. & Smithline, H. A. (2000). Patient care by physician assistants and by physicians in an emergency department. Journal of the American Academy of Physician Assistants, 13(12), 39–40, 49–50, 53–54, 81.

introduced in an effort to off-load some of the surgeon's workload. During this period of PA use, the injury severity scores increased 19%, transfer time to the operating room decreased 43%, transfer time to the ICU decreased 51%, and transfer time to the floor decreased 20%. The length of stay for admissions decreased 13%, and the length of stay for neurotrauma ICU patients decreased 33% (Exhibit 7-33). Some of the procedures performed by PAs included chest tube insertion, admit and discharge summaries, central venous and

EXHIBIT 7-33
Trauma Service Summary, 1994–1996

	1994	1995	1996
MECHANISM OF INJURY (PERCENT)			
Blunt	64	64	63
Penetrating	26	23	25
Burn	10	11	10
INJURY SEVERITY SCORE			
All admissions	10.0	12.0	10.8
Critical care	13.4	16.25	16.0
Stepdown	7.3	8.5	8.4
Floor	5.6	7.1	5.1
TRANSFER TO (HOURS)			
Operating room	2.3	2.0	1.5
Step/intensive care unit	5.9	5.1	2.9
Floor	4.9	4.8	3.9
LENGTH OF STAY (DAYS)			
All admissions	5.4	5.1	4.7
Critical care	9.3	7.8	6.2
Stepdown	3.1	3.2	2.9
Floor	6.4	3.2	3.8

Modified from Miller, W., et al. (1998). Use of physician assistants as surgery/trauma house staff at an American College of Surgeons–verified level II trauma center. Journal of Trauma, 44(2), 372–376.

EXHIBIT 7-34
Level of Training, Wound Care Practices, and Infection Rates

Emergency Department Practitioner and Wounds per No. of Cases Sutured	Wound Infection Rate (%)
Medical student (0/60)	0
All resident physicians (17/547)	3.1
PAs (11/305)	3.6
Attending physicians (14/251)	5.6
Junior practitioners (medical students and interns) (8/262)	3.1
Senior practitioners (PAs, residents, attending physicians) (34/901)	3.8

Modified from Singer, A. J., et al. (1995). Level of training, wound care practices, and infection rates. American Journal of Emergency Medicine, 13(3), 265–268.

p = .58, not significant for any difference.

pulmonary artery catheter placements, and subclavian catheterizations (Miller et al, 1998). The authors concluded the decreased length of stay in critical care units and in the hospital as a whole resulted in significant savings by the employment of these two trauma PAs.

Few studies comparing the outcomes of ED care provided by PAs versus that provided by physicians have been undertaken. One prospective, nonrandomized descriptive study compared the traumatic wound infection rates in patients based on level of training in ED practitioners. Wounds were evaluated in 1,163 patients using a wound registry and a follow-up visit or phone call. Exhibit 7-34 demonstrates the results on wound care. There was no significant difference in level of training and wound care rates between medical students, interns, PAs, resident physicians, and attending physicians. The authors concluded that the delegation of wound management to PAs is a safe one and that they perform similarly to physicians in the same setting (Singer et al, 1995).

A 10-year analysis of the roles of PAs and NPs in emergency medicine was undertaken by Hooker, Cipher, and Cawley (2008). The data source was the National Hospital Outpatient Medical Care Survey for Emergency Medicine spanning 1995 through 2004. The most frequently seen diagnoses were abdominal pain, otitis media, upper respiratory infections, chest pain, and acute pharyngitis (Exhibit 7-35). The mean number of prescriptions written by doctors, PAs, and NPs over this same period was very similar (Exhibit 7-36), suggesting convergence of approaches to similar patients.

PAs and NPs are also employed in EDs in Ontario and Manitoba, Canada. The PAs are all formally trained and are a mix of Canadians and Americans. Outcome studies in Ontario are comparing PAs, NPs, and doctors in the care they receive.

The development and use of PAs in England has produced some theoretical ways of their deployment. To determine the amount of time senior house officers (SHOs) spent performing tasks that could be delegated to a technician or administrative assistant (and therefore to quantify the expected benefit that could be obtained by employing PAs),

EXHIBIT 7-35
Most Frequently Seen Diagnoses by Type of Prescriber, 1995–2004

	Physician	PA	NP	p*
Abdominal pain, unspecified	33,215,742 (3.47%)	1,552,137 (2.65%)	341,470 (1.93%)	0.0001
Otitis media	31,146,225 (3.25%)	1,862,565 (3.18%)	796,764 (4.51%)	0.039
Upper respiratory infection	27,731,523 (2.89%)	1,759,089 (3.00%)	589,812 (3.34%)	0.594
Chest pain, unspecified	25,041,151 (2.61%)	951,978 (1.62%)	300,080 (1.70%)	0.0001
Acute pharyngitis	19,970,835 (2.08%)	1,655,613 (2.82%)	589,812 (3.34%)	0.0001

*p value from design-corrected Pearson chi-square.

Data from Hooker, R. S., et al. (2008). Emergency medicine services: Interprofessional care trends. Journal of Interprofessional Care, 22(2), 167–178.

EXHIBIT 7-36
Mean Number of Prescriptions Written by Type of Emergency Medicine Provider for 1995–2004

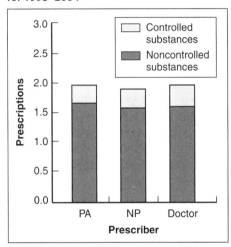

Data from Hooker, R. S., et al. (2008). Emergency medicine services: Interprofessional care trends. Journal of Interprofessional Care, 22(2), 167–178.

SHOs working in the ED were observed for 1 week by pre-clinical students who had been trained to code and time each task performed by SHOs. Activity was grouped into four categories: clinical, technical, administrative, and other. Those activities in the technical and administrative categories were those that could be performed by a PA.

The results showed that SHOs worked 430 hours in total; 86% of the time was accounted for by various codes. The process of taking a history and examining patients accounted for an average of 22% of coded time. Writing the patient's notes accounted for

an average of 20% of coded time. Discussion with relatives and patients accounted for 5% of coded time and performing procedures accounted for another 5% of coded time. On average across all shifts, 15% of coded time was spent doing either technical or administrative tasks. The authors concluded that an average of 15% of coded SHOs' working time was spent performing administrative and technical tasks, rising to 17% of coded time during a night shift. This is equivalent to an average time of 78 minutes per 10-hour shift per SHO. Most tasks included in these categories could be performed by PAs, thus potentially decreasing patient waiting times, improving risk management, allowing doctors to spend more time with their patients, and possibly improving doctors' training (Mitchell, Hayhurst, & Robinson, 2004).

Profile

In a survey undertaken by the AAPA, 2,651 PAs in emergency medicine responded (Exhibit 7-37). The average age was 40, and females were 52% of the cohort. Of respondents, 33% worked in a single specialty physician group practice, 37% worked in a hospital, 6% were self-employed (such as contracting their services), and the remainder were employed by different groups or agencies. Most (85%) worked in an urban setting. The majority (85%) worked full time (at least 32 hours per week). Approximately one-third were salary-based (36%) and 63% were paid an hourly wage. The average salary in 2008 was $99,635 (AAPA, 2008a). This higher salary differential from other specialized PAs may

EXHIBIT 7-37
Emergency Medicine Physician Assistants, 2008

Total survey respondents	2,651
Age (mean years)	40
Female	1,356 (52%)
Self-employed	155 (6%)
Solo physician practitioner	8 (0%)
Single specialty physician group practice	865 (33%)
Multispecialty physician group practice	140 (5%)
Hospital	970 (37%)
Minor surgical procedures	2,130 (80%)
Years in clinical practice	9
Work in urban setting	85%
Precept PA students	48%
Work more than 32 hours per week	85%
Mean income	$99,635

Data from American Academy of Physician Assistants. (2008a). 2008 AAPA Physician Assistant Census Report. Alexandria, VA: Author.

reflect that many emergency medicine PAs are shift workers.

Professional Society

The Society of Emergency Medicine Physician Assistants (SEMPA) maintains a website at http://www.sempa.org and has a membership of over 3,000 PAs. An annual survey is undertaken by SEMPA.

Endocrinology (and Diabetology)

Endocrinology involves the study of the biosynthesis, storage, chemistry, and physiological function of hormones and the cells of the endocrine glands and tissues that secrete them. Such organs include the thyroid, parathyroid, pancreas, ovaries, testes, adrenal, pituitary, and hypothalamus. Most endocrinologist work is with diabetes, thyroid disorders, and bone metabolism.

Role

The PA in endocrinology may manage patients with endocrinopathies such as thyroid disease, metabolic syndrome, vitamin deficiencies, and bone mineral metabolism, or may choose to focus on patients with type 1 or type 2 diabetes mellitus. Almost all endocrinology PAs work

with an endocrinologist, but a diebetology PA may be part of an internal medicine practice.

History

Diabetes is considered the domain of endocrinologists and primary care. The American Diabetes Association recognizes that a diabetologist is anyone who is involved with the diagnosis and management of diabetes and its complications.

The early PA programs stressed that PAs be trained in the insulin management of diabetes. The Diabetes Trust Fund in Birmingham, Alabama, established the only known diabetes PA program in the late 1960s. This 2-year program offered a certified diabetes PA degree and approximately six individuals matriculated through the program (Sadler, 1972). Little is known about this program other than that the graduate was a PA trained in diabetes management. One book has been written detailing diabetes management in HMOs using primarily PAs (Power, Bakker, & Cooper, 1973).

Profile

In a survey undertaken by the AAPA, 116 PAs in endocrinology responded. Eleven were pediatric oriented and three were with the Veterans Health Affairs (Exhibit 7-38). The average age was 42, females were 83% of the cohort, and 29% worked in a single specialty physician

EXHIBIT 7-38
Endocrinology Physician Assistants, 2008

Total survey respondents	116
Age (mean years)	42
Female	96 (83%)
Solo physician practitioner	30 (26%)
Single specialty physician group practice	33 (29)%
Multi-specialty physician group practice	21 (18)%
Years in clinical practice	10
Work in urban setting	94%
Precept PA students	30%
Work more than 32 hours per week	88%
Mean income	$78,956

Data from American Academy of Physician Assistants. (2008a). 2008 AAPA Physician Assistant Census Report. Alexandria, VA: Author.

group practice. Almost all (94%) worked in an urban setting. The majority (88%) were full time (worked at least 32 hours per week) and 92% were salary-based. The average salary in 2008 was $78,956 (AAPA, 2008a).

Forensic Medicine, Coroner, Medical Examiner

Forensic medicine is a broad spectrum of sciences used by the judicial system to answer questions concerning a crime or a civil action. It is a multidisciplinary specialty that provides impartial scientific evidence for use in the courts of law. As a discipline, it draws principally from chemistry, biology, physics, geology, psychology, and the social sciences. A coroner is an appointed official responsible for investigating deaths and determining the cause of death. Depending on the jurisdiction, the coroner may determine the cause himself or herself, or act as the presiding officer of a special report conducted by other appointed experts dictated by the case. *Medical examiner* is a frequently used alternative title; however, unlike a coroner, a medical examiner is typically a licensed pathologist.

Role

Forensic medicine PAs are employed as investigators in a number of jurisdictions. Examples include the medical examiner offices in Suffolk County, New York; Pueblo, Colorado; New Hampshire; Washington, DC; and New York City. For some PAs, these jobs are full time; for others, their role is part time.

Qualifications vary by state, but it is not unusual for a public coroner to be a PA, although the role of coroner is largely investigative in many jurisdictions. The coroner examines the crime scene, records what is present at the scene, and then makes determinations as to whether an autopsy, judicial hearing, or coroner's inquest is necessary. Whereas a board-certified pathologist (preferably a forensic pathologist in criminal cases) undertakes the autopsy, the medical examiner can be a PA with a good background in pathology (Howard, 2000b).

History

That PAs would be attracted to forensic medicine is interesting because there seems to be little emphasis on forensic pathology as a potential area of practice in the current PA education curriculum (Cardenas, 1993). As one coroner put it, "Forensic medicine requires many of the same skills looked for in applicants to PA school. It has to be someone who is interested in medicine, someone with the ability to make decisions, someone who can communicate and is compassionate, firm, and fair. And, of course, you have to have the ability to understand scientific data" (Wright & Hirsch, 1987).

The role of a forensic medical examiner can be broad and involves solving crimes, protecting public health, exposing unsafe consumer products, and addressing questions related to insurance claims. Other roles that come into play involve assisting clergy, funeral directors, and embassies. The examiner is called to answer who, what, when, where, and why (Gerchufsky, 1996).

A medical legal investigator tracks the circumstances that led to a violent, unexpected, suspicious, or unattended death; the death of a child; or the death of someone in government custody. Sometimes the death could affect public health, such as with bubonic plague or tuberculosis, or the victim is involved in a "medical misadventure," such as poisoning.

The Philadelphia College of Osteopathic Medicine offers an advanced degree in forensic medicine. This graduate program is designed for the working professional, combining weekend (Friday/Saturday or Saturday/Sunday) classes with online courses that culminate in the degree of master of science in forensic medicine.

Professional Society

Physician Assistants in Forensic Medicine is a special interest group founded in 2000. It focuses its activities on educating PA students in forensics, participating with law enforcement agencies in forensic-based activities, reviewing the literature, and presenting about forensic medicine.

Gastroenterology

Gastroenterology is the study and management of the digestive system and its disorders from the mouth to the anus. Although principally an internal medicine specialty, important advances have contributed to the enteroscopic management of esophageal, intestinal, liver, pancreatic, and biliary tree diseases (hepatology or hepatobiliary medicine).

Role

PAs working in gastroenterology are part of a rapidly widening internal medicine field. They may have procedure-oriented roles such as performing endoscopies (primarily flexible sigmoidoscopies and colonoscopies) or liver biopsies (van Leeuwen, 2002). Other roles include assessing and managing patients with celiac sprue, esophagus disease, gastric disease, biliary disease, inflammatory bowel diseases, irritable bowel syndrome, and other intestinal disorders (Gunneson et al, 2002). Additionally, hospitals with large gastroenterology centers may use a PA for procedures, monitoring treatment for hepatitis C, and routine maintenance of certain diseases (Neighbors, 2007).

History

From 1972 to 1976 a technician-type PA program in gastroenterology operated briefly at the University of Washington and the VA hospital in Seattle. This 12-month federally funded program trained about 12 PAs to perform rigid sigmoidoscopies, blind biopsies of the esophagus, and manometry; to process tissue; and to assist in other aspects of endoscopy, all of which preceded the development of flexible fiberoptic instruments. Although this program did not survive long, the role of the PA in various endoscopic procedures has persisted. Several screening flexible sigmoidoscopy programs have relied on PAs, NPs, and RNs for more than a decade (Cargill et al, 1991; Schroy et al, 1988; Weissman et al, 1987). The question of sanctioning independent endoscopy has been debated in the literature (Palmer, 1990; Smith, 1992). Currently, PAs are trained formally and informally in flexible sigmoidoscopy, colonoscopy, and gastroscopy (Horton et al, 2001).

The benefit of a PA in one gastroenterology setting included improved staff efficiency, improved house staff education, and ability to perform an increased number of procedures with existing staff over a 3-year period (Lieberman & Ghormley, 1992) (Exhibit 7-39). It is probably no coincidence that this study was done at a VA center because of the historical role they have played in developing the PA concept and because the large scale of these medical centers allows them to experiment with alternatives to physician-directed services.

Researchers at Harvard Vanguard Medical Associates, a large multispecialty medical group, assessed NPs and PAs who perform screening flexible sigmoidoscopies. Data from 9,500 screening procedures were evaluated. The authors concluded that, in comparison

EXHIBIT 7-39

Impact of a Gastroenterology Physician Assistant on Procedure Workload

	Procedures per Year			Percent Change 1987 to 1990
	1987 (before PA)	1989 (after PA)	1990	
Sigmoidoscopy	313	386	442	(+) 41
Panendoscopy	646	810	821	(+) 27
Colonoscopy	373	437	439	(+) 18

Data from Lieberman, D. A., & Ghormley, J. M. (1992). Physician assistants in gastroenterology: Should they perform endoscopy? American Journal of Gastroenterology, 87(8), 940–943.

EXHIBIT 7-40
Gastroenterology Physician Assistants, 2008

Total survey respondents	372
Age (mean years)	39
Female	283 (77%)
Single specialty physician group practice	216 (59%)
Hospital	16%
Years in clinical practice	8
Work in urban setting	95%
Precept PA students	24%
Work more than 32 hours per week	86%
Mean income	$84,268

Data from American Academy of Physician Assistants. (2008a). 2008 AAPA Physician Assistant Census Report. *Alexandria, VA: Author.*

with gastroenterologists, trained PA and NP endoscopists performed screening flexible sigmoidoscopy with similar accuracy and safety but at lower cost. The implications were that screening flexible sigmoidoscopy performed by PAs and NPs increased the availability and lowered the cost of flexible sigmoidoscopy for colorectal cancer screening (Horton et al, 2001).

Profile
In a survey undertaken by the AAPA, 372 PAs in gastroenterology responded (Exhibit 7-40). Most (98%) of these PAs see adult patients; however, 17 were pediatric-oriented. The average age was 39, females were 77% of the cohort, and 59% worked in a single specialty physician group practice. Most (95%) worked in an urban setting. The majority (86%) worked full time (at least 32 hours per week). Almost all were salary-based (94%) and the remainder were paid hourly. The average salary in 2008 was $84,268 for adult gastroenterologists (AAPA, 2008a).

Professional Society
The website for Gastrointestinal Physician Assistants (GIPA) is http://www.gipas.org.

Geriatric Medicine

Geriatrics is the branch of internal medicine that focuses on health promotion and the prevention and treatment of disease and disability in later life. Gerontology is the study of the aging process and the research surrounding the delivery of services to elders.

Role
PAs working in geriatrics may work with a geriatrician or in a nursing home or long-term care setting. Typically, they perform a geriatric assessment and elicit significant information regarding living situations, activities of daily living, and psychosocial and other functional status information that may be helpful to rehabilitation professionals. The PA can provide the therapy team (which may include a physical therapist, an occupational therapist, a physiatrist, a rehabilitation nurse, and a psychologist) with an overview of the patient's chronic and acute medical problems, level of disability, level of cognitive impairment, drug history (including current therapy), and other factors that may impact formulation or progress of a rehabilitation program (Brugna, Cawley, & Baker, 2007). Rehabilitative team members working in geriatrics may encounter a PA acting as a primary medical caregiver utilizing (or not utilizing) a geriatric care model; a specialty care provider working with an orthopedist, neurologist, or physiatrist; an administrator; a clinical researcher; or as a direct member of a rehabilitation team in a multidisciplinary approach.

The specific role of a geriatric PA presents many unique clinical challenges, in part because geriatric patients require a substantial amount of coordination of care. "The health care of elders in the United States presents the clinician with social, medical, spiritual and political challenges that cut across the full spectrum of race, religion and social standing" (Alliance for Aging Research, 2003). Multisystem medical problems become even more challenging in the context of ethical and social dilemmas of providing compassionate care. PAs need to know when to refer patients for physical or occupational therapy services, and what information to provide to help therapists effectively provide rehabilitative services. Contact with families, lengthy discussions surrounding end-of-life care, and the coordination of care between many specialists is time consuming and critical in appropriate medical management of geriatric patients. Physicians commonly lack the time required to perform these vital functions. PAs could be very effective at this coordination and liaison role, especially in a solo or small group medical practice.

PAs can also have an important preventive role in the care of geriatric patients (Woolsey, 2005). Most nursing homes and long-term care facilities do not have a full-time medical staff. Physicians typically visit such facilities on a weekly basis. Patients with acute problems are generally treated over the phone or sent to an emergency department. Having a full-time PA on staff at a nursing home or long-term care facility can translate into patients being evaluated sooner and can prevent transfer to the hospital in many cases. In fact, one study found that employment of PAs and NPs in nursing homes was associated with a lower hospitalization rate (Intrator, Zinn, & Mor, 2004).

History

PAs were recognized as effective providers of quality care in geriatric care facilities as early as 1979 (Isiadinso, 1979), and since the late 1980s, most PA programs have tended to include gerontology (Aaronson, 1991; Kane et al, 1991; Aaronson, 1992; Ouslander & Osterweil, 1994). Although geriatric medicine is currently identified by only a small percentage of PAs as their primary specialty area, a significant number, 1,170 or 5.6% of all clinically active PAs, report that they see patients in a nursing home or other long-term facility (AAPA, 2007a). A large number of PAs report treating elderly patients, arbitrarily defined as those 65 years of age or older. In the 2006 AAPA census, PAs reported treating many patients for disorders seen primarily in the elderly population. For example, PAs reported performing approximately 3,584,959 visits for Alzheimer's disease; 6,697,969 visits for osteoporosis; and 4,306,698 visits for overactive bladder/urge incontinence (AAPA, 2007d). However, it is necessary to distinguish between PAs caring for people older than age 65 years and those PAs providing

comprehensive geriatric care. A geriatric care model has a holistic perspective, focusing on function, cognition, and special needs of patients typically 75 years of age or older.

The demographic shift toward an aging population has created a great need for PAs competent in caring for the elderly. In a study analyzing data from the 2005 National Ambulatory Medical Care Survey, 32% of all patients seen by a PA for an outpatient visit were age 65 or older (Cherry, Woodwell, & Rechtsteiner, 2007). Segal-Gideon, a PA in geriatric practice, notes that:

> PAs can act as key facilitators in caring for geriatric patients with multiple chronic, complex, interrelated problems and also in identifying acute problems that may arise. The physician-PA team at my facility coordinates an interdisciplinary approach to geriatric care and rehabilitation, ensuring that patients are medically stable for rehabilitation services and communicating information to therapists and other team members regarding patient's medical status. (Segal-Gidan, 2002)

Despite it being an issue that has been recognized for years, preparing a healthcare workforce for the "aging" of the population in the United States has not been well planned. The elderly represent a large group of Americans with unmet healthcare needs (Alliance for Aging Research, 2006). Recruiting and training PAs to provide services to geriatric populations is recognized as an avenue to address the currently unmet healthcare needs of the elderly population (Frary et al, 2000). Including more content specific to geriatric medicine in PA program curricula can create a PA workforce better prepared to provide needed services in a relatively short time. Curry, Fasser, and Schafft (1987) reported on an increased focus on geriatrics in PA training curricula and reviewed evidence that PAs can provide quality care and improve patient outcomes in ambulatory and institutionalized geriatric patients (Curry, Fasser, & Schafft, 1987).

PAs are well positioned to function on interdisciplinary teams because they are trained to provide care in a team model. The American Geriatric Society's position paper on Geriatric

Rehabilitation supports an interdisciplinary approach, and specifically includes the PA as a provider along with the doctor and NP:

> Rehabilitative or restorative care for older persons with complex needs is therefore optimally provided by an interdisciplinary approach, which may involve physical, speech, occupational and recreational therapists, physicians, nurses, social workers, and/or other health professionals. For specific needs, patients may be well served by the provider (physician, NP, PA) and one or more therapists. (American Geriatrics Society Position Statement, 1999)

Caring for elders usually requires greater clinician time than other patient populations, and past reimbursement constraints and low levels of reimbursement for PA services set by the Centers for Medicare and Medicaid Services (CMS) may have constrained the PA from choosing to practice geriatric medicine (Brunga, Cawley, & Baker, 2007). Recent gains in reimbursement and practice authority for PA services by the CMS have helped improve the climate for PA geriatric practice. Services provided by PAs are reimbursable by Medicare and Medicaid in all patient care settings, including home visits. Under recently expanded CMS guidelines, PAs may participate in telemedicine services and order durable medical equipment (Crane, personal communication, 2006, AAPA comment on proposed CMS rulemaking).

More than 20 studies on the use of PAs in geriatric medicine have been published. The consensus is unanimous: PAs are very effective in patient management and care in geriatric facilities, contributing to quality care by allowing more patients to be seen and relieving the physician of fewer pressing problems. More than one study has demonstrated shorter hospitalization and overall lower medical costs using PAs in geriatric institutional settings (Tideiksaar, 1986). A study by the Rand Corporation demonstrated improvements in care and outcomes when PAs and NPs were introduced into nursing homes. Both nursing home administrators and directors in the demonstration model expressed

higher levels of satisfaction with the process of care (Buchanan, Kane, & Garrard, 1989). Caprio (2006) argues that only by utilizing PAs and NPs in nursing homes will the needs of this special population be met.

In one study on the impact of adding a PA to a large nursing home, the hospitalization rate was dramatically altered. A 6-year case series examined hospital events of one nursing home before and after a PA joined a 92-bed teaching hospital in central Georgia. After the PA started, the number of annual hospital admissions fell by 38%, and the total number of hospital days per 1,000 patient years fell by 69%. The number of nursing home visits increased by 62% (Ackermann & Kemle, 1998) (Exhibit 7-41).

Historically, both medical school and PA program curricula were slow in emphasizing geriatrics (Yturri-Byrd & Glazer-Waldman, 1984; Tideiksaar, 1986). With the revision on Medicare and Medicaid reimbursement for nursing homes, geriatric health care became center stage, and with it came the renewed interest in and the cost-effectiveness of PAs (May, 1988). The increase in the geriatric population and the growing medical concerns of this population have increased the need for more PAs in this area (Dychtwald & Zitter, 1988; Schafft & Cawley, 1987). Virtually all studies on the aging population of both the United States and the world agree that the healthcare needs of the elderly will continue to increase. The opportunities for PAs in new and expanded roles in geriatric medicine and administration are predicted to increase dramatically in the decades to come (Dieter & Fasser, 1989).

Profile

In a survey undertaken by the AAPA, 162 PAs in geriatrics responded (Exhibit 7-42). The average age was 45, females were 78% of the cohort, and 19% worked in a single specialty physician group practice. Approximately 88% worked in an urban setting. The majority (83%) worked full time (at least 32 hours per week) and 87% were salary-based. The average salary in 2008 was $85,973 (AAPA, 2008a).

EXHIBIT 7-41
Hospital Use Rate Before and After Introduction of a Physician Assistant in a Nursing Home

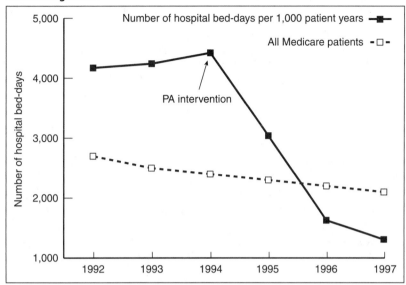

Data from Ackermann, R. J., & Kemle, K. A. (1998). The effect of a physician assistant on the hospitalization of nursing home residents. Journal of the American Geriatrics Society, 46(5), 610–614.

EXHIBIT 7-42
Geriatric Physician Assistants, 2008

Total survey respondents	162
Age (mean years)	45
Female	125 (77%)
Solo physician practitioner	16 (10%)
Single specialty physician group practice	30 (19%)
Multispecialty physician group practice	20 (12%)
Nursing home or long-term care facility	31 (19%)
Years in clinical practice	13
Work in urban setting	89%
Precept PA students	27%
Work more than 32 hours per week	83%
Mean income	$85,973

Data from American Academy of Physician Assistants. (2008a). 2008 AAPA Physician Assistant Census Report. Alexandria, VA: Author.

Professional Society

The Society of Physician Assistants Caring for the Elderly (SPACE) was started in 1997 by a group of PAs interested in enhancing care for the elderly. One of the goals is to promote education and training of all PAs in geriatric health care. Their website is http://www.geri-pa.org.

Global Medicine

Although global medicine is not an official specialty designation for doctors or PAs, the diverse opportunities for the PA who wants to travel abroad to work with international populations must be mentioned.

Role

Global opportunities abound for PAs. PAs in global medicine become skilled in administering immunizations, handling refugees, dealing with sanitation, providing rural remote health and primary care, and treating diseases unique to endemic areas. Various countries have been recruiting PAs for roles in PA demonstration projects. Some of these PAs are assisting educators and healthcare analysts to implement PA programs. Specifics about this trend are discussed in Chapter 18.

The *AAPA News* (and its successor *PA Professional*) have profiled a number of PAs working overseas in various roles over the past decade. Some of these PAs have been recognized as Humanitarian PA of the Year by the AAPA.

Chidley (1997a) offers an example of a PA working in global medicine. To practice in Kenya, the PA had to apply for a reciprocal license as a "clinical officer," a designation more or less equivalent to the U.S. designation of PA, but she was allowed to function autonomously 6 miles from the Tanzanian border on the shore of Lake Victoria. She was the highest ranking clinician in the area. (The nearest physicians were a 1-day's drive over a difficult road.) She oversaw 18 Kenyans who had been trained informally by previous U.S. staff. She supervised the staff, provided most of the administration, and saw patients (Chidley, 1997a).

History

Today, more than 40 agencies recruit volunteer PA, physician, nurse, and allied health personnel to work in underdeveloped countries. Most stints range from 1 to 2 years (Kuhns, 2002). Usually, transportation and a small stipend are provided for the volunteer. Employers of PAs include the U.S. government, with agencies such as the Peace Corps, U.S. Agency for International Development, and the State Department; nongovernmental organizations such as Doctors Without Borders; and nongovernment organizations (NGOs) or private corporations.

One of the easiest ways for PAs to work outside the borders of the United States is through corporations that specifically employ PAs along with other health workers. For example, Seavin is a health unit that employs over a dozen PAs in Egypt who work in remote areas to provide health care to American and Egyptian personnel.

Profile

A survey of PAs working overseas was undertaken in 2001, and the resulting list of countries in which PAs have worked is extensive (Exhibit 7-43). Obstacles and advantages to working in global medicine are outlined in Exhibits 7-44 and 7-45, respectively.

EXHIBIT 7-43
Partial List of Countries Where Respondent Physician Assistants Have Worked or Volunteered

Afghanistan	Guinea-Bissau	Papua New Guinea
Albania	Guyana	Peru
Angola	Honduras	Philippines
Australia	India	Republic of Georgia
Belize	Indonesia	Russia
Brazil	Iraq	Saipen
China	Jamaica	Samoa
Columbia	Kazakhstan	Saudi Arabia
Cuba	Kenya	Sierra-Leone
Dominican	Kosovo	Solomon Islands
Republic	Laos	Sudan
East Timor	Mexico	Tanzania
Ecuador	Mongolia	Thailand
El Salvador	Mozambique	Togo
Egypt	Nepal	Tonga
Great Britain	Nicaragua	Vietnam
Guam	Nigeria	
Guatemala	Pakistan	

Data modified from Rogers, S. E. (2002). Physician assistants working and volunteering abroad: A survey. *Unpublished doctoral dissertation, Arizona School of Health Sciences Physician Assistant School, Mesa, Arizona.*

Professional Society

Physician Assistants for Global Health (PAGH) is a network organization for PAs with international experience. Their website provides a list of items to consider when seeking a job as a PA overseas as well as a list of job opportunities and organizations. Their website can be found at http://www.pasforglobalhealth.org/pas.htm.

Infectious Disease, Immunology, Immunodeficiency

Infectious disease specialists address disease-causing organisms likely to be transmitted to people through the environment. Most of these specialists are trained in internal medicine and work in hospital and outpatient settings.

Role

PAs who are infectious disease specialists commonly work in both inpatient and outpatient settings. Some PAs have assumed the

EXHIBIT 7-44
Significant Obstacles of International Physician Assistant Work

Obstacles Listed by Respondents	Percentage of Respondents
Language barriers	37.0
Sub-standard facilities	10.9
Lack of equipment or medicine	21.7
Competition with local doctors	2.2
Financial support	15.2
Transportation to medical facilities	2.2
Lack of knowledge of the PA profession	23.9
None	2.2
Lack of follow-up	4.4
New medicines	2.2
Governmental security	4.4
Patients' limited education in Western medicine	2.2
Lack of supervising doctors	4.4
Cost of travel	2.2
Cultural beliefs	4.4
Finding a medical team	2.2
No support from the American Academy of Physician Assistants	2.2
Lack of respect for female clinicians	2.2
Getting time off work	4.4
Time away from family	2.2

Data modified from Rogers, S. E. (2002). Physician assistants working and volunteering abroad: A survey. *Unpublished doctoral dissertation, Arizona School of Health Sciences Physician Assistant School, Mesa, Arizona.*

role of the communicable disease nurse in hospital settings. Others consult with patients seeking advice regarding travel or see patients with immune deficiencies. This latter role commonly involves infectious disorders such as human immunodeficiency viremia (HIV) and acquired immunodeficiency syndrome (AIDS). How these roles are formalized and in what capacities they are performed have not been detailed in the literature.

History

To compare the quality of care provided by NPs and PAs with that provided by physicians, a cross-sectional analysis of 68 HIV care sites in 30 different states was undertaken. These care sites were funded by the Ryan White Comprehensive AIDS Resources

EXHIBIT 7-45
Significant Advantages of International Physician Assistant Work

Significant Benefits Listed by Respondents	Percentage of Respondents
Learning about another culture	37.0
Giving health care to those in need	37.0
Self-growth	15.2
Appreciation for the United States	4.4
New friends	10.9
Patients' eagerness for help	4.4
Travel	8.7
Challenge of clinical skills	19.6
Learning a new language	6.5
More medicine and practice options	6.5
Teamwork	2.2
Demonstrating compassion	4.4

Data modified from Rogers, S. E. (2002). Physician assistants working and volunteering abroad: A survey. *Unpublished doctoral dissertation, Arizona School of Health Sciences Physician Assistant School, Mesa, Arizona.*

Emergency (CARE) Act Title III. The authors surveyed 243 clinicians (177 physicians and 66 NPs and PAs) and reviewed medical records of 6,651 persons with HIV or AIDS. Eight quality-of-care measures were assessed by medical record review. After adjustments for patient characteristics, six of the eight quality measures did not differ between NPs and PAs and infectious disease specialists or generalist HIV experts. Adjusted rates of purified protein derivative testing and Papanicolaou smears were statistically significantly higher for NPs and PAs (0.63 and 0.71, respectively) than for infectious disease specialists (0.53 [$P = 0.007$] and 0.56 [$P = 0.001$], respectively) or generalist HIV experts (0.47 [$P < 0.001$] and 0.62 [$P = 0.025$], respectively). NPs and PAs had statistically significantly higher performance scores than generalist non-HIV experts on six of the eight quality measures. For the measures examined, the quality of HIV care provided by NPs and PAs was similar to that of physician HIV experts and generally better than physician non-HIV experts. The authors concluded that NPs and PAs can provide high-quality care for persons with HIV. Preconditions for this level of performance include high levels of experience, focus on a single condition, and either participation in teams or other easy access to physicians and other clinicians with HIV expertise (Wilson et al, 2005).

Professional Society

The Physician Assistant AIDS Network (PAAN) is an AAPA Ethnocultural Caucus for PAs involved in HIV/AIDS direct care, education, or research. The network was developed in association with the AAPA in 1995 and was designed to facilitate access to current information and the exchange of ideas among PAs who serve people with HIV/AIDS. PAAN's mission is focused on enhancing communication and clinical expertise among PAs with substantial involvement with HIV/AIDS care, education, and research. PAAN accomplishes this mission through education, information dissemination, and the development of professional networks.

Maritime Physician Assistant

Maritime medicine is the care of sick and injured patients on various seafaring vessels in remote areas of the world. The scope of this field of medicine is broad and includes patients of all ages, with every conceivable form of illness or traumatic injury. The unique aspects of maritime medicine are a result of the characteristic problems encountered by those at sea, the logistical difficulties of assessing and treating these patients on the vessel, and the difficulty in arranging and monitoring definitive care.

History

The U.S. Public Health Service Hospital at Staten Island, New York, developed a 12-month PA program for former military medical corpsmen who wanted to continue their medical careers. It was operational briefly in the late 1960s as a technical-type PA program for the Merchant Marine fleet. Graduates were referred to as *marine PAs* and were stationed on ships that employed large crews to oversee their health and safety (DeMaria, Cherry, & Treusdell, 1971; Sadler, Sadler, & Bliss, 1972). The duration of this program and why it closed are not known.

Role

PAs who have served as medical officers on ships such as luxury ocean liners found the experience interesting despite some technical challenges (e.g., having to obtain an unusual medication that a passenger forgot). PAs serving as a ship's medical officer have two basic responsibilities: to care for passengers and crew. Anecdotal reports are that few medical problems came up that a PA was unable to handle.

PAs have also worked for Maritime Medical Access, an institution that provides a link to appropriate medical care for shipping vessels, aircraft, yachts, and teams in remote locations. In operation since 1989, Maritime Medical Access offers worldwide telemedicine advice in addition to clinical case management, repatriation, training, and recommendations for medical equipment and medicine chests. The institution is affiliated with the George Washington University and provides 24-hour access to teams of board-certified emergency physicians and PAs, which has enabled companies to reduce unnecessary medical expenses and the risk of liability. Such formal arrangements with an academic emergency medical center ensures current, state-of-the-art medical practices and case management for ill or injured crewmembers. Information about Maritime Medical Access is available at http://www.gwemed.edu/maritime.htm.

Nephrology

Nephrology is a subspecialty of internal medicine and involves the study and clinical care of kidney diseases. It is based both in the inpatient hospital setting, the office setting, as well as in specialized settings such as transplant units and outpatient dialysis clinics.

Role

PAs in nephrology provide a wide variety of clinical functions including staffing chronic kidney disease clinics, end-stage renal disease (ESRD) dialysis management, vascular access for dialysis management, hospital rounds and reports, and transplant patient management. Almost three-quarters (71%) of responders see

EXHIBIT 7-46
Nephrology Physician Assistants, 2008

Total survey respondents	152
Age (mean years)	40
Female	111 (74%)
Single specialty physician group practice	77 (51%)
Multispecialty physician group practice	22 (15%)
Hospital	30 (20%)
Years in clinical practice	10
Work in urban setting	91%
Precept PA students	22%
Work more than 32 hours per week	91%
Mean income	$80,842

Data from American Academy of Physician Assistants. (2008a). 2008 AAPA Physician Assistant Census Report. Alexandria, VA: Author.

office patients, with a mean of 23 office visits per week. The vast majority (92%) of nephrology PAs manage dialysis patients, with a mean number of 110 seen per week.

Profile

In a survey undertaken by the AAPA, 12 PAs in nephrology responded (Exhibit 7-46). The average age was 41, females were 74% of the cohort, and 51% worked in a single-specialty physician group practice. Approximately 91% worked in an urban setting. The majority (91%) worked full time (at least 32 hours per week) and 96% were salary-based. The average salary in 2008 was $80,842 (AAPA, 2008a).

Professional Society

The American Academy of Nephrology Physician Assistants (AANPA) is the organization representing PAs in this field. The AANPA was founded in 1997 with the purpose of supporting the professional growth, development, training, education, and networking of PAs within the specialty practice of nephrology. It is an officially recognized chapter of the AAPA and maintains an affiliation with the National Kidney Foundation. The organization's website is http://www.aanpa.org/.

Neonatology

Neonatology is a subspecialty of pediatrics involving the medical care of neonates,

especially premature neonates and neonates who require special medical care because of conditions such as low birth weight, intrauterine growth retardation, congenital malformations, sepsis, or birth asphyxia. It is a hospital-based specialty and is usually practiced in neonatal intensive care units (NICUs).

Role

Most neonatal PAs work in large hospitals or medical centers as full-time employees and are oftentimes supervised by a neonatologist. They may take charge of a baby's case immediately based on the baby's birth weight or condition and hospital policies (Otterbourg, 1986). For example, most hospitals with NICUs have a policy that says something along the lines of, "If the baby is sick enough to need intensive care or is significantly premature, it must be taken care of by the hospital neonatologists." Typically, PAs working in neonatology do not see patients in a private office outside of a hospital, although there are exceptions. The role of the neonatal PA has rapidly expanded since the early 1990s because neonatal units have grown faster than the number of pediatric staff members qualified to work on them.

History

The use of nonphysician providers in the neonatal unit has been endorsed in some form since the early 1980s. The Committee on Fetus and Newborn of the American Academy of Pediatrics published a statement on the roles of the NP and PA in the care of hospitalized children, which strongly supported their roles as members of a care team in the neonatal ICU (American Academy of Pediatrics, Committee on Hospital Care, 1999).

Formal postgraduate neonatology programs for PAs exist at the University of Kentucky (Reynolds & Bricker, 2007). Two other residency programs trained the pediatric PA in neonatology: Norwalk Hospital and the Wolfson Children's Hospital in Jacksonville, Florida. The Norwalk program closed in 1996.

Evidence suggests that using neonatal PAs and NPs in the intensive care setting

EXHIBIT 7-47

Pediatric Resident Questionnaire About Working with Neonatology Physician Assistants and Nurse Practitioners

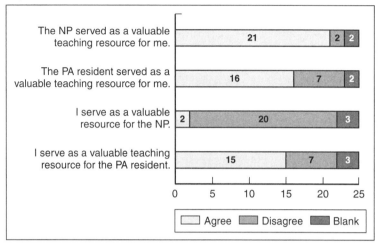

Data from Reynolds, E. W., & Bricker, T. J. (2007). Nonphysician clinicians in the neonatal intensive care unit: Meeting the needs of our smallest patients. Pediatrics, 119(2), 361–369.

is an effective alternative to using pediatric residents. No significant differences in management, outcome, or charge variables can be demonstrated when comparisons are made between patients cared for by either provider at Wolfson Children's Hospital in Jacksonville, Florida (Carzoli et al, 1994; Schulman, Lucchese, & Sullivan, 1995). At the Bronx Municipal Hospital Center, the phasing in of PAs and neonatal NPs overlapped the phasing out of pediatric residents. A study on the survival by birth weight comparing both pediatric residents and neonatal PAs and NPs failed to find any difference between the providers. Additionally, after a period of adjustment to the PA and NP staff, the authors found work rounds required less time with the PA and NP staff than with the residents. The number of errors in ordering parenteral alimentation solutions (as noted by the hospital pharmacy) had fallen as well (Schulman, Lucchese, & Sullivan, 1995).

When the University of Kentucky was unable to recruit PAs and NPs to staff the neonatal ICU, they created a postgraduate training program that drew on the presence of a university-based PA program. A 3-year physician fellowship was altered into a 1-year

PA fellowship in which the objective was to gain experience and knowledge in patient management and technical skills. The program involved 8 months of "hands-on training" in the NICU, 1 month in the neonatal nursery, and three 2-week elective rotations with specific goals developed for each rotation. During the first few years of this effort, a questionnaire was circulated among the pediatric residents asking how they perceived the value and role of the neonatal PA or NP (Exhibit 7-47). The authors concluded that gaps in the neonatal workforce are growing and that neonatal PAs offer an opportunity to help bridge some of the gaps. Without formal PA postgraduate programs, PA graduates are unlikely to select neonatology. The neonatal PA or NP appears to be interchangeable, but some differences do emerge (Reynolds & Bricker, 2007).

Neurology

Neurology is a branch of medicine dealing with disorders of the nervous system. Physicians in neurology investigate, diagnose, and treat neurological disorders of the brain or peripheral nervous system. Pediatric neurologists work with children with congenital disorders, attention deficit disorders, and convulsive disorders.

Role

PAs in neurology perform complete physical and neurological examinations and diagnose and manage patients with multiple sclerosis, movement disorders such as Parkinson's disease, seizure disorders, sleep disorders, and other conditions. They are involved in developing treatment plans for neurological conditions within their scope of practice and in conjunction with the neurologist. They also implement therapeutic interventions when appropriate. PAs in neurology practice in primary care settings as well as with neurologists.

History

A 1987 study of members of the American Academy of Neurology revealed that 29% of respondents to the survey used PAs or nurse clinicians (NCs) in their practices. Institutionally

based neurologists were more likely to use PAs and NCs than those in private practice (Gunderson & Kampen, 1988). At the time of this study, many of these physicians were bringing their office PAs and NCs into the hospital. Unfortunately, this study did not define what a PA was, so presumably these were medical assistants and doctor's assistants.

Taft and Hooker (1999) conducted a telephone survey of 46 full-time neurology PAs working in neurology offices (mostly group practices) (Exhibit 7-48). They found that the range of conditions seen by neurology PAs was similar to that of neurologists (Exhibit 7-49). Most PAs performed lumbar punctures (63%) and initiated multiple sclerosis therapy (50%). Other procedures that were usually reserved for neurologists were also done by PAs (Exhibit 7-50). Half were involved in clinical research studies. Clearly, PAs in neurology practices are performing a wide range of services that are probably not appreciated by physicians who do not work with PAs (Taft & Hooker, 1999).

EXHIBIT 7-48
Practice Setting Characteristics of Neurology Physician Assistants, 1998

PRACTICE SETTING	NUMBER		
Group practice	26		
Hospital-based practice	12		
Solo practice	6		
Health maintenance organization	2		
TOTAL	46		

CHARACTERISTICS	Mean	Range	N
No. of years as a PA	13.5	1–25	46
No. of years working in neurology	7.2	1–25	46
No. of years employed in current neurology practice	5.7	2–19	46
No. of neurologists in your practice	4.2	1–20	46
If you see hospitalized patients, how many do you see in a typical week?	26	4–120	36
If you are in an outpatient practice, how many patients do you see in a typical week?	43	12–100	33
Hours employed to see patients	43.8	16–55	46
Do you see patients in nursing home?	Yes = 7	—	—
Do a you "take call?"	Yes = 17	—	—

Data from Taft, J. M., & Hooker, R. S. (1999). Physician assistants in neurology practice. Neurology, 52(7), 1513.

EXHIBIT 7-49
Conditions Managed by Neurology Physician Assistants in Order of Frequency

- Headaches (all types)
- Cerebral vascular accidents
- Parkinson's disease and other movement disorders
- Seizure disorders
- Multiple sclerosis
- Low back pain
- Peripheral neuropathies
- Chronic pain syndromes (fibromyalgia, focal myofascial pain, and others)
- Dementia, Alzheimer's disease, and others
- Head injuries

NEUROMUSCULAR DISORDERS (CONGENITA0L AND ACQUIRED)

- Neurovascular disorders
- Motor neuron disease
- Myasthenia gravis
- Muscular dystrophies
- Hereditary sensory motor neuropathy
- Radiculopathies (cervical and lumbar)
- Neck pain
- Spinal cord injuries
- Postpolio syndrome

Data from Taft, J.M., & Hooker, R.S. (1999). Physician assistants in neurology practice *Neurology*, 52 (7), 1513.

EXHIBIT 7-50
Procedures Performed By Neurology Physician Assistants by Percentage *N* = 46

Procedure	Percent
Lumbar punctures	63
Initiate multiple sclerosis therapy	50
Tender point injection	14
Nerve conduction studies	14
Initiate and monitor tissue plasminogen activator	11
Nerve blocks	11
Evoked potentials	7
Quantitative sensory testing	2
Botulism injections	2
Interpret electroencephalograms	2

Data from Taft, J. M., & Hooker, R. S. (1999). Physician assistants in neurology practice. Neurology, 52(7), 1513.

EXHIBIT 7-51
Neurology Physician Assistants, 2008

Total survey respondents	161
Age (mean years)	41
Female	118 (74%)
Solo physician practitioner	29 (18%)
Single specialty physician group practice	57 (36%)
Multispecialty physician group practice	26 (16%)
Hospital	23%
Years in clinical practice	8
Work in urban setting	97%
Precept PA students	20%
Work more than 32 hours per week	88%
Mean income	$81,762

Data from American Academy of Physician Assistants. (2008a). 2008 AAPA Physician Assistant Census Report. Alexandria, VA: Author.

Profile

In a survey undertaken by the AAPA, 161 PAs in neurology responded (Exhibit 7-51). The average age was 41, females were 74% of the cohort, and 36% worked in a single specialty physician group practice. All (97%) worked in an urban setting, the majority (88%) worked full time (at least 32 hours per week), and 92% were salary-based. The average salary in 2008 was $81,762 (AAPA, 2008a).

Occupational and Environmental Medicine

Occupational and environmental medicine (also known as *occupational medicine, industrial medicine,* and *corporate medicine*) is a cross-disciplinary area concerned with the safety, health, and welfare of workers. As a secondary effect, occupational and environmental health services may also protect coworkers, family members, employers, customers, suppliers, nearby communities, and other members of the public who may be impacted by the workplace environment. Occupational and environmental medicine is one of the three subspecialties of preventive medicine; the other two are general preventive medicine and aerospace medicine.

Role

The PA in occupational and evironmental medicine delivers physical, mental, and emotional health care and practices preventive medicine. Although health promotion and disease prevention are stressed, much of the PA role encompasses primary care. Activities include occupational health and safety, stress reduction, smoking cessation, and wellness. PAs perform annual employee physical examinations, exercise stress testing, occupational health education, drug screening, and treatment of work-related injuries.

History

Occupational and environmental medicine used PAs as early as 1971, and the specialty has been an optional rotation within many PA programs. One early use of PAs in this field was on the Alaska Pipeline Project in the 1970s. Involvement of PAs in occupational and environmental medicine escalated in 1978 as industry responded to cost-containment pressures. Work settings initially focused on underserved areas; today they include plant sites, private industrial medicine clinics, and corporate medical administration.

In Canada, retired military PAs from the Canadian Forces have found work in such locations as oil and gas extraction sites and refineries. Many of these industries are located in remote areas such as Northern Alberta.

The delivery of routine physical examinations for industries and insurance companies by PAs can result in substantial savings compared with the cost when this service is performed by a physician, which makes the PA particularly attractive. Industrial health studies conducted primarily by PAs, instead of physicians, have been a trend in certain sectors for the past three decades (Harbert, 1978; Romm et al, 1979; Elliott, 1984a; Elliott, 1984b).

Hooker (2004) undertook an administrative study of PA activities in occupational and environmental medicine and compared them with physicians in the same setting. The study took place in 1999 at a large industrial medicine clinic where 30 physicians and 15 PAs provided care to industrially employed patients. The results revealed that PAs work more hours and thus see more patients per year than physicians. Characteristics of the patients seen by each provider were similar in age, gender ratio, and severity of injury. Physicians saw, on average, 2.8 patients per hour; PAs saw 2.5. The average charge per patient visit and total charge for an episode of care were similar. Differences between PAs and physicians were on the duration of limited duty prescribed: PAs prescribed, on average, 15 days and physicians 17 days. PAs were likely to refer a patient to an outside provider 19.7% of the time, whereas a physician referred 17.4% of the time. The salary of a physician was approximately twice as much as a PA. The conclusion was that the use of PAs in occupational and environemental medicine may represent a cost-effective advantage from an administrative standpoint (Exhibits 7-52 and 7-53) (Hooker, 2004).

An editorial that accompanied the Hooker study identified approximately 3,000 doctors in U.S. occupational medicine and 1,500 PAs. Because PAs are demonstrating their ability to manage relatively uncomplicated cases presenting to occupational medicine, the authors offered that opportunities are present to create new roles of doctors in overseeing PA-directed activities and to improve productivity and efficiency (Bunn, Holloway, & Johnson, 2004)

An innovative development in PA education that sought to expand PA services through formal training occurred at the University of Oklahoma's PA program. At one time the program sponsored a graduate occupational health program that trained and granted a master's degree in public health and industrial medicine.

Profile

In a survey undertaken by the AAPA, 580 PAs in occupational and environmental medicine responded (Exhibit 7-54). The average age was 48 and females were 43% of the cohort. One-fourth (25%) worked in a hospital. Most (89%) worked in an urban setting. The majority

EXHIBIT 7-52

Comparison of Occupational and Environmental Medicine Physician Assistants and Physicians by Outcomes of Episodes of Care

	PA Average	Physician Average	Overall Average	P	SD	95% CI
Average no. of days of limited activity assigned	15.6	17.4	16.8	0.015	48.2	16.1–17.5
Likely to refer a patient to an outside provider	19.7%	17.4%	18.2%	0.0001		17.6–18.7
Average no. of patient visits per hour	2.5	2.9	2.8	0.008	1.9	2.8–2.8
Average charge per visit	$284.77	$302.53	$296.72	NS		294.50–298.93
Average total charges for episode of care	$565.98	$608.13	$594.33	NS		583.91–604.75
Average severity score of problems treated (mild, 1; moderate, 2; severe, 3)	1.92	1.93	1.93	NS	0.33	1.93–1.94
% of male patients	74.3%	72.5%	73.1%	0.007		72.5–73.2
Average age of patients	35.3	35.5	35.5	NS	11.2	35.3–35.7
Probability patients likely to keep their appointment	81%	76%	79%	0.0024	1.04	78.0–80.9

Data from Hooker, R. S. (2004). Physician assistants in occupational medicine: How do they compare to occupational physicians? Occupational Medicine (Oxford, England), 54(3), 153–158.

EXHIBIT 7-53

Occupational and Environmental Medicine Provider Characteristics

	No.	Average Age	Gender	Average Salary	Average No. of Visits per Day
Physicians		50	18 males, 6 females	$143,056	
PAs		45	7 males, 5 females	$74,208	
Average	32.72				23.31

Data from Hooker, R. S. (2004). Physician assistants in occupational medicine: How do they compare to occupational physicians? Occupational Medicine (Oxford, England), 54(3), 153–158.

(83%) worked full time (at least 32 hours per week) and 78% were salary-based. The average salary in 2008 was $92,323 (AAPA, 2008a).

Professional Society

The American Academy of Physician Assistants in Occupational Medicine was founded in 1981 to develop continuing medical education programs and educate industry and the public about PAs in occupational medicine (Ramos, 1989; Ramos, 2003). Later, the American College of Occupational and Environmental Medicine (ACOEM) replaced the AAPA organization and became the

professional society for PAs in this discipline. ACOEM meets twice per year and has 20 special interest sections. The physician-PA section has a vote on critical issues that affect PAs and physicians working in those fields. The section gives PAs a voting seat as long as this section maintains at least 50 dues-paying members.

Oncology

Oncology is the branch of medicine that studies cancers and seeks to understand their development, diagnosis, treatment, and prevention. Most oncologists are also hematologists.

EXHIBIT 7-54
Occupational and Environmental Medicine Physician Assistants, 2008

Total survey respondents	580
Age (mean years)	48
Female	247 (43%)
Solo physician practitioner	7%
Single specialty physician group practice	17%
Multispecialty physician group practice	11%
Hospital	24%
Years in clinical practice	16
Work in urban setting	89%
Precept PA students	16%
Work more than 32 hours per week	83%
Mean income	$92,323

Data from American Academy of Physician Assistants. (2008a). 2008 AAPA Physician Assistant Census Report. Alexandria, VA: Author.

Role

The role of the oncology PA is diverse and is divided into four categories: medical (adult), pediatric, radiation, and surgical. The PA, depending on the specialization, may be employed in a large center or a smaller outpatient group practice. In almost all instances, the oncology PA will be part of a broad-based team that includes doctors, nurses, social workers, pharmacists, and others (Polansky, 2003).

History

Major academic centers, such as the M. D. Anderson Cancer Center in Houston, Texas, employ more than 100 PAs in oncology (Ross, 2008). The Fred Hutchinson Cancer Research Center in Seattle, Washington, employs more than 50 PAs. The Oncology Center at the Johns Hopkins Hospital in Baltimore, Maryland, employs a large cadre of PAs in multiple roles. A postgraduate program for PAs in oncology started in 2001 at the M. D. Anderson Cancer Center (Polansky, 2007). All of these efforts have centered PAs in divisions of labor and economy of scale that provides value added in the delivery of complex care (Tabachnick, 2006).

Such increased use of PAs and NPs in oncology tends to improve practice efficiency. According to a survey of members of the American Society of Clinical Oncology by Erikson and colleagues (2007), 54% of oncologists already work with PAs or NPs. On average, the practice was able to handle a higher volume of weekly visits because of the collaboration with PAs and NPs. Results also indicated that productivity is highest for physicians who regularly use PAs and NPs for advanced activities such as assisting with new patient consults, ordering routine chemotherapy, and performing invasive procedures. Additionally, the practitioner survey suggested that physicians who work with PAs and NPs believe that using PAs and NPs improves efficiency and patient care as well as professional satisfaction (Erickson et al, 2007).

An observational study was undertaken to determine the ability of a PA to insert a peripheral subcutaneous implanted vascular access device (VAD) in an ambulatory setting as well as the ability to transfer this training from one PA to another. Also evaluated were the performance and complications associated with this new device. The peripheral access system (PAS) port catheter was inserted in patients who required long-term (greater than 3 months) vascular access for infusion therapy. The first PA (PA-1) successfully inserted 57 of 62 devices (92%) in 10 patients after gaining experience with the technique (success rate, 5 of 10 [50%]; $P = 0.003$). The second PA (PA-2) was successful in 8 of 10 initial attempts (80%) and 25 of 30 overall (83%). Complications were few and limited to phlebitis, thrombosis, and a low infection rate (0.2 per 1,000 catheter days). The authors concluded that PAs can be taught to insert a peripheral subcutaneous implanted VAD. This technique is transferable from one PA to another, and the device studied is appropriate for outpatient VAD programs (Rubenstein et al, 1995).

Ross (2008) undertook a survey of 54 oncology PAs and their roles at M. D. Anderson Cancer Center. More than one-half of those surveyed had never worked in another field outside of oncology and came directly to M. D. Anderson out of a PA program (although all had rotated through the center as students). A distribution of where PAs worked is illustrated in Exhibit 7-55.

EXHIBIT 7-55
Distribution of Oncology Physician Assistants at M. D. Anderson Cancer Center by Departments

	Number	Percent
Surgical oncology	9	16.7
GI medical oncology	8	14.8
Radiation oncology	6	11.1
Leukemia	5	9.3
Anesthesiology and pain management	3	5.6
Cardiology	3	5.6
Head and neck surgery	3	5.6
Lymphoma	3	5.6
Bone marrow transplantation	2	3.7
Melanoma medical oncology	2	3.7
Plastic surgery	2	3.7
Urology	2	3.7
Cardiovascular surgery	1	1.9
Dermatology	1	1.9
Head and neck medical oncology	1	1.9
Orthopaedics	1	1.9
Genitourinary medical oncology	1	1.9
Gynecological radiation oncology	1	1.9
TOTAL	54	100.0

Data from Ross, A. C. (2008). The role of physician assistants in oncology. Advances for Physician Assistants, 12*(3), 46–49.*

Profile

In a survey undertaken by the AAPA, 479 PAs in oncology responded (Exhibit 7-56). The average age was 39 and females were 84% of the cohort. Almost all (93%) worked in an urban setting. The majority (91%) worked full time (at least 32 hours per week). The average salary in 2008 was $84,336 (AAPA, 2008a).

Professional Society

The Association of Physician Assistants in Oncology (APAO) is a nonprofit specialty organization affiliated with the AAPA. It consists of PAs working in the field of oncology, in both clinical and research settings. Their website is http://www.apao.cc/.

EXHIBIT 7-56
Oncology Physician Assistants, 2008

Total survey respondents	479
Age (mean years)	39
Female	400 (84%)
Single specialty physician group practice	155 (33%)
Hospital	204 (43%)
Years in clinical practice	8
Work in urban setting	93%
Precept PA students	37%
Work more than 32 hours per week	91%
Mean income	$84,336

Data from American Academy of Physician Assistants. (2008a). 2008 AAPA Physician Assistant Census Report. Alexandria, VA: Author.

Ophthalmology

Ophthalmology is the branch of medicine that deals with the diseases of and surgery for the visual pathways, including the eye, brain, and areas surrounding the eye, such as the lacrimal system and eyelids. Most opthalmologists are surgeons.

Role

The PA in opthalmology tends to be office-based more than surgically based, but all such PAs work with opthalmologists. They deal with acute injuries; diseases of the eye such as infections, uveitis, and glaucoma; débridement of foreign bodies; surgical excision of lid ptosis; postsurgical wound dressings; seeing patients postoperatively; and preparing patients for surgery. Some states have provisons that prohibit PAs from performing duties that overlap with optometry.

History

Currently, there are no formal ophthalmology programs that teach PAs to be clinicians in ophthalmology. Two programs were developed in the 1960s to train PAs in the management of eye diseases: the Georgetown University Hospital in Washington, DC, and Columbia-Presbyterian Medical Center in New York. Each had a 2-year certification program. Both programs are defunct. Graduates of these ophthalmology programs could perform refractions as well as assist in surgery and manage uncomplicated nonsurgical ophthalmologic problems such as eye infections (Sadler, 1972).

Profile

Approximately 50 PAs who are members of the AAPA report that their primary responsibilities are in ophthalmology. Most are employed in large practices that specialize in cataract and radial keratotomy procedures (Wilson, White, & Murdock, 1990). The role of PAs in ophthalmology is not viewed positively by optometrists who would like to have expanded roles in eye disease care for themselves but are usually prohibited by narrowly defined state laws.

Pathology

Pathology is the study and diagnosis of disease through the examination of organs, tissues, cells, and body fluids. The term encompasses the medical specialty, which uses tissues and body fluids to obtain clinically useful information, as well as the related scientific study of disease processes.

Role

The roles and responsibilities of a pathologists' assistant include histopathology, surgical frozen sections, and general autopsies. They perform specific tasks and duties under the direction and supervision of a licensed pathologist. Pathologists' assistants interact with pathologists in the same manner that formally trained PAs perform their duties under the direction of physicians in medical and surgical specialties (Grzybicki & Vrbin, 2003; Grzybicki et al, 2004).

History

Pathologists' assistants are commonly referred to as *PAs*. Although they are a type of PA, they differ from typical PAs because they are not trained in primary care. They are formally trained in pathology. Additionally, pathologists' assistants do not have an association with the AAPA or the Physician Assistant Education Association.

Pathologists' assistants programs at the University of Alabama and Quinnipiac College in Connecticut have been active since 1971. Both are 2-year master's degree programs and have seen more than 200 individuals graduate. The Quinnipiac College program is affiliated with the Veterans Administration Medical Centers in West Haven and with Yale University School of Medicine. Other programs are at Duke University, University of Maryland, and Finch University of Health Sciences, which has offered a master's of science in pathologists' assistant since 2000.

Grzybicki and Vrbin (2003) obtained attitudes and opinions of pathology residents about pathologists' assistants in anatomic pathology practice. They wanted to assess the implications of resident attitudes and opinions in regards to pathology practice and training. A self-administered, mailed, voluntary, anonymous questionnaire was distributed to a cross-sectional sample of pathology residents in the United States (2,531 pathology residents registered as resident members of one of the national pathology professional organizations). The questionnaire contained (1) items relating to resident demographics and program characteristics, (2) Likert-scale response items containing positive and negative statements about pathologists' assistants, (3) a multiple-choice item related to the scope of practice of pathologists' assistants, and (4) an open-ended item inviting additional comments. Quantitative and qualitative analysis of responses was performed.

The overall response rate was 19.4% (N = 490); 50% of the respondents were women, and 77% reported use of pathologists' assistants in their program. Most respondents were 25 to 35 years old and in postgraduate years 3 through 5 of their training, and most were located in the midwestern United States. The majority of residents expressed overall positive attitudes and opinions about pathologists' assistants and felt that pathologists' assistants enhanced resident training by optimizing resident workload. A minority (10% to 20%) of residents expressed negative attitudes or opinions about pathologists' assistants

(Exhibit 7-57). Additionally, some residents reported a lack of knowledge about pathologists' assistants' training or roles. The authors concluded that increased resident education and open discussion concerning pathologists' assistants may be beneficial for optimizing resident attitudes about and training experiences with pathologists' assistants (Grzybicki & Vrbin, 2003).

Professional Society

The American Association of Pathologists' Assistants (AAPA—not to be confused with the American Academy of Physician Assistants, which is also abbreviated as AAPA) is the professional association for pathologists' assistants and is the primary provider and repository of continuing education credits for pathologists' assistants. The AAPA offers an annual continuing education conference designed for PAs featuring lectures and workshops by outstanding and nationally recognized speakers. The AAPA states it has grown to over 1,000 national and international members. The website for this society is http://www.pathologistsassistants.org/.

Psychiatry and Mental Health

Psychiatry is a branch of medicine that treats mental disorders and has a theory base for its existence. The clinical application of psychiatry has been considered a bridge between the social world and those who are mentally ill. Because psychiatry's research and clinical applications are considered interdisciplinary, various subspecialties and theoretical approaches exist. Psychiatrists specialize in the doctor-patient relationship, using unique classification schemes, diagnostic tools, and treatments.

The mental health field also includes nonphysician therapists who provide psychosocial services. Most of these workers are psychologists, social workers, chemical and addiction counselors, nurses, and mental health counselors.

Role

PAs in the mental health setting are unique because they can see patients who need psychiatric or psychological services, prescribe psychotropic medication, and provide general medical services. Most mental health PAs are in roles delegated by a psychiatrist. They primarily work in mental health offices within the community, in psychiatric offices, corrections institutions, or as outpatient workers associated with psychiatric hospitals. PAs also have a cost-effective role in providing primary care and nonpsychiatric inpatient care in psychiatric settings (Morreale & Chitradon, 1977). Additionally, a role for PAs in the psychological aspects of oncology has been described (Tabachnick, 2006).

History

The first documented use of a PA functioning in a psychiatric role was in 1977 (Greenlee, Levy, & Allen, 1977). Since then, a few studies have demonstrated how well PAs perform in the mental health field. One clinical assessment study found that psychiatric evaluation interviews conducted by PAs were comparable to those of physicians for all items, including those thought to require the most clinical and medical judgment (Coryell, Cloninger, & Reich, 1978).

Another study found PAs could successfully identify the medical disorders that accompany psychiatric disorders, which caused the psychiatric symptoms (Mathew & Stevens, 1982). In a third study, PAs detected nearly three times as many physical illnesses as the psychiatrist. The psychiatrists were significantly more likely to miss diagnoses among older patients and women (D'Ercole et al, 1991). These findings suggest that sometimes the PA provides a role as the primary care clinician, managing most of the medical needs of the patient in a mental health setting.

Trained specialist PAs have also demonstrated value in filling critical shortages in state hospitals. One institution's addition of PAs to the mental health staff significantly increased the time that psychiatrists had in which to plan and implement treatment. There was a high degree of acceptance of the PAs in this setting (Matthews & Yohe, 1984).

The Association of Postgraduate Physician Assistant Programs approved a psychiatric PA program at the University of Texas Medical

EXHIBIT 7-57
Pathology Residents Attitudes About Pathologists' Assistants

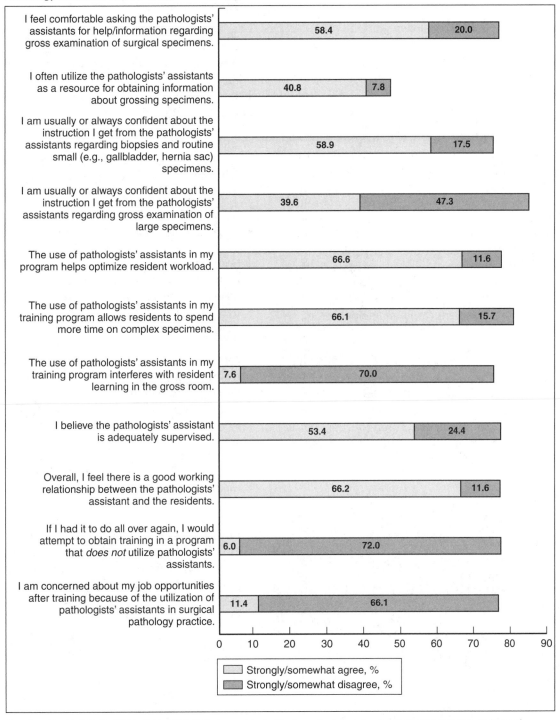

Data from Grzybicki, D. M., & Vrbin, C. M. (2003). Pathology resident attitudes and opinions about pathologists' assistants. Archives of
Pathology & Laboratory Medicine, 127(6), 666–672.

Branch Managed Care Health Service in 1998. This program provides residency-style, on-the-job training to PAs who are interested in enhancing their knowledge and therapeutic skills in caring for the mentally ill (Rose, 2001). Students who sucessfully complete the program are eligible to receive a certificate of completion from the university.

Another postgraduate mental health program for PAs is located in Cherokee, Iowa. The stated goal of the program is to train PAs in the field of psychiatry in order to extend the psychiatric care provided by psychiatrists. The program is 12 months in duration and concentrates on providing PA residents with advanced skills in differential diagnosis and medical management of psychiatric conditions with psychotropic medications. PA residents also learn the fundamentals of the interpersonal process. Areas of focus include adult and child/adolescent inpatient services as well as outpatient case management.

Profile

In a survey undertaken by the AAPA, 256 PAs in psychiatry responded (Exhibit 7-58). The average age was 46, females were 64% of the cohort, and 12% worked in a single specialty physician group practice. Three-fourths (78%) worked in an urban setting. The majority

EXHIBIT 7-58
Psychiatric Physician Assistants, 2008

Total survey respondents	256
Age (mean years)	46
Female	163 (64%)
Solo physician practitioner	33 (13%)
Single specialty physician group practice	31 (12%)
Multispecialty physician group practice	6 (2%)
Hospital	90 (35%)
Community health center	39 (15%)
Years in clinical practice	12
Work in urban setting	78%
Precept PA students	30%
Work more than 32 hours per week	80%
Mean income	$85,361

Data from American Academy of Physician Assistants. (2008a). 2008 AAPA Physician Assistant Census Report. Alexandria, VA: Author.

(80%) worked full time (at least 32 hours per week) and 87% were salary-based. The average salary in 2008 was $85,361 (AAPA, 2008a).

Professional Society

A group of mental health PAs was formed in the late 1990s, and in 1998 the House of Delegates of the AAPA granted specialty organization recognition to the Association of Psychiatric Physician Assistants (APPA) at their meeting in Salt Lake City, Utah.

The APPA is organized for educational, research, publication, and charitable purposes. Accordingly, the purposes of this association are the following:

- Assist the members of this organization in sharing and communicating information that leads to professional development and current concepts involved in the treatment of patients suffering from mental and emotional problems.
- Assist in defining the professional role of the Psychiatric Physician Assistant.
- Assist in the development of professional training opportunities for Psychiatric Physician Assistants.
- Assist in publicizing and promoting the professional role and capabilities of Psychiatric Physician Assistants.
- Assist in obtaining and maintaining official recognition from other professional medical organizations and professionals.
- Serve as an information gathering and sharing site for Psychiatric Physician Assistants, Physician Assistant Training Programs, American Academy of Physician Assistants, and other disciplines related to the training, professional roles, and standards for Psychiatric Physician Assistants.

More information about the APPA is available on their website at http://www.psychpa.com/.

Public Health and Preventive Medicine

Public health is the study and practice of addressing threats to the health of a community. The field pays special attention to the social context of disease and misery and focuses on improving health through society-wide measures such as immunizations or the fluoridation of drinking water. The field is occupied by doctors, nurses, PAs, NPs, and many allied health disciplines.

Role
The role of the public health PA includes primary care, epidemiological research, public health promotion, and disease prevention (Mullan, 1989). The public health PA works in various clinic settings or in field offices for the various branches and agencies of state and federal government (see Chapter 17). For example, many PAs are employees of the uniform and nonuniform branches of the U.S. Public Health Service (USPHS), including the Coast Guard, the National Oceanic and Atmospheric Administration, the Centers for Disease Control and Prevention, the Food and Drug Administration, the Federal Aviation Administration, Health and Human Services, the Office of Health Promotion/Disease Prevention, the Health Services and Resources Administration, the Bureau of Prisons, and the National Centers for Health Statistics. As commissioned officers they wear a Navy uniform and retain a Navy rank. The highest ranking PA in the U.S. Public Health Service is an admiral.

History
The impact of a PA as manager on full-time public health coverage was first examined in 1980 when a PA became the public health director of a region in Connecticut (Jekel et al, 1980). This experience in Connecticut demonstrates that the public health world does not need to rely solely on physicians. In fact, in this setting the level of care improved when a PA assumed the role of health director (Atwater, 1980).

Profile
In a survey undertaken by the AAPA, 40 PAs in public health responded (Exhibit 7-59). The average age was 44, females were 57% of the cohort, and 38% worked in community health centers. Most (82%) worked in an urban

EXHIBIT 7-59
Public Health Physician Assistants, 2008

Total survey respondents	40
Age (mean years)	44
Female	23 (58%)
Community health center	20 (51%)
Correction systems	8 (21%)
Other facility	7 (18%)
Years in clinical practice	11%
Work in urban setting	82%
Precept PA students	38%
Work more than 32 hours per week	85%
Mean income	$81,387

Data from American Academy of Physician Assistants. (2008a). 2008 AAPA Physician Assistant Census Report. Alexandria, VA: Author.

setting. The majority (85%) worked full time (at least 32 hours per week). The average salary in 2008 was $81,387 (AAPA, 2008a).

Professional Society
U.S. Public Health System PAs are eligible to join the Veteran Affairs Physician Assistant Association (VAPAA), a society for federally employed PAs. Their website is http://www.vapaa.org/.

Radiology
Radiology is the medical specialty that uses imaging technologies to diagnose and, sometimes, treat diseases. Originally, radiology was the aspect of medical science dealing with the use of electromagnetic energy emitted by x-ray machines or other such radiation devices for the purpose of obtaining visual information. Today, another aspect of radiology—interventional radiology—involves using fine catheters to reach organs for diagnosis or treatment.

Role
The role of PAs in radiology include performing histories and physical examinations for referring doctors and presenting the results to the radiologist. In some instances, they perform fluoroscopic tests and procedures, provide fine needle biopsies and angiography, insert and remove central and peripheral venous

catheters, or provide initial interpretations of studies. In other instances they may perform pre- and postprocedure evaluations and postprocedure follow-up as well as write discharge summaries. PAs may administer conscious sedation, and they commonly provide first-assist services in the operating or procedure room. PAs in radiology may also write medical orders and interpret laboratory tests.

History

A program to train experienced radiologic technologists to become PAs in diagnostic radiology (PA-DRs) was initiated at the University of Kentucky Medical Center in 1970. This 2-year program was underwritten by the federal government and was designed to improve the efficiency of radiologic procedures. Approximately 30 individuals graduated before the program closed after withdrawal of support by the American College of Radiology.

Despite the small number of graduates from the program, six studies have examined the use of PAs in diagnostic radiology. In one study of work activities a radiologist would have performed, which included examinations and radiograph screening for disease, the PAs performed these activities "accurately and acceptably." Each PA-DR averaged a savings of 34% of the employing radiologist's time (Kiernan & Rosenbaum, 1977). Duties were wide ranging and included fluoroscopic procedures, excretory urography, and chest radiographic screening (Thompson, 1974). Another study trained primary care PAs to perform competently in screening radiographs, IV pyelograms, and brain scans. The authors concluded that the PA-DRs performed as well as radiologists (Thompson, 1971, 1972).

At the Johns Hopkins Hospital, PAs on the interventional radiology staff perform histories, physical examinations and Doppler pressures, schedule laboratory work and admissions, answer referring physicians' calls, and obtain preliminary patient information (White et al, 1989). The addition of PAs decreased the mean length of stay for patients undergoing various procedures and increased the capacity for interventional procedures (White et al, 1988).

As PAs entered the radiology specialty, surveys of chiefs of radiology departments were generally favorable when asked if they were willing to delegate traditional radiologist tasks to PAs (Thompson, 1971). When private practice radiologists were surveyed, however, at least 60% showed reluctance to delegate these tasks (Parker, McCoy, & Connor, 1972). These studies are in need of repeating to reflect current trends.

A study on mammograms interpreted by PAs found that the interpretations were more sensitive and as specific as those made by six HMO radiologists who interpreted the same cases and were as effective as those by radiologists described in the literature. The study concluded that mammogram interpretations by PAs were similar to those made by radiologists, took less time, and cost less than those performed by radiologists (Hillman et al, 1987).

In 1991, a controversial editorial called for renewed interest in training PAs to work in radiology (Ellis, 1991; McCowan et al, 1992). In 1996, the subject was reviewed again after describing a few PAs who provide radiology services in some different settings. PAs who are involved in interventional radiology use fine catheters to reach and destroy tumors in deep organs (McCowan et al, 1992).

In an interview with three PAs in radiology, the AAPA found that one group of 20 radiologists hired a PA to help out generally in the group and specifically to assist an interventional radiologist who was setting up new programs. In addition to assisting the neuroradiologist, the PA focused on posttreatment rounds and consults. A positive experience with the first PA led to the hiring of another PA to conduct histories and physical examinations, perform and assist with invasive procedures, and write discharge summaries. The physicians also wanted the PAs to perform fluoroscopies. In that state the radiologists could delegate to the PAs anything within their scope of practice, except final interpretations of scans and x-ray films.

In another state, an interventional radiology practice hired a PA who started out doing all the first-assisting duties with one physician. Eventually, the practice added three physicians: one fellow and two residents. Because the fellow and residents took over the first-assisting duties, the PA was asked to take on a new role. She took over most of the communicating with referring physicians and performing case evaluations, including such duties as determining whether patients needed antibiotics, IV orders for hydration, and insulin management.

Another PA working in interventional radiology at a major teaching hospital said he spent most of his time running the outpatient department. He performed histories and physical examinations and wrote laboratory orders, assisted on some procedures, and followed up with patients. This particular practice had a high percentage of patients with liver disease with biliary tubes. The PA provided patient education on dealing with the tubes, assisted with placement and maintenance of tubes, and removed 95% of the Hickman catheters. He also provided coordination and consultation by phone with patients who needed help with their tubes and with family physicians who needed to know about caring for the patient's tubes.

As interventional radiologists develop busier and busier practices, there is less time to spend with individual patients. PAs represent an excellent way to improve clinical patient care. Stecker, Armenoff, and Johnson (2004) described what PAs are and how they work together with radiologists at Indiana University. The authors illustrated differences between PAs and other physician extenders and described the duties that may be delegated to PAs in the interventional radiology setting.

The authors described how the PAs provided an opportunity to improve clinical patient care. The interventional radiology PAs were involved in daily morning inpatient rounds with the radiology fellows and residents rotating on the radiology service. In this capacity, they evaluated abscess, urinary, and biliary drainage catheters to ensure proper function and monitored patient progress. They also performed and monitored compliant chart documentation for all inpatients being followed by the interventional radiology service. In conjunction with the house staff, the PAs communicated with referring services as needed and helped triage

queries and consultation requests during these rounds (Exhibit 7-60). In addition, the interventional radiology PAs provided a major role in billing for inpatient evaluation and management services, a process that tended to be overlooked by the staff. The authors concluded that revenue generated by two interventional radiology PAs at this academic medical center covered the costs of their employment (Stecker, Armenoff, & Johnson, 2004).

Radiology Practitioner Assistants

A radiology practitioner assistant (RPA) is a midlevel healthcare professional technician who performs many radiological procedures

EXHIBIT 7-60
Procedures of Interventional Radiology Physician Assistants

- Venous access
- Temporary central venous catheters (infusion, apheresis, dialysis)
- Peripherally inserted central catheters
- Tunneled catheters (infusion, apheresis, dialysis)
- Troubleshooting of venous access devices
- Drainage catheters (biliary, urinary, abscess, and other)
- Catheter exchanges
- Troubleshooting of drainage catheters
- Resuturing of dislodged catheters

OUTPATIENT VISITS
- New patient consultations (including history and physical examination)
- Vascular malformations
- Symptomatic uterine fibroids
- Liver tumors
- Portal hypertension
- Established patient follow-up
- Wound checks (port placement, removal)
- Post-(chemo)embolization follow-up
- Post–arterial angioplasty/stent treatment
- Valuation and tracking of dialysis access performance
- Evaluation and management billing

INPATIENT CARE
- Daily patient visits
- Morning rounds
- Communication with other medical service teams
- Evaluation and management billing

under the supervision of radiologists. This technical role is sometimes confused with NCCPA-certified PAs in radiology. The RPA is an extension of the radiologic technologist, and must maintain certification and continuing education requirements. The scope of practice of the RPA is defined by the supervising radiologist. The RPAs' responsibilities include conducting radiologic patient assessments, participating in patient management, and separating normal from abnormal imaging exams. The majority of RPAs work in hospital radiology departments and imaging centers. The differences between RPAs and PAs are outlined by Stecker and colleagues (2004).

One research focus was to determine RPAs' accuracy in recognizing abnormal image patterns and their ability to independently perform gastrointestinal fluoroscopic procedures. The results support previous research indicating that technologists with additional education and training and radiologist supervision can detect abnormal image patterns and perform fluoroscopy successfully (Van Valkenburg et al, 2000).

Profile

In a survey undertaken by the AAPA, 262 PAs in radiology responded (Exhibit 7-61). The average age was 40, females were 56% of the cohort, and 56% worked in a single specialty physician group practice. Almost all (97%) worked in an urban setting. The majority (93%) worked full time (at least 32 hours per week). The average salary in 2008 was $95,214 (AAPA, 2008a).

Research

Almost as soon as there were more than a handful of PAs, there were researchers to study them. At first, medical sociologists, behaviorists, economists, and health services researchers examined the nascent profession and everything that PAs did (Hooker, 1994). Within a few years, PAs became part of investigative teams as well as the subjects of research. Since the early 1970s the PA research agenda has been shaped not only by health researchers interested in the profession, but also by PAs formally or informally trained in the social research disciplines (Jarski, 1988). These medical, social, and health services research activities involved PAs at five levels: (1) supplying information about ongoing activities as providers, (2) helping to develop new data, (3) participating in data analysis, (4) assisting in research design, and (5) coauthoring papers that result from research.

In clinical investigations, PAs participate in drug trials and biochemical research. They assume roles previously occupied by a physician (Morian, 1986). Many PAs around the country conduct clinical trials in settings ranging from private firms to university research clinics.

The role of the PA in research is expected to grow as the demand for clinical trials increases and the need for skilled clinicians who can be employed at less cost than a physician also increases. Many PA programs on the master's level have a research component as part of the curriculum, which is likely to stimulate further research.

Rehabilitation Medicine and Physiatry

Physical medicine and rehabilitation, or physiatry, is a branch of medicine dealing with functional restoration of a person affected by physical disability. A physician specializing in restoring optimal function to individuals with injuries to the muscles, bones, tissues, and nervous system (such as cerebral vascular accident victims) is a physiatrist.

EXHIBIT 7-61
Radiology Physician Assistants, 2008

Total survey respondents	262
Age (mean years)	40
Female	146 (56%)
Single specialty physician group practice	146 (56%)
Multispecialty physician group practice	26 (10%)
Hospital	77 (30%)
Years in clinical practice	8
Work in urban setting	97%
Precept PA students	31%
Work more than 32 hours per week	93%
Mean income	$95,214

Data from American Academy of Physician Assistants. (2008a). 2008 AAPA Physician Assistant Census Report. Alexandria, VA: Author.

Role

PAs are found in many rehabilitative roles, including employment in hospitals and rehabilitative units. They function essentially as physiatrists, helping to diagnose and treat patients with chronic pain disorders and spine problems, and as directors of rehabilitative care. Some have mastered nerve conduction studies and electromyographic skills. Others provide medical care along with management for paralyzed patients—those with spinal cord injuries in specialty units.

History

Anectodatal observations have shown that some PAs in this specialty were physical therapists before becoming PAs. A few were formally trained as athletic trainers, naturopathic physicians, or chiropractors.

Rheumatology

Rheumatology is a subspecialty of internal medicine and pediatrics involved in the diagnosis of and therapy for rheumatic diseases. Rheumatologists mainly deal with problems involving the joints and the allied conditions of connective tissue as well as pathogenesis of major rheumatological and autoimmune disorders. Better understanding of the genetic basis of rheumatological disorders makes rheumatology a specialty that is rapidly developing based on new scientific discoveries. New treatment modalities are based on scientific research on immunology, cytokines, T lymphocytes, and B lymphocytes. Future therapies may be directed more toward gene modulation.

Role

The role of the rheumatology PA includes the diagnosis and management of autoimmune and inflammatory diseases. Although the majority of these diseases are systemic, the PA in rheumatology is also skilled in medical orthopedics. Rheumatology PAs provide a broad range of services, including evaluating new patients, monitoring drug administration, performing procedures such as joint injections and muscle biopsies, and performing rounds in the hospital. Some PAs expand

their roles to include pain management, sports medicine, bone metabolic disorders, and primary care (Hooker, 2007).

Although a small contingent of AAPA members consistently cite their primary medical responsibility as rheumatology, their role is only now being documented (Hooker, 2008). In one study of rheumatology referrals in an HMO, a PA and two rheumatologists shared approximately equally all of the consultations for that year (Hooker & Brown, 1985).

With the demand for rheumatology service increasing and the number of training programs for rheumatologists relatively flat, it seems that this is an unfilled niche for PAs (Deal et al, 2007). This observation resulted in a role delineation study. Of 112 PAs identified, 58 agreed to participate (rate of return of 54%). Females comprised 71% of both the survey participants and the total list of PAs (Exhibit 7-62). The mean number of years in rheumatology practice was 7.5 (range, 2 to 21 years). The mean number of years since graduating from a PA program was 23 (range, 2 to 28 years). All but three of the respondents acquired their skills through on-the-job training and continuing medical education; three were graduates of a 12-month postgraduate fellowship (Hooker & Rangan, 2008).

The office arrangements where PAs are employed varied, with 29% in solo practice (one doctor), 16% in partnership (two doctors), 29% in group practice (three or more doctors), 16% in medical schools and universities, and the remaining in government service (Exhibit 7-63). The average number of rheumatologists with whom PAs worked was 2.7 (range, 1 to 17). In clinical practice, the number of rheumatology PAs and NPs they worked with was three (range, zero to five).

A total of 69% of the respondents spent 80% to 100% of their work week caring for patients; 31% worked less than 32 hours per week. Three-quarters (76%) provide the initial consultation for new patients (Exhibit 7-64). A total of 27% of patient visits were doctor-assigned; the remaining were either undifferentiated (no triage), patient preference, or nurse-assigned. Of the respondents who answered the question about whether they initiated disease-modifying

EXHIBIT 7-62
Characteristics of Physician Assistants in Clinical Rheumatology

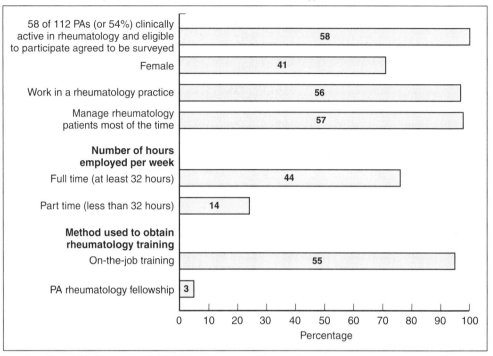

Data from Hooker, R. S., & Rangan, B. V. (2008). *Role delineation of rheumatology physician assistants.* Journal of Clinical Rheumatology, 14(4), 202–205.

EXHIBIT 7-63
Characteristics of Rheumatology Clinic Setting Where Physician Assistants Are Employed

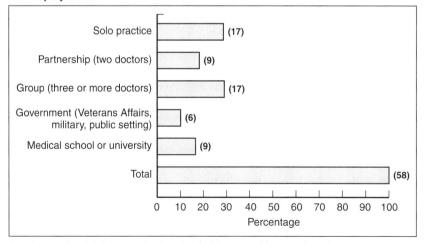

Data from Hooker, R. S., & Rangan, B. V. (2008). *Role delineation of rheumatology physician assistants.* Journal of Clinical Rheumatology, 14(4), 202–205.

EXHIBIT 7-64
Roles of Rheumatology Physician Assistants

	Number	Percentage
CLINIC TIME SPENT IN RHEUMATOLOGY		
Full time (at least 32 hours per week)	44	76
HOW PATIENTS ARE ASSIGNED		
Randomly, no-triage	42	73
Some assignment (supervising doctor, nurse, or patient preference)	16	27
First contact or consultation for a first patient visit	44	76
NUMBER OF PATIENTS WHERE YOU ARE THE FIRST CONTACT (PROVIDE THE INITIAL CONSULTATION)		
Average per 4 weeks	20	
Range per 4 weeks	0–50	
MEDICATIONS INITIATED FOR PATIENTS WITH RHEUMATOID ARTHRITIS		
Disease-modifying antirheumatic drugs	55	95
Biologicals (aTNFs, abatacept)	55	95
Antiosteoporitic (bisphosphonates, calcitonin)	54	93
MAXIMUM NUMBER OF RETURN-VISIT PATIENTS SEEN ON A DAILY BASIS		
Average	12	
Range	7–25	
Injections (intra-articular and soft tissue)	51	88
Knees	51	88
Shoulder impingement syndrome	48	83
Other joints	49	85
Number that participated in clinical research	37	64

Data from Hooker, R. S., & Rangan, B. V. (2008). Role delineation of rheumatology physician assistants. Journal of Clinical Rheumatology, 14(4), 202–205.

anti-rheumatic drugs (DMARDs), biologicals, or antiosteoporotics, 95% said they did. The study also revealed that 64% participated in research (of which 39% were in clinical trials or drug studies). More than 88% of the respondents administered joint or soft tissue injections.

The majority (84%) of the PA respondents did not know of any practice difficulties with insurance reimbursement (Exhibit 7-65). In regards to membership in professional societies, 93% of the respondents said they belonged to the AAPA, 87% to the American College of Rheumatology/Association of Rheumatology Health Professionals, 83% to the Society for Physician Assistants in Rheumatology (SPAR), and 59% to their local state organizations.

Questions about job and career satisfaction were the few areas that did not produce full participation. Of those who answered, the vast majority (93%) were satisfied or very satisfied with their current clinical role in rheumatology, yet only two-thirds (68%) were satisfied/very satisfied with their current career. Narrative contributions were few and not useful. The difference between clinical role and career satisfaction results was primarily about dissatisfaction with salary, benefits, office structure, or relationships, but not on being in rheumatology as a discipline (Hooker & Rangan 2008). Industry sources in early 2008 said they had identified 367 rheumatology PAs and NPs; about one-third being PAs. This observation suggests that the preceding role delineation study is representative of all rheumatology PAs.

EXHIBIT 7-65
Administrative Elements of Rheumatology Physician Assistants

NUMBER OF RHEUMATOLOGISTS IN YOUR PRACTICE		
Average	2.7	
Range	1–37	

NUMBER OF RHEUMATOLOGY PAs AND NPs IN YOUR PRACTICE		
Average	3	
Range	1–5	

Professional Organization Memberships	Number	Percentage
Arthritis Related Health Professionals	31	53
Society for Physician Assistants in Rheumatology	48	83
American College of Rheumatology	1	4
American Academy of Physician Assistants	54	93
Other (state chapter of PAs)	34	59
SATISFACTION LEVEL OF CURRENT CLINICAL ROLE IN RHEUMATOLOGY (TOTAL 31)		
Extremely satisfied	13	42
Satisfied	16	51
Neutral	0	0
Dissatisfied	1	3
Very dissatisfied	1	3
SATISFACTION LEVEL OF CURRENT CAREER (TOTAL 40)		
Extremely satisfied	14	35
Satisfied	13	33
Neutral	9	23
Dissatisfied	3	7
Very dissatisfied	1	2
"HAVE YOU EXPERIENCED INSURANCE REIMBURSEMENT DIFFICULTIES?" (OPEN-ENDED QUESTION THAT WAS SUMMARIZED AS "NO" OR NEGATIVE ANSWERS)	49	84

Data from Hooker, R. S., & Rangan, B. V. (2008). Role delineation of rheumatology physician assistants. Journal of Clinical Rheumatology, 14(4), 202–205.

Profile

In a survey undertaken by the AAPA, 86 PAs in rheumatology responded (Exhibit 7-66). The average age was 40, females were 73% of the cohort, and 40% worked in a single specialty physician group practice. Almost all (97%) worked in an urban setting. The majority (85%) worked full time (at least 32 hours per week). The average salary in 2008 was $81,224 (AAPA, 2008a).

Professional Society

SPAR was formed in 2003 and counts over 75 PAs who provide rheumatology services. Their website is http://www.aapa.org/spar/.

EXHIBIT 7-66
Rheumatology Physician Assistants, 2008

Total survey respondents	86
Age (mean years)	40
Female	63 (73%)
Solo physician practitioner	19 (22%)
Single specialty physician group practice	34 (40)%
Multispecialty physician group practice	24 (28%)
Hospital	7 (8%)
Years in clinical practice	9
Work in urban setting	97%
Precept PA students	23%
Work more than 32 hours per week	85%
Mean income	$81,224

Data from American Academy of Physician Assistants. (2008a). 2008 AAPA Physician Assistant Census Report. Alexandria, VA: Author.

Sports Medicine

Sports medicine specializes in preventing, diagnosing, and treating injuries related to participating in sports and exercise. The sports medicine "team" includes specialty physicians and surgeons, athletic trainers, physical therapists, coaches, other personnel, and, of course, the athlete. Because of the competitive nature of sports, a primary focus of sports medicine is the rapid recovery of patients, which is the driving force behind many state-of-the-art innovations in healing injuries.

Many PAs provide care in sports medicine clinics, are team health providers, and function in a variety of roles that transcend orthopedics and rehabilitation medicine. Identifying these PAs is difficult because there is no formal designation for PAs in sports medicine and many list their specialty as family medicine or orthopedics. Some PAs come to this specialty having been athletic trainers. Others enter the field because they are (or were) athletes.

Tissue Procurement

Organ retrieval is an ideal role for PAs because of their training and because they can directly replace doctors providing the same service. In one 30-month study involving a PA replacing a physician, the total number of kidneys procured increased threefold, the number of usable kidneys increased dramatically, the number of referral hospitals increased threefold, and the number of kidneys shared with other transplant centers tripled as compared with any period before initiation of the PA approach (Schmittou, 1977). Historically, the tissue procurement PA will follow the organ back into the operating room to assist the surgeon in the transplantation. Other PAs are involved with monitoring transplant recipients for tissue rejection and other related illnesses (Joyner & Easley, 1984).

Urology

Urology is the branch of medicine that focuses on the urinary tracts of males and females, and on the reproductive system of males. Urologists diagnose, treat, and manage patients with urological disorders. The organs covered by urology include the kidneys, ureters, urinary bladder, urethra, and the male reproductive organs (testes, epididymis, vas deferens, seminal vesicles, prostate, and penis).

Role

Urology PAs tend to be more office-based than surgical. They often provide initial consultations, perform cystoscopies, evaluate and perform biopsies on the prostate, and manage impotent patients. An expanded role for PAs in this field is in sexology.

The urology PA tends to work in an office with one urologist or a group of urologists but sometimes extends into the surgical suite to perform lithotripsy procedures and assist in other roles. Women are increasingly employed in this traditionally male-dominated field. A female PA thus increases the availability and choice of providers for patients.

History

One of the first descriptions of an American PA was of a technician who functioned as a PA in a urology practice (Crile, 1987). Later, a role for the PA in urology was developed at a time when a number of emerging technologies were requiring a special person trained to manage the tools and instruments of this specialty. In 1970, a program in Cincinnati, Ohio, trained PAs in urology to administer IV pyelograms, obtain detailed voided specimens, assist in methods to snare renal stones, perform cystoscopies, and analyze renal calculi. Although there is plenty of opportunity for PAs to continue in this vein, the outpatient urology PA (an office-based PA who does not participate in surgery) has emerged.

Profile

In a survey undertaken by the AAPA, 339 PAs in urology responded (Exhibit 7-67). The average age was 40, females were 58% of the cohort, and 48% worked in a single specialty physician group practice. Almost all (93%) worked in an urban setting. The majority (91%) worked full time (at least 32 hours per week) and 94% were salary-based. The average salary in 2008 was $90,462 (AAPA, 2008a).

EXHIBIT 7-67
Urology Physician Assistants, 2008

Total survey respondents	339
Age (mean years)	40
Female	197 (58%)
Single specialty physician group practice	162 (48%)
Multispecialty physician group practice	40 (12%)
Hospital	84 (25%)
Years in clinical practice	9
Work in urban setting	93%
Precept PA students	28%
Work more than 32 hours per week	91%
Mean income	$90,462

Data from American Academy of Physician Assistants. (2008a). 2008 AAPA Physician Assistant Census Report. Alexandria, VA: Author.

Professional Society

The AASPA includes a special section for urology PAs. Their website is located at http://www.aaspa.com/urology.asp. In addition, a relatively new specialty society for PAs is the Urological Association of Physician Assistants. Their website is http://www.uapanet.org/membership.html. This association has approximately 50 urologic PA members.

Veterinary Medicine

Although we know of no study on PAs formally employed in veterinary medicine, anecdotes abound about rural PAs providing care for large domestic animals and small animals. These services include casting fractures, castrating, immunizing, administrating antibiotics, and delivering foals. This service should be viewed as only an occasional and informal tradition of the rural general practitioner and should not be taken as an erosion of the domain of the professional animal doctor.

Research and Specialization

The literature about the deployment of PAs in nonprimary care is mixed; in some areas it is being developed (e.g., rheumatology, neurology) and in other areas almost nothing is known (e.g., orthopedics, urology). A review of this literature reveals large areas missing and large questions unanswered. Following is a brief list of areas in need of research attention.

- **Case reports:** Writing about PAs in specialty care provides a view of what a PA in training can expect. Case reports can show what a specialty care PA does and what a typical day is like. Each specialty needs a case report.

- **Role delineation:** Role delineation studies are needed every 5 years or so to identify the skill sets and activities of PAs in different roles. These need to be undertaken for all types of PAs, including those in urban and rural settings, those in large multispecialty clinics, and those in solo practices.

- **Organizational arrangements:** How do large multispecialty groups arrange the care of a defined population and utilize PAs? What are the trade-offs organizations make in employing PAs and NPs? What are the overlaps in care by doctors, PAs, and NPs in the same setting?

- **Economics:** What is the overlap between the doctor, PA, and NP in each specialty role? Is this a substitution or a complementary effect?

- **Breadth of knowledge:** How does a specialty PA obtain his or her knowledge set once in practice? Does the acquisition of knowledge have different trajectories depending on age, gender, and experience?

- **Career selection:** Do PAs in some specialty area have different expectations and aspirations than those in other specialties?

- **Procedures:** What are the procedures that a PA in anesthesia (or any other specialty) needs to know to be considered competent?

- **Ratios:** What are the ratios of PAs and NPs to doctors in various specialties? What contributes to these differences?

- **Retention:** What are the factors that contribute to retention or attrition of PAs in orthopedics (or any other specialty)?

■ **Education:** How do PAs in a specialty come to that specialty and how are they trained to carry out their roles? Do they build on some fundamental set of skills or do they have a formal indoctrination?

SUMMARY

One of the major rationales for the development of the PA profession was to augment the supply of medically trained providers in those specialties in greatest need of assistance. The diversity of employment settings is an indication of the maturity of the profession. Although the primary care role of the PA is the root of the profession and remains the basis of PA education, the profession has become much more specialized since the mid-1990s, primarily the result of economic pressures. These areas of specialization are where the jobs are and where the role of the PA may be more enhanced. Specialty PAs are widely dispersed throughout the spectrum of medical disciplines and have become well integrated. Many PAs enjoy membership status in physician specialty societies or professional specialties of their own making. These specialty pathways involve PA residencies, master's degrees in clinical and nonclinical disciplines, and entry into other fields through experience and formal training. Specialization will remain an important component of the PA program, and with the exception of surgery, no one specialty is likely to dominate.

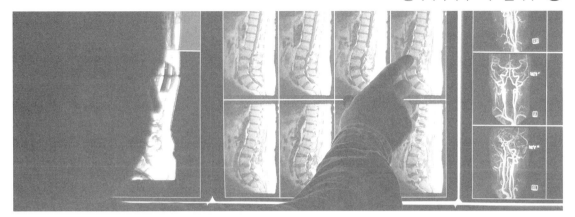

CHAPTER 8

PHYSICIAN ASSISTANTS IN HOSPITAL SETTINGS

RODERICK S. HOOKER ■ JAMES F. CAWLEY ■ DAVID P. ASPREY

How many desolate creatures on the earth have learnt the simple dues of fellowship and social comfort, in a hospital?
—Elizabeth Barrett Browning, English poet, political thinker, and feminist (1806–1861)

ABSTRACT

When the role of the physician assistant (PA) emerged in America, characterized by its clinical flexibility, it was in many respects a natural fit for hospital practice. PAs were intended to be general-purpose extenders of physician practices. As a result, PAs have been utilized in a wide range of hospital roles, serving in emergency medicine, intensive care units, labor and delivery units, and infection control, or as hospitalists and surgical first assistants. In fact, several of the first graduates of the Duke PA program took positions in the Duke University hospital. PAs in the Netherlands are trained almost exclusively in hospitals and practice primarily in this setting.

A shrinking pool of postgraduate medicine trainees and an economy of scale for reliable specialized medical and surgical labor continues to create demand for inpatient PAs. Paramount to hospitals is the number of medical, nursing, and allied health staff available. The use of postgraduate trainees has been one of the chief mainstays of this labor force, but with expansion of hospitals and population demands, inpatient services are highly reliant on PAs to step into the breech. Publicly and privately owned hospitals are striving to meet the needs of patients and the PA has emerged as a perfect fit for this activity—more so than the transient resident. The effect of financing and culture has a profound impact on the organization of hospital beds and this element is predicted to drive more PA demand.

INTRODUCTION

In his masterful history of the U.S. hospital system, *The Care of Strangers: The Rise of America's Hospital System,* Charles Rosenberg argues that it is not possible to understand medicine and the medical care system without a full appreciation of the role played by hospitals. Hospitals have become a major workplace for most healthcare professionals, including physician assistants (PAs).

Most of us begin our lives in a hospital and all too sadly many of us will end our lives there as well. The latter may contribute to the widely disproportionate share of healthcare spending in the last 30 days of one's life. Many

Americans have never come to accept death as have other cultures and when coupled with a troubled medico-legal system, end-of-life decisions are often handled poorly.

At the start of the new millennium there were a little more than 6,000 hospitals in the United States; by 2008 the number of registered hospitals had decreased to 5,747. A number of explanations for this decrease are at hand. Economy of scale meant that small hospitals could not survive, and newer, modern hospitals were needed due to marketing and other pressures. Hospitals also needed to be reengineered for efficiency and safety. In spite of the shrinking number of stand-alone hospitals, the number of beds has grown. In 2006 there were 947,421 hospital beds in the United States (American Hospital Association, 2006). Each bed patient requires a doctor and a nurse to oversee care or have some responsibility for the outcomes of care. Like many places in the world, the demand for physician services has exceeded the supply. Dispersed widely, PAs work in major teaching hospitals, medium-size hospitals, small community and rural hospitals, and other types of inpatient care institutions (Exhibit 8-1). As of 2007, approximately 23,504 clinically active PAs have some connection with a hospital in some capacity (American Academy of Physician Assistants [AAPA], 2007a).

According to findings from a sample of 1,690 PAs employed in hospitals who responded to a national survey, 45% of these PAs were serving as house officers, although that term is becoming more and more difficult to clearly define. More than 90% of the respondents held formal medical staff privileges and were credentialed under hospital bylaws. Since 1992, the percentage of hospital PAs with written job descriptions has grown, permitting them to write diagnostic and therapeutic orders within the institution. A national study of 116 teaching hospitals reported a 62% use of PAs and/or nurse practitioners (NPs) in at least one of their departments (which could include outpatient settings). In these hospitals, PAs were used to perform some tasks previously done by physician residents. Of the 178 departments using PAs in roles traditionally reserved for physicians, 42% were surgical, followed by primary care (25%) and medical specialties (21%). PAs were more likely than NPs to work in surgery and emergency departments (EDs), although NPs were more likely than PAs to work in pediatrics and neonatal care (Riportella-Muller, Libby, & Kindig, 1995).

The role of PAs in inpatient settings tends to be focused in specialty and subspecialty areas such as neonatology, surgery, intensive care, and other specialties. (Mathur et al, 2005). Of the 10% of employed PAs, one-half

EXHIBIT 8-1
Physician Assistants in Hospitals

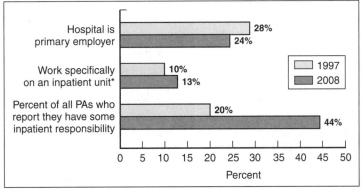

*Inpatient units include intensive care units and critical care units.
Data from American Academy of Physician Assistants. (2008a). 2008 AAPA Physician Assistant Census Report. Alexandria, VA: Author.

work in inpatient units and critical care units. About 22% (3,500) are in outpatient units, and 27% (4,300) are in EDs. Another 21% (3,300) work primarily in the operating room (AAPA, 2007). Hospital-employed PAs also work in primary care or ambulatory care departments, in community outreach clinics, and in the hospital employee health center at remarkably high levels (Hooker & McCaig, 1996; Lin et al, 2002).

Hospital experiences with PAs on inpatient services demonstrate they provide a high level of safety, skills, and clinical efficacy. Usually, these reports verify the capabilities of PAs to assume tasks commonly performed by resident physicians or attendings in a given clinical specialty or unit. Published reports attest to successful experiences of PA use in inpatient internal medicine (Frick, 1983), surgical and surgical subspecialty (Heinrich et al, 1980), and pediatric services (Silver & McAtee, 1984; Mathur et al, 2005). In addition, PAs have been found to be effective and are employed in critical care units (Dubaybo, Samson, & Carlson, 1991; Grabenkort & Ramsay, 1991; Kleinpell, Ely, & Grabenkort, 2008); subspecialty services, such as diagnostic radiology (White et al, 1988); neonatal intensive care units (Reynolds & Bricker, 2007); and EDs (Goldfrank, Corso, & Squillacote, 1980; Sturmann, Ehrenberg, & Salzberg, 1990; Hooker & McCaig, 1996). The addition of PAs to inpatient medical staffs reveals high levels of acceptance by employing physicians and patients, a favorable cost-benefit margin to the institution, and maintenance of high levels of patient care quality (McKelvey, Oliver, & Conboy, 1986).

PHYSICIAN ASSISTANTS AS HOUSE STAFF

PAs work in positions in which they assume the essential roles of physician residents (house officers or house staff) because of their skills in clinical assessment, diagnostic acumen, medical and pharmacologic management, and procedural skills. Most PA programs train students in the hospital setting and in such circumstances students work alongside residents. A growing body of literature documents that teaching hospitals have favorable experiences using nonphysician providers (NPPs) on the wards, in critical care, in surgery, and in a growing variety of other specialties and hospital units (Cawley, 1988; Cawley & Perry, 1988; Russell, Kaplowe, & Heinrich, 1999; Duffy, 2003; Kleinpell, Ely, & Grabenkort, 2008).

The use of PAs has been particularly widespread in surgery to fill positions once filled by residents. In fact, some residency programs have lost accreditation because they lacked sufficient cases to provide adequate clinical experience (Foreman, 1993). PAs have been thus utilized to provide essential preoperative and postoperative care, thereby freeing residents to obtain the required operative case experience necessary to meet residency requirements. Increasingly in modern medicine, PAs are assuming considerable clinical responsibility for preoperative and postoperative care, obtaining histories, conducting physical examinations, and performing invasive as well as noninvasive clinical procedures. One early example of an institution adopting widespread utilization of PAs as house staff was Butterworth Hospital in Grand Rapids, Michigan, where PAs serve in cardiothoracic surgery, neurosurgery, urology, orthopedics, and numerous other medical and surgical specialties. Large PA house staffs, with numbers of anywhere from 100 to 250 PAs, are now seen in such major academic teaching institutions such as the Johns Hopkins Hospital, the Mayo Clinic, the University of Iowa Hospitals and Clinics, Yale-New Haven Hospital, Brigham and Women's Hospital, Grady Memorial, Duke University Hospital, Wake Forest University/Baptist Hospital, M. D. Anderson Hospital, and numerous other major centers.

Under certain circumstances, PAs may be preferable to residents (Exhibit 8-2). Some faculty would rather work with PAs who, research studies have demonstrated, have a lower turnover rate, greater familiarity with departmental procedures, and more clinical experience than first- and second-year residents (Silver & McAtee, 1988; Mitchell,

EXHIBIT 8-2
Advantages of Utilizing Physician Assistants in Resident Substitute Roles

Advantage	Reference
Provide the full range of clinical services required	Riportella-Muller, Libby, & Kindig, 1995; Russell, Kaplowe, & Heinrich, 1999
No decline in quality of care	Reynolds & Bricker, 2007; Dhuper & Choksi, 2009
Enhance the educational experiences of residents	Mathur et al, 2005
Provide continuity of care to inpatient services	Rosenfeld, 1997; Dhuper & Choksi, 2009
Cost effective	Frick, 1983; van Rhee et al, 2002
Support the team model	Mathur et al, 2005; Dacey, 2007

EXHIBIT 8-3
Hospital-Based Doctor Nomenclature

Because some confusion arises when using terms for hospitals and their employees, a brief set of definitions and terms used for hospitals in North America is offered:

Attending doctors: The journeyman doctors employed by the hospital to have ultimate responsibility for the patient. They are the senior doctors in charge of the residents and are involved with their education. Generally they countersign the notes of the trainees.

Chief resident: A member of the medical staff who is employed, usually for 1 year, to oversee the residents. They are not trainees but may take a fellowship after serving as a chief resident.

Fellowship: The period after a residency during which a physician is trained in a subspecialty.

Hospitalist: An attending physician who devotes at least three-quarters of his or her time overseeing acutely ill, hospitalized patients.

House staff/house officers: Doctors in postgraduate training. The term is held over from when resident house staff were given room and board to live in a hospital for their internship and additional training.

Internship: The first year of postgraduate training. A residency may follow the internship year or include the internship year as the first year of residency. At one time, only graduates of medical school did an internship before starting a general medical practice.

Medical and PA students: Students who are assigned to a team of doctors. The team may be composed of an attending doctor, a senior resident, an intern, and a student.

Medical staff: Physicians and other clinicians who are granted privileges to admit patients to the hospital and perform a range of defined duties and responsibilities in patient care, such as surgery and obstetrics.

Residency: A stage of postgraduate medical training certification in a primary care or referral specialty. In the United States and Canada, a resident physician has received a medical degree (MD, MBBS, MBChB, or DO) and mainly cares for hospitalized or clinic patients, mostly with direct supervision from senior physicians.

Hayhurst, & Robinson, 2004). Using PAs is a strategy to ensure that residents have richer educational experiences. For example, a time-and-motion study of residents at three Minnesota teaching hospitals found that residents spent 12% of their time inserting catheters and drawing blood, procedures that can be done by PAs (Lurie et al, 1989). Because these tasks lose their pedagogical value after a certain number of repetitions, delegating them to PAs freed residents to focus on more complex cases.

Because the American and Canadian medical nomenclature may differ from terminology in other countries, a brief taxonomy is offered in Exhibit 8-3.

Demand for Hospital-Based Physician Assistants

PA utilization on inpatient teaching services is increasing due to the Accreditation Commission on Graduate Medical Education (ACGME)-imposed work hour limitation on physician resident work hours. Resident work hour limitations, which became effective on July 1, 2004, has led GME programs to consider alternative staffing arrangements. The combined effects of the U.S. hospitalist movement, the employment of PAs as hospitalists, and in particular,

adjustments of residency training programs to the ACGME regulations, likely has increased the utilization of PAs in hospital settings and in resident-substitute and hospitalist roles. In a 5-year span beginning in 2000, the resident working hour limitation resulted in a swell of hospital-based PAs (Exhibit 8-4). Employment of inpatient and hospitalist PAs increased from 2000 through 2006 (Cawley & Hooker, 2006).

This AAPA-generated data revealed that the number of PAs in inpatient settings rose from 1,322 to 1,848. The likely actual number in 2010 is much higher. At the same time, the number of PAs in critical care units increased slightly (403 to 405), and the number of PAs working in hospital operating rooms fell from 1,629 to 1,488 (Exhibit 8-5).

Perceived Barriers

Clinical, financial, and practical criticisms have been raised about using PAs to assume the role of residents. Although PAs may work well as substitutes for first- and second-year residents, some suggest they may require additional training to assume responsibility for more complex cases that call for more

EXHIBIT 8-4
Number of Physician Assistants in Select Hospital Settings, by Year

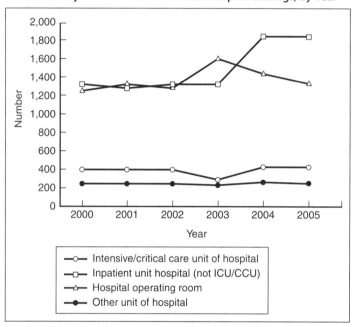

Data from Cawley, J. F., & Hooker, R. S. (2006). The effect of resident work hour restrictions on physician assistant hospital utilization. Journal of Physician Assistant Education, 17(3), 41–43; and the American Academy of Physician Assistants Census Reports, 2000–2005.

EXHIBIT 8-5
Trends in Physician Assistants Working in Hospital Settings, 2003–2008*

	Percentage (and Number) of all AAPA Census Respondents			
	2003 *(N = 18,155)*	*2005* *(N = 19,951)*	*2006* *(N = 21,023)*	*2008* *(N = 25,174)*
All hospital work settings	17.9%	18.1%	18.6%	19.0%
Intensive care/critical care unit	1.5% (280)	2% (403)	2.1% (446)	2.3% (590)
Inpatient unit	7.4% (1,335)	9.3% (1,848)	9.8% (2,059)	10.3% (2,595)
Operating room	9% (1,629)	6.8% (1,350)	6.7% (1,408)	6.4% (1,608)

*Respondents working in hospital outpatient units and emergency departments were not included.
Data from the American Academy of Physician Assistants Census Reports, 2003–2008.

advanced medical decision-making or greater technical skill. However, in a study by Riportella-Muller, Libby, and Kindig (1995), this concern was not the case in teaching hospitals. In this national sample, PAs and NPs were filling positions that had been filled by junior and senior residents (Exhibit 8-6). On the other hand, leaders in medical education have made the point that the complexity of modern medicine may require PAs to possess advanced educational training and skills (Whitcomb, 2007b). This view has led to the development of an increasing number of hospital-based PA postgraduate residency programs where graduate PAs obtain additional formal training in inpatient medical and surgical disciplines.

Two other barriers to using more PAs arise from time to time. One is the view that PAs are more expensive to hire than residents and work fewer hours. For example, the 2008 median total salary for PAs was $89,898 compared with an average stipend of about $50,000 for second- and third-year residents. Residents are likely to work more than 50 or 60 hours per week, whereas PA house officers tend to work fewer than 45 hours per week. Stipends for PAs in postgraduate residency program are roughly similar to physician residents.

The other argument against using PAs is reimbursement. One of the chief financial issues when trading resident services for PA services in the United States is federal remuneration. Physicians in training, or residents, bring GME payments (through Medicare) to the institution. Hospitals, on the other hand, do not always receive an explicit payment for the services of the PA, depending on how they bill insurers. Currently, Medicare pays practices and services employing PAs for hospital-delivered services under Medicare Part B when such services would be covered if furnished by a physician, including assistant-at-surgery services, inpatient hospital care, and assisting-at procedures. Specifically, for all billable service in the hospital, Medicare will cover PAs at 85% of the physician fee schedule, if the service would have been covered if performed by a physician (Medicare Transmittal AB-98-15).

However, counterarguments to these perceived barriers are offered by hospital employers of PAs. The main argument is that PAs employed by hospitals may be more economical than salary figures suggest because they may be more efficient than residents, use fewer resources than residents, and require less faculty supervision. In the long run, the

EXHIBIT 8-6
Distribution of Departments Where Physician Assistants Are Performing Some Tasks Previously by Resident Physicians

Specialty	Physician Assistant Only		Nurse Practitioner Only		Both		Total	
	No.	%	No.	%	No.	%	No.	%
General surgery	20	17.2	0	0.0	9	14.5	29	11.4
Surgical specialties	36	31.0	14	19.2	9	14.5	59	23.1
Internal medicine	16	13.8	11	14.3	11	17.7	38	14.9
Pediatrics	1	0.9	13	16.9	4	6.5	18	7.1
Other primary care	5	4.3	8	10.4	7	11.3	20	7.8
Emergency	14	12.1	2	2.6	3	4.8	19	7.5
Neonatal	0	0.0	15	19.5	2	3.2	17	6.7
Other specialty	14	12.1	6	7.8	5	8.1	25	9.8
Unspecified	10	8.6	8	10.4	12	19.4	30	11.8
TOTAL	116	100	77	100	62	100	255	100

Data from Riportella-Muller, R., Libby, D., & Kindig, D. (1995). The substitution of physician assistants and nurse practitioners for physician residents in teaching hospitals. Health Affairs, 14(2), 181–191.

cost utility to the institution may be less when the PA house officer, as a permanent employee, does not need to be retrained each year (or every few months), is knowledgeable about the system, and operates at a higher level of visibility with the staff. An annual transition to new staff and scheduling arrangements takes time and money.

Models for PA-Resident Integration

At least three models exist for PA-resident integration: (1) a fully integrated model with PAs and residents sharing responsibilities for the same group of patients, (2) a separate but equal model, and (3) a partially integrated model. A model of the effective use of PAs in a typical community hospital setting is presented in Exhibit 8-7. Trade-offs of these models include the need for institutional commitment; the influence of local circumstances; the need to emphasize partnership, not competition, between PAs and residents' value of an educational component; the need to build a cohesive program; and the importance of effective PA leadership (Russell, Kaplowe, & Heinrich, 1999).

Expanding and contracting work demand creates job inequality. Residents with limited exposure to PAs and their capabilities may view the PAs as their assistants and relegate tasks that don't fully utilize the PAs' skills. Thus, the fully integrated model is subject to whim and misuse or underuse of skills. At the other end of the labor spectrum is the separate but equal PAs and residents model. With this model, services are often duplicated and separate policies and skills apply to different types of providers. The partially integrated model has the residents and PAs "cross-cover" for each other when needed and stratifies junior and senior resident services. Over time, the residents and the PAs come to see the advantage of each other's roles and seek the availability of each other's services when the hospital census is high. The main difference in roles is that the resident's role is to learn and move on, whereas the PA's role in the hospital is a career.

At one major teaching institution in the Northeast there are three grades of PAs. These grades are based not on their clinical experience, but on the nonclinical responsibilities they take on in addition to their work with patients. Some work on continuing education programs, whereas others work on hospital-wide PA grand rounds. One PA works in the organizational area of patient satisfaction and has been doing quality improvement projects related to satisfaction with the PA program. Another PA conducts chart reviews and looks at readmission rates, and one PA works as a liaison between the hospital and the group, working on qualifications and credentialing issues. One physician/administrator predicts that by 2016 one-half of all inpatients will be taken care of by PAs or NPs (Callahan, 2007).

Benefits of Hospital-Based Physician Assistants

PAs have been shown to be effective serving in hospital roles where they assume responsibilities similar to residents and house officers (Frick, 1983; Duffy 2003). The use of PAs on inpatient staffs addresses a number of issues in modern GME. In addition to helping meet service needs brought about by the limitation of resident working hours, there is the need for programs to protect residents' educational experiences and to maintain standards of hospital care (Dhuper & Choksi, 2009). PAs are not only capable of fulfilling a substantial portion of the clinical duties required on inpatient services (Knickman et al, 1992; Mitchell, Hayhurst, & Robinson, 2004), they also provide patient care continuity and promotion of medical education goals for physician residents (Mathur et al, 2005). In fact, incorporating PAs allows in-house coverage of patients, preserves the educational integrity of the physician residency programs, allows time for residents' conferences and clinics, and prepares junior doctors for practice on multidisciplinary teams (Samuels et al, 2005).

Typically, the roles of house staff PAs encompass a fairly standard list of functions (Exhibit 8-8). Duties may go beyond the basic job description, depending on the PA's experience and training and the approval of the hospital credentials committee. House staff PAs

EXHIBIT 8-7
A Community Hospital Model of Physician Assistant Utilization

Northwest Hospital Center (NWHC) is a 240-bed, nonteaching community hospital located in the Baltimore metropolitan area. The hospital is part of the LifeBridge Health system, which also contains a large tertiary academic medical center, Sinai Hospital of Baltimore. NWHC serves a suburban and urban patient base and treats primarily adult patients. The institution is one of the more successful hospitals in Maryland from both a financial and growth perspective.

The hospital opened in the late 1960s and employed its first PA in 1974 to serve as an assistant in the operating room. NWHC also served as one of the first preceptor sites for the then newly formed Essex Community College PA program (now the Towson/CCBC PA Program). Over the next several years, additional PAs were employed to provide operating room assistance, admission support, and coverage of the acute care floors in performing minor procedures such as inserting nasogastric tubes and catheters. The impetus to provide these services was in part due to the growth of the facility, but also at the request of the attending medical staff, who expected services at par with those facilities with resident staff.

In 1984, changes in Medicare policy prohibited hospitals from including physician charges in their rates, and the clearer distinction of Part A and Part B billing caused many facilities to rethink the role of their house staff. NWHC, which in addition to PAs had a number of house doctors, recognized that they would not be able to recoup those expenditures through the new physician charge system. The decision was made to decrease the component of physician staff serving in this role and to expand the PA coverage around the clock, giving PAs more responsibilities for assisting with patient management. Initial skepticism that PAs could replace physicians faded as communication improved and customer service satisfaction rose, due in large part to the PA staff.

Throughout the 1990s, PAs at NWHC continued to gain experience and respect from many skeptical physicians. During this time, under new leadership, PAs at NWHC were cross-trained in the medical and surgical disciplines. Capitalizing on this PA plasticity model provided management efficiency by requiring flexibility of the PA staff. Shifting staff to the areas of greatest need without being restricted by specific discipline boundaries is considered a highly principled management tool. As a consequence, management, under a PA manager, developed into a department of PAs (as opposed to having PAs in departments). As additional staff members were hired, the PA division's responsibility grew to include employee health and occupational health services.

Another period of growth followed the federal Balanced Budget Act in 1997, which allowed for reimbursement of PA services. NWHC significantly increased its operating room PA staff, at the same time recovering the majority of expenses through first-assisting fees. As the PA program at NWHC grew, the attending surgical staff endorsed this improved service by redirecting their patients to NWHC. The reason most often cited was because of the reliability of and satisfaction with the surgical service.

At the turn of the century NWHC underwent an internal analysis of its staffing and expenses utilizing a prominent healthcare consulting firm. After extensive review and piloting of programs, the PA department was one of the few areas that increased staff. By assigning a PA directly to each patient zone (20 beds), NWHC demonstrated improved efficiency with a reduction of length of stay by nearly one-third.

In 1999, a hospitalist program was inaugurated at NWHC. PAs were quickly incorporated into teams of doctors and PAs. The service integrated the hospitalist physicians with PAs to afford greater efficiency of both components. After a decade of experience, the Hospitalist/PA service alone accounts for the management of 35% of all hospital admissions.

In summary, NWHC is a metropolitan hospital with a sizeable PA staff. It has grown from four PAs in the 1970s to 30 full-time equivalent PA staff. The constant pulse-taking of its operation, using 360-degree analysis techniques, allows service and quality to be assessed. The high results from patients, staff, management, and employees endorse this staffing strategy. Overall, for 2008, the Hospitalist/PA service achieved a 99th percentile on both patient and physician satisfaction surveys. The relationship with nursing and other professional staff remains "outstanding." PA employment retention is high and job satisfaction equally high. Finally, the trust of the attending physicians and administration suggests the strategy of utilizing a flexible and talented team of doctor, nurse, and PA has spelled financial and management success at NWHC (R. Rohrs, PA-C, Director of Hospital Medicine, Northwest Hospital, personal communication, May 2008).

within internal medicine departments have assumed a wide assortment of duties including bone marrow aspiration, thoracentesis, lumbar puncture, coronary angiography, joint injections, liver biopsies, invasive radiological procedures, and numerous other technical procedures.

House staff PAs are also involved in clinical research activities, which may include duties such as collecting specialized data on patients, monitoring therapeutic effects, participating in the analysis of clinical data, and overseeing professional communication. If the hospital is

EXHIBIT 8-8
Basic Job Description of a House Staff Physician Assistant

As a member of the healthcare team, the PA will provide medical and/or surgical support to the hospital's attending physicians, nurses, and patients and may perform the following:

- Review patient records to aid in determining health status.
- Take patient histories, perform physical examinations, and identify normal and abnormal findings on histories, physicals, and commonly performed laboratory studies.
- Perform developmental screening examinations on children.
- Record pertinent patient data in the medical record.
- Carry out or relay a physician's orders for diagnostic procedures, treatments, and medication in accordance with existing drug laws.
- Transcribe the orders on the patient chart as a verbal or telephone order from the physician and then sign it. Orders written by PAs may be reviewed by the physician.
- Collect specimens for commonly performed blood counts and laboratory procedures.
- Assist in surgery, fulfilling all requirements of a surgical assistant.
- Provide preoperative and postoperative surgical and medical care.
- Provide patient education, health promotion, and disease prevention instructions.
- Screen patients to determine the need for medical attention.
- Perform other duties as delegated by the physician and approved by the credentials committee and the bylaws of the institution.

a teaching institution, the house staff PA may participate in teaching rounds; assist in the training of residents, medical students, and PA students; and be involved in other medical educational activities.

Hospitals and institutions that employ 6 to 12 PAs tend to have PAs cover 50 to 150 beds that were previously covered by physician residents and attending physicians. Sometimes PA house staff duties encompass periods of emergency medicine or outpatient clinic duties, depending on service and institutional needs. In one hospital that involved a rapid response team led by PAs, the myocardial infarction mortality rate was substantially decreased (Dacey et al, 2007).

Knickman and colleagues (1992) addressed the clinical potentials for several types of PAs and NPs to fulfill resident roles. Although the estimates of PA-specific capacities for resident substitution are not precise, these data offer insight by comparing the proportion of levels of PA capabilities to assume physician resident inpatient clinical duties in teaching hospitals. The exercise is useful in addressing current workforce issues related to PA roles in the downsizing of GME programs (Exhibit 8-9).

In their time-and-motion study examining the clinical activities of two NPs and eight internal medicine residents in two New York City teaching hospitals, researchers documented the time taken by physicians versus other types of healthcare personnel in performing inpatient medical care tasks traditionally done by physician residents. They compared those times estimated using physicians and nonphysicians under a revised inpatient staffing model. To determine the time per task activity potential for resident substitution, inpatient clinical, educational, personal, and administrative activities were classified by (1) tasks that had to be done by physicians, (2) tasks that were educational only, and (3) tasks that could be done by PAs/NPs or other healthcare personnel.

A total of 1,726 specific activities were recorded. Under scenario 1, the traditional model in which the physician serves as the primary medical manager of the patient, about one-half of a resident's time was spent

EXHIBIT 8-9
Personnel Who Could Perform Physician Resident Activities: Two Staffing Scenarios, by Percent Time

	Traditional Model		PA/NP Model	
	No.	*%*	*No.*	*%*
Physician only	6,248	46.7	2,693	20.0
None (education activities)	2,778	20.7	2,778	20.8
None (personal time)	1,800	13.3	1,800	13.4
Nurse	588	4.5	449	3.4
Laboratory technician	160	1.2	160	1.2
Unskilled personnel	822	6.1	822	6.1
PA/NP	988	7.4	4,681	35.0
TOTAL	13,384	100.0	13,383	100.0

Modified from Knickman, J. R., et al. (1992). The potential for using non-physicians to compensate for the reduced availability of residents. Academic Medicine, 67(7), 429–438.

in activities that must be performed by a physician. The alternative model was one in which a PA or NP assumed an appropriate level of clinical responsibility for day-to-day patient monitoring; only 20% of activities required a physician. The authors concluded that the potential for PAs and NPs to assume inpatient medical tasks is substantial, that only 20% of each resident's lost time must be replaced with other physicians' time, and that to achieve this level of clinical efficiency, inpatient hospital staffing models would need to be restructured to allow for the contributions of nonphysicians to augment physician services (Knickman et al, 1992).

One surgical program observed that the use of PAs met the hospital's expectations for in-house coverage of surgical patients, protected the educational integrity of the physician residency program in surgery, protected time for residents' conferences and clinics, and prepared residents for future practice in multidisciplinary teams. In this instance, duties were assigned to avoid overlap between services of the PAs and services of the residents. Both services were teaching services, which motivated PAs to be committed to the service and fostered equality. The PAs' and the program's goals were determined to have been achieved, including protecting time for residents' education and maintaining humane on-call schedules for

residents. Issues were job satisfaction, turnover, the financial realities of paying for PAs' salaries, benefits, and educational programs, as well as the loss of Medicare, direct medical education (DME), and indirect medical education adjustment (IMEA) reimbursement when a PA replaces a resident (Mathur et al, 2005).

Growth of Inpatient Physician Assistants

In 2003, the AAPA, recognizing that an expanding sector of their membership were identifying themselves as inpatient specialists and aligning themselves with hospitalists, created a category called "Hospital-Employed PAs." The growth of these inpatient specialists has been surprising and continues to grow. Whether this growth is due to policy changes in resident hours, the increased number of beds in American hospitals, more specialized care, or population growth has not been delineated fully. Clearly, there has been substantial growth of PAs in hospital roles (Cawley & Hooker, 2006).

The distribution of hospital-based PAs differs depending on geographic location. In 2008, the AAPA asked members to describe their location of practice and whether they were hospital employed. On average, 21% answered that they were located in a hospital setting. In the Northeast, 41% of PAs worked in a hospital setting. In the South Central and

West, fewer than one in six PAs was hospital based (Exhibit 8-10).

The expanding roles of hospital-based PAs have caught the attention of health policy analysts, and various explanations for this phenomenon have been advanced. One leading reason for such expansion is the disproportionally high use of international medical graduates as house officers on the East Coast. The increasing difficulty in filling these resident positions has led to replacement by PAs. This trend began in the early 1980s and seems to be increasing.

Another explanation for the difference in geographic distribution is the type of training programs on the East and West Coasts. The Medex model that began in Seattle was strictly outpatient based, both in training and in practice of its early graduates. The Duke model, on the other hand, began in the university hospital setting and continues to expose its students to an inpatient role. Many of the programs that sprang up in the Midwest and on the East Coast have followed the Duke model.

A third hypothesis that explains regional role differences for PAs is that the need for rural providers is far greater in the south

central and western parts of the United States than in most other regions of the country. The PA seems to be better suited to fill roles in these regions than in inpatient settings. Further research will concentrate on to what extent the PA who identifies a hospital as his or her location of practice actually provides inpatient services (Exhibit 8-11).

Case Studies of Physician Assistants in Hospitals

Duke University Hospital was the first hospital to employ PAs, including several of the first graduates of the Duke PA Program. A few years later, Montefiore Medical Center in Bronx, New York was among the first hospitals to use PAs as a means to augment inpatient medical and surgical house staff. Beginning in 1971, PAs were hired for house staff roles on surgical wards at Montefiore to offset reductions in the number of surgical residents. To provide a steady supply of inpatient surgical PAs, Montefiore instituted the first PA postgraduate residency program. Today, the institution employs more than 150 PAs, not only in surgical areas but also in internal

EXHIBIT 8-10
Hospital-Employed Physician Assistants by Region in the United States, 2008

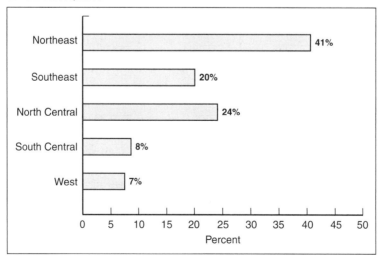

Data from American Academy of Physician Assistants. (2008a). 2008 AAPA Physician Assistant Census Report. Alexandria, VA: Author.

EXHIBIT 8-11
Number of Physician Assistants Employed by Select Major Medical Centers, 2008

Columbian Presbyterian Hospital	175
The Johns Hopkins Hospital	110
University of Iowa Hospital and Clinics	75
University of Michigan Health System	48
M. D. Anderson Cancer Center	110
Duke University Hospital	150
Dallas VA Medical Center	60
University of Texas Southwest Medical Center	60
Cleveland Clinic Hospital System	220

medicine, the medical subspecialties, emergency medicine, obstetrics and gynecology (OB/GYN), employee health services, transplantation services, burn units, and a broad range of administrative, education, and research roles.

Geisinger Medical Center, a 577-bed referral facility located in rural northeastern Pennsylvania, began employing PAs in the mid-1970s and now has PAs serving in primary care as well as in specialty and subspecialty roles. Like many institutes, Geisinger uses PAs and NPs to staff family medicine clinics and the ED, in addition to using them in general medical internal medicine specialties, general surgery and surgical subspecialties, high-technology diagnostic and therapeutic service areas, and roles in outpatient clinics at satellite settings (Walters, 1986; Harbert, Shipman, & Conrad, 1994).

Hurley Medical Center in Flint, Michigan, established a trauma program in which PAs fill the roles normally held by surgical residents. A study reported in the *Journal of Trauma* showed that despite an increase in patient acuity, in its first 2 years the program resulted in a 23% decrease in transfer time to the operating room, a 51% decrease in transfer time to the trauma intensive care unit (ICU), and a 20% decrease in transfer time to the surgical floor. Length of stay for neurotrauma ICU patients decreased by 33% (Miller et al, 1998).

Yale-New Haven Hospital officials describe their hospitalist service as, "A model partnership with Yale-New Haven Hospital, the Yale University School of Medicine Department of Medicine, and private physicians, physician assistants, and nurse practitioners in the community." With more than 21 internists and 16 PAs, hospitalists are available around the clock, caring for more than 50% of the general medicine patients. The program is a tremendous success, with shorter lengths of stay for patients and high patient satisfaction scores. Community physician and nursing satisfaction with care is similarly high.

Cleveland Clinic employs 222 PAs in nearly all specialties: 152 on the main campus and 70 in the system's seven other hospitals and clinics. Mark Harrison, MD, chair of medical operations for the Cleveland Clinic, says he would "be thrilled to double" the number of PAs there. He and other physicians throughout the institution speak glowingly of PAs' qualifications and of their contributions. The presence of PAs enables each medical team to treat more patients, and provides continuity of care that gives physicians more time to focus on research and writing.

M. D. Anderson Cancer Center in Houston, Texas, has employed PAs for decades and has a strong history in PA education. More than 130 PAs work in inpatient and outpatient settings within the institution. M. D. Anderson Cancer Center places a premium on teamwork. Most departments hold weekly multidisciplinary meetings at which patients' treatment options are analyzed by all of the professionals involved in their care. Both physicians and PAs at this institutition say that the single greatest contribution PAs make is the continuity of care they provide. A key to successful integration of PAs has been allowing each department the flexibility to define the PA role to meet its needs.

Other major institutions that employ substantial numbers of PAs include Brigham and Women's Hospital in Boston, Duke University Medical Center, Geisinger Health System in Pennsylvania, Johns Hopkins Hospital, Massachusetts General Hospital, the Mayo Clinic, New York Presbyterian University Hospital, Stanford University Medical Center University of Florida, University of Iowa, University of Medicine and Dentistry of

New Jersey, University of Michigan Health Systems, University of Pittsburgh Medical Center, and University of Utah. PAs are well integrated into 13 of the nation's top 18 hospitals identified by *U.S. News and World Report* in 2007 (AAPA, 2008b).

HOSPITAL CREDENTIALS

Although the PA is a dependent practitioner, he or she must develop and exercise a degree of independent clinical judgment to be effective. The parameters for the application of PA clinical judgments are usually first defined by existing state statutes on PAs and their scope of practice. Since 2007, all states and most territories have laws regulating PAs. Beyond state regulations, hospitals develop their own institutional guidelines for employed PAs through amendments to the medical staff bylaws (the policies laid out by the hospital board of directors that act as a type of governance for the conduct of the hospital). Such documents spell out important procedures and standards to which members of the hospital must adhere. Ultimately, physicians and PAs must be credentialed by the hospital under the bylaws if they are to have the privilege of entering the hospital for professional purposes.

Credentialing is a process of validating the background and assessing the qualifications of professionals to provide healthcare services in medical institutions (Exhibit 8-12). This process involves the evaluation of a person's current licensure, training or experience, competence, and ability to perform the privileges requested. *Privileges* are authorizations granted by the governing body of an institution to provide specific care services within defined limits. Granting of privileges is based on a person's licensure, education, competence, health status, and judgment (Calabrese, Crane, & Legler, 1997).

The primary purpose of credentialing providers is to protect healthcare organizations and institutions from the legal liability that could result from the actions of unqualified providers. To be credentialed by a hospital the

EXHIBIT 8-12

Information Collected for Credentialing and Privileges of Physician Assistants

- Address (home and work)
- Social Security number
- License or registration number
- National Commission on Certification of Physician Assistants certification
- State prescribing number
- Drug Enforcement Administration number
- Degrees and certificates
- Additional training (e.g., advanced cardiac life support, advanced trauma life support)
- Professional experience, including names of employers
- Teaching appointments
- Past and current privileges
- Legal and administrative actions taken against an individual:
  - By employers, hospitals, other institutions
  - By government agencies
  - By professional societies
  - By other monitors of professional conduct
- Professional liability:
  - Current liability coverage
  - Past and current claims and suits
  - National Practitioner Databank information
- Personal health
- References
- Practice-related information

Data from Calabrese, W. J., Crane, S. C., & Legler, C. F. (1997). Issues in quality care. The two-sided coin of PA credentialing. *Journal of the American Academy of Physician Assistants, 10*(5), 121–122.

institution must review and approve the qualifications and backgrounds of healthcare professionals before granting specific privileges. Since 1980, a wide variety of nonphysician healthcare professionals have been awarded medical staff privileges by hospitals, including PAs, NPs, certified nurse-midwives, optometrists, podiatrists, psychologists, and other members of the healthcare delivery system.

Typically, the credentials committee of the medical staff develops guidelines delineating the duties of a PA. These guidelines take into consideration the intended duties, the specific needs and requirements of the medical attending staff, the expected training and qualifications of the PA, and provisions regarding supervision and monitoring of the PA's performance. An important part of these guidelines is the PA job description, which is usually developed for each type of service for which PAs work (e.g., medicine, surgery, and pediatrics). The PA's job description must accommodate common tasks and the specific duties on a given service. Basic methods of delineating clinical privileges include the following:

■ Job description
■ List of procedures each practitioner is likely to perform
■ Categorization of a clinical situation according to severity of illness, level of training required, or degree of required supervision
■ Primary or supervising physician of the PA

Most hospitals use the same form or process for PAs that they use for physicians in granting privileges—usually proctoring until competence is shown. The AAPA document "Guidelines for Amending Hospital Staff Bylaws" includes the major issues that a PA may encounter in seeking hospital privileges and typical hospital responsibilities. Each state's enabling legislation may also contain PA credentialing guidelines that specify which type of educational and professional qualifications a PA must have to receive privileges. Typically, a PA candidate is required to be:

■ a graduate of an ARC-PA-accredited PA training program,
■ eligible for or have passed the national certifying examination administered by the National Commission on Certification of Physician Assistants (NCCPA), and
■ hold a current license from the appropriate medical licensing board.

Evaluation of an organization's credentialing program features prominently in surveys by the Joint Commission and the National Committee for Quality Assurance. By ensuring that providers are qualified, credentialing also promotes quality care. Although the major emphasis of credentialing is to judge the qualifications of physicians, other providers, such as PAs, who participate in the delivery of medical services and who may be legally liable for the quality and safety of the procedures performed are also being credentialed (Calabrese, Crane, & Legler, 1997). The AAPA has a member liaison on the Joint Commission's Hospital Professional and Technical Advisory Committee, which develops and critiques standards in survey process. The AAPA monitors the Joint Commission's activity on a routine basis to ensure that PAs are represented on key issues. Recent examples would be the Anesthesia Task Force and the Credentialing and Privileging Task Force.

Appointment to the medical staff of a hospital usually is term-limited (i.e., 2 years), and is subject to review prior to renewal. For reappointment, staff members must typically update the information on their original application, provide evidence of continuing education, and document any professional training that may be pertinent to a proposed modification of their privileges. PAs adhere to the same standards of quality, competence, and patient satisfaction that are expected of a physician. One PA who is a 35-year member of the medical staff of a major urban hospital advocates that PAs, as full members of the staff, must insist on involvement in all aspects of the administration of hospital credentialing (Condit, 2000).

HOSPITAL SPECIALTY ROLES

Inpatient PAs are on the staff in many medical and surgical specialties and subspecialties (e.g., cardiology, pulmonary medicine, gastroenterology, nephrology, rheumatology, infectious disease, and oncology), in addition to pediatrics, internal medicine, and geriatrics. In these disciplines, PAs not only assist physicians in routine patient care duties but also perform many technical procedures. PAs who work in cardiology, for example, perform exercise stress tests, coronary angiography, and similar invasive and noninvasive diagnostic evaluations. A PA in Parkland Memorial Hospital in Dallas, Texas, performs most of the liver biopsies and is a specialist in liver diseases.

Hospital-based PAs are also involved in renal transplant teams, burn units, critical care units, intensive care units (ICUs), cardiac transplant teams, and neurology and neurologic units, as well as many specialty-oriented technical procedures. A small, but growing, number of PAs work in anesthesiology, and some PAs who specialize in cardiothoracic surgery have obtained additional formal training and certification in cardiac bypass pump technology. In a 1987 study, PAs performing coronary angiograms had a lower rate of complications than did cardiology fellows (DeMots et al, 1987). A second study in 2001 validated these findings (Krasuski et al, 2003). PAs are extensively deployed in neonatology and pediatric ICUs (DeNicola et al, 1994; Reynolds & Bricker, 2007). For such PAs, a handful of university centers provide extended specialty training programs. Some of the many other specialties that PAs have entered include neurology; neurosurgery; ophthalmology; dermatology; urology and urodynamics; renal dialysis; geriatrics; radiology; pathology; allergy and immunology; ear, nose, and throat; and infectious diseases.

In an effort to describe the roles of PAs in inpatient specialty roles, McKelvey, Oliver, and Conboy (1986) surveyed 23 PAs employed by the University of Iowa Medical Center. Using written questionnaires and personal interviews, they found that four PAs were in general medicine, one in general surgery, and the rest in various subspecialties (four in cardiothoracic surgery, two in pediatric cardiology, three in hematology, and one each in radiology, psychiatry, occupational health, gynecologic oncology, urology, burn care, and cardiology) (McKelvey, Oliver, & Conboy, 1986). Two other PAs were in urologic oncology. The role activities of these providers and the mean percentage of time spent in each activity covered the following five areas:

- Patient care (59%)
- Technical/procedural (18%)
- Administration (11%)
- Medical education (6%)
- Research (5%)

Patient education was identified as an important component of PA patient care activities, ranging from 25% of all patient care time in surgical specialties to 55% of patient care time in pediatrics. Interestingly, when PAs' estimates of their activities were compared with their physician supervisors' estimates, more than 75% of the physicians significantly underestimated PA activity in patient education (McKelvey, Oliver, & Conboy, 1986).

Results of a 1995 survey showed that 60% of teaching hospitals had experience with either replacing house staff or augmenting the residency programs with nonphysician providers (Riportella-Muller, Libby, & Kindig, 1995). As one study stated, "It makes more sense from a public policy perspective to encourage the use of such persons who will be available for an entire career, as opposed to residents who work for only 3 years before going to the already existing surplus of practicing physicians" (Knickman et al, 1992).

Surgery and Trauma

Since the early days of the PA profession, PAs have worked as surgical first assistants and have provided preoperative and postoperative care to patients as members of surgical teams in hospitals (Rosenfeld, 1997). Twenty-three percent (25,187) of the nearly 70,000 clinically practicing PAs work in surgical specialties or subspecialties (orthopedics, cardiovascular/thoracic surgery, neurosurgery, general surgery, and all the surgical subspecialties). The majority of these PAs work in hospitals. The American College of Surgeons and the Society of Thoracic Surgeons recognize PAs as qualified first assistants.

PA roles in cardiothoracic surgery have grown at particularly rapid rates, and it is estimated that there are more than 1,000 PAs in this field alone. Nearly all of these PAs are hospital based (typically in academic medical centers or large community medical centers) and perform a wide range of duties. Their duties include preoperative evaluation and preparation of the patient, intraoperative assisting (harvesting the saphenous vein, establishing cardiopulmonary bypass, controlling bleeding, and wound closure), postoperative management of the patient in both the ICU and later on the surgical ward, and a variety of other clinical, teaching, and administrative functions (Willams et al, 1984).

PAs are assets to surgical teams because of their versatility and because of the fact that third-party payers cover physician services provided by PAs. Surgeons at Hurley Medical Center in Flint, Michigan, found that when they incorporated PAs in surgery the transfer time to the operating room decreased 43%, the transfer time to the ICU decreased 51%, and the transfer time to the floor decreased 20%. This came at a time when the injury severity scores increased 19% over the previous year's scores. The length of stay for admissions decreased 13% and the length of stay for neurotrauma ICU patients decreased 33%. They concluded that Hurley Medical Center's trauma surgeon–PA model is a viable alternative for verified trauma centers unable to maintain a surgical residency program. Consistency and high-quality of care indicated by shortened length of stay is a hallmark of such a model (Miller, Craver, & Hatcher, 1978; Miller & Hatcher, 1978a).

The overall supply of general surgeons is declining in the United States. Over a quarter of a century (1981–2005), the general surgeon ratio declined steadily from 7.7 to 5.7 per 100,000 population. The overall urban ratio dropped from 8.0 to 5.9 per 100,000. The average age of rural surgeons increased compared to their urban counterparts (Lynge et al, 2008). These findings have substantial implications for the delivery of health care in general and the role that surgical PAs are likely to play over the next two decades.

Neonatal Intensive Care Units

PAs and NPs are increasingly being recruited to fill roles traditionally performed by neonatal residents and fellows (Little, 1996). For example, downsizing of a pediatric residency program prompted phased replacement of house staff in a 26-bed neonatal intensive care unit (NICU) in the Albert Einstein College of Medicine-Montefiore Medical Center in Bronx, New York. Subsidized education for neonatal NPs, recruitment of PAs, and leadership took place over 18 months, at which time all house staff functions were assumed by PAs or NPs. The cost to establish this program, the impact on the hospital revenue under New York's prospective reimbursement system, and quality of care were evaluated. Using 1995 dollars, the net start-up cost for the program was $441,000 ($722,000 for education, salaries, staff replacement, and recruitment, partially offset by a New York State workforce demonstration project grant). Ongoing costs of the program are $1.2 million per year (including salaries, off-hours medical backup, recruitment, administrative overhead, and loss of indirect and direct medical education reimbursement, partially offset by recaptured house staff salaries and ancillary expense reductions). Access to care was maintained. Quality of care was assessed during the last 6 months of house staff being in service and during the first 6 months of full PA and NP staffing, revealing similar rates of survival of low-birth-weight neonates and an improvement in documentation and compliance with immunization and blood use guidelines during the PA and NP period.

In the long run, PAs and NPs are expensive in comparison with house staff when only salary is examined. However, in the study, revenue was minimally adversely affected and access to NICU services and quality of care were preserved and, in some cases, enhanced. The authors concluded that in the context of GME reform, staffing problems such as this hospital experienced will occur increasingly in inpatient subspecialty settings (Schulman, Lucchese, & Sullivan, 1995).

Another study was undertaken to compare patient care delivery by neonatal PAs and NPs with that of pediatric residents in the ICU setting. This study differed from the Schulman study (1995) in their use of retrospective chart review after developing specific performance criteria (namely, patient management, outcome, and charges). Charts for 244 consecutive admissions to an NICU in Jacksonville, Florida, were reviewed. Patients were cared for by one of two teams: one staffed by residents and the other by neonatal PAs and NPs. The two teams cared for similar patients as determined by patient background characteristics and diagnostic variables. Performance of the two teams was assessed by comparing patient management, outcome, and charges. Management variables included data on length of critical care and hospital stay, ventilator and oxygen use, total parenteral nutrition use, number of transfusions, and the performance of various procedures. Outcome variables included the incidence of air leaks, bronchopulmonary dysplasia, intraventricular hemorrhage, patent ductus arteriosus, necrotizing enterocolitis, retinopathy of prematurity, and infant death. Charge variables included hospital and physician charges. The results demonstrated no significant differences in management, outcome, or charge variables between patients cared for by the two teams. This study underscores other observations that neonatal PAs and NPs are effective alternatives to residents for patient care in the NICU (Carzoli et al, 1994).

A recent example of the effective utilization of PAs in specialized inpatient service comes from the Department of Pediatrics at the University of Kentucky. At this institution, as with most academic institutions, the limitation of resident work hours combined with the increasing demands on physicians' time and a growing number of patients in the NICU led to a relative workforce shortage in the NICU. The facility attempted to meet their staffing needs by expanding PA and NP coverage, but they were unable to recruit and retain enough qualified individuals to provide complete coverage of the NICU. The university had a PA training program that had been an untapped resource for the NICU. Realizing that PA training is in general primary care practice, it was obvious that any PA hired would not have the knowledge base or skills required for competent practice in the NICU.

A residency was developed to provide neonatal experience. The faculty developed a 1-year curriculum of clinical experience that is combined with didactic lectures. The program covers the entire clinical component of a neonatology fellowship in 1 year instead of 3 years—the current standard for physicians. A clinical curriculum consists of 8 months of hands-on training in the NICU, 1 month in the neonatal nursery, 1 month of high-risk obstetrics, and three 2-week electives on other services.

Each rotation for this program has specific goals. In general, the focus of the NICU months is to gain experience and knowledge in patient management and technical skills. Experience in the neonatal nursery for the PA resident provides opportunities to examine normal newborns and, thus, makes the PAs able to recognize abnormal findings. The goals of the obstetric and elective rotations are to learn how these services interact with neonatology and affect the patient in the NICU and how the NICU affects other services.

While in the program, the PA residents take in-house calls during the residency, and they are on-call with a resident and an attending physician. Initially, the pediatric residents provide an excellent resource for the PA. As the PAs gain more experience, they soon serve as a resource for the pediatric residents. The on-call schedule is necessary because it provides the PA resident with a greater opportunity to learn the skills required for a career in the NICU.

The didactic curriculum of the training program consists of lectures that are usually arranged for the neonatology fellowship program. Because of the volume of material that must be covered, additional lecture time for the PA residents is also arranged. These lectures are on disease-specific or clinically oriented topics and follow an outline that combines several study guides for neonatology fellowship. Research topics are not included in the curriculum, but accommodations are made if a particular resident is so inclined. The PA residents also attend regional or national clinical conferences. Training needs of the PA residents are met through bedside teaching rounds and small didactic sessions during clinical rotations (which do not require additional

EXHIBIT 8-13
Pediatric Resident Survey of Physician Assistants and Nurse Practitioners in the Neonatal Intensive Care Unit

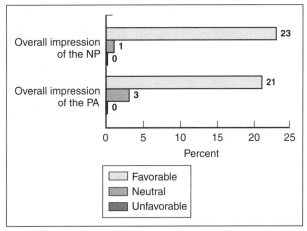

Data from Reynolds, E. W., & Bricker, J. T. (2007). Nonphysician clinicians in the neonatal intensive care unit: Meeting the needs of our smallest patients. Pediatrics, 119(2), 361–369.

commitments from the faculty), the regular didactic lectures designed for the fellowship program (also, not requiring additional commitments from the faculty), and PA resident-specific sessions, usually requiring 1 extra hour per week divided among the faculty. Graduates of the PA residency program command salaries similar to NPs. At the discretion of the institution, they may be able to bill for some services that would offset some of the cost of their employment (Reynolds & Bricker, 2007).

After 3 years of experience and surveying pediatric residents of their satisfaction with the PA neonatal resident, Reynolds and Bricker concluded that the gaps in the neonatal workforce were growing and the neonatal PA offered an opportunity to bridge some of those gaps (Exhibit 8-13).

Intensive Care Units

The use of PAs as providers of care in a medical ICU has also been established. Modern ICUs present unique challenges to physician administrators in the current healthcare environment (Kleinpell, Ely, & Grabenkort 2008). Several models of care (e.g., open vs. closed ICUs and PAs in the ICU) are used throughout the country with varying degrees of success. Although all care models may work, the ideal model for a given ICU can be found only through ongoing performance improvement (Stradtman, 1989).

An early model of successful PA utilization in an ICU setting was described by Dubaybo and colleagues (1991). After 3 months of rigorous training, two PAs were assigned to the ICU. Their performance and the operation of the ICU over a 2-year period were evaluated and compared with the preceding 2 years when it was operated by house officers (residents). There were no changes in occupancy, mortality, or the rate of complications. Evidence for more careful evaluation of patients before admission and discharge, manifesting as slightly fewer admissions and slightly longer duration of hospitalization, was also documented. The authors concluded that properly trained PAs may have a role in providing health care in intensive care settings.

Bone Marrow Transplantation

Bone marrow transplantation is another one of the many subspecialties that has used PAs. Operating without residents or fellows in continuous attendance, the University of Iowa Hospitals and Clinics Pediatric Bone Marrow Transplant Unit used PAs to assume primary responsibility for patients and to ensure continuity of care. Major tasks assigned to the PAs included performing evaluations and assessments, writing notes and orders, and following up in clinics. Basic PA training in pharmacology, physiology, and pathology proved a sufficient background, supplemented by extensive on-the-job training. Knowledge of hematology was considered helpful (Trigg, 1990).

Interventional Radiology

Another emerging area for PAs is the inpatient admitting service, which includes interventional radiology. One example involving interventional radiology demonstrated improved service by developing a clinic and hiring a PA. The service, which began in 1982, was managed by a senior radiologist and fellows. Because of increasing admissions (from a mean of 52 per year from 1982 through 1985 to 110 per year from 1985 through 1987), a half-day, twice-weekly clinic was created in 1985 to evaluate new patients and perform follow-up examinations. In 1986 a PA was hired to assist in the clinic and during patient admissions. Use of the clinic and the PA streamlined patient flow and management during hospitalization, resulting in a decrease in mean length of stay for patients undergoing angioplasty (from 3.74 days in 1982 and 1983 to 2.41 days) and a decreased mean cost savings for the hospital under the prospective payment system. Other benefits included improved physician-patient relationships and follow-up, new patients for colleagues (15% of patients had anatomy unsuitable for interventional procedures and were referred to staff surgeons), and increased professional fees (Stecker et al, 2004).

Psychiatry

Psychiatry reports critical shortages in the availability of trained specialists. One of the earliest studies on PAs in hospitals was a report on the use of PAs in a state mental hospital. In many state hospitals the number of patients and patient care episodes per psychiatrist is very high, particularly in comparison with the situation at private psychiatric hospitals. PAs are typically used in psychiatric settings to provide medical care to psychiatric patients. In the study, the addition of PAs to the staff significantly increased the time that psychiatrists had to plan and implement treatment, enabling the institution to remain open. Other clinical disciplines showed a high degree of acceptance of the PAs in this setting. One report suggested that psychiatry is a promising area for employment of PAs and PAs are probably underused (Matthews & Yohe, 1984). Such promise has not transpired except for experiences in specialized hospitals, as there are less than 1% of all PAs working in psychiatry.

Hospitalists

One of the shifts in hospital-based medicine has been the introduction, or more precisely, the rise of the hospitalist. This discipline is concerned with the medical care of hospitalized patients rather than a specialty organized around an organ system (as with gastroenterology or a disease such as diabetes) or a patient's age (geriatrics). The term "hospitalist" was coined by Wachter and Goldman (1996). Hospitalist activities may include patient care, teaching, research, and leadership related to hospital care. Hospitalists manage patients throughout the continuum of hospital care, often seeing patients in the ED, admitting them to inpatient wards, following them as necessary into the critical care unit, and organizing postacute care. Hospitalists are typically board certified in internal medicine, family medicine, or pulmonology.

Hospital medicine has been an emerging opportunity for PAs (Ottley, Agbontaen, & Wilkow, 2000). Anecdotal information identifies PAs as part of many hospitalist teams (Kessler & Berlin, 1999). Other reports are that this work tends to attract internal medicine matriculants who are looking to bridge some time until they can enter a fellowship. As a result, there has been doctor turnover in some

EXHIBIT 8-14
Hospital Medicine Physician Assistants, 2008

Total respondents	421
Age (mean years)	39
Females	274 (66%)
University hospital	83 (20%)
Other hospital	211 (50%)
Multispecialty physician group practice	39 (9%)
Years in clinical practice	8
Work in urban setting	88%
Precept PA students	38%
Work more than 32 hours per week	92%
Mean income	$87,550

Data from American Academy of Physician Assistants. (2008a). 2008 AAPA Physician Assistant Census Report. Alexandria, VA: Author.

hospitals, leaving the PA as the staff member in place for continuity in care.

Profile

In a survey undertaken by the AAPA, 421 PAs in hospital medicine responded (Exhibit 8-14). The average age was 39, females were 66% of the cohort, and 70% were employed by the hospital. Almost all (88%) worked in an urban setting. The majority (92%) worked full time (at least 32 hours per week). The average salary in 2008 was $87,550 (AAPA, 2008a).

Emergency Departments

A telephone survey of 250 healthcare facilities offering emergency services was conducted by Ellis and Brandt (1997). They described current practice regarding the use of PAs and NPs in EDs. Of the EDs surveyed, 21.6% were using a PA and/or an NP at the time of the survey, and of those not using PAs and/or NPs, 23.5% intended to do so within the next 2 years. Those using PAs and NPs had been using them for a mean duration of 3.5 years (Exhibits 8-15 and 8-16).

To understand trends in emergency medicine visits in the United States, and interprofessional roles in delivering this care, Hooker and colleagues (2008) analyzed a 10-year period (1995–2004) by provider, patient characteristics, and diagnoses. The analysis focused on how doctors, PAs, and NPs shared emergency medicine visits. Data taken from the National Hospital Ambulatory Medical Care Survey produced over 1 billion (1,034,758,313) "weighted" ED visits for 1995 to 2004. The majority of patients were female (53.2%); the mean age of all patients was 35.3 years old. By 2004, physicians were the provider of record for emergency visits at 92.6%, with PAs at 5.7% and NPs at 1.7%. ED visits increased for all three providers over the 10 years. However, patients seen by PAs increased significantly when compared with those seen by physicians or NPs. Medications were prescribed for three-quarters of the visits and were consistent in the mean number of prescriptions written across the three prescribers. Controlled substances accounted for 29.8% of prescriptions written by physicians, 29.3% by PAs, and 26.9% by NPs. No significant differences emerged when urban and rural settings were compared (Exhibits 8-17 and 8-18).

Factors that may explain the expansion of the roles and interprofessional care provided by PAs may include increasing acceptance, clarification of legal and regulatory aspects of practice, staffing adjustments for overcrowded patient care circumstances, shortages of fully trained doctors, and the limitation of working hours of physician postgraduate trainees. Emergency department visits are forecasted to increase to a degree greater than the population increase, with PAs and NPs being used in greater numbers. In view of an increasing demand for emergency medical services and a continuing shortage of physician personnel, policies are needed for workforce planning to meet the demand (Hooker et al, 2008).

Rural Hospitals

The employment of PAs and NPs by rural hospitals is rising. In 1991, approximately 10% of nonmetropolitan hospitals employed a full-time PA and almost 9% employed an NP. In 1993, 16% employed a full-time PA and nearly 11% a full-time NP (American Hospital Association, 1992, 1994). This rise in employment may be because of the need to improve

EXHIBIT 8-15
Procedures and Evaluations Performed by Physician Assistants and Nurse Practitioners in Emergency Departments

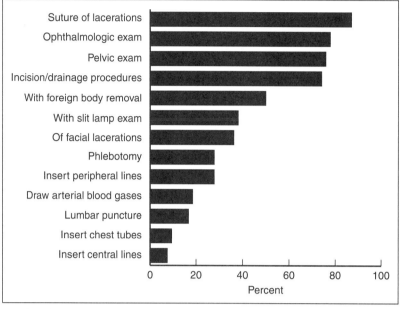

Data from Ellis, G. L., & Brandt, T. E. (1997). Use of physician extenders and fast tracks in United States emergency departments. American Journal of Emergency Medicine, 15(3), 229–232.

or maintain access to healthcare services and the inability to recruit or retain primary care physicians (Drozda, 1992).

One study on rural hospital PA employment described and compared 407 sites spread over 8 northwestern states (Minnesota, North Dakota, South Dakota, Iowa, Montana, Idaho, Oregon, and Washington). The results show that rural hospitals are important employers of PAs and NPs, and there is a greater demand than supply for these providers and for physicians (Krein, 1997a).

Rural hospitals tend to use PAs and NPs to enhance their delivery of outpatient services. An additional factor related to the employment of PAs and NPs in rural areas is that their employment is a requirememt of the rural health clinic (RHC) program. PAs and NPs are also considered cost-effective or more economical for rural areas (Krein 1997a; Krein 1997b) (Exhibit 8-19).

COSTS AND FINANCING ISSUES

It is no coincidence that the period of rapid growth of employment of PAs, beginning in the early 1980s, closely parallels the time when hospitals were coming under increasing pressure to contain costs. Even before the introduction of diagnosis-related groups (DRGs) in 1982, many hospitals were faced with the problems of inadequate staffing, rising costs of physician and nursing staffing, and loss of physician residency training programs. For many hospital administrators the use of PAs in a restructured staffing pattern was an attractive solution to these problems.

Salaries

Most PAs who work in hospitals are salaried employees, with wages dependent on the type of service or department, the type of hospital, and the hours worked. The salary of PA house

EXHIBIT 8-16
Survey of Use of Physician Assistants and Nurse Practitioners in Emergency Departments

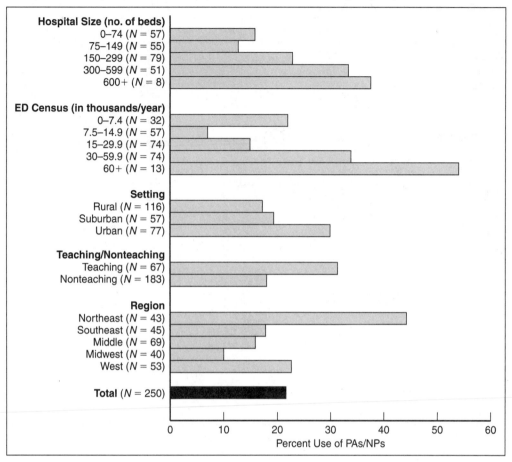

Data from Ellis, G. L., & Brandt, T. E. (1997). Use of physician extenders and fast tracks in United States emergency departments. American Journal of Emergency Medicine, 15(3), 229–232.

officers is approximately twice as high as salaries paid to interns and residents, but it is far below what a fully licensed physician or a hospitalist commands. Hospitals have found that by adjusting the mix of attending physicians, residents, and PAs, they can reduce overall salary costs for inpatient staffing while preserving adequate levels of medical care. Before 1987 payment for services delivered in inpatient hospital settings by PAs was made either retrospectively on the basis of cost or prospectively on the basis of DRGs. Hospitals paid PAs as salaried employees, and there was no statutory provision under Medicare for or against payment of PA services when they were employed by hospitals.

Reimbursement

In late 1986, Congress enacted the Omnibus Budget Reconciliation Act (Public Law [PL] 509), which for the first time permitted Medicare reimbursement to hospitals for services rendered by PAs. The act modified Medicare reimbursement policies and authorized coverage of PAs assisting at surgery at a level of 65% of a physician's reasonable charge and 75% for PAs employed by hospitals.

EXHIBIT 8-17

Demographic Variables of Patients Seen by Physicians, Physician Assistants, and Nurse Practitioners in Emergency Departments from 1995 to 2004

	Physician	PA	NP	Total Percent
GEOGRAPHIC REGION				
Northeast	190,395,530	13,141,431	4,656,412	20.12%
Midwest	242,029,969	14,590,092	3,932,082	25.18%
South	350,990,020	18,108,270	5,070,316	36.16%
West	174,977,631	12,727,527	4,139,033	18.54%
METROPOLITAN STATUS				
MSA	770,067,137	48,944,068	14,279,665	80.53%
Non-MSA	188,429,489	9,623,252	3,414,702	19.47%
Age (median)	35.64	33.61	31.71	—
GENDER				
Female	509,411,517	30,939,274	9,519,776	53.14%
Male	448,981,632	27,731,523	8,174,591	46.86%
ETHNICITY				
Hispanic/Latino	89,680,565	4,715,164	2,403,809	10.47%
Not Hispanic/Latino	102,544,549	5,691,171	2,690,372	10.72%
Blank	739,645,242	45,425,890	13,348,382	77.16%
RACE				
White	732,194,982	45,322,414	13,658,810	76.46%
Black/African American	198,777,072	11,589,293	3,621,654	20.68%
Asian or Native Hawaiian/ Other Pacific Islander	18,418,698	1,241,710	382,861	1.94%
American Indian/Alaskan Native	5,277,267	258,690	72,433	0.54%
Other	3,000,799	98,302	43,460	0.30%

Data from Hooker, R. S., et al. (2008). Emergency medicine services: Interprofessional care trends. Journal of Interprofessional Care, 22(2), 167–178.

EXHIBIT 8-18

Trends in Patient Contact by Type of Emergency Medicine Provider

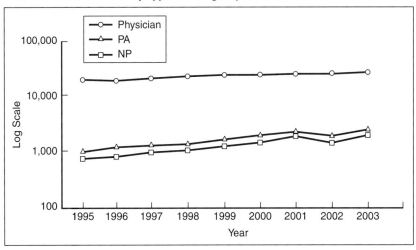

Data from Hooker, R. S., et al. (2008). Emergency medicine services: Interprofessional care trends. Journal of Interprofessional Care, 22(2), 167–178.

EXHIBIT 8-19
Characteristics of Rural Hospitals That Use Physician Assistants and Nurse Practitioners

Hospital and Community Characteristics	Physician Assistants*		Nurse Practitioners*	
	Use (N = 216)	*Do Not Use (N = 191)*	*Use (N = 125)*	*Do Not Use (N = 282)*
Hospital beds	49 (45)	42 (34)	60§ (53)	39 (31)
Full-time hospital employees	122‡ (150)	96 (102)	164§ (177)	86 (94)
Physicians on active staff	20 (32)	15 (22)	30§ (39)	12 (19)
No. of specialty types on active staff	4 (4)	4 (4)	6§ (5)	3 (3)
Primary care physicians on active staff†	9 (11)	8 (8)	12§ (13)	7 (7)
Hospital admissions	1,509‡ (1,962)	1,183 (1,334)	2,101‡ (2,362)	1,026 (1,170)
Outpatient visits (emergency and other)	22,621 (25,033)	18,544 (21,566)	31,283§ (31,655)	16,020 (16,910)
Surgical procedures (inpatient and outpatient)	1,138 (1,739)	867 (1,232)	1,654§ (2,079)	725 (1,092)
Percent of revenue from Medicare	54% (14.5)	54% (13.4)	51%‡ (13.9)	55% (13.8)
Owns or manages a rural health clinic	35%§	16%	30%	24%
Education site for PA/NP/CNM/CRNAs	28%	14%	22%	21%
Currently recruiting for a physician	66%	68%	74%	64%
Population of the hospital's service area (38,914)	26,731 (33,571)	23,558 (44,993)	35,559§ (31,056)	20,690
Road miles to a city of 50,000 population	92 (60)	92 (65)	95 (60)	90 (63)

*Mean values with standard deviations in parentheses.

†*Primary care* is defined as general practice, family practice, internal medicine, and pediatrics.

‡$P < 0.05$ (compared with hospitals that do not use the practitioner).

§$P < 0.001$ (compared with hospitals that do not use the practitioner).

Modified from Krein, S. L. (1997). The employment and use of nurse practitioners and physician assistants by rural hospitals. Journal of Rural Health, 13(1), 45–58.

Title 42 of the U.S. Annotated Code—Public Health & Welfare, Section 1395x(s)(K)(i)—notes the statutory coverage of PAs in the hospital practice setting. The Centers for Medicare and Medicaid Services' (CMS) regulations for PAs make no distinction between hospital inpatient, outpatient, and ED practice settings. Generally, all services for which Medicare would pay if provided by a physician are also covered when performed by a PA. In the 1986 revisions to the Medicare Hospital Conditions of Participation (Federal Register 51, no. 116, [17 June 1986]: Section 482.12[c]) that refer to the ability of the physician to delegate patient care responsibilities to the PA, CMS states that the use of the term *physician care* is "not intended to restrict the ability of doctors of medicine or osteopathy to delegate tasks to appropriately qualified health care personnel such as physician assistants . . . in accordance with state law."

In the 1997 Balanced Budget Act (BBA), the level of payment for PA services was set at 85% of the customary payment for a physician in the same setting. The BBA legislation made PAs even more attractive to hospitals and hospital-based physicians during an era when PA utilization in such settings was already beginning to flourish. Recognition of the value of PA services by Medicare was a long-sought-after goal for the PA profession because this policy not only allows PAs to firmly justify their roles in institutional settings, but also has promoted the expanded use of PAs by hospitals that were previously reluctant to employ them. Because most third-party payers emulate the Medicare program in terms of reimbursement policies, they tend to reimburse PA services as well.

Medicare follows the PA regulations established in each state regarding the degree of physician supervision required in hospitals.

The physician supervisor need not be physically present with the PA in the hospital when a service is being furnished to a Medicare patient, unless required by state law or by the hospital's regulations. However, if the physician supervisor (or physician designee) is not physically present with the PA, he or she must be immediately available to the PA for consultation purposes by telephone or other effective, reliable means of communication (AAPA, 2008b).

Billing in Hospital Settings

Medicare Part A (also known as *hospital insurance*) covers inpatient hospitalization, nursing facility care, home health care, and hospice care (such as facility fees and supply costs). Part B (supplemental medical insurance) covers professional services provided by physicians, PAs, and certain other authorized practitioners in the office, clinic, hospital (including emergency room), and nursing facility.

In the past, Medicare gave hospitals two options for covering services by hospital-employed PAs. Services provided by PAs could be billed under Medicare Part B as a professional service, or the PA's salary could be included in the hospital's cost reports and covered under Medicare Part A. Because of Medicare's shift to prospective payments, the option of including the PA's salary in the hospital's cost reports is no longer an appropriate method of coverage. It appears that many Medicare carriers are not fully aware of this policy change and may still allow Part A coverage. AAPA will engage in educational efforts with PAs and hospitals to make sure that all parties are aware of Medicare's requirements.

Rules for Evaluation and Management Services

Traditionally, Medicare rules for hospital (inpatient, outpatient, or ED) billing required that the practitioner who provided the majority of professional service to the patient be the one that bills for the service. That is, if the PA did the majority of the work for the patient, the service should be billed under the PA's

personal identification number (PIN) and reimbursement would be at 85% of the fee schedule. Some mistakenly believed that the service could be billed by the physician at 100% if the physician was on-site, cosigned the patient's chart, and/or provided some minor service to the patient. Likewise, the "incident to" billing concept is never applicable in the hospital setting.

From September 2001 through September 2002, Medicare suggested that a concept known as "split billing" be used to separately bill for evaluation and management (E/M) services provided by PAs and physicians when both provided care to the same patient on the same day in the hospital setting. After being made aware of the administrative and billing difficulties that this concept would cause for both practitioners and Medicare carriers, the split billing concept was rescinded.

As of October 25, 2002, new rules championed by the AAPA give PAs and their physicians increased latitude in hospital billing for E/M services. The new requirement (Medicare Transmittal 1776; see Appendix L) will allow PAs and physicians who work for the same employer or entity to share visits made to patients with the combined work of both billed under the physician at 100% of the fee schedule. That is, if the PA provides the majority of the service for the patient and the physician provides any face-to-face portion of the E/M encounter, the entire service may be billed under the physician. This new rule does not extend to procedures performed in the hospital. The practitioner who does the majority of the procedure is the one under whom the procedure should be billed.

For reimbursement of a PA's service the following guidelines must be in place:

- The PA and the physician must work for the same entity (e.g., same group practice, same hospital, or PA is employed by a solo physician).
- The regulation applies to E/M services, but not procedures or consultations.
- The physician must provide at least some face-to-face part of the E/M visit. Simply

reviewing or signing the patient's chart is not sufficient.

■ The PA and physician must see the patient on the same day.

If the physician does not provide some face-to-face portion of the E/M encounter, then the service is appropriately billed at the full fee schedule amount under the PA's PIN with reimbursement paid at the 85% rate.

Consultations as Shared Visits

The CMS issued Transmittal #788, dated December 20, 2005, which states that consultations may not be billed as shared visits. Other office and hospital evaluation and management services continue to be eligible for shared billing.

If the PA performs the majority of the consultation, the consult is appropriately billed under the PA's name and Medicare number with payment at 85% of the physician fee schedule, even if the physician provides some level of care to the same patient on the same day. If the physician repeats enough of the consultation (history of present illness, examination, medical decision-making), then the consultation could be billed under the physician at 100% of the fee schedule.

The AAPA held discussions with CMS and argued that consults should be included as eligible shared visit services. CMS did not agree with the AAPA's position. For more information, the transmittal is available at http://www.cms.hhs.gov/transmittals/downloads/R788CP.pdf.

Medicare Support of Health Professions Education

For the training of physicians, financial support through Medicare is provided directly to the teaching hospitals sponsoring the clinical specialty training of physicians after medical school. The 3- to 8-year process of GME takes place largely in teaching hospital settings and comprises clinical educational experiences in which physicians complete their medical professional preparation and obtain qualification for state medical licensure and specialty board certification. Medicare finances a large proportion of physician residency training (i.e., GME) by reimbursing hospital charges through a direct cost "pass-through" mechanism and by allowing for an indirect cost educational adjustment for payments to hospitals eligible for reimbursement for educational activities under Medicare Part A DRG payments. Medicare's direct medical education (DME) and indirect medical education (IME) adjustment payments are based on hospital eligibility criteria relative to levels of noncompensated care. The total amounts paid by Medicare to supplement the training of physicians totals more than $10 billion annually. Medicare payments, however, do not cover PA-delivered clinical services even when augmenting physician residency services in teaching hospital settings.

In the 1986 Consolidated Omnibus Budget Reconciliation Act (PL 99-272 Sec 9202), Congress fixed certain limits on the allowable cost per physician resident in an attempt to slow the growth of physician residency programs in certain subspecialties perceived to be overcrowded. The act established new incentives for the expansion of primary care residency training and contained mild disincentives for the training of future subspecialists at then current levels.

In an effort to assess the financial impact of resident cutbacks stemming from the limitation on resident work hours per week in teaching hospitals in New York state, a number of options were examined. Two options for hospitals included enlisting attending physicians to replace residents or hiring licensed physicians to serve as house officers, both expensive options. A staffing mix using PAs with physician residents was determined to be far less costly in providing necessary coverage levels for inpatient services than the former option ($160 vs. $85 million). Yet the adoption of such an approach would have required about 1,300 additional PAs for New York teaching hospitals alone, when the annual supply of PAs at the time was 2,000 and many hospitals already had difficulty in attracting sufficient numbers of PAs (Foreman, 1993).

Hospitals employing PAs as general medical house staff or in GME substitution roles are believed to be using one of two existing financing methods to obtain reimbursement to cover costs of inpatient PA staffing:

- by incorporating their costs into per diem charges that are billed and reimbursed under Medicare Part A DRG-based payments, or
- by billing for the clinical services performed by PAs through eligibility under Medicare Part B, which allows payment when PA services are performed in certain settings.

Before Part B eligibility (PL 99-509, OBRA, 1986), hospitals employing PAs typically covered their employment costs by building them into the per diem charges billed under Medicare DRG-based Part A allowances. The general observation is that most hospitals continue to finance their use of PAs through this mechanism, rather than by billing for PA services under the Medicare Part B option.

COST-EFFECTIVENESS OF HOSPITAL-BASED PHYSICIAN ASSISTANTS

Teaching hospitals have relied heavily on house staff to provide inpatient care over the past century. However, beginning in the early 1990s changes in hospital financing and residency training and the emergence of managed care prompted the development of new cost-effective models of healthcare delivery. Regulations governing residents' work hours and required shifts in the site of residency from inpatient to outpatient settings decreased the availability of residents to staff inpatient wards (Thorpe, 1990; Knickman et al, 1992). These decreases in resident physician labor worsened the house officer-patient ratio.

With ongoing changes in the medical environment, hospitals are struggling to meet inpatient needs in a cost-effective manner while maintaining a high level of quality. To meet this challenge, hospitals tend to use PAs and NPs as willing providers who are mobile

and able to adapt to change. For example, as a result of new medications for infectious disease, patient care is moving toward outpatient rather than inpatient care, and the PA's flexibility allows for adaptation to this change.

Economists generally regard the services of a resident as neutral or negative because efficiency is less than that provided by a permanent staff house officer and the educational commitment to train and pay the resident is expensive (Kearns et al, 2001; Nasca et al, 2001). However, hospitals pay salaries to PAs to be house officers with the expectation that greater continuity and coordination of care will contribute to better outcomes, shorter length of stay, and savings.

In one randomized trial comparing two inpatient staffing models, a PA was incorporated. The study was undertaken to compare the clinical and financial outcomes for general medicine inpatients assigned to resident (teaching) or staff (nonteaching) services. The staff service used a PA and four physicians. When the unit was fully staffed and operational, patients admitted to the staff service had a 1.7-day lower average length of stay than patients admitted to the resident service, lower average total charges, and significantly lower laboratory and pharmacy charges. No differences emerged in mortality rates or readmission rates. Although the personnel costs were higher on the staff service, the staffing arrangement was financially viable because of the more efficient pattern of care. Shorter length of stay was translated into cost savings and increased revenue that offset the higher salary costs (Simmer et al, 1991).

In a similar but retrospective study, van Rhee and colleagues (2002) compared the use of resources and length of stay between patients cared for by PAs or residents. This study drew its sample from patients admitted to internal medicine attending physicians who rotate between the PA and resident services over 1.5 years. A mixed model analysis was used for each of the five DRGs to test for significant differences in resources used and length of stay (Exhibit 8-20). The results of this study revealed no significant differences in usage of resources except for pneumonia, which was significantly lower in the PA group than the resident group. There were no significant differences in the length of stay.

In 1990, Thorpe surveyed all New York state hospitals to evaluate the financial implications of capping residents' work schedules. Thorpe estimated that reducing resident physicians' schedules to 80 hours per week would require 424 full-time equivalent (FTE) personnel to maintain existing patient care in New York hospitals. Internal medicine was noted as needing the largest amount of substitution—231 FTEs. Physician replacement for all specialties was estimated to cost $159.6 million, PA replacement was $56.9 million, and a mix of physicians and PAs was estimated at $85.1 million. Physician replacement for internal medicine was estimated at $23

million, PA replacement at $9.2 million, and a mixed replacement at $13.8 million. By allowing PAs to contribute to filling the gap in care, New York state hospitals estimated savings of $74.5 million and internal medicine would potentially save $9.5 million (Thorpe, 1990). Hospitals were quick to recognize that by adjusting the mix of attending physicians, resident physicians, and PAs it was possible to reduce overall salary cost for inpatient staffing, while preserving adequate levels of medical care (Schafft & Cawley, 1987).

With multiple changes occurring in the staffing and cost arrangements of hospitals in the new century it seems that hospitals, at least teaching hospitals, may want to consider incorporating PAs to serve as adjuncts to staff services and teaching services. By doing so

EXHIBIT 8-20
Outcomes of Patients Managed by Physician Assistants and Medical Residents

Diagnosis-Related Group	Variable	PA Service Mean (SD)	Resident Service Mean (SD)
CVA/stroke	Total RVUs	695.41 (389.53)	803.63 (475.42)
	RAD RVUs	192.37 (207.24)	241.63 (281.18)
	LAB RVUs	149.13 (83.39)	182.30 (96.67)*
	LOS	5.93 (2.15)	5.75 (2.68)
Pneumonia	Total RVUs	480.41 (331.89)	626.31 (378.73)[†]
	RAD RVUs	79.69 (71.81)	98.35 (82.29)
	LAB RVUs	208.77 (102.83)	271.01 (145.73)[†]
	LOS	5.80 (2.68)	6.16 (2.21)
AMI, discharged alive	Total RVUs	785.46 (300.96)	789.95 (279.05)
	RAD RVUs	33.28 (21.46)	30.68 (31.97)
	LAB RVUs	188.17 (83.31)	200.55 (94.43)
	LOS	5.05 (1.76)	4.97 (1.42)
Congestive heart failure	Total RVUs	454.67 (260.75)	501.53 (245.50)
	RAD RVUs	67.69 (75.71)	62.81 (52.25)
	LAB RVUs	200.43 (87.95)	236.97 (111.87)[†]
	LOS	5.12 (2.42)	5.44 (2.41)
GI hemorrhage	Total RVUs	506.86 (310.50)	491.45 (244.58)
	RAD RVUs	48.31 (100.42)	53.02 (77.16)
	LAB RVUs	246.71 (146.00)	240.94 (101.31)
	LOS	3.96 (2.00)	3.84 (1.77)

*$P < 0.05$
[†]$P < 0.01$

Key: AMI, acute myocardial infarction; CVA, cerebrovascular accident; GI, gastrointestinal; LAB, laboratory; LOS, length of stay; RAD, radiology; RVU, relative value unit; SD, standard deviation.

Data from Van Rhee, J., Ritchie, J., & Eward, A. M. (2002). Resource use by physician assistant services versus teaching services. Journal of the American Academy of Physician Assistants, 15(1), 33-42.

they are promoting team management of patients and providing another skill level that residents might not obtain elsewhere.

SATISFACTION WITH HOSPITAL PHYSICIAN ASSISTANTS

The efficiency with which PAs can see patients and the quality of the health care they can deliver is commonly determined by the cooperation of the nursing staff with whom they work. To evaluate nurses' attitudes toward PAs, Erkert (1985) conducted a survey in two hospitals, one of which employed no PAs. The results of the study indicated that nurses who have experience working with PAs or have an understanding of the role of the PA in the healthcare system have more positive attitudes toward them than those nurses who do not have such knowledge or experience (Exhibit 8-21). In a study of a hospital that transitioned from resident house officers to PA hospitalists, the patient satisfaction was the same. Almost all (95%) of the patients were satisfied with the thoroughness of care given by house officers from 1996 to 1998 and PA-hospitalists from 1998 to 2000 (Dhuper &

EXHIBIT 8-21
Physician Assistants at the Johns Hopkins Hospital

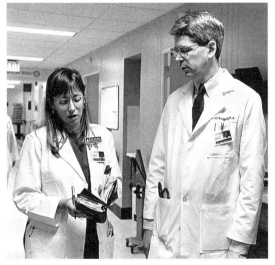

Courtesy of the American Academy of Physician Assistants.

Choksi, 2009). Other longitudinal studies show that there are no issues in terms of acceptance of PAs by patients in the hospital setting (Russell, Kaplowe, & Heinrich, 1999).

Most of the literature on supervising PAs in the hospital is concerned with clinical management. One area of concern that has been overlooked is compliance with quality assurance, continuing education, legal and regulatory requirements, and the normal personnel matters that occur with any employee. The policies and procedures that have evolved along with the use of PAs are areas that have only been touched upon superficially.

Research and Hospital-Based Physician Assistants

The literature about PAs employed in hospitals is limited and somewhat outdated. A review of this literature reveals large areas missing and important questions unanswered. Select research questions that might contribute to the successful deployment of PAs in hospital-based operations are offered.

- **Case reports:** Writing about PAs in inpatient settings provides a view of what a PA in training can expect. Case reports can show what a hospital-based PA does and what a typical day is like. Each defined role in a hospital needs a case report.

- **Role delineation:** Role delineation studies are needed every 5 years or so to identify what skill sets and activities are required of PAs serving in intensive care medicine and emergency medicine services and of those serving as hospitalists. These studies need to be undertaken for PAs in urban and rural settings, in large and small hospitals, and compared.

- **Organizational arrangements:** How do hospitals use their PAs? What are the overlaps in hospitalist care by doctors, PAs, and NPs in the same setting?

- **Economics:** Does the use of PAs on a hospitalist team produce some synergy that is missing if two doctors are working in parallel as hospitalists? Does the addition of a PA provide a substitution or a complementary effect?

■ **Breadth of knowledge:** How does a PA in an ICU obtain his or her knowledge set once in practice? Does the acquisition of knowledge have different trajectories depending on age, gender, and experience?

■ **Career selection:** How do PAs in neonatal care units come to their jobs? Do they take hospital-based care as a choice or a trade-off? How long do they remain in this career setting?

■ **Procedures:** What are the procedures that an emergency PA (or any other specialty) needs to know to be considered competent?

■ **Ratios:** What are the ratios of PAs and NPs to doctors in various types of hospitals? What contributes to these differences? Are the differences due to shifting policy regarding residents and fellows? Are there management advantages to using one practitioner over the other?

■ **Retention:** What are the factors that contribute to retention or attrition of PAs in neonatal intensive care (or any other specialty)?

■ **Education:** How do PAs in hospital-based specialties come to that specialty? How are they trained to carry out their role? Do they build on some fundamental set of skills or do they have a formal indoctrination?

SUMMARY

Expansion of the roles of PAs into the hospital setting has been the most significant recent trend in health care's use of these professionals. Initially intended to be primary care providers, PAs have moved into the institutional setting with ease and in large numbers to assume roles as medical and surgical inpatient house staff and as assistants to specialists and subspecialists. This trend is a manifestation of the even larger trend of PA specialization. In most instances, PAs have adapted to these types of roles without postgraduate training. PAs in hospitals maintain or improve the existing level of quality and access to medical care, are cost-effective in the delivery of inpatient services, and display extensive clinical versatility among the various medical disciplines.

The use of PAs in hospitals emerged from changing forces in the healthcare personnel supply pool and mandated adjustments in the patterns of GME. Employing PAs has permitted hospitals to cost-effectively maintain the required level of patient care, has allowed residency programs to balance the number of specialty-trained physicians, and thereby has contributed to a more balanced supply of specialists in overcrowded fields. The use of PAs has also contributed to increasing the continuity of care on hospital services and to measures that enrich the quality of residency education for physicians in training.

To accommodate PAs as inpatient providers, amended medical staff bylaws now recognize the education and expertise of PAs and provide the institutional sanction necessary to perform inpatient duties under the supervision of physicians. Accrediting groups, such as the Joint Commission, have acknowledged and standardized the roles of PAs as inpatient healthcare providers and have set requirements regarding their employment and regulation in hospitals.

Federal legislation amending the Medicare program has clarified and established policies whereby employing hospitals are now reimbursed for services provided by PAs. The significance of these actions is the recognition by major third-party payers of the value of PAs in rendering quality clinical services in various settings. Such measures solidify the role of the PA as an important member of the healthcare team.

No longer overlooked by health workforce experts, the demand for PAs in a broad variety of inpatient settings is likely to continue. Employment trends indicate a strong demand for PAs among hospitals and not enough PAs to fill available positions. Much of this trend is the result of new technology, the limitation on resident work hours, and the appreciation of PA clinical adaptability and flexibility.

The successful incorporation of PAs in the inpatient hospital setting indicates that these providers are well accepted by physicians, administrators, and patients. This acceptance has been earned by PAs who, working with physicians, have adapted to the demands of the hospital environment. There is every reason to believe that PAs will continue to function successfully in the hospital setting.

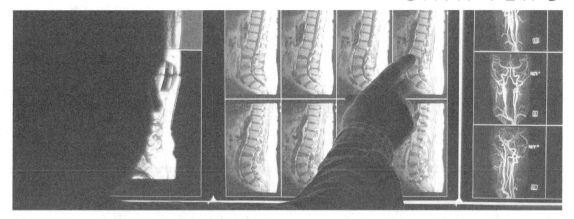

CHAPTER 9

PHYSICIAN ASSISTANTS
IN RURAL HEALTH

RODERICK S. HOOKER ■ DAVID P. ASPREY ■ JAMES F. CAWLEY

The public health infrastructure in rural America is not well understood but is potentially the most fragile aspect of the rural health care continuum.
—Thomas C. Ricketts, 1999

ABSTRACT

Physician assistants (PAs) play a key role in increasing access to primary care in rural areas. Proportionally they are more likely to provide primary care in rural locations than doctors, and they do so with lower labor costs. In many of the nonmetropolitan facilities where they are deployed, PAs provide a wide range of services for patients ranging from newborns to the elderly, and treat a diversity of illnesses and emergencies. The adaptability of PAs to their surroundings and their ability to fit in has endeared them to many communities in the United States. This adaptability will be more visible as their presence expands globally. In many instances, PAs have come from rural areas and have returned home to practice. This trend appears in a few western and southwestern communities and Alaska. Some of this is the result of federal incentives for rural health clinics to employ at least one PA, nurse practitioner, or nurse-midwife, and offering loan repayment programs for bonded rural service. The continued staffing of rural locations with an adequate supply of providers is a challenging policy for state governments.

INTRODUCTION

Most industrialized nations have faced the issue of having insufficient numbers of health-care providers who are willing to work and live in rural areas. Access to health care in nonurbanized areas in the United States, Australia, Canada, and South Africa depends on a sufficient supply and distribution of primary care doctors and nurses (Exhibit 9-1). These countries are singled out as making a concerted effort toward developing physician assistants (PAs) to manage healthcare needs. However, other countries, such as those in eastern Europe, sub-Saharan Africa, and Asia, have adopted policies that require physicians to serve some period of time working in rural and underserved regions or have introduced some form of PA to address the shortage of doctors (Hooker, Hogan, & Leeker, 2007; Mullan & Frehywot, 2007).

In spite of the efforts on four continents to meet the needs of citizens, the rural people of the world are left wanting (Dal Poz et al,

EXHIBIT 9-1
Population Statistics—Doctors and Physician Assistants, 2007

	Population	No. of PAs	No. of Doctors	Doctor/Population Ratio	Percent Rural Population
Australia	20,264,082	2	47,875	2.6/1,000	7%
Canada	33,098,932	170	66,583	2.1/1,000	19%
England (UK)	60,609,153	26	133,641	2.3/1,000	11%
Netherlands	16,491,461	75	50,854	3.2/1,000	33%
Scotland	5,062,011	12	12,738	2.5/1,000	20%
South Africa	47,391,900	0	30,740	0.7/1,000	32%
United States	301,000,000	65,000	650,000	2.1/1,000	14%

Data from Hooker, R. S., Hogan, K., & Leeker, E. (2007). The globalization of the physician assistant profession. Journal of Physician Assistant Education, 18(3), 76–85.

2006). Nor is the public health infrastructure in rural America well understood. Ricketts (1999) bluntly summarizes the lack of providers in rural America by stating, ". . . it is potentially the most fragile aspect of the rural health care continuum."

The issues for rural healthcare delivery are fairly universal:

- Delivery of needed health resources is underserviced due to a maldistribution of resources, infrastructure, economics, or labor.
- The needed population for economic viability of a doctor or clinic is often too small.
- Specialty services tend to be scarce and barriers to specialty care can be economical or geographical.

The devolution of responsibility for health care, income security, employment and training programs, and social services from the U.S. federal government to the states has been gradual but has left general and rural areas within states struggling for infrastructure resources. Rural communities are experiencing changes caused by many of the same forces that are affecting urban areas. Due to the arrangement of the healthcare system, the characteristics of the population, and other realities of rural life that differ in significant ways from the urban experience, the market and policy effects of these forces in rural areas can be quite different from the effects in urban areas. Whereas approximately 20% of North Americans live in rural areas, less than 10% of doctors practice there. Therefore, it is important to consider explicitly the impact of competitive forces and public policy developments on rural healthcare systems and the patients and communities they serve.

The reasons for leaving rural health are similar: workload (working long hours and being on call frequently), lifestyle (social interaction, education, and leisure), professional concerns (lack of collegial interaction, limited access to technology, lack of health and infrastructure), and economics (inadequate income or professional amenities). North America is hardly unique and other countries suffer similar if not worse statistics.

Changes in the healthcare sector are threatening many rural and urban settings. The failure of a provider, whether it is a health facility or a health professional's practice, is potentially greater in rural areas. Because alternative sources of care in the community within reasonable proximity are scarce, each provider likely plays a critical part in maintaining access to health care in the community. For this reason, in most rural communities all providers should be considered part of the healthcare safety net—if not directly through their care for vulnerable populations, then indirectly through their contribution to the stability of the community's healthcare infrastructure. Moreover, the healthcare infrastructure in a rural community is likely to be a mainstay of the community's economy. Closure of a rural hospital, in particular, can represent a serious threat not only to health but also to the economic well-being of the community (Ormand, Wallin, & Goldenson, 2000).

The ability of rural communities to maintain healthcare services for their residents in a changing healthcare environment is a challenge. In addition to the constantly evolving healthcare marketplace, factors that influence the structure and strength of the rural healthcare safety net include demography, geography, and policies at the federal, state, and local levels. The safety net in rural areas generally includes most local providers. Therefore, maintaining the safety net in rural communities strengthens the entire healthcare infrastructure.

In the United States, doctors, PAs, nurse practitioners (NPs), certified nurse-midwives (CNMs), dentists, and a host of nonphysician healthcare professionals play key roles in delivering this care. Although physician supply and distribution have been the focus of this problem, in the late 1980s attention began shifting to PAs and NPs as alternatives when it became apparent that many of them were successfully filling these rural provider roles (Office of Technology Assessment [OTA], 1990).

Family physicians are the principal health providers for rural America and Canada. In Australia, South Africa, and the United Kingdom these physicians are termed *general practitioners*.

The discipline of family medicine is the only medical specialty in which the ratio of physicians to population is greater in rural than in urban areas (Exhibit 9-2). Even pediatric visits to physicians are higher in rural areas than in urban areas (Probst et al, 2002). In the United States, there are more PAs in family medicine than any other medical specialty; however, the percentages are falling.

The medical specialties of primary care make up the majority of PAs in general and in rural areas in particular (Exhibit 9-3). Family medicine makes up the bulk of rural practice PAs.

Approximately one-third of PAs practice in communities with populations of 50,000 or less, and 7% are in rural areas with less than 20,000 people (American Academy of Physician Assistants [AAPA], 2008a). In work on the state level, researchers in North Carolina, Washington state, California, and other states have found that PAs are in high levels of visibility in small communities when compared with doctors (Martin, 2000; Jones & Hooker, 2001; Grumbach et al, 2003). Jones analyzed the 254 counties of Texas by population, persons per square mile, and specialty for clinically active doctors and PAs in 2007. A total of 60 counties (24%) were populated with six or fewer people per square mile—thus meeting the federal guideline of "frontier" county. In frontier counties there were 32 PAs and 75 primary care physicians, or 1 PA per 2.3 physicians. Fourteen of the 32 PAs (44%) were female. Seventeen Texas counties (exceeding the land mass of Connecticut, Vermont, and

EXHIBIT 9-2
Distribution of Urban and Rural Visits by Specialty of U.S. Doctors, 1996–1997

	Percent of Visits All Patients			
	Family Practice	*General Practice*	*Internal Medicine*	*Pediatrics*
Urban	34.2	8.9	29.9	27.0
Rural	60.3	9.3	22.1	8.3
	Patients Ages 14 Years and Younger			
Urban	16.0	5.0	2.0	77.0
Rural	53.0	4.0	2.0	41.0

Data from Probst, J. C., et al. (2002). Rural-urban differences in visits to primary care physicians. Family Medicine, 34(8), 609–615.

EXHIBIT 9-3
Distribution of U.S. Physician Assistants in Rural Primary Care, 2008

	Family Medicine	General Internal Medicine	Pediatrics	Obstetrics and Gynecology (Women's Health)
Number who responded to a survey	6,339	1,303	1,069	590
Percent of all PAs	23.7	4.7	3.9	2.1
Mean age	43	43	40	39
Percent female	64	70	80	97
PERCENT RURAL DISTRIBUTION OF PRIMARY CARE PHYSICIAN ASSISTANTS				
Nonmetropolitan population 20,000 to 1 million	9.9	9.8	5.6	3.6
Nonmetropolitan population 2,500 to 20,000	14.9	5.5	5.3	3.3
Nonmetropolitan population < 2,500	5.3	0.7	0.3	0.5

Data from American Academy of Physician Assistants. (2008a). 2008 AAPA Physician Assistant Census Report. Alexandria, VA: Author.

Rhode Island) had no licensed physician (Jones, 2008).

Because physicians, PAs, nurses, and other workers are needed in rural areas, the U.S. government has created a national policy of promoting health provider relocation to rural and underserved areas through the National Health Service Corps (NHSC). This program, set within the federal Bureau of Health Professions of the Health Resources and Service Administration, has implemented a number of strategies to employ more physicians, PAs, and NPs in primary care and rural areas. These strategies include service commitments to a designated health professional shortage area (HPSA) through loan repayment and scholarships.

Although the NHSC program has had success in the deployment of providers to rural and medically underserved areas, the NHSC experience is not always ideal in terms of nonphysician providers such as PAs. NHSC scholarship recipients have identified various underlying problems with the current system which lead to poor PA provider retention:

- Too few potential placement sites are made available from the outset.

- NHSC placement deadlines do not allow enough time for making the best possible placement.
- Many community health centers (CHCs) are not highly supportive of or invested in the program.
- NHSC efforts to support the development of local medical providers from within underserved regions are inadequate.
- NHSC officers working with nonphysician providers do not demonstrate a high degree of commitment to achieving an optimal provider-site match.

Changes in the NHSC program based on these five problems are recommendations to improve the retention of nonphysician providers in this important program (Earle-Richardson & Earle-Richardson, 1998).

Improving Rural Health Access

The use of PAs and NPs to improve the access of rural people to health care has been advocated since the 1970s. Early in the development of PAs and NPs, this hypothesis was tested in a remote rural area of southern Appalachia served by a network of three clinics that were staffed by PAs, NPs, and doctors.

During the first 3 years of operation, 76% of the geographically defined target population of 5,500 received services. PAs and NPs provided care in one-half of the 40,252 medical encounters and 89% of their patient contacts were managed without consultation with or referral to the doctor. The PAs or NPs managed 36% of first-year visits, 51% of second-year visits, and 54% of third-year visits. Concurrent with this shift in patient care responsibility to the PA or NP, differences in the types of conditions managed by the three providers decreased with time. Population surveys indicate that consumer satisfaction is high and that health care from this system is perceived as being more accessible than care from alternative sources. Experience suggests that, as members of a healthcare team, PAs and NPs can manage most problems encountered in rural primary care with a high level of consumer satisfaction and improved access (Blake & Guild, 1978).

Because primary care and rural health were the two driving reasons for developing the PA concept, early on, the central government thought PAs could be a vital part of the healthcare infrastructure that supports ambulatory and institutional care in rural areas. In 1977, the U.S. Congress enacted the Rural Health Clinics Act (Public Law [PL] 95-210) to encourage the use of PAs, NPs, and CNMs in rural areas. This decision was based on a growing realization that many small communities could no longer support doctors. PL 95-210 facilitated this goal by entitling various health providers to receive reimbursement from Medicare and Medicaid on a cost basis. This policy continues into the 21st century with modifications enabling rural health clinics (RHCs) to remain in operation as characteristics of staffing and populations change.

Beyond providing temporary staffing, NHSC clinicians contribute to the long-term growth of the non-NHSC physician workforce of the communities they serve; although some worry that NHSC clinicians compete with and impede the supply of other local physicians. Pathman and colleagues (2006) assessed the long-term changes in the non-NHSC primary care physician workforce of rural underserved counties that have received NHSC staffing

support relative to workforce changes in underserved counties without NHSC support. Using data from the American Medical Association (AMA) and NHSC, they compared changes from 1981 to 2001 in non-NHSC primary care physician to population ratios in two subsets of rural whole-county HPSAs. The focus was on (1) 141 counties staffed by NHSC physicians, PAs, and NPs during the early 1980s and for many of the years since, and (2) all 142 rural HPSA counties that had no NHSC clinicians from 1979 through 2001. What was found was that from 1981 to 2001, counties staffed by NHSC clinicians experienced a mean increase of 1.4 non-NHSC primary care physicians per 10,000 population, compared with a smaller, 0.57 mean increase in counties without NHSC clinicians. The finding of greater non-NHSC primary care physician to population mean ratio increased in NHSC-supported counties remained significant after adjusting for baseline county demographics and healthcare resources ($P < 0.001$). The estimated number of "extra" non-NHSC physicians in NHSC-supported counties in 2001 attributable to the NHSC was 294 additional physicians for the 141 supported counties, or two extra physcians, on average, for each NHSC-supported county. Over the 20 years, more NHSC-supported counties saw their non-NHSC primary care workforces grow to more than 1 physician per 3,500 persons, but no more NHSC-supported than nonsupported counties lost their HPSA designations. The authors concluded that the NHSC contributed positively to the non-NHSC primary care physician workforce in the rural underserved counties where its clinicians worked during the 1980s and 1990s (Pathman et al, 2006).

WHY RURAL HEALTH CARE IS UNIQUE

Many factors associated with rural areas impact the health of rural citizens. For example, economic factors and access to providers are common healthcare obstacles in rural areas. Also, research has shown that certain healthcare issues tend to be more prevalent in rural areas (Exhibit 9-4).

EXHIBIT 9-4
A National Rural Health Snapshot, 2005

Characteristic	Rural	Urban
Percentage of U.S. population	25%	75%
Percentage of U.S. physicians	10%	90%
No. of specialists per 100,000 population	40.1	134.1
Population aged 65 and older	18%	15%
Population below the poverty level	14%	11%
Average per capita income	$19,000	$26,000
Population who are non-Hispanic whites	83%	69%
Adults who describe health status as fair/poor	28%	21%
Adolescents (ages 12–17) who smoke	19%	11%
Male death rate per 100,000 (ages 1–24)	80	60
Female death rate per 100,000 (ages 1–24)	40	30
Population covered by private insurance	64%	69%
Population who are Medicare beneficiaries	23%	20%
Medicare beneficiaries without drug coverage	45%	31%
Medicare spent per capita compared to U.S. average	85%	106%
Medicare hospital payment-to-cost ratio	90%	100%
Percentage of poor covered by Medicaid	45%	49%

Data from *Eye on Health* by the Rural Wisconsin Health Cooperative, and from an article entitled, Rural Health Can Lead the Way, by Tim Size, Executive Director of the Rural Wisconsin Health Cooperative.

Economic Factors

Rural economies may be based on agriculture, mining, manufacturing, oil and energy, tourism, or forestry. In some rural areas, the largest single employer is the local school system. Residents in these areas tend to be poorer. On average, 1999 per capita income was $7,417 lower than in urban areas, and rural Americans were more likely to live below the poverty level. In fact, one analysis determined that even though only 22% of Americans lived in rural areas in 2001, 31% of food stamp beneficiaries lived in rural areas (National Rural Health Association [NRHA], 2007). Also, the rural poor are less likely to be covered by Medicaid benefits than poor residents of urban areas.

Access

Access to care is limited in rural areas. Less than 10% of physicians practice in rural America. There are 2,157 rural and frontier areas of all U.S. states and territories classified as HPSAs compared with 910 HPSAs in urban areas (Gamm et al, 2003). Even if clinics are available, they may be difficult to access because of distance or barriers such as mountains, rivers, gorges, and lakes. Jones (2008) identified that in 2007 PAs were more likely to be the providers of care in some of the most remote areas of Texas than doctors. Pedersen and colleagues found that PAs in Utah were more productive in rural clinics than those in urban Utah (Pedersen et al, 2008).

Health Trends

When certain healthcare issues of urban and rural areas are compared, some trends concerning the healthcare needs of rural residents emerge. For example, death and serious injury accidents account for 60% of total rural accidents versus only 48% percent of urban accidents, and two-thirds of all deaths related to motor vehicle accidents occur on rural roads. Additionally, one report determined that the rates of cerebrovascular disease and hypertension were higher in rural areas than urban areas, and the suicide rate among rural men is significantly higher than in urban areas, particularly among adult men and children (Gamm et al, 2003). Rural residents are also at a significantly higher risk of death by gunshot than urban residents (NRHA, 2007).

Alcohol use, including underage drinking, is also an issue in rural areas. The rate of arrests for driving under the influence is significantly greater in rural areas compared with urban areas, and 40% of rural 12th graders claimed to have consumed alcohol while driving compared to 25% of their urban counterparts (Gamm et al, 2003).

A number of rural health sources of information are provided in Exhibit 9-5.

RURAL HEALTH PHYSICIAN ASSISTANTS

Rural health PAs are self-defined as those who identify their location of employment, either by some policy definition or the characteristics of their employer (designation, geographic location, etc.) as rural. PAs who work in rural health do not necessarily need to live in these locations. In its annual census, the AAPA identifies PAs by population density. Nonmetropolitan areas are generally under 50,000 in population and rural is considered less than 10,000 in population.

In a statewide survey of PAs and NPs in Georgia, rural providers tended to be older and have less graduate years of education, to possess fewer specialty credentials, and to be employed longer when compared with comparable urban providers. Of the providers who preferred smaller communities, more were likely to mention the importance of community dynamics, whereas providers who preferred larger communities were more likely to mention professional contact as important for a work setting (Strickland, Strickland, & Garretson, 1998).

However, the future for rural employment of PAs may be bright. Two studies by Shi and others suggest that the demand remains fairly strong in rural areas (Shi et al, 1994; Shi & Samuels, 1997). These observations found no difference in demand between PAs and NPs.

EXHIBIT 9-5
Rural Health Information Sources

Rural Healthy People 2010—*Healthy People 2010: A Companion Document for Rural Areas,* is a project funded with grant support from the federal Office of Rural Health Policy. Documents are available on the Web at http://www.srph.tamhsc.edu/centers/rhp2010/publications.htm.

The WWAMI Rural Health Research Center, funded by the Federal Office of Rural Health Policy, works with various entities in the states of Washington, Wyoming, Alaska, Montana, and Idaho to perform policy-oriented research on issues related to rural health care. Their study is described in: Baldwin, L. M., et al. (2004). Quality of care for acute myocardial infarction in rural and urban U.S. hospitals. *Journal of Rural Health, 20*(2), 99–108. Additional information is available on the Web at http://depts.washington.edu/uwrhrc/.

OTHER LINKS AND RESOURCES
- Ricketts, T. C., III (Ed.). (1999). *Rural Health in the United States.* New York: Oxford University Press.
- Centers for Disease Control and Prevention, National Center for Health Statistics. (2001). *Health, United States, 2001 with Urban and Rural Health Chartbook.* Washington, DC: Government Printing Office.
- Rural Information Center Health Service (RICHS): http://www.nal.usda.gov/ric/
- National Rural Health Association: http://www.ruralhealthweb.org/
- Health Resources and Services Administration (HHS): http://www.hrsa.gov/
- National Association of Rural Health Clinics: http://www.narhc.org/
- Rural Assistance Center: http://www.raconline.org/
- The Frontier Education Center: http://www.frontierus.org/
- Technical Assistance and Services Center (TASC) for the Rural Hospital Flexibility Program: http://www.ruralcenter.org/tasc/
- The National Rural Recruitment and Retention Network (3R Net): http://www.3rnet.org/
- National Association for Rural Mental Health (NARMH): http://www.narmh.org/
- The Kaiser Commission: Health Insurance Coverage in Rural America and The Kaiser Commission: The Uninsured in Rural America: http://www.kff.org/uninsured/4093.cfm

At the time of this study the interpretation reinforced other observations that the demand was similar for both providers regardless of the setting (Shi et al, 1993).

Clinical Activities

What PAs do and how often they provide care has been based more on assumption and less on documentation. However, some literature does exist, particularly from the first two decades of the profession, during which work was done in several key states that demonstrated the capabilities and advantages of PAs in clinical practice settings located in rural communities. A survey of Iowa family practice PAs was undertaken to identify the clinical activities they provided and how these skills and procedures compared with family practice physicians in the same state (Dehn & Hooker, 1999). The undertaking was an effort to understand what skill set a PA would require when entering rural health care. Fifty-five Iowa PAs responded and all reported a wide range of activities: patient education, prescribing and dispensing medication, interpreting radiographs, and evaluating and referring patients (Exhibit 9-6). In this study, it was shown that PAs possess a wide range of skills and procedures and seem to use these frequently. One of the findings of this study was that rural PAs regard themselves as generalists and place a fair amount of pride in their ability to be versatile.

Asprey (2006) found in a survey of PAs practicing in rural Iowa that the most commonly performed skill was dispensing medications (Exhibit 9-7). This trend was presumably due to the lack of available pharmacy services in the small rural communities in which the clinics were located. Other commonly identified skills included obtaining cervical screening smears, teaching breast self-examinations, performing venipuncture, and administering injections. Such findings underscores that PAs practicing in rural settings are responsible for providing a wide array of clinical services, including those that in many larger settings may be performed by other clinical personnel. In addition, the rural practicing PAs reported cardiopulmonary resuscitation, suturing, and field-block anesthesia as the most important skills for their practices (Exhibit 9-8).

The deficit of primary care providers in rural environments has the potential to increase the role of PAs. Yet little is known about the conditions, sites, and patterns of practice of PAs and their distribution in Pennsylvania, the state with the largest rural population. To learn more about these providers in rural and urban settings and their willingness to practice in underserved areas, Martin (2000) conducted a census of all PAs with a Pennsylvania license. Survey results revealed significant differences in socio-economic, demographic, and practice profile parameters between rural and urban providers. For example, providers in rural areas are more likely than urban counterparts to practice in a primary care setting, see more patients per week, and are the principal provider of care for a higher percentage of their patients. A rural PA is more likely than an urban PA to practice in an underserved area—at least in Pennsylvania (Exhibit 9-9). For rural and urban PAs who practice primary care, significant differences were noted in their willingness to practice in a rural underserved area compared with PAs who do not practice in primary care (Martin, 2000).

Rural Health Clinics

RHCs are any outpatient medical center located in a nonmetropolitan area. Certified RHCs are usually located in HPSAs, medically underserved areas (MUAs), or a governor-designated shortage area. Federally certified "independent" RHCs are reimbursed on a cost basis for their Medicare and Medicaid patients and designed by the government to provide care that would not otherwise be available through enterprise or the market place. Since the early 1980s, RHCs make up one of the largest outpatient primary care programs for rural underserved communities and one of the fastest growing Medicare programs. By law they must be staffed by PAs, NPs, or CNMs at least one-half of the time the clinic is open.

EXHIBIT 9-6
Activities Performed by Iowa Family Practice Physician Assistants by Frequency (N = 55)

Clinical Skill	Mean*	(SD)	Clinical Skill	Mean*	(SD)
Patient education	3.95	(0.30)	Neonatal checks	1.19	(1.02)
Dispense medication	3.44	(1.23)	Primary treatment of psychiatric illness (e.g., bipolar disorder, schizophrenia)	1.16	(1.10)
Make patient referrals directly to specialists	3.39	(0.68)			
X-ray film interpretation	3.19	(1.18)	Nasal packing for epistaxis	1.13	(0.71)
Electrotherapy or cryotherapy of the skin	2.92	(0.81)	Incise and drain external hemorrhoid	1.07	(0.77)
Counseling for contraception	2.91	(0.83)	Provide care to patients in a home setting (house calls)	1.00	(1.03)
Manage depression by drug therapy	2.82	(0.88)	Perform audiometry	0.87	(1.18)
Counseling for smoking cessation	2.80	(0.88)	Low-risk prenatal care	0.85	(1.15)
Repair and close laceration	2.75	(0.83)	Bladder catheterization	0.79	(0.57)
Counseling for stress management	2.61	(0.76)	Administer pulmonary function test	0.78	(1.15)
Electrocardiographic interpretation	2.60	(0.87)	Joint injection	0.68	(0.83)
Manage depression by counseling	2.53	(1.03)	Perform cardiopulmonary resuscitation	0.65	(0.62)
Removal of small skin lesions	2.43	(0.82)	Perform advanced cardiac life support	0.65	(0.73)
Psychological counseling	2.42	(1.13)	Bartholin cyst drainage	0.64	(0.52)
Fluorescein eye examination or foreign body removal from eye	2.36	(0.65)	Reduce fractures and dislocations	0.64	(0.73)
Perform vision screening	2.33	(1.39)	Diaphragm fitting	0.57	(0.64)
Use a microscope	2.15	(1.60)	Arthrocentesis	0.55	(0.72)
Incision and drainage of abscess	2.09	(0.66)	Perform advanced trauma life support	0.55	(0.69)
Counseling for alcohol abuse	1.93	(0.80)	Nasogastric tube placement	0.33	(0.58)
Provide care to patients in nursing homes	1.85	(1.47)	Endotracheal intubation	0.32	(0.51)
Evaluate wet mounts or potassium hydroxide stains	1.84	(1.50)	Arterial blood gas draw	0.31	(0.63)
			Use a slitlamp	0.30	(0.64)
Involved in personal management activities	1.81	(1.49)	Perform breast mass aspiration	0.28	(0.49)
Splinting and casting	1.78	(0.88)	Norplant insertion/removal	0.25	(0.43)
Skin biopsy	1.73	(0.99)	Perform Gram stain	0.11	(0.37)
Removal of ingrown toenail	1.71	(0.99)	Central venous line placement	0.06	(0.23)
Counseling for human immunodeficiency virus testing	1.63	(0.94)	Chest tube placement	0.04	(0.19)
			Paracentesis or thoracentesis	0.04	(0.19)
Perform urinalysis	1.56	(1.74)	Lumbar puncture	0.02	(0.14)
Regional block with local anesthesia	1.49	(1.20)	Suprapubic tap on infants	0.02	(0.14)
Counseling for drug abuse	1.46	(0.88)	Colposcopy	0.00	(0.00)
Venipuncture	1.25	(1.24)	Flexible sigmoidoscopy	0.00	(0.00)
			Obstetric ultrasonography	0.00	(0.00)

*Mean frequency of reported activity on a relative scale of 0 to 4. Never = 0; a few times a year = 1; at least once a month = 2; at least once a week = 3; daily = 4.

Physician-owned RHCs make up almost one-half of the clinics. Hospitals and public and private companies own the rest (Exhibits 9-10 and 9-11). Over two-thirds of RHCs employ one or more PA or NP (Gale & Coburn, 2003).

Although RHCs are required to employ a PA, NP, or CNM, they may receive a waiver of this requirement for up to 1 year. Approximately one-fifth of clinics have operated without a PA, NP, or CNM for some period and many clinics have problems retaining a PA,

EXHIBIT 9-7

Most Frequently Performed Skills in Communities of Less Than 10,000 (N = 94)

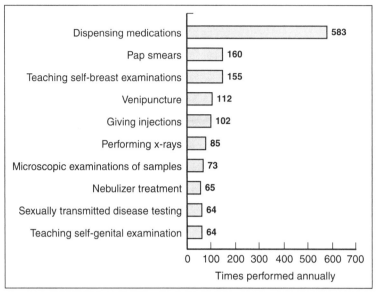

Data from Asprey, D. (2006). Clinical skills utilized by physician assistants in rural primary care settings. The Journal of Physician Assistant Education, 17(2), 45–47.

EXHIBIT 9-8

Skills Assigned Greatest Importance in Communities of Less Than 10,000 Population (N = 94)

Rank	Skill	Average Level of Importance*
1.	Cardiopulmonary resuscitation	4.9
2.	Suturing	4.8
3.	Field block anesthesia	4.7
3.	PAP smear	4.7
3.	Sexually transmitted disease testing	4.7
3.	Self-breast examination	4.7
7.	Splinting of digits or extremities	4.6
7.	Casting	4.6
9.	Four items tied for ninth: Cardioversion, intubation, incision and drainage of abscesses, microscopic wet smears	4.5

*Scale utilized is 1 = low, 5 = high.

Data from Asprey, D. P. (2006). Clinical skills utilized by physician assistants in rural primary care settings. Journal of Physician Assistant Education, 17(2), 45–47.

NP, or CNM. This is not surprising since at least one-third of RHCs reported difficulty retaining healthcare professionals in general.

It is increasingly evident that PAs who remain in rural areas differ from urban-based PAs. Studies indicate that PAs practicing in rural areas place considerably more importance on autonomy in selecting the location of their practice than other PAs, perhaps because they spend more time away from their supervising physician. They also have a significantly higher level of satisfaction with role and professional acknowledgment than urban-based PAs (Pan et al, 1996; Singer & Hooker, 1996; Larson, Hart, & Ballweg, 2001; Henry & Hooker, 2007).

Yet the retention of PAs in some rural practices is quite striking. In a survey by Larson and colleagues (1999), PAs listed all of the places where they had practiced since completing their PA training, making it possible to classify the career histories of PAs as "all rural," "all urban," "urban to rural," or "rural to urban." The study examined the retention of PAs in rural practice at several levels: in the

EXHIBIT 9-9
Characteristics of Rural and Urban Physician Assistant Respondents

Characteristic	Urban (N = 491)	Rural (N = 190)	Test of Differences Between Samples	Statistical Significance (P)
Age	39.40 (7.87)*	39.29 (8.14)*	F = 0.030	0.863
GENDER			Chi-square = 10.603	
Male	37.6 (183)[†]	51.3 (97)[†]		0.001
Female	62.4 (304)	48.7 (92)		
RACE			Chi-square = 6.395	
White	92.1 (452)[†]	97.4 (185)[†]		0.011
Nonwhite	7.9 (39)	2.6 (5)		
Income	$53,545 ($17,188)*	$49,534 ($12,255)*	F = 8.215	0.004

*Mean (standard deviation).

[†]Percentage (number).

Data from Martin, K. E. (2000). A rural-urban comparison of patterns of physician assistant practice. Journal of the Academy of Physician Assistants, 13(7): 49–50, 56, 59, 63–66, 72 passim.

EXHIBIT 9-10
Distribution of Rural Health Clinic Ownership

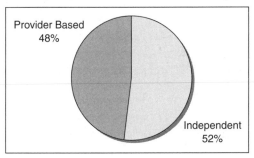

Provider Based 48%

Independent 52%

Data from Gale, J. A., & Coburn, A. F. (2003). The Characteristics and Roles of Rural Health Clinics in the United States: A Chartbook. Portland, ME: University of Southern Maine, Edmund S. Muskie School of Public Service.

first practice, in rural practice overall, and by predominantly rural states. PAs who started their careers in rural locations were more likely to leave them during the first 4 years of practice than urban PAs, and female rural PAs were slightly more likely to leave than their male counterparts. Those starting in rural practice had high attrition and left for urban areas (41%); however, a significant proportion of the PAs who started in urban practice settings left for rural settings (10%). Because the proportion of urban PAs is so much larger than rural PAs, this movement kept the total proportion of PAs in rural practice at a steady 20%. Although 21% of the earliest graduates of PA training programs have had exclusively rural careers, only 9% of PAs with 4 to 7 years of experience have worked exclusively in rural settings (Exhibit 9-12). At the state level, generalist PAs were significantly more likely to leave states with practice environments unfavorable to PA practice in terms of prescriptive authority, reimbursement, and insurance (Larson et al, 1999).

Because the U.S. government is expanding the capacity of CHCs to provide care to underserved populations, Rosenblatt and colleagues (2006) set out to examine the workforce shortages that may limit CHC expansion. They used a questionnaire to survey all of the 846 federally funded U.S. CHCs within the 50 states and the District of Columbia that directly provided clinical services in 2004. The chief executive officer of each grantee completed the questionnaire. Information was supplemented by data from the 2003 Bureau of Primary Health Care Uniform Data System and weighted to be nationally representative. The overall response rate was high (79%) and revealed staffing patterns and vacancies for major clinical disciplines by rural and urban location, use of federal and state recruitment

EXHIBIT 9-11
U.S. Rural Health Clinic Ownership

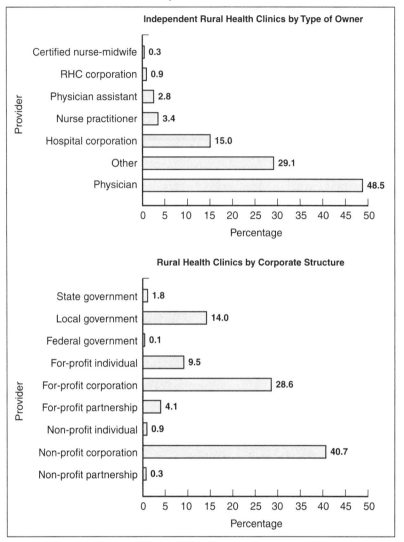

Data from Gale, J. A., & Coburn, A. F. (2003). The Characteristics and Roles of Rural Health Clinics in the United States: A Chartbook. *Portland, ME: University of Southern Maine, Edmund S. Muskie School of Public Service.*

programs, and perceived barriers to recruitment. Primary care physicians made up 89% of physicians working in the CHCs, the majority of whom were family physicians. In rural CHCs, 46% of the direct clinical providers of care were nonphysician clinicians compared with 39% in urban CHCs. There were 428 vacant funded full-time equivalent (FTE) positions for family physicians and 376 vacant FTEs for registered nurses. Rural CHCs had a higher proportion of vacancies and longer-term vacancies and reported greater difficulty filling positions compared with urban CHCs. Physician recruitment in CHCs was heavily dependent on NHSC scholarships, loan repayment programs, and international medical graduates with J-1 visa waivers.

Major perceived barriers to recruitment included low salaries and, in rural CHCs, cultural isolation, poor-quality schools and

EXHIBIT 9-12
Current Practice Location and Specialty by Total Experience

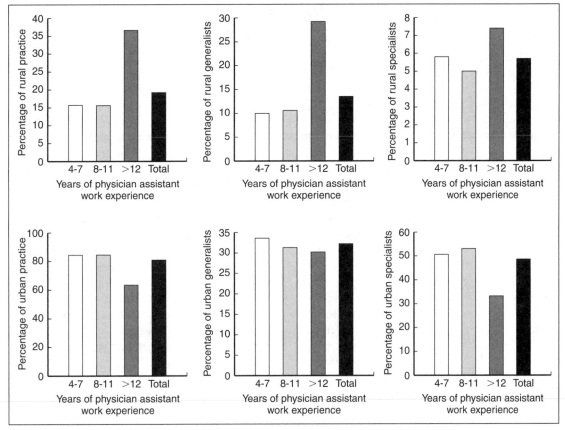

Data from Larson et al (1999). Dimensions of retention: A national study of the locational histories of physician assistants. Journal of Rural Health, 15(4), 391–402.

housing, and lack of spousal job opportunities. The authors concluded that CHCs face substantial challenges in recruitment of clinical staff, particularly in rural areas. The largest numbers of unfilled positions were for family physicians at a time of declining interest in family medicine among graduating medical students. The success of the current U.S. national policy to expand CHCs may be challenged by these workforce issues unless PAs and NPs are considered in the staffing mix (Rosenblatt et al, 2006).

Redfield Rural Health Clinic
The Redfield Rural Health Clinic is the only medical clinic in the town of Redfield (population 883), located in the rural southwestern corner of Iowa. The last full-time physician at the clinic died suddenly in October 1985. Ed Friedman, PA, moved to Redfield in November of 1985 to work with physicians from the University of Osteopathic Medicine in Des Moines, 35 miles away to keep the clinic open. The clinic served as a site to train medical and PA students in rural medicine. Although the number of patients seen at the clinic had doubled, by July 1988 the University decided to close the clinic as it continued to lose money.

Friedman and his wife, Libby Coyte, PA, decided to try to keep the clinic open. A surgeon and general practice physician from Des Moines who had a part-time office in a neighboring town was willing to provide medical supervision if he did not have to be responsi-ble for the clinic finances and management. He already had a busy practice in Des Moines and in the neighboring town. In 1988, the only way a PA-run clinic could receive Medicare and Medicaid coverage was by becoming a federally certified RHC.

When the previous owner announced the closure of the Redfield clinic, Friedman and Coyte received phone calls from worried patients asking where they would get their medical care. One 90-year-old lady with a dri-ver's license restricted to the Redfield area said having to go to a neighboring city for her medical care was "like driving to the far side of the moon." Young families with only one car used by a parent to commute to a job dur-ing the day were concerned about how they would be able to take a sick or injured child for medical care. Ambulance trips for many emergencies are not covered by insurance and pose a large financial burden for families just getting started and for the poor. Low-income families frequently have unreliable vehicles that don't always start, especially in Midwest winters. The cost of gas poses another barrier.

The purpose of the RHC program is to increase access to medical care in rural, med-ically underserved areas by providing cost based Medicare and Medicaid reimbursement to practices that utilize PAs or NPs at least 50% of the time the clinic is open to see patients. To become an RHC a HPSA designation was obtained for the Redfield Clinic service area and the facility passed the required Medicare inspection. The clinic reopened as a PA staffed RHC August 1988. Since that time, the clinic has operated with one full-time PA and a supervising physician who is accessible by phone and visits the clinic periodically (as required by law and to review the care provid-ed). Since 1999, the clinic registers 4,000 to 5,300 patient visits a year. The clinic PA sees patients in three different nursing homes and provides several home visits every month to patients who can't travel. In 2007, 52% of vis-its were for Medicare or Medicaid patients with another 8% from Medicare advantage plan patients. About 10% of Redfield's patients have no insurance. The clinic admin-isters paperwork for about 50 patients without insurance to obtain medications from various pharmaceutical companies at no charge. PA students from both the University of Iowa and the Des Moines University PA programs rotate through the clinic to experience practice in a small town. The Redfield RHC employs three full-time and three part-time employees.

Having a RHC in Redfield proves beneficial. For example, a typical house call involved an 89-year–old woman, who lived alone. She sud-denly developed right facial paralysis and she and her family were worried about a stroke. Treatment was initiated for Bell's palsy with medicines from the clinic, and the patient was able to remain at home. A trip to the ER at night, costing at least four times as much as a RHC visit and an ambulance ride ($500) was avoided. Similar situations occur regularly in Redfield. Lacerations are sutured, broken bones are x-rayed, pneumonia, and streptococcal infec-tions diagnosed and treated in a timely fashion. Life threatening anaphylaxis and myocardial infarctions are stabilized prior to evacuation. The RHC is the only source of prescription medicines in Redfield as there is no pharmacy nearby.

The people of Redfield visit the clinic in suf-ficient numbers to keep it financially viable, for now. Yet Redfield has changed little since the clinic reopened in 1985 and the population unchanged in number and age strata for 25 years. As an agricultural-based census tract, the town has a feed store, a volunteer fire department, post office, a library, a couple of bars, two small diners, an insurance agent, and a convenience store but no grocery store or pharmacy. A high school, once a large employ-er, has closed. Redfield is surrounded by corn-fields and scattered single-family farmsteads. The cost-based reimbursement for Medicare and Medicaid patients and economized staffing costs of utilizing a PA remains the only way this clinic has been able to survive finan-cially over the past decade (E. Friedman, per-sonal communication, June 2009).

DEFINING RURAL HEALTH

Because census tracts may not reflect details of rurality, the rural-urban commuting area (RUCA) codes were devised. RUCA codes are detailed and flexible schemes for determining the degree of a rural or urban location, and have been updated using data from the 2000 decennial census. These codes are based on the same theoretical concepts used by the Office of Management and Budget (OMB) to define county-level metropolitan and "micropolitan" areas. Similar criteria are applied to measures of population density, urbanization, and daily commuting to identify urban cores and adjacent territory that is economically integrated with those cores. The creators of the RUCA codes adopted OMB's metropolitan and micropolitan terminology to highlight the underlying connections between the two classification systems.

High commuting areas (designated as codes 2, 5, and 8) are areas in which the largest commuting share was at least 30% to a metropolitan, micropolitan, or small-town core. Many micropolitan and small-town cores (and even a few metropolitan cores) have high enough out-commuting to other areas to be coded 2, 5, or 8; typically these areas are not job centers themselves, but serve as bedroom communities for a nearby, larger city. Low commuting (codes 3, 6, and 9) refers to cases in which the single largest flow is to a core, but is less than 30%. These codes identify "influence areas" of metro, micropolitan, and small-town cores, respectively, and are similar in concept to the "nonmetropolitan adjacent" codes found in other Economic Research Service (ERS) classification schemes (U.S. Department of Agriculture, 2004).

The 10 RUCA codes offer a relatively straightforward and complete delineation of metropolitan and nonmetropolitan settlement based on the size and direction of primary commuting flows. Demographers can use these codes to identify where health providers work, the communities they serve, and areas of scarcity and demand.

PHYSICIAN ASSISTANTS IN UNDERSERVED AREAS

Because so little is known about the types of providers and their propensity to care for underserved populations, Grumbach and colleagues (2003) focused their research on

two state populations: California and Washington. Both states have significant rural populations and both states have a long history of using PAs and NPs in rural areas (Exhibit 9-13).

The research team focused on primary care clinicians (family physicians, general internists, general pediatricians, PAs, NPs, and CNMs). PAs ranked first or second in each state in the proportion of their members practicing in rural areas and HPSAs. In California, PAs also had the greatest proportion of their members working with vulnerable populations (Grumbach et al, 2003).

Retention

Understanding why someone chooses a lifestyle and career path is complex, but one phenomenon that reoccurs in medical workforce research is that a small, but substantial, cadre of PAs remain in rural areas providing health care. Larson and colleagues (1999) studied the location histories of a representative national sample of PAs. The intent was to observe locational behavior for recruitment and retention of PAs in rural practice. Through a survey, PAs listed all the places they had practiced since completing their education. The information obtained made it possible to classify their career histories as "all rural," "all urban," "urban to rural," or "rural to urban." The study examined the retention of PAs in rural practice at several levels: in the first practice, in rural practice overall, and in states. PAs who started their careers in rural locations were more likely to leave them during the first 4 years of practice than urban colleagues, and female rural PAs were slightly more likely to leave than men. Those starting in rural practice had high attrition to urban areas (41%); however, a significant proportion of the PAs who started in urban practice settings left for rural settings (10%). This trend kept the total proportion of PAs in rural practice at a steady 20%. Whereas 21% of the earliest graduates had exclusively rural careers, only 9% of PAs with 4 to 7 years of experience worked exclusively in rural settings. At the state level, generalist PAs were significantly more likely to leave states with practice environments

EXHIBIT 9-13
Percentage of Clinicians Practicing in Underserved Areas, by Type of Underserved Area

	Rural Area	Vulnerable Population Area	Primary Care Health Professional Shortage Area
California	13.0	39.0	28.0
Family physician	13.2	30.5	24.2
General pediatrician	6.2	31.0	18.6
General internists	5.9	31.5	17.9
Obstetricians/gynecologists	6.3	28.3	16.9
Nurse practitioner	15.0	34.4	26.3
Physician assistants	21.7	47.7	35.2
Certified midwives	15.5	41.1	35.3
Washington	24.0	40.0	38.6
Family physician	23.6	45.6	43.5
General pediatrician	14.3	43.5	32.8
General internists	13.8	54.5	28.4
Obstetricians/gynecologists	13.7	52.9	31.6
Nurse practitioner	19.7	51.8	37.3
Physician assistants	27.8	50.3	42.1

Data from Grumbach, K., et al. (2003). Who is caring for the underserved? A comparison of primary care physicians and nonphysician clinicians in California and Washington. Annals of Family Medicine, 1(2), 97–104.

unfavorable to PA practice in terms of prescriptive authority, reimbursement, and insurance at the time of the study (Larson et al, 1999).

One of the typical views of PAs in rural towns was of a male who was in a solo practice with another older male, working in a clinic. In this setting, the two clinicians shared patients and responsibilities. Henry and Hooker (2007) examined whether this stereotype endured. They chose one particular type of clinician: the autonomous PA who functioned primarily as the sole practitioner in small and remote towns. PAs in Texas were sought who could meet a set of criteria outlined in Exhibit 9-14. Thirty-eight PA-town dyads were screened and eight were selected. Town size, geographic region, and type of industry in the county provided the diverse settings for this qualitative study.

Using workforce specialists and medical anthropologists, the towns were visited by the team. Those residing in the town as well as the PA were interviewed. The results were surprising; only one of the eight PAs was raised

in a small town—the rest grew up in large urban areas. Those with families were there primarily for the amenities of a small town and, as one PA said, "So my child could ride his bike down the main street and if [he was]

EXHIBIT 9-14
Criteria for Retention of Rural Physician Assistants Study

- The PA must be working autonomously in a rural health clinic with no more than 8 hours per week with the supervising doctor.
- The PA must be employed as the sole primary care practitioner in the community.
- The PA must have worked in the community for more than 24 months prior to being interviewed.
- The town (or census tract) is smaller than 5,000 persons and was in Texas.
- Town residents had no other primary care options within a 40-km radius.
- The PA and the town leaders were willing to be interviewed.

Data from Henry, L. R., & Hooker, R. S. (2007). Retention of physician assistants in rural health clinics. *Journal of Rural Health, 23*(3), 207–214.

hurt someone would take care of him." All but one PA lived in the town where they worked (the eighth lived in a nearby town that had a high school for his children). Most of the PAs were civic leaders (e.g., a member of the Lions Club), and all socialized with the residents of the town. Most of the towns were quite remote (Exhibits 9-15 and 9-16) and the commuting distance to a larger town was quite long. None were close to a major highway. Seven of the eight PAs were not bound by a contract or other links to the town and were free to move away if desired. Two of the PAs were female, and all eight were married.

Interviewing townsfolk about the PA revealed that only two-thirds had used the PAs' services. The main reason cited for not using the PA or the clinic was that they had a relationship with a doctor in some other town. Almost all said they would like to have a doctor instead of a PA, but that a PA was better than no medical care provider. For some parents, the presence of a health clinic, regardless of the type of provider, was the reason they remained in the town. If the clinic were not available, some parents of young children said they would move closer to an urban area.

EXHIBIT 9-15
Characteristics of Rural Towns Served by Physician Assistants

	Town A	Town B	Town C	Town D	Town E	Town F	Town G	Town H
Population	637	2,235	241	2,589	844	2,424	800	740
RUCA code*	5	5	10.5	10.5	5	10	10.6	10
Distance from nearest town (miles)	30	25	60	32	25	30	80	25
Median age	40.4	39.3	46.1	37.8	38	38.7	43	42.7
Median household income	$28,333	$42,098	$28,281	$41,686	$20,278	$24,712	$23,594	$27,778

*Rural-Urban Commuting Area (RUCA, Version 2.0) codes. RUCA codes range from 1 to 10.6, with 1 being the most urban and 10.6 being the most rural. A RUCA code of 5 means that the census tract is strongly tied to a large town, with primary flow 30% or more to a large town. A RUCA code of 10 means that the town is considered an isolated small rural census tract, with less than 5% primary flow to a larger town. A RUCA code of 10.6 is slightly more rural than a code of 10.

Data from Henry, L. R., & Hooker, R. S. (2007). Retention of physician assistants in rural health clinics. Journal of Rural Health, 23(3), 207–214.

EXHIBIT 9-16
Age and Years in Rural Health Location of Texas Physician Assistants

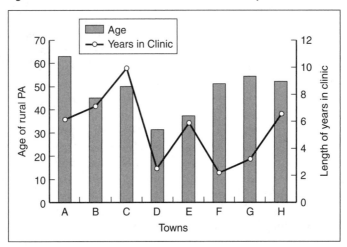

Data from Henry, L. R., & Hooker, R. S. (2007). Retention of physician assistants in rural health clinics. Journal of Rural Health, 23(3), 207–214.

Most of the PAs in this rural and autonomous study were employees of a hospital system some distance away. Almost all were dissatisfied with the hospital, primarily due to inefficiencies, bureaucracies, or reimbursement errors. Yet all of the PAs were satisfied with their careers and their relationships with their towns. They liked their clinic staff and had a good relationship with their supervising doctor. They maintained contact with the doctor primarily via phone, but the doctor could also be contacted by beeper or e-mail. Texas State Board of Medical Examiners policy requires the supervising doctor to work in the same clinic with the PA at least 8 hours every 2 weeks. Both the supervising doctor and the PA adhered to this policy requirement and commented positively about seeing each other on a periodic basis for professional reasons (Henry & Hooker, 2007).

Perceptions

Although some literature cites the differences in rural and urban physicians' perceptions of the role and practice of PAs, NPs, and CNMs (nonphysician providers), the available data are not extensive or conclusive. A study was undertaken to compare differences between rural and urban primary care physicians' perceptions of the role and practice of nonphysician providers. Despite a 16% response rate using a mail-out survey in South Carolina, data from 681 rural and urban primary care physicians were returned. The results indicated that nonphysician providers possess the necessary skills and knowledge to provide primary care to patients. Furthermore, these providers were an asset to a clinic, freed the doctor's time to handle more critically ill patients, and increased revenue for the practice. However, they also indicated that nonphysician providers increased the risk of patient care mistakes and the physician's time spent in administrative duties. Urban physicians' mean scores were higher for perceiving that nonphysician providers are able to see as many patients in a given day as a physician but experience impediments in the delivery of

patient care. Such results may be useful in clarifying physicians' perceptions regarding the role and practice of nonphysician providers to reduce impediments to patient care access (Burgess et al, 2003).

Isberner and colleagues (2003) surveyed rural Illinois physicians to identify incentives and constraints that influence their receptivity to utilization of PAs. Receptive physicians reported six incentives related to appointments, workload, productivity, education/counseling, complex cases, and patient satisfaction. Unreceptive physicians identified four constraints related to perceived patient opposition, malpractice risk, overstepping authority, and continuity of care. Receptive physicians also identified perceived patient opposition as a constraint. PA educators need to inform PA students about incentives and constraints influencing physician and patient receptivity, especially in rural and underserved communities (Isberner et al, 2003).

Community Acceptance

Baldwin and colleagues (1998) explored community acceptance of PAs and NPs in rural, medically underserved areas. Community acceptance in the context of this study implied not only satisfaction with the care received, but also willingness of the community to support an NP or a PA practice through its infrastructure and encourage members to initially seek and continue to receive care from an NP or PA. Five focus groups were conducted in each of five rural, medically underserved communities. The two most pervasive findings were the lack of previous exposure to NPs and PAs and the general belief that PAs and NPs would be accepted in these communities if certain conditions could be met. The theme of conditional acceptance included personal and system factors. Personal factors included friendliness, competence, willingness to enter into the life of the community, and the ability to keep information confidential. System factors considered critical for acceptance included service type, integration with the existing healthcare system, cost, geographic proximity, and availability. The results of this study offer insight into community attitudes and suggest marketing strategies for those who plan to introduce NP or PA services into rural communities (Baldwin et al, 1998).

Reimbursement

Another important issue for rural PAs is favorable reimbursement policy. Because state-to-state variability in compensation and Medicaid reimbursement laws affect PA deployment, increased efforts should be directed toward tailoring state policies to compensate PAs adequately (Pan et al, 1996).

Unique to the United States is the patchwork quilt of health insurance plans (more than 160), along with federal and state medical care entitlements, free clinics, and other policies. Reimbursement is the repayment or settlement for services met. For the first three decades of development, PAs had difficulty being consistently reimbursed for their services (Anonymous, 2002). After 1997, this situation began to change and since 2000 has largely been addressed in most areas of the country.

As long as recruitment and retention of physicians in sparsely populated areas remains difficult, PAs will be sought in greater numbers to help fill this growing void, particularly in primary care. Federal and state initiatives are likely to increase recruitment of PAs to fill the needs of medically underserved America. Retaining them after economic incentives expire present some of the formidable challenges.

Reimbursement is also considered a critical indicator of output and is commonly used as a benchmark for productivity. Evidence based on productivity measures, salaries, and costs of medical education indicates that PAs and NPs are cost-effective (Hooker, 2002). Managed care suggests that health maintenance organizations (HMOs) tend to utilize these professionals effectively and at high levels (Roblin et al, 2004).

Other studies suggest underserved rural areas utilize PAs and NPs to not only improve

access to health care but provide a revenue source for hospitals (Krein, 1999; Henry & Hooker, 2007). To test this hypothesis two other researchers examined the role of payment sources in the utilization of PAs and NPs using the 1994 National Hospital Ambulatory Medical Care Survey (NHAMCS) conducted by the National Center for Health Statistics, U.S. Centers for Disease Control and Prevention. Rural versus urban results were compared. The study found that significant rural-urban differences exist in the relationships between payment sources and the utilization of PAs and NPs. Also found was that the source of payment (Medicare, Medicaid, third party insurance) varied for physicians, PAs, and NPs that saw outpatients in hospital settings. Surprisingly, prepaid group practices and HMO types of reimbursements tend to have no relationship with PA and NP utilization; this finding is the same for rural and urban patient visits. After controlling for other influences, the study showed that all three providers (doctors, PAs, and NPs) are each as likely as the other to be present at a rural managed care clinic visit (Anderson & Hampton, 1999).

Caring for the Poor and Uninsured

After more than 40 years of having the PA profession in America, mounting evidence now can address the social question of whether the creation of PAs produces a social good. Using 5 years of data from the National Ambulatory Medical Care Survey—a cross-sectional survey of doctors' offices—Staton and colleagues (2007) demonstrated that patients who paid medical expenses out of pocket (the poor and uninsured) were visiting PAs more than patients with insurance who were more likely to see doctors for their care. This observation was further amplified when patients in rural areas were assessed and found to be more likely to visit PAs than those living in urban areas. Without PAs, one can suggest that a segment of the nation as a whole would not be able to receive care because of cost or lack of access. It demonstrates that PAs are providing care where doctors are not, and the benefits are immeasurable.

Rural Hospitals

Krein's study (1997a) on PAs and NPs by rural hospitals in an eight-state region in the northwestern tier of the United States (Minnesota, North Dakota, South Dakota, Iowa, Montana, Idaho, Oregon, and Washington) centered on how different market and organizational factors influenced the employment of PAs and NPs by rural hospitals. Rural hospital administrators (N = 407) were interviewed by telephone. Data obtained were then analyzed using descriptive tables and logistic regression. Krein's work revealed a number of observations. First, there is greater demand than supply of both types of practitioners. Moreover, there are several differences in the characteristics of hospitals that employ the different types of practitioners. Rural hospitals use PAs and NPs to enhance the delivery of outpatient services, and a major factor related to their employment is the RHC program; yet few of the hospitals reported that PAs or NPs have admitting or discharge privileges, although PAs appear to provide a more expanded scope of services in rural hospitals. In the aggregate, rural hospitals seem to employ PAs and NPs for similar reasons:

- to extend care, assist physicians, or increase access to primary care;
- because physicians are unavailable or too difficult to recruit;
- because PA and NPs are considered cost-effective or more economical for rural areas; and
- for RHC certification.

Krein also undertook a longitudinal design and pooled cross-sectional study of rural hospitals across the United States to examine the response of rural hospitals to various market and organizational signals by determining the factors that influence whether they establish a provider-based RHC. The study found that PAs and NPs play a crucial role in this development. Key variables included measures of competitive pressures (e.g., hospital market share), physician resources, NP or PA practice regulations, hospital performance pressures (e.g., operating margin), innovativeness, and institutional pressure (i.e., the cumulative force of RHC adoption). The author's principal finding was that adoption of provider-based RHCs by rural hospitals appears to be motivated less as an adaptive response to observable economic or internal organizational signals than as a reaction to bandwagon pressures.

Another conclusion was that rural hospitals with limited resources tend to have an inadequate ability to fully evaluate strategic activities for remaining viable. One strategy for remaining viable is to employ PAs and NPs, which serves as a cost-effective strategy for a hospital referral base. Additionally, because PAs and NPs are more flexible than doctors, they are easier to employ in outlying rural clinics (Krein, 1999). Although the author concluded that such activity could have a harmful effect on some providers and some rural residents, evidence of harm has not been demonstrated in the decade since the study was conducted.

Bergeron and colleagues (1999) used survey data from 285 small rural hospitals and case studies of 36 of these hospitals to answer questions about the extent to which PAs and NPs provide primary care in small, rural hospitals; the benefits that they might bring to the hospitals; and the reactions of the public to such providers. The data were collected as part of an evaluation of the hospitals, which received Rural Health Care Transition grants from the Health Care Financing Administration in 1993 and 1994. Most of the hospitals used these nonphysician providers; 70% used NPs, 30% used PAs, and 20% percent used both. There were some negative reactions to the use of PAs and NPs, but overall they were accepted. The hospitals benefitted in the form of reduced recruitment costs, increased revenues, and increased service offerings. Bergeron researchers concluded that practitioners are beneficial to rural hospitals, and mechanisms to encourage their acceptance should be developed and implemented.

Productivity in Rural Areas

Larson (2001) wanted to understand the contribution to generalist care made by PAs and NPs in underserved rural areas. His group addressed the following questions:

■ What is the total contribution to generalist care made by PAs and NPs?
■ What is the role of PAs or NPs in providing generalist care in rural HPSAs?
■ What proportion of the total generalist care is provided by women doctors, PAs, and NPs?

An important issue in health workforce analysis is how to count the contribution of each provider and each provider type to patient care. Simple head counts of providers are unlikely to produce realistic estimates of the actual supply of health care available to a population (Ricketts, Hart, & Pirani, 2000; Larson, Hart, & Ballweg, 2001; Pedersen et al, 2008). Differences in training, location, specialty, inpatient care activities, experience, scope of practice, and full-time/part-time status create large differences in the number of visits that a given clinician is likely to perform during a week. If, for example, an average family physician provides 105 ambulatory patient visits each week, a general pediatrician 95, and a general internist about 65, then we have some idea of productivity by specialty. If estimates of available care are to include PAs and NPs, then basing estimates of available care on head counts becomes yet more doubtful because so little is known about the productivity of PAs and NPs and their total contribution to care.

Estimating the Supply of Generalist Ambulatory Visits

To estimate the total supply of ambulatory visits available from different types of providers in rural and urban areas in Washington state, Larson and colleagues (2001) converted the role and productivity of family physicians to a FTE, or a 40 hour work week. This produced fairly dramatic effects by converting from unadjusted head counts, to estimated head counts, to physician FTEs.

The licensing/survey data identified 4,124 generalist physicians, but outpatient visit productivity data indicated that those physicians were providing the visits that could be supplied by 2,781 family physician FTEs. An estimated 699 NPs provided 330 family physician FTEs and 581 PAs provided 411 family physician FTEs. In short, an estimated 5,469 generalist providers in Washington state provided approximately 3,522 family physician FTEs of outpatient visits. Generalist physicians make up 76.6% of the generalist providers in Washington state and provide 78.9% of the generalist FTEs; NPs provide 9.4% and PAs provide the remaining 11.7%.

There are some differences in the contribution to care made by PAs and NPs in rural versus urban areas of Washington state. Overall, PA and NPs provide 24.7% of the total generalist outpatient visits in rural areas (10.3% by NPs, 14.4% by PAs) compared with 20.1% in urban areas ($p = 0.014$). In rural and urban settings, NPs provide about 10% of the outpatient visits; the rural-urban difference in contribution is primarily attributable to the larger proportion of total visits provided by rural PAs (Exhibits 9-17, 9-18, and 9-19). The range of PA and NP contribution to generalist care in rural HPSAs is quite wide.

The preceding analysis indicates that nonphysician clinicians provide about 21% of the generalist ambulatory visits performed in Washington state, with their contribution slightly higher in rural parts of the state (24.7% compared with 20.1% in urban areas). These estimates are improvements over those based on unadjusted head counts because they are based on actual productivity data (when available, and imputed estimates when not available) and actual differences in specialty distribution. Converting estimated head counts into FTEs also revealed the difficulties with estimating available care from head counts. There were productivity differences both within and across professions that, when applied to head counts and converted to FTEs, result in steep downward productivity adjustments.

Although this study is of one state, it is not an exception. Observations throughout the

EXHIBIT 9-17
Active Generalist Providers in Washington State, 1998–1999

	Generalist MD/DOs	Generalist PAs	Generalist NPs	Total
Count	4,124 (81.6%)	485 (9.6%)	442 (8.8%)	5,051 (100.0%)
Mean age	46.7	45.4	47.1	46.6
% female	28.9	38.8	92.7	35.5
% practicing in rural HSAs	19.4	27.8	19.7	20.2
% practicing in geographic health professional shortage areas	0.8	2.0	3.1	1.1
PHYSICIAN SPECIALTY				
% family physician/general practitioner	56.3	—	—	46.0
% general internal medicine	28.2	—	—	23.0
% general pediatrics	15.3	—	—	12.6

Data from Larson, E. H., et al. (2003). The contribution of nurse practitioners and physician assistants to generalist care in Washington state. Health Services Research, 38*(4), 1033–1050.*

EXHIBIT 9-18
Active Identified and Imputed Generalist Providers by Rural/Urban Location in Washington State, 1998–1999

	Generalist Doctors Count (%)	Generalist PAs Count (%)	Generalist NPs Count (%)	Total Count (%)
Rural	811.2 (73.9)	152.7 (13.9)	133.9 (12.2)	1,097.8 (100.0)
Urban	3,377.8 (77.3)	428.1 (9.8)	565.5 (12.9)	4,371.4 (100.0)
TOTAL	4,189.0 (76.6)	580.8 (10.6)	699.4 (12.8)	5,469.2 (100.0)

Data from Larson, E. H., et al. (2003). The contribution of nurse practitioners and physician assistants to generalist care in Washington state. Health Services Research, 38*(4), 1033–1050.*

EXHIBIT 9-19
Generalist Provider Supply (in FTEs) in Rural Geographic Health Professional Shortage Areas (HPSAs), Washington State, 1989–1999

	Generalist Doctors Count (%)	Generalist PAs Count (%)	Generalist NPs Count (%)	Total Count (%)
Rural HSAs with no HPSA population (25 HSAs)	320.3 (77.4)	51.8 (12.5)	41.6 (10.1)	413.7 (100.0)
Rural HSAs with 1% to 33% of population in HPSAs (12 HSAs)	170.5 (74.6)	34.1 (14.9)	23.8 (10.4)	228.4 (100.0)
Rural HSAs with 34% to 100% of population in HPSAs (15 HSAs)	64.4 (67.4)	20.6 (21.6)	10.5 (11.0)	95.5 (100.0)
TOTAL	555.2 (75.3)	106.5 (14.4)	75.9 (10.3)	737.6 (100.0)

Data from Larson, E. H., et al. (2003). The contribution of nurse practitioners and physician assistants to generalist care in Washington state. Health Services Research, 38*(4), 1033–1050.*

Pacific Northwest as well as other locations (such as Utah, Arizona, New Mexico, California, and Texas) suggest that PAs (and NPs) are providing care disproportionately more than doctors in rural areas. When broken down by the presence of PAs and NPs in rural geographic HPSAs, they appear to be more abundant per capita than in non-HPSAs. In fact, in Washington state, the PAs appear to make a larger contribution in HSAs with large HPSA populations, compared to non-HPSA HSAs. In Utah, the PAs are approximately 10% more productive than doctors in rural primary care (per annum) when using the standard that one FTE provider produces 105 visits per week (Pedersen et al, 2008).

Female Providers in Rural Settings

Although women make up an increasing part of the generalist physician workforce and are the providers of choice for many female patients (Rourke, Rourke, & Brown, 1996), rural medicine has been relatively unattractive to women physicians (Doescher, Ellsbury, & Hart, 2000). Work by Larson and colleagues (2003) found that in rural settings, female PAs and NPs represent a larger share of the care provided by women than female doctors; combined they provide 51% of the FTEs provided by women (Exhibit 9-20). In rural settings, female physicians provided less than one-half (49%) of the FTEs provided by women. In contrast, female physicians provided 63.5% of the generalist care provided by women in urban settings. Not surprisingly, in both rural and urban settings, NPs make up the majority of female PA and NP FTEs (Larson et al, 2003).

RURAL HEALTH GLOBALLY

No two countries define rural health quite the same way. For some countries, it is a definition of geographic location or population density. For example, Australia uses the term "remote" to define a uniquely isolated community, whereas the United States uses the term "frontier counties" to designate boundaries containing less than one person per square mile. The islands and highlands of Scotland can present difficulties to access. Most demographers define "rural" as sparsely clustered communities and not metropolitan. Oftentimes the term needs to be parsed to allow publicly funded programs to assist rural populations.

Australia

The medical workforce shortage in Australia is significant, but is particularly evident in rural and remote areas (Hooker, Hogan, & Leeker, 2007; O'Conner & Hooker, 2007; Jolly, 2008). As Australia has thought about strategic ways to extend care with a limited cadre of doctors the PA model has emerged. The appeal is that the PA is under the supervision of a medical officer in a delegated practice model. Taking a cue from the United States and Canada—that they are trained by doctors in medical schools and can assume as much as

EXHIBIT 9-20
Female Generalist Providers by Provider Type (in FTEs) by Rural/Urban Location, Washington State, 1998–1999

	Doctor Count (%)	PA Count (%)	NP Count (%)	Total Count (%)
Rural	98.6 (49.3)	37.8 (18.8)	63.8 (31.9)	200.2 (100.0)
Urban	599.3 (63.5)	115.1 (12.2)	228.8 (24.3)	943.2 (100.0)
TOTAL	697.9 (61.0)	152.9 (13.4)	292.6 (25.6)	1,143.4 (100.0)

Data from Larson, E. H., et al. (2003). The contribution of nurse practitioners and physician assistants to generalist care in Washington state. Health Services Research, 38(4), 1033–1050.

90% of the general practice visit safely—their skills may be particularly adapted to rural and remote settings where their team orientation to care can be highly leveraged.

One of the most important reports addressing this shortage is the *Report on the Audit of Health Workforce in Rural and Regional Australia,* published in 2008. This report by the Australian Government Department of Health and Aging addresses shortages, compares the medical shortages in other countries with those in Australia, discusses the use of international medical graduates, and identifies areas for improvement, which includes the use of PAs.

In addition, Jolly's assessment (mentioned previously) that PAs would fit in the Australian medical workforce was delivered to Parliament in 2008. The report, an extensive review of the PA literature, was positive and endorsing of the PA concept, especially for rural areas (Jolly, 2008). Additionally, two public health policy papers by O'Connor and Hooker (2007) discuss specific roles that the PA could undertake within rural Australian society. Some of these settings include hospitals, general practices, and indigenous health clinics.

Murray and Wronski (2006), two rural health medical observers, argue there is compelling evidence for the success of the "rural pipeline" (rural student recruitment and rurally based education and professional training) in increasing the rural workforce. The nexus between clinical education and training, a sustained healthcare workforce, clinical research, and quality and safety needs greater emphasis. As senior academic leaders, both authors state that a "teaching health system" for nonmetropolitan Australia requires greater commitment to teaching as a core business, as well as provision of an infrastructure, including accommodation and access to the private sector. Because workforce flexibility is mostly well accepted in rural and remote areas, there is room for expanding the scope of clinical practice by nonmedical clinicians, such as PAs and NPs, in an independent codified manner with flexible local medical delegation (e.g., practice nurses, Aboriginal health workers, and therapists). In the end, Murray

and Wronski call for the imbalance between subspecialist and generalist medical training to be addressed. Improved training and recognition of Aboriginal health workers, as well as continued investment in programs that will allow entry of indigenous people into other health professional programs, such as PA programs, remain policy priorities.

Demonstration projects introducing PAs into rural Queensland and urban South Australia began in 2009. James Cook University, which was established with a rural mandate for improving health care to Northern Queensland, is committed to a similar PA program in 2011. The University of Queensland has a traditional role in dispersing medical students into rural areas for clinical training. This tradition is extended to the University of Queensland PA program, which started in 2009.

The Mount Isa Centre for Rural and Remote Health is an extension of James Cook University. Located in a remote part of central Australia, this setting has access to indigenous people and isolated communities and fosters opportunities for a wide range of health professionals in their clinical phase of education to spend time in this community. PA students are now included in this activity.

Canada

Information on PAs in Canada in general and in rural areas is emerging. From 1984 to 2008, the development of PAs was largely by the Canadian Forces for use in the Canadian Forces Medical Group. As PAs finished their military careers and retired, many sought roles in the civilian sector. Because no legislation existed until Manitoba enacted theirs in 2000, most former PAs either gave up healthcare work or sought employment in the civilian sector as health and safety officers in industry—sometimes in remote locations.

In 2008, the Ontario Ministry of Health and Long-Term Care enacted a demonstration project to recruit PAs from Canada and the United States to work in emergency medicine, hospitals, and community health clinics. This impetus has allowed other provinces to consider

PAs for their more rural and indigenous populations. Manitoba, a province with very remote populations and large indigenous groups, enacted a PA program to try to address the shortages of medical care to rural communities. New Brunswick will employ PAs in 2010.

Great Britain

Although Great Britain is not known for its rural locations, at least 50 small towns are considered rural and difficult to service. These areas include parts of Ireland, Scotland, and many outlying islands. The evaluation of U.S.-trained PAs working in the National Health Service (NHS) in England and a similar project in Scotland delivered by NHS Education for Scotland (NES) has identified a number of benefits with PA deployment (Woodin et al, 2005; Farmer et al, 2009). English-educated PAs will ultimately replace recruitment of American PAs and deployment to less urban areas is expected to result from this activity.

South Africa

The huge tracts of wilderness and distances between small towns and villages present challenges to the South African government. In clinics, whether they are in the outlying areas or in townships, the ratio of doctor to patient is quite low. On top of this issue, the number of professionals, including doctors, leaving South Africa is burdensome (Mullan & Frehywot, 2007). To overcome this handicap, South Africa is looking for solutions (Hugo, 2005). Implementing PAs is one of the first steps in dealing with low doctor-to-population ratios. A PA program is being developed at the University of the Witwatersrand (Hugo & Mfenyana, 2007). Other universities are involved with similar efforts. The intent is to train PAs for both urban and rural deployment.

INNOVATIONS IN RURAL HEALTH EMPLOYMENT

The deployment of PAs to U.S. areas of medical need is attributed to policies initiated by the federal government. Meeting the needs of rural populations has roots in 200 years of priorities—going back to the development of the North American agrarian society. At the beginning of the 20th century, 70% of the American population was based in agriculture and lived outside of urban centers. As of the 21st century, 3% of Americans farm or grow items for consumption (yet this population produces almost all of the food for the rest of the country). The percentage of Americans who are considered rural is 14%. Federal congress and state legislatures have created policies to address the disparities of rural people, and those policies have direct effects on PAs. Some of these innovations are outlined below.

Telemedicine and Rural Health

Clinical telemedicine uses interactive video technologies and telecommunications networks to deliver medical consultations to distant patients and their primary care providers. Because telemedicine provides real-time access to specialists whose services might not otherwise be available in rural or medically underserved areas, this technology is seen as a means for connecting providers to centers of medical care specialization. Although there has been dramatic growth in the use of telemedicine, there is little evidence that telemedicine as a patient care delivery system has been incorporated into the medical school curriculum. However, the current status of telemedicine in medical curricula has been adopted in various PA education operations, such as the University of Iowa PA program (Asprey, Zollo, & Kienzle, 2001).

Education

A PA education program rural track was developed to improve nonmetropolitan PA placement. Graduates (1997–2003) of this rural track were interviewed about the community and area of health care in which they practiced and their admission files were reviewed to identify previous rural community exposure. At the time of the survey, of the 19 graduates with rural backgrounds, 58% were practicing in rural communities, while 56% of those with little or no rural background were also serving in rural areas. Changes to the clinical and didactic curriculum increased student exposure to rural settings and provided courses more appropriate for rural practice. By emphasizing rural placement, this PA program successfully integrated a rural track into its existing curriculum and increased the percentage of graduates practicing in rural areas, independent of previous exposure to rural communities (Ruff et al, 2006).

Information via Computers

Information systems for rural practice may assume that rural clinicians have different information-seeking needs, but studies have not directly compared rural and nonrural information needs using common methodology. Gorman (2004), a medical informatics doctor, compared rural and nonrural information needs, information seeking, effectiveness of information seeking, and use of information resources. Through observation and interviews during one half-day of office practice (with telephone follow-up 2 to 10 days later), primary care providers were assessed. The providers included 39 physicians, 42 NPs, and 22 PAs in ambulatory practices in rural and nonrural Oregon. Overall, rural clinicians tended to practice in smaller groups, but were otherwise similar to nonrural clinicians. During half-day interviews, clinicians cared for an average of 8.2 patients (95% CI 7.5–8.8) and asked an average of 0.83 questions via the computer per patient seen (95% CI 0.73–0.92). At follow up, they had obtained an answer, on average, to 47% of their questions (95% CI 40%–53%), and reported being successful in finding an answer to 77% of those they pursued (95% CI 70%–84%). There were no statistically significant differences between rural and nonrural clinicians for any of these variables. The authors concluded that rural and nonrural clinicians had similar information needs, information seeking, knowledge resource use, and effectiveness at finding answers to their questions. Human consultants, digital resources, and library-based resources were less available, but these differences in availability had little impact on their use (Gorman, Yao, & Seshadri, 2004).

Educational Development Grants

The Health Professions Assistance Act of 1963 was designed, in part, to stimulate the growth of PAs through funding of Title VII, section 747 of the Public Health Service Act. Policy planners were striving to supply providers for underserved populations with nurses and assistants to doctors (Vangsnes, 2005). Borne out of the progressive times of President Johnson's Great Society, change was in the wind; the plight of the poor and underserved was a force to be reckoned with and needed to be addressed in creative ways (R. Smith, former Assistant Surgeon General, personal communication, May 5, 2006). The concept of PAs, as they are known today, was not part of American medicine's infrastructure and no one envisioned they would grow as they have. However, the policymakers of the 1960s believed if the right social strategy could be created then all of America could be lifted from its impoverished roots. Although policy tends to be a blunt instrument for change, Title VII served as that mechanism for transformation of medical care delivery in unforeseen ways.

The emphasis of Title VII funding was to promote the preparation of PAs for roles working with primary care physicians and for deployment to medically underserved areas. Incentives in Title VII grant awards encouraged PA programs to educate practitioners with an orientation in primary care. They have also fostered methods of deployment of PA graduates to enter primary care/ambulatory practice and to locate in medically underserved areas. A high proportion of federally funded PA educational programs have developed curricular components that identify clinical training sites and affiliations in rural and medically underserved areas. Qualifications require students to serve a portion of clinical training in such sites.

Rural Health Service Loan Repayment

Education loan repayment is one of the strategies to entice PAs and other providers to rural healthcare locations. In exchange for qualifying service, usually in a health personnel shortage area or a state designated area of unmet healthcare need, participants may receive funds to repay qualifying graduate-level, federal loan debt. The maximum of any state or federal loan repayment is $100,000. The loan has some obligations. Once the first payment from this program is received and processed, the participant is obligated to satisfy the minimum practice requirement or pay a penalty equal to 150% of the program benefit received.

For PAs and NPs the annual payments equal to 25% of the total qualifying loan principal for a minimum service obligation of 3 years and maximum program participation of 4 years. Two years of employment is required to avoid penalties. Students may apply for the program during the last year leading to the professional degree.

National Health Service Corps

The NHSC is a federal program that places healthcare professionals in more than 500 areas (neighborhoods to rural areas) that are suffering from critical shortages of primary healthcare providers. The Health Resources and Services Administration (HRSA) Bureau of Primary Health Care administers the NHSC.

A number of recruitment funds support programs that offer financial help for PAs and other medical care professionals in exchange for professional services. These programs include scholarships, the Federal Loan Repayment Program, the NHSC State Loan Repayment Program, and the Commissioned Officer Student Extern Program (COSTEP).

Economic Incentives for Rural Health Placement

A number of initiatives are created by states to encourage relocation to and retention in rural practices. These come in the form of loan repayment similar to the federal government system, tax incentives (usually in the form of deductions), mortgage assistance in the form of low-cost loans subsidized by the state, and cash incentives.

Enabling State Legislation

Legislation on the state level has been instrumental in expanding PA development and deployment into rural areas. This legislation involves three important components: enabling legislation, prescribing, and reimbursement. Expanding the authority of PAs to work with fewer restrictions than before allows for PA development in medically underserved areas.

At one time prescribing authority was a particularly troublesome barrier to PA practice effectiveness, and its presence in state law is reflected in the patterns of marketplace demand and utilization of PA providers. State prescribing authority can have a marked influence on the capacity and efficiency of PAs to contribute to healthcare delivery (Gara, 1989). One example was seen in Texas, where before the passage of PA prescriptive authority there were only 26 PA RHCs. By 1992, only 15 months after the passage of prescriptive authority for PAs in Texas, the number of PAs employed by these clinics had nearly quadrupled to 99. During the same period the percentage of Texas PAs practicing in rural areas tripled, increasing from 5% to 15% (Willis, 1993). The deployment in Texas is illustrative; proportionally more PAs are in rural and frontier locations than primary care doctors (Jones, 2008). Many PAs are in rural and remote locations where once there was a doctor but the economy could no longer support the doctor or the clinic (Jones & Hooker, 2001; Henry & Hooker, 2007).

Rural Health Clinics Act

The Rural Health Clinics Act (PL 95-210) in 1977 was an attempt to provide for the development of federally subsidized RHCs and to staff them appropriately. One proviso provides for the reimbursement of services to Medicare patients by PAs and NPs who practice in communities that are rural and/or underserved. A modification to the Rural Health Clinics Act in 1997 and the creation of the National Association of Rural Health Clinics (NARHC) have allowed the number of RHCs to grow from 600 in 1990 to more than 3,000 in 2005.

The Centers for Medicare and Medicaid Services (CMS) issued a rule relating to RHCs in 2003 that has had a significant impact on PAs and NPs. Much of this rule was adopted in response to statutory requirements signed into law in 1997 (under the Balanced Budget Act of 1997). Various components of the rule stipulate the following:

- All RHCs must be located in "currently" designated shortage areas.
- RHCs that can no longer meet the location requirements must apply for an exception to this requirement and continue to participate in the RHC program.
- There are limits for waivers of nonphysician provider staffing.

The rule also:

- codifies the definition of a "bed" for purposes of the RHC cap exception for hospitals with fewer than 50 beds;
- codifies the RHC payment limits previously extended to most provider-based RHCs;
- codifies PA/NP/CNM staffing requirement at 50% of the time the clinic is open to see patients;
- restricts PA/NP/CNM staffing waiver requests to already certified RHCs; and
- mandates the establishment of a Quality Assessment Performance Improvement initiative by RHCs.

The impact of these policies continues to be felt because of the requirement for RHCs to employ a PA, NP, or CNM. More importantly, these policies emphasize that PAs and NPs are valued in these settings (Exhibit 9-21).

Shortage Area Designations

The designation of healthcare shortage areas is used to direct public money to areas of greatest need. Although they are more broadly stated

EXHIBIT 9-21
Physician Assistant in Rural Health Clinic in West Virginia

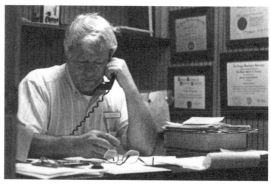

Courtesy of the American Academy of Physician Assistants.

than specific for rural locales, these designations nonetheless cover most of the concerns of access to health care for individuals in rural areas. Three designations emerged from this policy: (1) health professional shortage areas (HPSAs), (2) medically underserved areas (MUAs), and (3) medically underserved populations (MUPs). By creating these designations, geographers and health workforce economists have identified the areas of need, the barriers to this care (geographical, political, economic, and social), and policies that may be used to improve the situation.

Retaining Rural Health Clinic Certification

Although rules and policies are in place to create RHCs, the criteria are sometimes difficult to adhere to because of shifting resources and demographic changes. In order for a shortage area (HPSA, MUA, or a governor-designated area) to be considered current, the area must have been designated or updated within the 3-year period prior to RHC certification or recertification.

For a facility to retain its RHC certification, despite no longer being located in a valid shortage area, the RHC must demonstrate that it is an "essential provider." The new rules identify four types of essential providers: (1) sole community provider, (2) major community provider, (3) specialty clinic, or (4) extremely rural community provider. This policy has a number of implications. It allows a facility to retain the RHC designation, allows some clinics to make the economic transition from federally subsidized to a more market-driven clinic operation, and allows the retention of staff who otherwise might be released due to funding shortages.

Other Rural Health Clinics

Two additional federally funded clinics that impact employment of PAs in rural areas are community health clinics and migrant health centers. Both of these clinics have tripled in their expansion since the early 1990s.

Migrant Health

Given the fact that migrant farm workers' health status is below that of the average American and that availability of and accessibility to health care is limited by financial, cultural, and social barriers, a study assessed the capacity of healthcare providers in selected counties in east Tennessee to provide primary care to this population. The attitudes of these providers toward migrants were also examined. The first half of the survey assessed the providers' opinion in three areas: awareness of migrants' health needs, options for delivering care, and desirability of migrants as patients. The second part requested information regarding the type of provider (physician, NP, or PA), type of agency (private or community/public health), type of practice (primary care, obstetrics/gynecology, or pediatrics), number of encounters with migrants, and the provider's ability to speak Spanish. Also, the respondents were given a list of primary care services and asked to identify those provided directly, formally referred, or not provided.

The results revealed that both groups of providers were not very knowledgeable about migrants' health needs, but providers expressed a willingness to learn more about their health needs and to support local initiatives toward the amelioration of migrants' conditions. Also, providers were in favor of extending Medicaid to migrants and accepting referrals or contractual agreements to provide the care. Physicians generally were less inclined to approve of the federal government subsidizing the care than PAs and NPs. Although both provider groups would treat migrants as any other patients regardless of legal status, the PAs and NPs were more willing to accommodate their schedules to fit the schedules of migrants. The majority of providers were found to deliver basic healthcare services, though deficiencies were noted in some health education areas, dental health, and issues related to pesticide exposure. The author concluded there was a need for major improvements in establishing linkages and cooperative agreements at the interagency level and between agencies and institutions of higher learning in meeting the health needs of migrants (Henning, Graybill, & George, 2008).

A research team led by Shi (1994) studied factors associated with the employment of nonphysician providers (PAs, NPs, and CNMs) in rural and urban community and migrant health centers. Results of the survey suggest that nonphysician providers primarily serve as physician substitutes and are more likely to be employed by health centers that are large and have affiliations with nonphysician provider training programs. Rural or urban location is not significantly related to the employment of nonphysician providers after controlling for center size. The fact that rural centers employ fewer nonphysician providers than urban centers can primarily be accounted for by the relatively small size of the centers rather than a lack of interest. These findings demonstrate that the use of nonphysician providers is an important way to achieve cost containment and improve access to primary care for migrants and those residing in medically underserved areas (Shi et al, 1994).

National Association of Rural Health Clinics

The NARHC is the only national organization dedicated exclusively to improving the delivery of quality, cost-effective health care in rural underserved areas through the RHC program. NARHC works with Congress, federal agencies, and rural health allies to promote, expand, and protect the RHC program. Through the association, NARHC members become actively engaged in the legislative and regulatory process.

The website for NARHC (http://www .narhc.org/) serves as an information resource for and about the RHC program. Because of remoteness and limited ability for various clinics to network this agency, the website provides valuable up-to-date information on issues affecting rural health clinics and the communities they serve. In addition, there are valuable links to other sites. The result is continuous improvement with rural health policy actions and initiatives.

Area Health Education Centers

Area Health Education Centers (AHECs) were developed by the Bureau of Health Professions to enhance access to quality health care, particularly primary and preventive care. They improve the supply and distribution of healthcare professionals through community and academic educational partnerships. Many of the AHECs are located in rural areas and serve to expose health professional students to rural health. For example, the Central Texas AHEC assists PA programs with placement of students in rural family medicine clinics. In some instances, the organization will arrange for the students' lodging and sometimes their transportation and per diem. The intent is to maximize the exposure of the students to rural healthcare delivery.

State Policy Enactments

Various strategies of state governments have resulted in proven policy initiatives for PA placement in rural areas. One strategy used in a number of states, such as Washington, California, Iowa, and New Mexico, is to underwrite public-funded PA programs that emphasize rural health. With this approach, state funds are used to subsidize the education of PAs in the hope that such students would practice in rural communities within the state upon graduation. Some states, such as Pennsylvania and Utah, have developed comprehensive health workforce plans that include PAs and other nonphysician providers as part of the strategy to improve service delivery and efficiency.

COMPARING NURSE PRACTITIONERS AND PHYSICIAN ASSISTANTS IN RURAL HEALTH

The education and regulation of PAs and NPs would suggest unique role differentiations and practice functions between the professions. One study explored to what extent the practice patterns of PAs and NPs in primary care actually differ. It was hypothesized that the primary care services provided by NPs would tend to be oriented to women's health, family health, health prevention and promotion, and servicing minority and socioeconomically disadvantaged patients, and that NPs would be less dependent on physician supervision than PAs. In contrast, the services provided by PAs would more likely be medical-surgical oriented; diagnostic, procedural, and technical in nature; located in rural areas; and more dependent on physician supervision than NPs. The study used patient data from the National Ambulatory Medical Care Survey and National Hospital Ambulatory Medical Care Survey. Although some differences emerged, the argument was not compelling to suggest strong, unique practice differences across all ambulatory care settings between the two types of providers. The specific type of ambulatory setting appears to influence the practice pattern for both provider groups. If practice patterns are less distinctive than previously believed, more opportunities for interdisciplinary education need to be explored, and health policies that promote a discipline-specific primary care workforce may need to be reexamined (Mills & McSweeney, 2002).

A descriptive cross-sectional study was undertaken to determine if a significant difference exists in perceived primary healthcare outcomes of rural clients treated by NPs and those treated by physicians or PAs. Primary healthcare outcomes were defined as (1) perceived satisfaction with care, (2) compliance with antibiotic medications, and (3) perceived health. The sample of 151 subjects were age 18 or older, could read and understand English, and lived in a predefined rural county. The majority of subjects were female, white, and married. There was no significant difference found in satisfaction with care or compliance with antibiotic medications among rural clients treated by an NP and those treated by a physician or PA. Clients of NPs had higher levels of perceived health, general health, and physical health than clients of physicians or PAs. Rural clients in this study were more satisfied with NPs in relation to general satisfaction, interpersonal manner, time spent with healthcare provider, and accessibility and convenience. Financially, rural clients in this study were more satisfied when treated by physicians and NPs when compared to PAs (Taylor, 2000).

Strickland and colleagues (1998) examined provider and practice characteristics, location preference, and reasons for location preference among Georgia PAs, NPs, and CNMs (N = 1,079). Data collected through a statewide survey revealed that providers were concentrated in urban areas. Rural providers tended to be older and less educated, to possess fewer specialty credentials, and to be employed longer than urban providers. NPs were significantly more likely to prefer small communities, and PAs were significantly more likely to prefer large communities. Providers who preferred small communities were likely to practice in rural and urban areas, but providers who preferred large communities were substantially more likely to practice in urban areas. Providers who preferred small communities were significantly more likely to mention the importance of community dynamics, whereas providers who preferred large communities were significantly more likely to mention professional context.

Research and Rural Health

The literature about PAs in rural health is limited. A review of this literature reveals missing information and unanswered questions. Select research questions that might contribute to the successful deployment of PAs into rural health are offered here.

- **Case reports:** Writing about individual roles and settings using 1 year's accumulation of data provides a foundation for others to build upon. Case reports describe rural and remote health, how it works, the community the clinic serves, and the role of the PA in this setting.

- **Role delineation:** What is the role of the PA in a rural health setting? How is this role shared between the PA and the supervising physician?

- **Organizational research:** How does a rural health clinic with a PA compare with a facility in an urban setting with a PA? Contrast and compare the practice setting, the population served, and the activity of each member of the team for each facility.

- **Economics:** How does a clinic in a rural setting staffed with a PA compare with a comparable clinic without a PA? What are the economies of scale and staffing patterns in both settings?

- **Epidemiology:** What are the frequency of diagnoses, the characteristics of patients seen, and the incidences of diagnoses in the community when comparing rural PAs with urban PAs?

- **Quality of care:** How does the quality of care in a rural clinic staffed with a PA compare with similar clinics without a PA? Does the inclusion of a PA change the quality of care?

- **Procedures:** What are the procedures used and the skills needed for a primary care PA in a rural setting?

- **Patient satisfaction:** Do patients have any different perceptions of PAs in rural settings versus those in urban settings?

- **Retention:** What are the social and economic factors that contribute to retention or attrition of PAs in rural locations?

- **Education:** Are there education strategies that can be a factor to successful deployment of PAs to rural settings?

SUMMARY

The rural healthcare system has changed dramatically since the new century because of a general transformation of healthcare financing, the introduction of new technologies, and the clustering of health services into systems and networks. The result has been the expansion of PAs into rural health in unprecedented moves. Despite these changes, resources for rural health systems remain relatively insufficient. Many rural communities continue to experience shortages of doctors, nurses, allied health professionals, and PAs. The proportion of rural hospitals under financial stress is much greater than that of urban hospitals. The healthcare conditions of selected rural areas compare unfavorably with the rest of the nation. Market and governmental policies have attempted to address some of these disparities by encouraging network development and changing the rules for Medicare and Medicaid payments to providers.

Rural health in Australia, Canada, Great Britain, and South Africa have similar challenges and are turning to PAs as one strategy among many to assist in addressing this social situation. Federal, state, provincial, and Health Authority rural bonding policies may come into play as public funds are used to underwrite PA education. As each of these countries experiments with doctor alternatives to rural health delivery, opportunities for innovation and creativity will merge with new technology to improve the health outlook of remote people throughout the world.

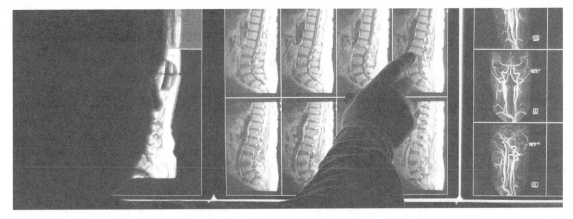

CHAPTER 10

OTHER PROFESSIONAL ROLES
FOR PHYSICIAN ASSISTANTS

JAMES F. CAWLEY ■ RODERICK S. HOOKER ■ DAVID P. ASPREY

We tell these tales, which are strictest true,
Just by way of convincing you
How very little, since things was made
Anything alters in any one's trade.
                    —*Rudyard Kipling (1865–1936)*

ABSTRACT

Mobility for a physician assistant (PA) differs no less than any other occupation, whether the change involves management, specialization, entrepreneurial development, or serves as a stepping stone for an out-of-the-ordinary line of work. For over four decades PAs have pioneered a wide range of roles that differ from the profession's clinical origins, including roles in management, the legal system, research, journalism, and owning and operating clinics. Some of the direction for reinventing the PA role arose from dissatisfaction with being clinicians and a desire to seek new challenges and personal growth. That PAs would seek such change identifies them more along the norm for people in general and no different from the doctors with whom they work closely.

INTRODUCTION

Physician assistants (PAs) are highly versatile clinicians and professionals. Throughout their careers such versatility allows for mobility that leads them in different directions. The 2008 American Academy of Physician Assistants (AAPA) Physician Assistant Census Report estimates that about 15% of all individuals who have graduated from PA educational programs are no longer in full-time clinical practice as PAs (AAPA, 2007a). However, with 85% of formally trained PAs in some PA-type role, this level of professional retention is higher than that noted for allied health and nursing occupations. Only physician retention is comparable.

It is not known how many of the 15% of PAs who are not clinically practicing still work within the PA profession or in the healthcare field in roles that do not involve patient contact. Some have obtained additional degrees in medically related fields (e.g., public health, healthcare administration, education, and research) and have developed various careers. A sizable number are faculty in PA programs and other academic settings. At least 70% of PA faculty members maintain part-time (average of 10 hours per week) clinical practices in addition to their educational duties; 62% of PA program directors remain in clinical practice (Physician Assistant Education Association [PAEA], 2007). Some PAs have combined their years of clinical experience and expertise with graduate degrees in administration and have evolved into roles in health services management. Others have assumed public health positions and roles in research and health policy (Exhibit 10-1). During the early development of the PA profession, about 2% of all persons educated as PAs went on to become physicians (Jones, 1994). That no longer seems to be the case.

EXHIBIT 10-1

Nonclinical Roles of Physician Assistants

- Attorney
- Academic educator/researcher
- Consultant for political candidates
- Forensic scientist/legal expert
- Hospital administrator
- Health facility owner/entrepreneur
- Health information management
- Health insurance management
- Health lobbying
- Health planner/regulator
- Health services administration
- Health services research/health policy
- Industrial hygienist
- Insurance reviewer
- Malpractice reviewer
- Medical editor/publisher
- Medical epidemiologist
- Naturopath
- PA educational faculty/administration
- PA service/house staff administrator
- Pharmaceutical representative
- Pharmaceutical medical liaison
- Politician
- Professional recruiter
- Public health officer
- Researcher, clinical and medical social

The 2008 AAPA Census Report asked respondents a series of questions about their status if they were in nonclinical roles or if they were working not as PAs (Exhibit 10-2). The largest group was PA educators who were primarily out of the clinical mainstream. A little less than half are represented in this exhibit. Another 500 or so were not employed by choice. Since a large proportion of this group is female between 25 and 50 years of age, we speculate they may be taking time to raise families. Another sizeable group of respondents are administrators, researchers, and other nonhealth professionals.

The PA credential is often recognized in the healthcare field as a valuable background permitting individuals to move into many types of expanded clinical and nonclinical roles, and attrition from the PA profession does not appear to be a major problem. One can argue that in any profession a predictable number of people will migrate to other related roles or explore new opportunities. Moreover, this is a positive feature that affords individuals in the PA profession a wide degree of career latitude if they decide to seek expanded or alternative roles. As PAs become increasingly visible in the healthcare field, more opportunities in administration, leadership, and research will surface. Schneller (1994) writes:

> The fact that some PAs are not satisfied with their level of autonomy and seek career advancement outside of the PA field has not been a concern for the profession. From its origins the PA occupation has been an "accelerator" occupation, allowing members to work to their potential and to aspire to the tasks performed by their supervisor. This is the essence of the occupation's design. A minority will realize that the PA occupation is not their final occupation destination. The one-life, one-career imperative is no longer active. Recall that the PA was designed by physicians and that, in the early years, the occupation was "managed" by medicine. PAs have now come to positions of great respect and power as educators and as members of organizations that represent PAs. These advocates for the PA must not become so attached to the desires of some portion of the membership that they jeopardize the most important features of the occupation.

EXHIBIT 10-2
Census Respondents by Current Professional Status*

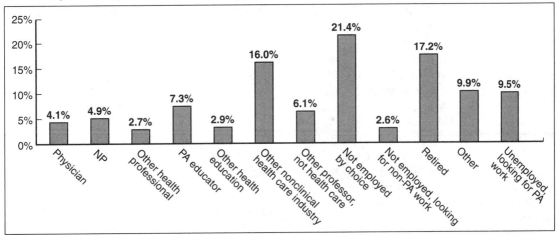

*Percentages do not sum to 100 because only select respondents were used for this exhibit. Respondents were instructed to mark all that apply in the questionnaire.

Data from American Academy of Physician Assistants. (2008a). 2008 AAPA Physician Assistant Census Report. Alexandria, VA: Author.

Although most people who become PAs do so because they want to work with patients, there are PAs who for various reasons have opted to no longer engage in clinical practice (Howard, 2000a). This role is similar to physicians becoming administrators and nurses taking on supervisory roles. Although including these formally trained PAs as part of the census is consistent with medicine and nursing head counts because their work undoubtedly contributes to healthcare delivery, it is difficult to understand the full spectrum of medical services doctors or PAs bring if they are doing work other than direct patient care. Nonetheless, many of these PAs remain active in the AAPA, contributing to development of the profession (Rogers, 2000). Not surprisingly, more than a dozen of the past presidents of the AAPA work outside of clinical practice.

The expanding roles for PAs are sorted into the following five categories:

- Business and management
- Legal and regulatory professions
- Academics, research, and public health
- Other professional clinicians
- Journalism, medical writing, and publishing

BUSINESS AND MANAGEMENT

Hospital Administrator

Rick Rohrs, PA, former AAPA and National Commission on Certification of Physician Assistants (NCCPA) president, recounts his personal career history in administrative medicine—one he believes is typical for many PA administrators. As a hospital-based clinician in internal medicine in Maryland, he gradually assumed additional administrative duties as the department grew. The opportunity to add skills in the management of PAs led to additional responsibilities over the years. Today, as Director of Hospital Medicine, Rohrs is responsible for more than 80 clinical staff, including PAs, physicians, and technicians in the areas of house staff, hospitalists, intensivists, and the operating room. Rohrs points out that, "More importantly than being a department director is the opportunity it affords me to participate in other hospital activities. This is the true benefit to the profession of PAs serving as administrators. Being at the table, whether in one's own practice setting or in the regulatory environment, is what has helped fuel our professional growth. The opportunity to present PAs as a potential solution has created many of today's new positions."

Mr. Rohrs is often asked how he learned his administrative role. He answers, "Frequently, PAs have had prior life experiences that afforded them those skills. Our military colleagues are a prime example of this. Others have gone on to obtain advanced academic credentials. I have long advocated a relationship between professional service and administrative expertise. These two elements often go hand-in-hand and build upon each other. I believe I am a far better administrator for having served in many PA professional roles. Testifying before a state or national legislative committee certainly prepares one for making a case within their own practice. Vice versa, preparing and managing a large budget in one's practice makes for a much more seasoned professional leader." After 30 years, Rohrs is part of the senior management team at his institution and well known as a PA house staff expert and advocate in the Maryland hospital sector.

Hospital administration is a natural progression for health workers interested in the management side of medical organization. Many PAs start by assuming some of the administrative roles associated with medical office or department management, typically balancing clinical activities with organizational roles. These roles include straight administration, health planning, utilization review/quality assurance, and budgeting. Others may pursue a management degree and move full time into these roles. Understanding the needs of employees by sharing a historical background in the same career improves the overall efficiency of management. Various attempts have been made within the AAPA to create a hospital administration coalition of PAs, but most PAs in these roles find their needs are better met by the professional societies devoted to healthcare organization and management.

Medical Office Administrator

There are thousands of PAs who take on management roles in the medical practices in which they work clinically. Some transition entirely to management responsibilities, while others retain a portion of their clinical duties. One PA who became a medical office administrator worked in orthopedic surgery for 9 years and then moved into the management side of the organization (Brotherton, 2000) (see Health Facility Owner/Director in this chapter). These job "evolutions" to management roles may come about as a result of attaining an advanced degree in a field relevant to medicine (such as an MBA) or as a result of a desire to leave clinical practice.

Financial Broker

A background in clinical medicine and pharmacology may be seen as an advantage in certain areas of stock trading and financing. Openings are few but do exist, with a couple of PAs working as stock analysts. They assess the market impact of certain drugs and devices under clinical trials and upon release by the Food and Drug Administration. Knowledge about a particular class of drugs, such as monoclonal antibodies, make them particularly valuable members of a brokerage house when the initial product offering is released.

Practice Management Consultants

Patient flow and satisfaction of providers are key ingredients to any organization. Some PAs serve as practice management consultants for health-oriented organizations. Their roles include advising senior managers how best to use the PAs and advanced practice nurses (NPs, certified nurse-midwives [CNMs], and certified registered nurse anesthetists [CRNAs]) within the organization. Sometimes the advisor role involves negotiating labor disputes and contracts with hospitals, emergency departments, and others, and negotiating with insurers to secure appropriate rates of reimbursement. In other instances the role may involve training support staff in public relations, developing policies and procedures for new clinics, evaluating staff members, and negotiating salaries for PAs and NPs (Blaser, 1993). PAs serve as consultants to groups to develop and deliver health promotions and provide health-risk analysis reports and analysis reports for the Center for Medicare and Medicaid Services (CMS). For example, Practice Management Resource Group, a medical organization consulting firm, was developed by an AAPA past president (Brotherton, 2000). Most of the work is in financial management and Medicare compliance. Having a clinical background is believed to help most consultants in healthcare management.

Health Facility Owner or Director

Some PAs have become owners of health facilities—usually small medical offices. Consider these historical scenarios: Two physician owners of a rural clinic hire a PA. After a time, one of the partners retires and the partnership half is offered to the PA. Later, the PA may even buy out the second physician or find another physician with whom to partner. In a variation on this theme, the PA owner hires a physician as an employee to act as his or her supervising physician. In northwest Washington state, a PA and doctor partner hired an NP because doing so involved fewer licensing issues than hiring another PA for the practice.

PAs have been developing or purchasing clinics in small rural towns to run for profit or purchasing part of the business, such as the office equipment or the building. Many times these PAs become the clinic's director or manager (Blaser, 1993). Barnes and Hooker (2001) examined these types of practices and found that the PA owners were very satisfied with this type of enterprise (Exhibit 10-3). Another enterprise in the 1980s was the development of a company made up of Medex-trained PAs. The corporation purchased small hospitals in rural areas and staffed the senior management with PAs.

Health Services Corporation Executive

Dan Konow, PA, MBA, joined RediMed in 1987 to work in urgent care. From there he transitioned into both clinician and manager

EXHIBIT 10-3

Satisfaction of Entrepreneurial Physician Assistants: A Comparison Between Self-Employed and All Physician Assistants

GENERAL CHARACTERISTICS	
Number of self employed	545
Percent of females	46%
Age (mean)	45
Years since graduating from PA school	13
Percent in clinical practice	100
Percent working in metropolitan areas	50%
Percent working full time	70%
CLINICAL SPECIALTY (PERCENT)	
Family/general medicine	35
Emergency medicine	25
Surgery/surgical subspecialties	13
STATES MOST LIKELY TO BE SELF-EMPLOYED (10TH PERCENTILE)	
Florida	
California	
Texas	
Arizona	
New York	

Data from Barnes, D., & Hooker, R. S. (2001). Physician assistant entrepreneurs. Physician Assistant, 25(10), 36–41.

and eventually the senior director. He has served as chief executive officer for the company since 2000. The business includes five urgent care clinics, two occupational medicine clinics, and four physical therapy clinics. Working as a PA was excellent preparation for his current job, Konow says. Along the way he learned strategic planning and budgeting, how to write policies and procedures, and contract negotiation skills. He now oversees 232 full-time employees, including 13 PAs (Kuttler, 2007a). "As a PA, we're trained to work as a team. It's the team approach to treating injuries and illnesses," Konow says. "As a CEO, I have to work with my team of managers, build consensus, and be able to communicate with different personalities and styles in resolving our operational problems" (Kuttler, 2007a).

Professional Society Executive

Greg Thomas, PA, MPH, is the vice president of Professional Education and Alliance Development at the AAPA. One of the important aspects of Thomas' affiliation with the AAPA has been to increase the PA professional staff at the organization. By doing so, he has helped the Academy develop from a small organization to a profitable and dynamic one.

After graduating from the Baylor College of Medicine PA Program and University of Texas School of Public Health, Thomas moved to Dallas for his first position as a member of the faculty of the University of Texas Southwestern Medical Center PA Program. Eighteen months later, he was recruited by the George Washington University Medical Center (GWUMC) in Washington, DC to become the assistant director of the newly created Office of Continuing Medical Education (CME)—a position that included clinical, teaching, and administrative components. During his 13 years at GWUMC, the aspects of the position changed dramatically, with the administrative responsibilities taking precedence. He became director of the Office of CME in 1988.

As director of the Office of CME at a major medical university, Thomas became involved in other aspects of CME and served on the board of directors for the Alliance for CME, a major national organization. This interest in CME and conference planning led to his first involvement as a volunteer with the AAPA. He served as a member and then chair of the Conference Planning Committee (1980–1989). In 1983, he was among a small group that established the AAPA Health Care Industry Advisory Council—a council for which he plans and executes an annual meeting. Through this sort of involvement, Thomas became connected with the organization. In 1992, he joined the AAPA staff on a full-time basis as director, industry relations—a position designed primarily to educate the pharmaceutical industry about the value and power of the PA profession. At that time, there were two other PAs on staff, Judi Willis (director, research) and Leslie Kole (editor, *Journal of the American Academy of Physician Assistants*).

In 1996, Thomas was promoted to vice president, Clinical Affairs and Education. Although outreach to the industry remained an important component of his portfolio, a new emphasis was placed on expanding the visibility and influence of the AAPA and the PA profession in clinical circles within the federal government and within other medical organizations. Starting in 2000, additional PAs were hired within the department to expand the presence and visibility of PAs within the organization.

Today, there are more PAs on the full-time staff of the AAPA; five are in the Department of Professional Education and Alliance Development, which is led by Thomas. The level of participation of AAPA staff PAs in meetings and deliberations of clinically oriented organizations and coalitions continues to expand.

As the AAPA has grown and matured, so too has the role Thomas has played within it. He is on the senior management team—a team of dedicated and tenured individuals. Additional responsibilities include developing and enhancing relationships with other medical organizations (specifically, physician specialty organizations) and creating high-quality, educational opportunities for PAs. Over the years, Thomas has held various positions on the National Commission of Certification of Physician Assistants. He represents the AAPA and the PA profession on committees and work groups of the American Academy of Family Physicians, the American Medical Association, and the American Academy of Dermatology. His involvement in issues related to CME has continued. During his career, he has chaired two major national conferences devoted to CME.

The decision to join the staff of AAPA over 15 years ago was the right one for me. Although leaving clinical practice completely was difficult at first, I believe that my overall contribution to the profession has been enhanced by the outreach that has been possible given my career with AAPA. Whether it is a meeting of CME professionals in which I am participating or the board of directors of the National Council on Patient Information and

Education (on which I represent AAPA), no one is able to ignore the interests of the PA profession when I am part of the discussion. (G. Thomas, personal communication, January 2008)

Medical Recruiter

Recruitment of PAs has become a thriving business for placement enterprises and recruitment consultants. Since the early 1990s, the demand for PAs has increased. This is in stark contrast to the late 1970s and early 1980s when PAs had to compete for the few jobs available. PA graduates enjoy a wide choice of employers in most geographic areas (Cawley et al, 2000; U.S. Department of Labor, Bureau of Labor and Statistics, 2007). In 2008, the marketplace for PAs is such that employers of PAs often utilize the services of recruitment firms. Demand has led some PAs to start businesses that provide assistance to medical practices and institutions to identify PAs as potential employees. These PAs essentially become businesspersons engaged in the identification and matching of PAs (and other health professionals) to employment opportunities.

Paul Moson, PA, one of the first Presidents of the AAPA, established and maintains a successful employment consulting service for health professionals.

Working with a recruiter can substantially ease, if not completely eliminate, certain out-of-pocket expenses associated with a job search, such as the costs of long-distance phone calls, printing, mailing, and faxing. These expenses can add up, particularly if the PA is willing to relocate and wishes to cast a nationwide net that includes as many potential employers as possible (Exhibits 10-4 and 10-5).

Insurance Management

PAs have been employees and managers in health insurance companies (other than HMOs) since the late 1980s. They help to review cases, assign discharge diagnoses (diagnostic-related groups), provide utilization review, analyze reports, summarize the medical literature, and provide advice on policy matters (Webster &

EXHIBIT 10-4
Information a Physician Assistant May Need From a Recruiter

- Is there a fee charged to the practitioner?
- How long has the individual been recruiting?
- Does the recruiter specialize?
- What is the recruiter's general knowledge about PAs, NPs, CNMs, physicians, and their relationships?
- Does the recruiter exhibit at professional meetings, and if so, which ones?
- How is the issue of confidentiality handled?
- What policies and procedures govern the dissemination of curriculum vitae, resumes, and references?
- What happens if the applicant finds a job through another recruiter?
- What if the candidate previously has been in contact with an employer?
- Is the PA seeking a job required to sign a contract?
- Does the recruiter have a contract with the employer being represented?

EXHIBIT 10-5
Information a Recruiter Will Need From You

- Curriculum vitae
- Home mailing address
- Phone numbers: home, business, and preference
- PA program attended and year of graduation
- Specialties
- Certifications (NCCPA, ACLS, ATLS, other)
- Work history (to include present and immediate past employers if applicable)
- Motivation for changing positions
- Current salary, benefits, options, and bonuses
- Desired salary
- Relocation availability and requirements
- Important criteria for selection of a new position
- Home ownership
- Family considerations (e.g., spouse's career needs, children's schooling requirements, parents' care-taking needs, and leisure-time interests)
- Interview availability
- Desired start date
- Employers you have previously contacted or positions previously applied for

Modified from Feichter. (1997). *AAPA News.* American Academy of Physician Assistants, Alexandria, VA.

Snook, 1990). In one large HMO, a PA had a collateral duty of reviewing the medical records of former members who wanted to return to the health plan.

There are more than a dozen PAs who have developed extensive leadership in state medical regulatory offices. One PA served as president of the North Carolina Medical Board and another PA was the executive director of a state board of medical examiners. Many PAs volunteer part time in state board regulatory affairs and leadership activities. For example, a PA is the chair of the health professions disciplinary board in New York. Another was the executive director of Arizona's medical board.

Ruth Ballweg, PA, MPA, is on the board of Group Health Cooperative (GHC) of Puget Sound and the past chair. The chair position involves negotiating contracts with the president and chief executive officer of GHC, developing policies, and being called on to give presentations and lectures. Ballweg is also chair of the Medex Northwest Physician Assistant Program, serves on many university committees, and is special consultant to the dean of the medical school. In 2006, Ballweg was able to develop a program, through her influence in GHC and Medex, to introduce dental therapists in Alaska.

Pharmaceutical Representative

PAs have served as manufacturer representatives for pharmaceutical companies since the 1980s—many for some of the largest firms in the world. Most major pharmaceutical companies have hired at least one PA for detailing products to prescribers. Sometimes they have remained in the area of sales, but others have found niches within pharmaceutical companies that allow them to specialize as research liaisons to clinical trials, region managers, and administrators.

Robert McKenna, MPH, PA, is a senior medical liaison with Merck Pharmaceuticals. He graduated from PA school in 1981 and after a few years working clinical, he was offered a position with industry. At first he worked as a sales representative calling on former colleagues. However, his knowledge about research and his ability to understand the scientific literature made him more valued in working with researchers. Eventually he rose to become a senior medical liaison overseeing a number of liaison personnel as they interface with academia and researchers. McKenna's presence at AAPA meetings contributes to the communication his company desires to maintain with a growing population of prescribers.

Clinical Researcher and Consultant

Early in the evolution of the PA profession PAs were employed to undertake clinical trials. For some private practice doctors interested in undertaking clinical trials, PAs were natural allies. As clinicians they would recruit patients, compile clinical data, perform examinations, and monitor responses to interventions being studied, such as drug therapy. In other settings, such as universities, PAs serve as clinical researchers, clinical coordinators, or project managers. They work with physicians and statisticians in the design, conduct, and production and publication of research studies. A few have become principal investigators. In a role delineation study of rheumatology PAs, 60% surveyed were involved in clinical research of phase II or phase III studies (Hooker, 2008a).

A few PAs have established small clinical research firms and consulting businesses. These entrepreneurial companies contract with pharmaceutical or research companies to conduct part of a clinical trial or recruit participants. They establish a contract with one or more physicians to be principal investigators, using their practice facilities and recruiting their patients into trials (Blaser, 1993). One PA-owned business maintains contracts with pharmaceutical firms in recruiting women interested in trying newer forms of oral contraceptives.

LEGAL AND REGULATORY PROFESSIONS

Attorney

Pursuit of legal education continues to be a career move for select PAs. Some PAs have become attorneys after experiences or encounters with the legal system (Blaser, 1993). Many have retained their identity as

PAs and membership in the AAPA, and several PA attorneys have returned to PA education and maintained an interest in medicine and risk management. A few have even returned to medicine after finding the role of a general practice lawyer to be too competitive. Some PA attorneys have found careers in PA leadership roles.

Politician

Every year PAs in the United States venture into the area of politics. Those who succeed have served at the local and state level. They function as mayors, city council members, and county commissioners; a few have become state representatives in their district (Simmons, 2000). For one PA, the political role came after being a professional lobbyist. Another PA entered politics because no one was running opposed. In some cases, the individuals are still practicing clinical PAs (Cornell, 2000b).

In 2009, the Speaker of the Assembly in California is Karen Bass. Ms Bass began her career as a PA and continues to advocate for healthcare expansion in California. This also puts her as the highest-ranking politician whose roots were as a clinical PA.

Health Lobbyist

Healthcare lobbying attracts health professionals, particularly those who had intense legislative experience working on behalf of their state PA chapters. Most are associated with a healthcare organization. Some PAs have become professional lobbyists. For many years, one PA was the chief health lobbyist for the American Academy of Family Physicians.

Forensic Scientist or Legal Expert

The role of the PA in forensic medicine has been documented on a few occasions (Golden, 1986; Wright & Hirsch, 1987; Cardenas, 1993; Sylvester, 1996). Sometimes these PAs function as city or county medical examiners or coroners; at other times they are called on to act as forensic scientists and experts in homicides (see the discussion of coroners in Chapter 7). There are a number of medical examiner offices, including those in New York,

Washington, DC, and other jurisdictions, who employ staffs of PAs. In addition, dozens of PAs provide expert witness services to law firms. These PAs review medical records, provide testimony, and appear at trials offering their view of the expected PA standard of care for either plaintiffs or defendants. There are several who have incorporated their legal expert witness operations, and there is also a professional organization, the American Academy of Physician Assistants in legal Medicine, that aims to serve as a resource to PAs in legal medicine, risk management, medical malpractice prevention, and medical legal consulting.

Disaster Management Expert

A significant number of PAs enter the PA profession with a background in emergency medical services (EMS). Following PA graduation, some of these individuals re-enter the field of emergency medicine in a combination of clinical and administrative roles; several have attained high-level EMS administrative posts in several jurisdictions and on the national level. One PA was a high-ranking EMS administrator for the District of Columbia. Other PAs have assumed roles in disaster management for public health agencies on local, state, and national levels.

Health Regulator

A good number of PAs participate in regulatory activities related to health occupations. These administrators work for agencies that write and enforce rules governing healthcare providers. Some PAs in health regulation are full-time, paid employees of regulatory agencies and boards, whereas hundreds of other PAs serve in part-time, volunteer roles on state medical regulatory boards or advisory committees. There is at least one PA who has been an officer of the national organization of medical regulators, the Federation of State Medical Boards (FSMB).

A PA has served in the role of chair of the medical licensing board in more than one state, and it is now commonplace for PAs (usually practicing clinicians who serve as volunteers) to chair and hold the majority of seats on state regulatory subcommittees overseeing PA practice or chair separate PA boards. One PA is the full-time executive director of a state medical board. PAs have also served as executives of major health professions and healthcare facility accrediting agencies.

Health Associations/Organizations

Over two dozen PAs have assumed positions serving on the professional staffs of health professions associations. In these roles, PAs work in various capacities, such as writing and maintaining public relations, governmental relations, and relations to industry, on behalf of a particular group or health profession. As mentioned earlier, a growing number of PAs are employed by the AAPA. PAs have also become leaders of health organizations and health-issue advocacy groups. For example, one PA obtained a law degree to enable her to head an organization advocating the right to euthanasia.

Consultant for Political Candidates

Since the early 1990s, most political candidates have found that they need to be particularly informed about health policy and healthcare reform. When establishing campaign strategies, many candidates and political office holders discovered they understood some of the issues affecting physicians, nurses, hospitals, and insurance but lacked understanding of other healthcare workers, such as PAs, NPs, podiatrists, psychologists, and nursing home employees. In some instances, PAs were involved in campaigns to help shape positions on health policy.

ACADEMICS, RESEARCH, AND PUBLIC HEALTH

Academic Educator

PAs now assume the majority of faculty roles in PA programs. Most PA programs have PAs in positions such as director, academic coordinator, and clinic coordinator. Because PA programs are set in academic institutions, the program directors and faculty usually have faculty rank ranging from lecturer to full professor. Dozens of PAs have attained the rank of full professor (see Chapter 4 for additional information on PA faculty).

Academic Dean

Randy D. Danielsen, PhD, PA, graduated from the Utah Medex Physician Assistant Program in 1974 and worked clinically for two decades, primarily in the Southwest United States. He was also in the Air Force and Army National Guard where, as a senior officer, he developed many of his leadership skills. Dr. Danielsen is now dean and professor of the Arizona School of Health Sciences in Mesa, one of the schools of A. T. Still University. Professor Danielsen provides leadership to the university with specific responsibilities in assessment, program accreditation, curriculum development, strategic planning, faculty enhancement, alumni relations, and overseeing the budget for the school.

As with most deans, Dr. Danielsen reports directly to the provost and, ultimately, the president. In turn, various department chairs or directors report to him. Says Dr. Danielsen, "The bottom line, as I see it, is the dean spends 40% of his or her time with the daily nuts and bolts of running a school. Sixty percent of the time is spent in strategic planning, budget management and development activities that benefit the entire university." Reflecting on what allows him to keep up with the multiple activities of a university, he says, "A good dean needs to look forever outward. To do that he needs a vice-dean and a few associate deans whose job is to focus inward."

Professor Danielsen offers that a PA fits nicely into this role if the academic has ascended from the ranks of faculty to department chair to dean. Interacting with other faculty members in other departments is part of that development process. The dean must understand and effectively articulate the needs of the school in order to effectively work together with other deans. All must have the university in mind as they advance their own agendas. Fundamental issues between schools and programs are the same:

enrollment, attrition, faculty enhancement, self worth, and budget.

Other needed attributes are scholarship (such as published research), communication skills, personal and professional relationships, organizational management, and the ability to recognize opportunities. Very few deans are anointed without a doctoral degree. The process of attaining a doctoral degree combined with the experience of moving up the educational ranks will prepare a PA to become a dean. As of 2009, six PAs are deans and another dozen are associate or assistant deans; one PA has risen to the rank of provost (Douglas Southard, PhD, PA-C, of the Jefferson College of Health Sciences). There are also PAs who have risen to senior academic ranks in major academic medical centers including at least a dozen tenured full professors, plus several department chairs and senior administrators.

Health Services Researcher

A handful of PAs work in health services research. Although it is difficult to break into this field without significant research background and experience, more and more PA programs are emphasizing this as an area of activity within their mission. As PA programs expand into graduate-level studies, undertaking research has taken on more importance for PAs.

Perri Morgan, PhD, PA, is the director of research at the Duke University Physician Assistant Program. She was a clinical PA for a dozen years until she qualified for a health policy fellowship at Duke. While working at Duke in evaluating medical workforce issues, she obtained her doctoral degree in health services research. Her work centers on evaluating policy issues as they involve the utilization of PAs, NPs, and doctors in the organization of healthcare services. Her evaluation of how national databases, such as that of the National Ambulatory Medical Care Survey (NAMCS), underrepresent PAs has drawn attention to how critical a role PAs play in off-setting physician visits (Morgan et al, 2007; Morgan et al, 2008).

Public Health Officer

Several PAs have obtained formal additional training in public health and serve in various roles in that field. One PA works as a state epidemiologist, and another has been chief health officer in several New England jurisdictions. There are a number of roles that PAs have assumed in the U.S. public health service, including senior management posts in the Food and Drug Administration, the Health Services Resources Administration, the National Health Service Corps, and the Bureau of Prisons, among others (see Chapter 17).

Medical Epidemiologist

The Centers for Disease Control and Prevention (CDC) invites PAs to qualify as health officers in epidemiology through an intensive Epidemic Intelligence Service course. PAs in this role are prepared to respond to disease outbreaks as members of a medical investigation team. A few PAs serve as medical epidemiologists at the CDC, Health Resources and Services Administration, and state level.

Biostatistician

Statisticians arise from almost any discipline: psychology, physics, economics, biology, business, education, sociology, engineering, or other disciplines that rely on higher order mathematics to demonstrate relationships and value. Some PAs who have obtained advanced degrees in public health or other disciplines have pursued roles working in research as public health professionals or other sciences using biostatistics for hypothesis-driven research. Typically, this level of research requires a master's or doctoral degree in public health with a strong interest in biostatistics. Several former PAs serve in the U.S. public health service as professional biostatisticians.

Linda McCaig, MPH, PA, is a U.S. public health officer and a senior researcher with the National Center for Health Statistics working with the NAMCS (McCaig & Burt, 2005). Her work is portrayed in large national studies and she has developed international stature for her analysis of antibiotic use (McCaig, Besser, & Hughes, 2002). McCaig's work with the NAMCS has also been useful in examining how PAs and NPs produce primary care visits (Hooker & McCaig, 2001).

Industrial Hygienist

Industrial hygienists are usually employed by business or large manufacturers to help with the health management of their employees. The petroleum companies were the first to use PAs in occupational health, and since the late 1970s many companies expanded their corporate goal of reducing worker-related injuries and illnesses by employing PAs as occupational hygienists. Their role combines the clinical aspects of the PA role with administrative duties such as overseeing the nurse and clinicians who are monitoring the health of the employees. Some of the Canadian military PAs have retired from active duty and become industrial hygienists for oil and mining companies.

OTHER PROFESSIONAL CLINICIANS

Physician

For a small number of PAs, the desire to become a physician motivates them to seek admission to medical school. About 4% of persons who have been trained as PAs have gone on to allopathic or osteopathic medical school. Typically, medical schools accredited by the Liaison Committee on Medical Education do not grant advanced standing to enrollees who are PAs. That only 4% of PAs have gone on to medical school is noteworthy. In the formative years of the PA profession, arguments were put forth about why this new health occupation would fail. Among these arguments was the idea that PAs would become frustrated in their role and leave the field for greener pastures. The sources of frustration envisioned by these critics included the stress and strain of being an "almost doctor," without the intrinsic or extrinsic rewards that society provides for physicians. Furthermore, the intrinsic rewards of professional autonomy in clinical practice would not be available because of the need for close supervision by a physician. However, the view that PAs would become frustrated because of a narrow and limited professional role is now considered untenable. Job and career satisfaction levels for PAs are extraordinarily high (Hooker, 1995).

Nurse Practitioner

Roughly 1% of PAs indicate that they are working as NPs. This percentage may represent individuals who completed a PA educational program that also has an NP track, allowing graduates to be eligible to become certified as either a PA or NP (AAPA, 2008a).

Chiropractor

There are at least 10 health professionals who have been trained dually as chiropractors and PAs. Some of these individuals indicate a level of dissatisfaction with chiropractic practice and seek to perform a wider range of patient care services working in a physician's practice. Others became PAs first then chiropractors to be able to perform manipulative medicine.

Counselor

Some PAs have become psychologists relying heavily on their clinical backgrounds to identify where psychosocial and medical issues overlap. Joe Marzucco, PA, MBA, PhD, is a mental health counselor. In 1973, he graduated from the Medex Northwest PA program and worked clinically first as a family medicine PA and then a urology PA. In the early 1990s, Marzucco obtained a doctoral degree as a mental health counselor and subsequently as a sex therapist. Although he maintains his PA credentials and lectures at two PA programs as an educator, he regards his career primarily as a counselor. Because insurance is problematic if a clinician has two clinical degrees, he does not work as a PA. However, Marzucco's PA credentials allow him to work as an adjunct faculty member in two PA programs and to provide medical education lectures for PAs in urology and sexual dysfunction.

Naturopath

PAs have formally trained as doctors of naturopathy (NDs). Sometimes they combine their roles to allow for prescription writing, and sometimes NDs have gone on to train as PAs. Although the role of ND is mostly clinical, many NDs provide education and counseling services.

Podiatrist

Similar to the circumstances with chiropractors, there have been a number of former podiatrists who seek a wider range of patient care duties as PAs.

Pharmacists

More than 50 PAs started their careers as pharmacists and then moved into a PA career. Sometimes they are able to combine these roles in the same setting, and sometimes they remain as pharmacists. A few are employed as researchers. One PA in New York works 4 days a week as an orthopedic PA and the fifth day as a pharmacist. He enjoys both roles but also finds dual jobs keeps his interest in both roles.

Veterinarians

In rural areas, some PAs will provide limited services to the health and maintenance of domestic animals. This is not the usual practice for PAs or for any human health professional, but with increasing shortages in large animal veterinarians and fewer rurally placed veterinarians, PAs sometimes step in to address the need.

JOURNALISM, MEDICAL WRITING, AND PUBLISHING

Publisher

David Mittman, PA, was a clinician with Health Insurance Plan in New York but felt burnt out from the stress of a clinical overload of patients. In 1983, while on the board of directors of the journal *Physician Assistant*, he took a job as an editor for the journal as a way to get into the publishing business. As he recalls it, "The second week there I accompanied a few salespeople to a pharmaceutical company and met with a product manager who doubted PAs prescribed. I took out my Rx pad and wrote him a prescription. I asked him to take the prescription to a pharmacy and if they filled it, we would get the advertising support the journal deserved. If not, we would never bother him again. Right there, he told us he would support the journal and a publishing career was born." Within his first year in the industry, Mittman won the Pharmaceutical Journal Advertising Representative of the Year Award for the work he did on *Physician Assistant*.

In describing the role of publisher, Mittman says, "The title 'publisher' is someone who is in charge of the development of all parts of a medical journal. It is heavily involved with sales, marketing, and less editorial than what people think. I took over *Physician Assistant* (the journal) and within a few years directed it in all facets, including a new editorial direction (although not as the editor)."

In 1990, Mittman, along with Joe Leahy and Tom Yackeren, PA, founded Clinicians Publishing Group (CPG). They launched *Clinician Reviews* in February 1991. *Clinician Reviews* was the first PA journal with PAs involved in its ownership and the first journal to publish for both the PA and NP professions. Within 1 year, the journal led the PA and NP publishing world in advertising, and within 2 years it led in readership. Mittman and Yackeren were New York State Academy PA past presidents and believed being involved in the profession allowed them a certain amount of credibility and leverage in approaching PAs and pharmaceutical firms.

In 1992, CPG launched *Neurology Reviews*, the first news publication for neurologists. Subsequently, almost every year thereafter CPG launched a journal for a physician specialty. In 1995, CPG also launched *Clinician News*, the first news publication for PAs and NPs. In that same time, CPG also purchased the Ithaca Center for CME and was able to grant physician CME credits and implement physician meetings and symposia.

In 2003, CPG was sold to Jobson Medical Education. When it was sold, the "old CPG" had a staff of more than 70 people, nine journals, and a number of other subsidiaries. After the sale, Mittman stayed on as a consultant for 3 years. In 2009, David Mittman returned to publishing with an online publication for PAs and NPs titled *Clinician 1*.

Research and Other Professional Roles

The literature about the deployment of PAs in other professional roles is sparse and usually confined to the lay press. Because descriptions of PA roles have focused mostly on clinical practice, there are large areas of data missing and many questions unanswered. A major question that is often asked but underexplored is the question of how PAs can use their clinical expertise and experience to advance their careers in medicine itself. A brief review of other areas in need of attention is provided here.

- **Case reports:** Writing about PAs in other professional roles provides alternatives to direct patient care. Case reports can describe the various types of PA roles that exist and the typical daily activities involved in those roles. Each role needs a case report.

- **Economics:** What are the trade-offs of leaving clinical medicine and working in a nonclinical role? Is salary a driving factor? What are the motivators for change?

- **Breadth of knowledge:** How does a lawyer (or any other professional) who started a career as a PA obtain his or her knowledge outside of law school? Does the acquisition of this new knowledge have different career trajectories depending on age, gender, and experience than clinically focused PAs?

- **Career selection:** Do PAs in some nonclinical roles have different expectations and aspirations than those in other roles? Why do some abandon working as clinicians, never to return?

- **Psychological profile:** Do PAs who become entrepreneurs share common characteristics?

- **Politics:** Do PAs in political office influence the development of the PA profession in any way?

- **Organizational staffing:** Do members of any PA professional organization perceive some value when the staff is composed of some percentage of PAs?

- **Clinical blending of degrees:** How do PAs who hold two clinical degrees (e.g., PA and DC) blend their degrees and clinical services?

- **Mixing careers:** What is the percentage of PAs with two degrees who began their careers as nonclinicians?

- **PAs as doctors:** What are the reflections of doctors who started their careers as PAs?

SUMMARY

Many PAs have expanded their professional positions in health care. Some have used their PA backgrounds and experience to branch into related fields, whereas others have acquired further formal education and taken on nonclinical roles. Employment opportunities and training have led many PAs into different, more complex roles. At one time, a small cadre of all PAs moved on to medical or osteopathic school, but this phenomenon has become almost nonexistent since the mid-1990s. Employment patterns for PAs are extremely variable, depending on the interests, capabilities, and personalities of the individuals involved. PA training offers a springboard to diverse professional roles.

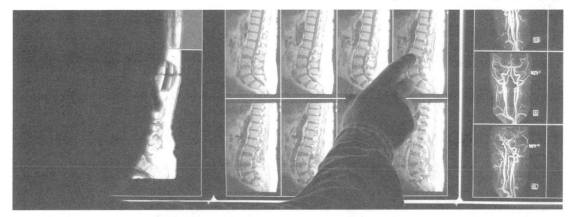

CHAPTER 11

ECONOMIC ASSESSMENT
OF PHYSICIAN ASSISTANTS

RODERICK S. HOOKER ■ JAMES F. CAWLEY ■ DAVID P. ASPREY

The introduction of physician assistants has been a responsible policy and . . . that many other innovations mediated by medical practitioners have gained widespread acceptance with much less rigorous prior evaluation than was given to . . . physician assistants.

—Walter O. Spitzer, 1984

ABSTRACT

Economics is the science that deals with the consequences of resource scarcity. This chapter deals with the roles of physician assistants (PAs) in delivering scarce resources: health care. The introduction of PAs into various societies has allowed labor, education, and organizational researchers to test some of the fundamentals of applied economics: substitution, complement, team effort, opportunity costs, and productivity. More than four decades of examination are available, and the findings are that PAs substitute for doctors at approximately 85% of the range of primary care tasks, produce approximately 2.4 times their salary in revenue, and are equally productive in outpatient visits. The opportunity cost of producing a PA is approximately 20% of a doctor and the PA produces approximately 5 years of healthcare services to society before a doctor is functioning

independently from postgraduate training. Although a PA is not a doctor, and should not be thought of as a doctor, at times the PA does produce a service that otherwise would not be supplied in the absence of a doctor.

INTRODUCTION

Are physician assistants (PAs) cost-effective? Are they productive enough to be considered replacements for doctors? If they are cost-effective, do the benefits of employing PAs accrue to the employer, the patient, or society as a whole? What happens to the output of a physician's practice (or inpatient service or outpatient clinic) when a PA is added to the clinical staff? Furthermore, what are the outcomes in terms of access to patient care services, level of quality of care, practice revenues, and productivity?

Although the practice contributions of PAs are determined by multiple influences, many of which are difficult to measure, a number of clinical performance characteristics have been described in the health services research literature. Many of the findings, some of which are from studies performed decades ago, remain valid well into the new century (Schneider & Foley, 1977; Greenfield et al, 1978).

Various studies over the past 40 years have shown that, within their spheres of practice competency, PAs provide lower cost health care that is comparable (and in some instances superior) to that provided by physicians (Office of Technology Assessment, 1986; Hooker, 2000; Morgan et al, 2008). Contemporary research has conclusively demonstrated that PAs are cost-effective in clinical practice (McKibbin, 1978), and substantial empirical and health services research evidence confirms the findings that they are cost-effective in almost all of the settings studied (Romm et al, 1979; Record et al, 1980; Record et al, 1981). Probably more significant is that the popularity of PAs and their use in clinical settings, after four decades, would be unlikely if they were not cost-effective.

Evidence indicates that the organizational setting is closely related to the productivity and cost benefits of PA use. Scheffler (1979) documented that PAs employed in institutional settings are more productive than those in private practice because they see more patients in the same period. Record (1981b) noted correlations among productivity, delegation of tasks, and organizational size and proposed that economies of scale and cost-saving incentives were the likely explanations for the observations of PA cost-effectiveness in the health maintenance organization (HMO) setting.

The performance of PAs in the delivery of medical care services has been under scrutiny since 1970. Initially, there was an interest in developing a more effective approach to the division of medical labor. Later, some researchers wanted to document the PA's effectiveness, whereas others thought the stories of PA use were overstated and needed to be refuted (Moore, 1994). Few professions just beginning have known such scrutiny (Spitzer, 1984).

The impact of PAs on access to healthcare services, quality of care, physician and patient acceptance continues to be measured with positive results, although the precise degree of productivity and cost-effectiveness of the use of PAs remains to be determined. It is the downstream benefits of PA employment that are unclear because the vast majority of PA productivity studies have viewed PAs as substitutes rather than members of interdisciplinary healthcare teams (Exhibit 11-1) (Scheffler et al, 1996; Hooker, 2001).

Almost all economic research on PAs has focused on cost-effectiveness of PA employment. Cost-effectiveness analysis is an economic technique designed to compare the positive and negative consequences of a specific resource allocation. The strategy is to measure the comparable benefit of a particular investment versus its cost. In health care, this technique is commonly applied to new medical technologies, diagnostic and laboratory tests, health facilities and delivery systems, and drug treatment and immunization programs.

The application of cost-effectiveness analysis to the delivery of medical care services and specifically to the provider of such services is a complex endeavor. It is difficult to measure accurately the content of a medical encounter, given variations in such factors as severity of illness, types of treatment, patient preferences, extent of use of diagnostic tests, level of provider training, and the site and mode of care delivery. Add to these factors the differences in the type of provider delivering a similar service and different styles of task delegation, and it becomes obvious that any efforts to determine cost-effectiveness tend to be methodologically difficult and quite expensive.

EXHIBIT 11-1
Physician Assistants on the Healthcare Team

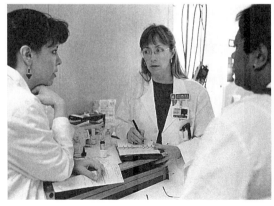

Courtesy of the American Academy of Physician Assistants.

PAs provide medical care services that overlap to a large extent with those services provided by physicians. Understanding what percentage of overlap exists constitutes the heart of the question for physician employers and health planners. Most studies suggest that PAs can substitute for (or complement) doctors in various ways. What is not clear is which services are included in these percentages and which are left out. The percentages vary considerably depending on practice setting and specialty, the degree of delegation of tasks by an individual physician to a PA, and the amount of supervision the PA requires or needs.

PHYSICIAN ASSISTANT COST-EFFECTIVENESS

Given satisfactory quality and patient acceptance, the substitutability of PAs for physicians depends on the volume of services delegated and the degree to which the PA's productivity matches that of the doctor in performing the delegated services. The delegation and productivity numbers can be combined to produce a physician-PA substitution ratio. For example, if half of the physician's services are delegated to a PA (or the PA's productivity is half that of the physician), it will take one PA to substitute for half of a physician, and the substitution ratio will be 0.5 physician:1 PA, or 0.5.

A review of the literature examining the issue of delegation identified 10 studies that used office visits as an output measure. The findings of these studies are summarized in Exhibit 11-2. In the aggregate, the range of delegation is extremely broad, 6% to 99%, with considerable overlap of the delegation level among the settings.

From the bulk of published studies evaluating PA performance, it is clear that most of the services performed by primary care physicians can be provided by PAs without consultation. The most rigorous of all PA economic

EXHIBIT 11-2
Delegation of Office Visits to Physician Assistants: Summary of the Literature

Reference	Study Period	Setting	Patients	Method of Triage	Level of Delegation
Record & Greenlick (1975)	1971–1973	HMO	200,000 health plan enrollees	By receptionist	79%
Record et al (1980)	1972	HMO	200,000 health plan enrollees	By receptionist	83%
Pondy, Jones, & Braun (1973)	1972	HMO group, solo (two), institution	Unknown	Not described	81% HMO, 36% group, 39% solo, 24% solo
Miles & Rushing (1976)	1971–1974	Solo	27,000 in rural Appalachia	N/A	33%
Henry (1974)	1971–1972	Satellite/independent	3,500 in rural Florida	All patients seen by PA	80%
Riess & Lawrence (1976)	1974	Satellite/independent	5,300 in rural Pacific Northwest	All patients seen by PA	90%
Watkins (unpublished data, 1978)	1977	Emergency department of an institution	200,000 health plan members	Triaged appropriate patients to PA	45%
Ekwo et al (1979)	1977–1978	Solo, group, and satellite	19 primary care practices in Iowa	By receptionist and independent	87%, 87% (satellite)
Weiner, Steinwachs, & Williamson (1986)	1975	Three HMOs	More than 300,000 health plan members	Varied by health plan	47%, 15%, 6%

Note: CHA, child health associate or pediatric PA.

Data from Hooker, R. S. (2000). The economics of physician assistant employment. Physician Assistant, 24, 67–85.

studies showed that the substitution ratio of traditional primary care medical office visits is 0.83, suggesting that it takes one PA to substitute for 83% of a physician in primary care ambulatory settings (Record et al, 1980). Other studies confirm that the clinical productivity of PAs in primary care ranges between 75% and 100% (Page, 1975; Scheffler, 1979; Mendenhall, Repicky, & Neville, 1980; McCaig et al, 1998).

If we accept the conservative assumptions that PAs are at least three-fourths as productive as physicians and are capable of managing at least 83% of all primary care encounters, and if we recognize that the mean salary of a PA is one-half that of a licensed primary care doctor, we can begin to appreciate the considerable cost-effectiveness that PAs bring to clinical practice. Unfortunately, these figures tend to become jumbled as a result of misunderstanding of the terms that economists use: practice arrangements, delegation, supervision, consultation, and cost-effectiveness. These terms, with explanations, are outlined in the following paragraphs.

Physician Assistants as Substitutes or Complements

Many studies have examined the role of the PA, and many authors have tried to determine whether PAs substitute for or complement physician services. In the classic economic definition, a *substitute* replaces a service with something in kind. For example, a kidney machine replaces a donated kidney, so both are substitutes for the original organ. A bicycle substitutes for an automobile (although not a perfect substitute, it is nonetheless a substitute). On the other hand, a *complement* is something that enhances the service being provided. For example, butter complements a piece of toast.

Feldstein (2004) points out that in medical care it is not always easy to know when an input is a complement or a substitute based just on the task to be performed. A PA may be as competent as a physician to perform certain tasks; if the PA works for the physician, and the physician determines the performance or directs the task, then the PA is a complement and will increase the physician's productivity. However, if the PA performs the same task and is operating relatively independently of the physician, then the PA is a substitute for the physician in providing that service. The essential element that determines whether an input is a complement or a substitute is who controls the use of that input.

Substitutability, as the term is used here, implies that quality of care is not threatened. In examining the literature on this question, Sox (1979) concluded that a PA should be able to "provide the average office patient with primary care that compares very favorably with care given by the physician."

Most studies examining cost-effectiveness of PAs have suffered some flaws based on the preceding constraints. For the most part, they have involved small sample sizes, analyzed experiences in only one type of ambulatory setting, compared nurse practitioners (NPs) and nurses instead of physicians, focused on primary care functions, and were incomplete in regard to revenue generation and cost data (Lawrence, 1978). Furthermore, most of these studies were performed in the 1970s, when the role of the PA was still developing.

Bearing in mind these limitations and recognizing that the published data are suggestive but not conclusive, it is asserted that the cost-effectiveness of PAs can be reasonably confirmed and measured to some extent by the data. Major studies of PA productivity and cost-effectiveness have shown that PAs usually generate practice revenue far beyond the costs of their salaries and overhead (Schneider & Foley, 1977; Mendenhall, Repicky, & Neville, 1980; Medical Group Management Association [MGMA], 2006). In addition, an important factor not commonly emphasized in major reviews is the nonmonetary contribution made by PAs to medical practice—a factor even more difficult to quantify than cost-effectiveness. Finally, even though one may never be able to precisely measure the cost-effectiveness in every practice setting and specialty, the fact that by 2009 more than 75,000 PAs (all countries) are clinically employed is significant empirical evidence for cost-effectiveness to some degree. Employers—physicians, federal agencies, clinics, and hospitals—would not hire PAs if they were not to some degree cost-effective.

Practice Arrangements

Practice arrangement is the organizational structure where the PA is employed. Studies have looked at estimates of PA productivity to try to determine the practice arrangements that best utilize the clinical services of PAs. Activity analyses used to develop a model of primary care practice organization and productivity consisted of listing the preponderance of tasks that fully describe most typical primary care practices. From this list, a model was developed that estimated that the introduction of a PA could increase medical practice productivity from 49% to 74%; that is, a physician usually producing 150 office visits per week may increase that number to 275 visits per week simply by hiring a PA. Nelson and colleagues (1975) also found that when PA providers were actually studied in medical practices, they increased practice productivity as measured by the number of office visits by 12% during the first year after their introduction, and 37% after their first year in the practice.

Reinhardt (1972) found that doctors who practiced in groups manage more patient care visits than those working in solo practices. He noted that medical care services delivered by physicians exhibited clear *economies of scale;* that is, showed patterns where the mean level of clinical productivity for each healthcare professional working in the practice served to increase the total productivity output of the practice as more personnel who could substitute for a portion of the physician were added.

Measures of PA productivity in the HMO setting are consistent with findings observed in studies in rural private practices, urban ambulatory care clinics, and geriatric settings (Frick, 1986; Hansen, Stinson, & Herpok, 1980). Scheffler (1977) found that PAs spend more of their time in patient care when working closely with three or fewer physicians in general medicine.

To estimate the savings in labor costs per primary care visit that might be realized from increased use of PAs and NPs in the primary care practices of a managed care organization, Roblin and colleagues (2004) analyzed 26 capitated primary care practices within a group model HMO. Data on approximately 2 million visits provided by 206 practitioners were extracted from computerized visit records for the years 1997 through 2000. Payroll ledgers were the source of annual labor costs per practice from 1997 to 2000. On average, PAs or NPs were the providers on record for one-third of adult medicine visits and one in five pediatric medicine visits. The likelihood of a PA or NP visit was significantly higher than average among patients presenting with minor acute illness such as acute pharyngitis. In adult medicine, the likelihood of a PA or NP visit was lower than average among older patients (Exhibit 11-3). Practitioner labor costs per visit and total labor costs per visit were lower among practices with greater use of PAs or NPs, standardized for case mix. The authors concluded that primary care practices that used more PAs or NPs in care delivery realized lower practitioner labor costs per visit than practices that used fewer PAs or NPs (Roblin et al, 2004).

Delegation

Delegation is a legal term and an economic term. In this chapter we refer to delegation as the percentage of primary care medical responsibilities that can be safely handled by a PA under optimal conditions. The term *delegability* was coined by Record to refer to the maximum level of delegation that can be achieved without threat to quality of care (Record et al, 1980; Record et al, 1981).

In one study at Kaiser Permanente, a large, prepaid group practice HMO, a multidisciplinary panel of health professionals developed a set of medical principles, focusing on the patient's complaint and medical history, for determining the limits of PA substitutability. An outpatient utilization database was examined for a year of clinical experience to identify the office visits that would have been

EXHIBIT 11-3

Percent Reduction in Primary Care Visit Costs With Increased Integration of Physician Assistants/Nurse Practitioners Into Primary Care

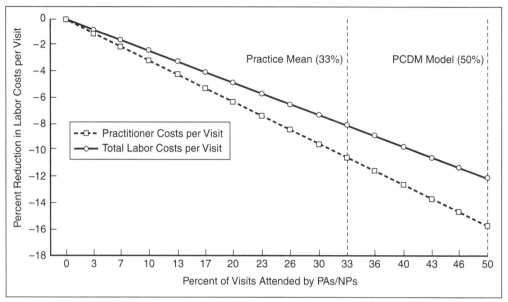

triaged to PAs had the panel's medical criteria been fully in effect. A number of conservative assumptions were used in undertaking this study. The theoretical construct was that the following would happen: significant illnesses such as cancer, renal failure, congestive heart failure, and similar progressive illnesses would be triaged away from PAs; all patients would be given a choice of a physician or a PA at the appointment; and no patient would be seen more than twice consecutively by a PA for the same diagnosis. PAs and physicians would be assigned the same number of appointments each day.

The research team found that the PA-appropriate medical office rate, or delegability, was 83% of the total in adult primary care during the study period (Record et al, 1981). This sentence, "PAs can take care of 83% of all primary care visits," has become something of an industry standard in medical workforce research. Even when other studies have shown that percent of primary care is higher, the 83% figure persists to this day.

Because of the economy of scale, large medical practices seem to be more likely to use PAs and NPs. These organizations, which include HMOs, the Department of Veterans Affairs, the military, and other vertically integrated systems, tend to experiment with new innovations in labor and technology. The other organizational trend in these settings is that doctors tend to delegate a larger percentage of medical services. By studying 70 primary care teams, Breslau and Novack (1979) found that a positive correlation occurs with size delegation. The larger the size of the practice the more delegation occurs. They found that delegation of technical tasks was greater by 24% and delegation of patient care tasks to be 6% greater in large medical organizations than in small office-based practices.

In a study of the potential for PAs substituting nonphysicians for resident physicians at two New York City hospitals, Knickman and colleagues (1992) conducted a time-motion study analyzing physicians' clinical tasks under two models: a traditional model in which the physician resident was the primary medical manager and an alternative model in which a PA or an NP performed baseline patient care monitoring. In the traditional model, residents spent almost half of their time on tasks they could not delegate. Under the alternative practice model, only 20% of the resident's time was nondelegatable.

The results of the hospital substitution study are applicable to many U.S. teaching hospitals. One survey of 144 teaching hospitals found that 60% of the medical directors reported experience with PA or NP substitution in their hospitals. One-third of the hospital departments said they were planning to increase the number of PAs and NPs (Riportella-Muller, Libby, & Kindig, 1995). Cawley and Hooker (2006) found an increase in PAs in hospital settings increased concurrently as resident hours were decreased.

Van Rhee, Ritchie, and Eward (2002) compared a sample of patients admitted to an internal medicine service where cases were compared between PA and teaching services. A total of 16 PAs and 32 postgraduate residents (with 1 to 3 years of training) in the internal medicine service were compared over a 180-month period in the mid-1990s (Exhibit 11-4). Resource use was measured using direct costs expressed as relative value units. The results revealed that PAs used fewer ancillary services for pneumonia, stroke, and heart failure. One of the conclusions was that PAs may be more efficient than residents in some hospital services.

Dhuper and Choksi (2009) demonstrated that when PA hospitalists replaced medical resident house officers, the results demonstrated that patient satisfaction and quality of care between the two groups remained unchanged. The case mix of the two providers was the same and the mortality rate during this 2-year study was significantly lower than the preceding 2 years. The authors concluded that the implementation of PAs as hospitalists was relatively easy.

Supervision

Supervision is a state-legislated term that has legal and economic implications. Competent supervision is essential for quality of patient care. However, sometimes restriction of delegated tasks can slow down productivity, such as interrupting the doctor to countersign all prescriptions. Loss of physician productivity can also occur if the employer's administrative tasks mean every chart needs to be reviewed and countersigned. How much time is devoted to supervision depends largely on the PA-physician relationship, yet little study

EXHIBIT 11-4

Summary of Sampling Scheme, Comparing Physician Assistants to Internal Medicine Residents on a Random Assignment of Patients to Two Separate Wards: January 1994–July 1995

Diagnosis-Related Group	Initial Sample Size		Number (%) Expired		Length of Stay Outliers (%)		Sample Size (%) for Study	
	PA	Resident	PA	Resident	PA	Resident	PA	Resident
Cerebral vascular accident/stroke	87	139	7 (8.0)	16 (11.5)	13 (16.3)	17 (13.8)	67 (77.0)	106 (76.3)
Pneumonia	126	132	16 (12.7)	6 (4.5)	16 (14.5)	15 (11.9)	94 (74.6)	111 (84.1)
Acute myocardial infarction, discharged alive	38	39	0 (0)	0 (0)	1 (2.6)	2 (5.1)	37 (97.4)	37 (94.9)
Heart failure	170	171	11 (6.5)	7 (4.1)	29 (18.2)*	14 (8.5)	130 (76.5)	150 (87.7)
Gastrointestinal hemorrhage	91	118	2 (2.2)	0 (0)	8 (9.0)	8 (6.8)	81 (89.0)	110 (93.2)

*$P < 0.05$ according to chi-square test.

Data from Van Rhee, J., Ritchie, J., & Eward, A. M. (2002). Resource use by physician assistant services versus teaching services. Journal of the American Academy of Physician Assistants, 15(1), 33–38, 40, 42 passim.

has been devoted to this important function. In 1992, the Department of Veterans Affairs surveyed approximately 100 supervising physicians of PAs and NPs (Alexander & Lipscomb, 1992). The average time assigned as the supervisor of a PA or NP in this system ranged from 9.2 to 16.1 hours per week based on a work week of approximately 30 hours of direct patient care (Exhibit 11-5). Although assigned the role of supervising the PA or NP, the supervising physicians were also engaged in patient care, usually in the same setting.

In one large HMO that employed PAs and NPs, the supervising physician's patient load was decreased by 10% per day. As a result, administrative time was inserted into the physician's schedule to compensate for supervising the PA or NP and reviewing medical records used by the PA or NP (Hooker & Freeborn, 1991).

Consultation

Consultation is the PA's decision to request a physician's assistance in a specific medical office visit. It differs from delegation, which is the doctor's decision to assign to the PA some subset of the physician's service. The consultation can be a part of the total delegated medical office visits for which the PA is responsible.

The *consultation rate* is the number of consultations of any kind over the total number of visits assigned to the PA in a given time. Many circumstances determine a consultation rate,

and consultations can take many forms, with varying time and cost results. For example, signing a prescription, verifying a radiograph finding, or approving a proposed medical management plan may take the PA's supervisor only a minute or two, but if a complicated case needs to be reviewed and the doctor needs to examine the patient, the consultation will take more time (Exhibit 11-6). The more time the physician spends consulting with the PA, the less time the physician has for his or her own tasks, thus decreasing the overall productivity of the PA-physician team. Another factor influencing consultation rate and duration is the experience of the PA. Generally speaking, a newly graduated PA will seek more consultations from a physician than a PA who has been practicing primary care for 20 years. Scope of practice as defined by a particular state may also influence consultation rates. One of the areas of inefficiency was to be a PA employed in a state that limited PA prescribing or dispensing. In this case, the PA had to consult with the physician on every patient who needed a prescription.

Consultation rates may be closely related to the level of delegation in a certain specialty or if the doctor wants to use the PA as his or her personal assistant. In other circumstances, willingness to delegate a broad range of services to a PA may be based on the assumption that consultation will be infrequent or that the PA needs little supervision. Other factors affecting consultation rates include the PA's

EXHIBIT 11-5
Physician Survey Mean Responses to Questions on Supervision of Physician Assistants and Nurse Practitioners

	Physician Supervises	
	*PAs (N = 75)**	*NPs (N = 34)**
Hours/week physician spends in direct care	33.0	29.7
Hours/week physician assigned to supervise the PA/NP	16.1	9.2
Percent time PA/NP takes first call for physician	20.2	26.4
Percent time supervision involves overseeing medical procedures	23.7	27.2
Checking orders with PA/NP	25.7	41.5
Other activities	50.6	31.3

*Number of responding physicians.

Data from Alexander, B. J., & Lipscomb, J. (Eds.). (1992). Physician Staffing for the VA. Washington, *DC: National Academy Press.*

Physician-Physician Assistant Consultation

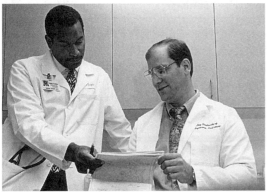

Photo courtesy of the American Academy of Physician Assistants.

relationship with the physician, the proximity to the physician (e.g., next door, down the hall, or upstairs), time, availability, and the patient mix. When the PA and physician share an office, the rate is undoubtedly higher than when they are separated by distances and office layouts that inhibit formal and informal consultations. Because consultations are usually informal, little has been documented about PA consultation rates. Time-motion studies documenting every minute of a physician-PA relationship would need to be conducted over a prolonged time to understand the importance of this labor assessment (Record et al, 1981).

Clinical Productivity

One of the first economists to study PA labor defined *productivity* this way:

> In theory, productivity is a simple concept: it measures changes in the total output that occur when small changes are made in one factor of production, with all other factors and circumstances held constant. Because these conditions can be met in the real world only rarely, productivity numbers are almost always rough estimates. Certainly that is the case with respect to [PAs]. (Record et al, 1981)

The findings on PA productivity reflect the changing policy concerns of the U.S. healthcare system. Initially, emphasis relied on documenting increased access to solo practice services in rural areas. Later investigations focused on costs and delegation in organized healthcare settings. An important contribution of health services research has been identifying the multifaceted effects of PAs on clinical productivity, meaning the overall output of a clinic or medical office when a PA is added to the medical staff. A common measure of productivity, one that can positively affect access to health care, is the number of patient visits performed in a clinical setting. The next question is whether the productivity of PAs compares favorably with that of physicians.

In virtually every study on productivity, PAs compare favorably with physicians (Crandall et al, 1984; Scheffler et al, 1996). In fact, there is evidence in some settings that PAs see more patients per unit time than physicians (Hooker, 1986; McCaig et al, 1998). PA productivity can be compared with physician productivity in two other ways: (1) on the basis of tasks PAs are qualified to perform, and (2) on the full range of tasks performed by a physician. The comparison of the range of these tasks is sometimes known as the *functional delegation* (Record, 1981a). For most practices, depending on the degree of task delegation, practice case mix, the healthcare delivery system, the context in which the PA performs the clinical service, and institutional policy, the use of PAs results in higher clinical productivity rates.

Nine medical practices that employed PAs were compared with control practices. The researchers found that the physician-PA team practices increased daily clinical productivity 4.4% (as measured by the number of office visits), whereas the control practices increased only 1.3% during the same time (Golladay, Miller, & Smith, 1973). Another study assessed the impact of a PA on the distribution of physician time in a small practice. After a PA was employed in primary care, a larger proportion of physician time was spent seeing older patients and seriously ill, hospitalized patients and communicating with patients (Nelson, Johnson, & Jacobs, 1977).

A small-scale study of the cost-effectiveness of nonphysician healthcare providers including PAs was conducted in another type of ambulatory care setting. This report describes the performance of four PAs and NPs and five family practice physicians, comparing measures of the practice costs of both types of healthcare providers working in a student health clinic, a type of prepaid system, and in a fee-for-service family practice clinic. Total hours worked, numbers of patients seen, revenue generated, and provider salaries were collected for the nine primary care providers over 49 weeks. In the student health clinic, the average cost for salaries to the clinic for each patient visit was $5.49 for NP and PA services, whereas it was $8.53 for each visit to the physician. In the family practice clinic, revenue generated per dollar of salary was $2.68 for NPs and $2.62 for family physicians (Hansen, Stinson, & Herpok, 1980).

Mathematical models have been developed to explore the most efficient contribution of healthcare personnel in different settings. The settings include private group practices, urban medical centers, military settings, and managed healthcare settings such as HMOs (Golladay, Miller, & Smith, 1973; Zeckhauser & Eliastam, 1974; Schneider & Foley, 1977; Cyr, 1985; McCaig et al, 1998; Ortiz et al, 2000) and tertiary care centers (Harbert, Shipman, & Conrad, 1994). Such models provide the documentation for the clinical productivity of PAs, with estimates ranging from 50% to 95% of physician productivity (where physician productivity equals 100%). These organizational and economic theories and carefully documented empirical approaches are similar in their assessment of PA clinical productivity. Hooker (1993) studied the hourly, daily, and annual productivity of PAs, NPs, and physicians in the primary care departments of internal medicine, family practice, and pediatrics and found that on an annual basis PAs see more patients than doctors in the same amount of time (29%). This difference is due in part to PAs being primarily outpatient based, whereas physicians had hospital or administrative responsibilities that took them away from the medical office (Exhibit 11-7). Patient visits to physicians and PAs tended to be similar in reason for visit in 90% of cases (the functional delegation level) but differed in illnesses associated with a hospitalization, such

EXHIBIT 11-7
Physician Assistant Clinical Productivity in an HMO Setting

Department	Patients per Hour	Patients per Day
FAMILY PRACTICE		
Physician	2.39	17.4
PAs	2.61	19.0
INTERNAL MEDICINE		
Physician	3.10	22.5
PAs	2.97	21.5
PEDIATRICS		
Physician	3.14	16.5
PAs	3.07	22.3

Data from Hooker, R. S. (1993). The roles of physician assistants and nurse practitioners in a managed care organization. In D. K. Clawson & M. Osterweis (Eds.), The Roles of Physician Assistants and Nurse Practitioners in Primary Care. Washington, DC: The Association of Academic Health Centers.

as for acute cardiac illnesses, cerebral accidents, and cancers (Hooker, 1993).

Whereas some practices employ PAs to meet increasing demand, others employ them to relieve physicians of excess workload. Some authors noted that after practices hired PAs, more patients in the practice were seen by appointment and more patients in the practice had specific plans for follow-up visits, suggesting more efficient patient flow (Kane et al, 1978; Kane, Olsen, & Castle, 1978; Olsen, 1978). Other researchers reached similar findings, which are displayed in Exhibit 11-8.

PA clinical productivity compares favorably with productivity levels of physicians, particularly in organized ambulatory care practice settings that use team approaches and structured division of medical care staffing. Although it seems likely that similar levels of PA clinical productivity exist for PAs working in other types of patient care settings, performance measures in newer practice areas, such as inpatient hospital settings, have not been performed. Additional studies examining levels of PA clinical performance characteristics are needed because the content of clinical care (the specific medical tasks) delivered by PAs differs within various clinical settings. It would be useful to know the number, content, and

EXHIBIT 11-8
Physician Productivity When a Physician Assistant Is Added to the Clinic

Study by First Author (Year of Publication)	PA-Physician Ratio	Productivity (%)*
Hooker (1993)	1:2	110.0
Cyr (1985)	1:1	80.1
Greenfield et al (1978)	1:1	92.0

*Productivity is defined as the percentage of patients seen in an outpatient setting compared with a physician's patient load.

patient outcomes of clinical services of PAs compared with those of physicians.

One of the many variables that is difficult to control in comparing productivity of PAs in different settings is the population base. Many significant differences exist between groups of PAs depending on the work setting, type of specialty, or years of experience. However, interesting findings emerge when some of these data are aggregated. Using data collected from the 1995 American Academy of Physician Assistants (AAPA) membership census, Kraditor (personal communication, 1996) examined the productivity of PAs in terms of number of outpatients seen per day, controlling for a number of variables.

Exhibits 11-9 and 11-10 present summary statistics on these measures of outpatient productivity for groups of PAs defined in terms of work setting, years of experience as a PA, and field of practice. All analyses used only data for PAs who reported being in full-time clinical practice and working for a single employer. Findings from this study include a statistically significant difference observed in the number of outpatients seen per day by work setting, with the largest differences reflected by PAs working in military facilities or correction facilities. When data on years of experience are examined, PAs with more experience see more patients per day than PAs with less experience. Field of experience also seems to make a

EXHIBIT 11-9
Outpatient Visits of Physician Assistants per Day by Work Setting, 2008

Specialty	No. of PAs in Practice	Mean Visits to a Typical PA per Week
Family/general medicine	20,554	88.8
General internal medicine	4,302	71.7
Emergency medicine	7,817	83.9
General pediatrics	1,891	94.2
General surgery	1,609	56.9
Internal medicine: cardiology	2,348	62.9
Other internal medicine subspecialities	5,310	59.9
Pediatric subspeciaties	1,311	53.0
Surgery: orthopedics	5,776	69.7
Surgery: cardiovascular/thoracic	2,134	41.7
Neurosurgery	1,457	52.5
Other surgical subspecialties	4,606	60.6
Obstetrics/gynecology (women's health)	1,723	69.4
Occupational medicine	1,974	80.4
Dermatology	2,872	102.2
Other	8,118	65

Data from American Academy of Physician Assistants, Research Division, 2008. Based on PAs reporting outpatient visits but no inpatient or nursing home visits. Data collected on the 2008 AAPA member census.

EXHIBIT 11-10
Mean and Standard Deviation of Outpatient Visits per Day by Years of Experience

Years of Experience	No. of Respondents	Mean	SD
Less than 1	139	18.6	7.2
1–3	821	20.8	8.8
4–6	505	21.9	10.1
7–9	341	21.2	8.5
10–12	410	21.6	8.6
13–15	371	22.5	10.2
16–18	343	22.8	10.5
More than 18	296	23.3	10.3
TOTAL	3,226	21.7	9.4

Data from American Academy of Physician Assistants, Research Division, 1996. Based on PAs reporting outpatient visits but no inpatient or nursing home visits. Data collected on the 1995 AAPA member census.

difference in terms of patients seen per day. The largest differences are found in emergency medicine, in which PAs report seeing 24.6 patients per day on average. Although these statistics are outdated they do reflect relative productivity of PAs.

When the PA work week was examined 10 years later (2007), the vast majority of PAs reported working an average of 44 hours per week. They reported, on average, seeing the following number of patient visits per week: general pediatrics (97), family medicine (90), and emergency medicine (88) (AAPA, 2007a).

The extent of PA productivity cannot be determined without reference to an array of interdependent variables, which, assuming that all of them can be identified, are difficult to evaluate. The classic conceptualization of how productivity should be measured—by observing what happens to total output when small homogeneous units of one input (in this case the PA) are added while other inputs and the larger context are held constant—is difficult to measure in a big practice and virtually impossible in a small one.

EDUCATIONAL COSTS

The cost of PA education in the United States varies widely and is influenced by many variables: public versus private school, undergraduate versus graduate, duration, and type of institution (community college vs. academic health center). For example, in 2000 the first-year tuition for a PA education ranged from $3,800 in the University of Texas system to $38,000 for the PA/MPH program at George Washington University in Washington, DC (Hooker & Warren, 2001). In comparison with medical student educational costs, however, the overall expense of PA training is relatively low. The average total cost for educating a medical student in 2008 is more than $150,000 (for residents of the state) in tuition on average; the tuition cost for educating an osteopathic medical student is estimated at $45,600 (Liaison Committee on Medical Education, 2001).

Student Costs

Student costs of a PA education include tuition and fees for the program, as well as required expenses such as medical equipment and textbooks. Also factored into student costs are the opportunity costs associated with pursuing PA education.

Tuition and Fees
A student draws tuition from a number of sources, including personal income, family income, debt, and/or financial aid. Although a large number of PA students receive some type of financial aid, it is usually in the form of loans that must be repaid upon graduation.

To assess the economic burden that PA students assume when they begin the education process, Hooker and Warren (2001) showed how PA programs compared in terms of tuition. Drawing from the theory of human capital, the authors looked at individual decisions regarding education and training. Although educational decisions can be influenced by love of learning, desire for prestige, and various other preferences and emotions, human capital theorists find it useful to analyze a schooling decision as if it were part of a business plan. The optimal length of education, from this point of view, is the number of years of school needed until the marginal revenue (in the form of increased future income) of an additional year of schooling is exactly equal to the marginal cost.

Data from 126 PA programs were analyzed. The total tuition cost of a PA education in 2000 ranged from $4,370 to $69,258. The mean cost of a publicly funded education was $14,366 and a private education was $38,846. At the time of this study, there were 58 master's programs and 68 undergraduate programs (bachelor's or certificate). The tuition burden of a master's program track was, on average, $32,531 (median $36,075; range $6,160 to $69,258) versus $22,685 (median $23,437; range $4,370 to $48,195) for an undergraduate track. The size of the entering class differed by type of institution. Private institutions averaged 40 (median 36; range 12 to 100) students per entering class, whereas public institutions averaged 35 students (median 32; range 10 to 80).

Because private institutions are believed to have more direct costs than public institutions, the total tuition revenue stream that a PA program would generate from the entering class was calculated. The gross tuition for the entering class for all 126 PA programs in 2000 was calculated as $61,385,864. For the 57 PA programs in public institutions, this averaged $251,293 (median $220,000; range $37,493 to $1,131,429). Gross tuition for the 69 classes entering private institutions averaged $682,060 (median $620,813; range $68,000 to $1,715,000).

The cost of a PA education shows almost a $65,000 difference from the least expensive tuition to the most costly in 1999. This sixteen-fold difference is found between public and private institutions, with state-supported programs being less expensive, on average, than private programs. Although this difference does shrink to a twelve-fold difference when duration of education is held constant, the difference still demonstrates a remarkable market demand for PA education. It also represents a large differential in the expected economic return to the educational investment (Hooker & Warren, 2001).

Respondent PA programs to the 2007–2008 PAEA survey estimated student tuition and educational expenses of PA classes entering programs in 2007 for the entire length of the program. These results are shown in Exhibit 11-11. (Incidental costs refer to living expenses, transportation, housing, food, etc.)

On average there was a $8,631 difference between state resident and nonresident tuition

EXHIBIT 11-11
Tuition and Expenses of Physician Assistant Students, 2007

	Mean	Range	*N*	Standard Deviation
TUITION FOR ENTIRE PROGRAM				
Resident (state) student*	$48,649	$11,362–$101,324	108	$22,007
Nonresident student	$57,280	$17,500–$101,324	106	$17,560
Books, fees, and equipment	$6,798	$950–$134,000	106	$14,711

*Students who live in the state where their publicly funded program is located usually pay a discounted rate over those from out of state. Private programs generally do not charge a differential fee.

Data from Physician Assistant Education Association. (2008c). Twenty-Forth Annual Report on Physician Assistant Educational Programs in the United States, 2007–2008. *Alexandria, VA: Author.*

among the 108 programs responding to the 2007 PAEA survey. Expenses associated with books, equipment, and fees averaged $6,798 per student for the entire professional training. The total expenses incurred by the typical student averaged $55,447 for residents and $64,078 for nonresidents. Tuition increased, on average, 9.4% per year over the past 21 years (PAEA, 2007).

Additional Student Expenses

PA programs were surveyed in 2008 to determine what purchases they require students to make. Medical equipment, supplies, and textbooks were required by more than 90% of the programs (Exhibit 11-12). Laptops and PDAs were required by about one-third of the responding programs. Fewer than 20% of programs required their students to purchase medical software or assessment materials. Other major purchases by students are shown in Exhibit 11-13.

Opportunity Costs

What is the rational trade-off between going on to graduate school and becoming a PA or remaining in one's current career? Because the cost of becoming a PA is more than the cost of tuition, economic reasoning for such a decision needs to include many factors. When these factors are aggregated, the result is an *opportunity cost.* Opportunity decisions are made every day, although they are not always made consciously or articulated. The economist puts a monetary value on this behavior as a means to calculate the trade-offs an individual makes.

When economists refer to the opportunity cost of a resource, they are referring to the worth of the next-highest-valued alternative use of that resource. If, for example, a person spends time and money going to a movie, they cannot spend that time at home reading a book, and technically cannot spend the money on something else. If the next-best alternative to seeing the movie is reading the book, then the opportunity cost of seeing the movie is the money spent plus the pleasure you forego by not reading the book. The opportunity cost of a PA education is the cost of a vocation foregone in order to obtain the education to embark on another career. It includes not only the tuition but also the earnings one would have if one remained a physical therapist or a paramedic instead of attending PA school.

EXHIBIT 11-12
Student Purchases Required by Physician Assistant Programs

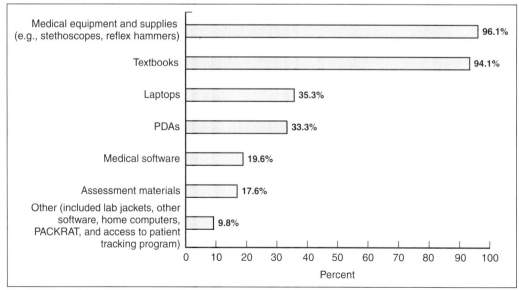

Data from Physician Assistant Education Association. (2008b). PA Programs' Purchasing Power Survey. Alexandria, VA: Author.

EXHIBIT 11-13
Other Major Purchases by Students

- *PACKRAT*
- *Health insurance*
- Malpractice insurance
- Transportation, parking, dues, etc.
- Housing at rotation sites
- Leasing fee for equipment/lab fees
- High speed Internet access
- Course manuals
- Scrubs
- Advance cardiac life support certification
- Lab coats
- Infection control certification
- Basic life support certification
- Memberships
- Clearances
- Patient tracking program access

Note: Items in italics had multiple entries.
Data from Physician Assistant Education Association. (2008b). *PA Programs' Purchasing Power Survey.* Alexandria, VA: Author.

The only study on opportunity costs of a PA education was undertaken by Philpot (2005), who examined the return to society by National Health Service Corps (NHSC) scholars who received training as PAs or NPs. By examining recipients of NHSC scholarships between 2003 and 2006 he was able to identify the payback potential between these two providers. The major findings were that (1) scholars repaid society's investment within 19 years after graduation, (2) PA scholars generated more tax revenue than NPs, (3) time to repayment was highly dependent upon scholarship debt, (4) NP students were required to forego an average of $5,216 more potential income than PAs during their training. The service period of NHSC scholars was not contingent on the amount of money invested in their scholarship (Philpot, 2005).

Makinde and Hooker (2009) examined the opportunity cost of a clinically active PA in his part-time studentship to obtain a doctorate in health sciences from Nova University (2004–2008). This activity was spread out over 4 years and involved traveling to and from the

university one to two times a year, tuition for online courses, purchasing texts, and other incidentals. In the aggregate, this individual was able to take vacations and extended weekends without having to take time off. The cost in 2008 dollars was $40,544 (Exhibit 11-14).

This case illustrates some economic trade-offs required for obtaining a higher degree. The value of earnings over a lifetime vary according to whether the time forgone involves lost wages or lost leisure. Personal career satisfaction and status are social benefits of such an endeavor but are also elusive attributes not easily captured in social research. What does the investment of a terminal degree such as a technical doctorate (DHSc) bring to the individual? Perhaps salary increases, administrative roles, independent research, or prestige. How this is weighed over a lifetime will depend largely on where the individual starts.

State Funding of Higher Education

State funding for higher education is related to the various policies the specific state is trying to promote. For example, in an effort to promote economic policies, states offer educational opportunities so that citizens will become educated, obtain higher paying jobs, and return something to the state in the form of higher taxable revenue. Although this approach is effective for undergraduate education, it is not necessarily the case with PA education. The debt incurred during PA education in terms of the opportunity costs (the income one foregoes and the debt one accumulates to obtain a higher paying degree) seems quite high for many programs. Many PA students are embarking on

EXHIBIT 11-14
Clinical Physician Assistant Obtaining a Doctoral Degree Costs

Item	Cost
Tuition	$28,260
Books, fees, housing, car rental, incidentals, etc.	$12,284
TOTAL	$40,544

Data from Makinde, J. F., & Hooker, R. S. (2009). PA doctoral degree debt. ADVANCE for Physician Assistants *17(3), 30–31.*

a second career. The return rate for some of the high-end PA educational programs may never be realized if a well-paying job is abandoned to become a PA student.

However, the potential benefit of state-supported education of PAs is that residents are then more likely to attend a state-supported school, thus remain in the state and offer a return to state taxpayers for their investment in higher education (Baer, Geslera, & Konrad, 2000).

Institution Costs for Physician Assistant Programs

What are the costs associated with starting and sustaining a PA program? These questions are at the heart of educational economics and are part of *human investment*. The students and the institution they attend are like firms—investing today for a return tomorrow. They are considered *investments in human capital*. Because these factors may be thought of as capital investments, the rate of return (educational costs) is viewed as an investment rather than the depletion of a resource.

Costs to Inaugurate a Physician Assistant Program

The cost to start up a PA program is expensive regardless of institution. Furthermore, costs are not easy to calculate because the analysis includes a number of variables and a number of unknowns. Some of the variables to consider are the following:

- Culture of the institution
- Whether the instititution is a medical school or a health sciences–based institution
- Whether the institution is private or public (private institutions have fewer rules and policies than public institutions, but have to fund internally; public institutions have more layers of administration and more policies and accountability, but may be eligible for state or provincial funds for start-up)
- Classroom and office space available
- Cost of faculty and supportive staff
- Cost of facilities such as clinical laboratories, simulations, and cadaver or autopsy laboratories

- Cost of a medical library
- Clinical education needs, such as clinical sites in the region and transportation and per diem cost for transportation, lodging, and meals for remote sites

To calculate start-up costs of a PA program a prototype PA program was created. PA educational trends over 5 years (2002 to 2006) and program costs were analyzed. The costs were part of data collected on 120 programs by the PAEA's annual survey. An *institutional cost model* was constructed. Built into the model were a set of assumptions of the program based on the experiences of the authors in consulting with new PA programs and the anticipated format of a new PA program in the year 2010 (Exhibit 11-15).

One of the assumptions built into this model is the purchase of clinical sites for clincal experience. Most American programs do not purchase clinical experiences, but programs outside of the United States do. A trend has emerged in which a few PA programs compensate their preceptors at $1,000 per 40-hour week, and others are likely to follow (Zayas, 1999; Kuttler, 2007b).

Because of the many variables not accounted for, we recommend setting aside a reasonable amount—2.2 million U.S. (2008) dollars—for the first 24 months of development prior to the first class entering the classroom. These are direct costs based on a public institution with a concentration in the health sciences.

Program Budgets and Expenses

In terms of the reported program budget, the cost of training the average PA student for 1 year of professional training can be roughly estimated by dividing the program budget by the total number of students enrolled. Thus, for the 2005 academic year, the cost for the typical program was approximately $11,320 to educate each student (mean budget of $990,527 divided by an average enrollment of 87.5 students/program at 27 months per student).

The mean total annual budget of 100 PA educational programs in 2006 was $873,977. There were wide ranges of total budgets ($105,598 to $2,993,000), depending on the size of the

EXHIBIT 11-15
Institutional Start-Up Costs for a Physician Assistant Program: Year 0–Year 6

ASSUMPTIONS
Existing building space
24 months from concept to first day of class
24-month program
20 students for first year
Add 5 students per year for 5 years: cap at 40 students per entering class
Sustain at 40 students per year
6 students per faculty
2 support staff per 10 faculty
Purchase clinical rotations at $1,000 per week per student (second year students)

Year	Activity	Costs (U.S. $, 2008)
0	Develop idea, assess needs, consensus meetings, travel, engage consultants, etc.	200,000
0.5	Employ project officer, education officer, finance officer. University leadership are brought on board and all are involved in many meetings.	200,000
1	Employ three faculty members and two staff (program director, medical director, academic coordinator, clinical coordinator) to organize curriculum. Have meetings and conferences. Recruit, travel, and enroll students.	1,200,000
2	Class I – 20 students Employ additional faculty.	600,000
3	Class I – clinical rotations Class II – 25 students	1,200,000
4	Class I – graduates Class II – clinical rotations Class III – 30 students	1,200,000
5	Class II – graduates Class III – clinical rotations Class IV – 35 students	1,200,000
6	Class III – graduates Class IV – clinical rotations Class V – 40 students	1,200,000

student body and the region of the country. The average cost per program to educate a PA student in 2006 was estimated to be $11,320 a year, a slight decline from the $11,500 figure reported in 2001 (Simon, Link, & Miko, 2001). The estimated cost per student is based on number of students enrolled and reported "program" budget. It should be noted, however, that these figures may exclude the following:

- Overhead costs provided by the institution
- Faculty, other than "core" program faculty (e.g., basic science faculty) that are supported by their respective departments
- Preceptors responsible for the clinical training of PA students

The primary source of internal financial support for most programs is the sponsoring institution. Based on 91 programs, they averaged $504,324 (median $476,000; SD $394,482; range $25,000 to $2,993,000). Federal grant awards to programs during 2000 ranged from $15,000 to $600,000, averaged $154,834 per program, and accounted for 18% of the total budget. Over the last decade when federal funding levels have remained constant at roughly $5 million a year, greater levels of internal support from sponsoring institutions have enabled programs to sustain operations and develop some measure of self-sufficiency. Other sources of support come from state grants (averaging $168,900 per program), research grants, program projects, hospital services, and practice plans (PAEA, 2007).

PA programs are periodically surveyed on their purchasing power and preferences. In 2008, a total of 139 program directors were surveyed; 53 responded (38%). PA programs spend an average of $32,488, primarily on the following five categories:

- Medical equipment and supplies
- Textbooks and other publications
- Nonmedical equipment such as laptops, personal digital assistants (PDAs), and smart boards
- Software
- Other major purchases

For the same categories, average student spending per program (for all students in the professional phase, a mean of 64) was $350,692. Exhibit 11-16 shows details of spending patterns of these programs and their students.

Other program purchases commonly reported by programs included simulators, training models, cadavers, office and classroom furniture, patient actors, and Physician Assistant Clinical Knowledge Rating and Assessment Tool (PACKRAT) standard examination fees. Technology, insurance, and consultation fees were also mentioned by some programs (Exhibit 11-17).

Programs were asked about major purchases planned for the next 3 years. Nearly two-thirds of the responding programs were planning to purchase clinical training models, simulators,

etc. in the next 3 years, and one-half of these programs have assessment materials in their 3-year purchasing plan. Exhibit 11-18 shows details of other planned purchases.

Efficiency of Physician Assistant Education

The theory side of educational economics asks whether PA education is efficient. As America increases its medical education system output in order to deliver more physicians, the efficiency of modern medical education comes into question. Does it require 7 or more years to adequately prepare physicians for a generalist role, particularly when PA education has shown that a similar task can be accomplished in far less time?

The seminal notion of Eugene Stead more than 60 years ago that gave rise to the PA profession concept was that physician education was too long and that medical education was distorted in its mission. Medical education, then as now, is characterized by a reductionist approach, where research and a singular biologic focus crowds out teaching, caring for patients, and addressing broader public health issues. Critics have called for a fundamental redesign of the content of medical training by, for example, placing greater emphasis on the social, economic, and political aspects of healthcare delivery and noting that "in academic hospitals, research quickly outstripped teaching in importance, and a 'publish or perish' culture emerged in American universities and medical schools."

EXHIBIT 11-16
Physician Assistant Program and Student Spending, 2008

	Medical Equipment and Supplies (e.g., stethoscopes, reflex hammers)	Textbooks and Other Publications	Nonmedical Equipment (e.g., laptops, PDAs, smart boards)	Software	Other Major Purchases
PROGRAM SPENDING					
Mean	$5,811	$3,202	$8,069	$2,998	$12,408
Median	$1,000	$1,000	$2,000	$2,500	$0
STUDENT SPENDING*					
Mean	$1,211	$2,408	$2,402	$70	$405
Median	$2,774	$5,503	$11,121	$130	$1,579

*Per student.

Data from Physician Assistant Education Association. (2008b). PA Programs' Purchasing Power Survey. *Alexandria, VA: Author.*

EXHIBIT 11-17
Other Major Purchases by Physician Assistant Programs

- *Simulators, training models*
- Charting desks
- *Cadavers*
- Diagnostic lab set up (exam tables, paper and supplies, blood pressure monitors, x-ray readers, desks, and lights)
- *PACKRAT/Standardized exam fee*
- Dry erase board
- *Office furniture*
- Wireless ports and electrical work to support laptops on student desks
- *Classroom furniture*
- Screens for projection
- Maintenance supplies
- Sonic foundry
- Casting supplies
- AV LED projector system
- Sutures
- Uniforms
- Needles
- Consultation for developing software for clinical rotations
- Linens
- Malpractice insurance
- Surgery tables
- Student gas cards for travel to distant rural clinical training sites
- Surgery scrub sink
- Conference travel
- Surgery lights
- Storage cabinets
- Standardized patients and assessment/testing materials

Note: Items in italics had multiple entries.
Data from Physician Assistant Education Association. (2008b). *PA Programs' Purchasing Power Survey.* Alexandria, VA: Author.

"Research productivity remains the metric by which faculty accomplishments are judged. Today's subordination of teaching to research, as well as the narrow gaze of American medical education on biologic matters, represents a long-standing tradition" (Cooke et al, 2006). Existing models that make the process shorter, more focused on the needs of society, and thus more efficient, deserve greater consideration.

These tenets comprise the heart of PA educational programs.

Many PAs participate in a 2-year post-bachelor education program, as compared with a 7-year post-bachelor program for internists, pediatricians, and family practice specialists. PAs receive much of their training on the job, having moved on with their lives and minimized their educational debt. In many practice settings, PAs and their nursing counterparts, NPs, function semiautonomously. Kindman (2006) asks: "Two years or 7 years—what can allopathic and osteopathic medical education learn from that?"

PA education has shown us that it is possible to train healthcare providers who are capable of most of the functions required of a generalist provider in a short timeframe. Harvey Estes, a major shaper of the profession during its first two decades, said, "The educational system producing physician assistants is more advanced, efficient, and cost-effective than that producing physicians" (1993).

Validation of this aspect of efficiency in education is seen in the choices that young people are making in terms of selecting health careers. Most faculty in PA education are familiar with the candidate who has the grade point average high enough to be admitted to medical school who chooses to enter PA training. These applicants have weighed the option related to the professional rewards and the length of training and have selected the PA profession. Estes and other contemporaries believed that medical educators must consider and incorporate the lessons learned from PA education and the profession itself (Estes, 1993). For example, Stead believed undergraduate medical education could be restructured to allow entering students to select a generalist track that would involve a shorter period of training versus a specialist track (Stead, 2001).

Comparing Physician Assistant and Medical Education Costs

Theoretic economic projections of the cost savings that could accrue under optimal conditions of nonphysician use are considerable, perhaps as much as $4 to $5 billion for PAs

EXHIBIT 11-18
Major Physician Assistant Program Purchases Anticipated Over the Next 3 Years

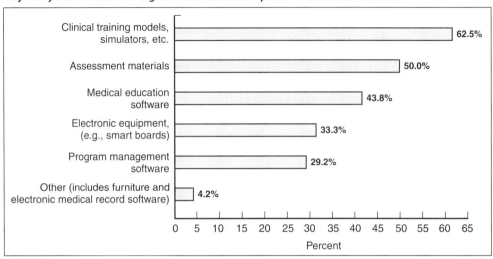

Data from Physician Assistant Education Association. (2008b). PA Programs' Purchasing Power Survey. Alexandria, VA: Author.

alone. For physicians, the three education-cost components are:

- medical school costs,
- graduate (resident) training costs, and
- opportunity costs.

The value of services to patients provided during medical training is often debated. There is a high cost of supervision and decreased productivity (at least in theory) because of this supervision, as well as staffing costs, inefficiencies in care, and overhead. Most economists tend to consider the value to society during the resident years (postgraduate years 1 through 3) as a net sum of zero in internal medicine and family medicine. More important, the opportunity cost (forgone years of practice) is large during this training period because "independent doctor" productivity is delayed until after the period of postgraduate training.

Because virtually no physician begins practice after medical school graduation, we must consider the cost of medical training as 7 years based on 4 years of medical school and at least 3 years of postgraduate residency. A PA chooses a different path of education that is approximately 2 years long. If

the medical student had chosen to be a PA, practice income would have begun after 2 years of professional training. Using the PA salary rather than the potential income of a 4-year medical school plus 3-year postgraduate-trained physician, we can estimate the cost differential of physicians and PAs.

Both the PA and the medical student start approximately from the same place academically. The average PA student has a baccalaureate degree, as does the medical student. Most have the same type of background with varying combinations of academic course work in their undergraduate years. Given the overlapping training periods for doctors and PAs, the opportunity costs for these two can be calculated and compared.

In Exhibit 11-19 the PA and medical students are assumed to begin education after completion of 4 years of undergraduate study (most enter medical school and PA school with a baccalaureate degree acquired after 4 years). The PA becomes fully productive after 2 years of education and the physician becomes a fully productive provider of care 5 years after the PA. Using the labor economic assumption that a provider is valued by his or her salary level, and that the PA salary is $65,000, the PA has delivered $325,000 ($65,000 × 5 years) worth of care before the physician begins practice. This figure is defined as the opportunity cost of additional medical education and training for the North American doctor. It is also the value of care that would have been delivered to society had the medical student chosen a PA training course.

Exhibit 11-19 also illustrates the opportunity cost of additional medical education and training. If direct training costs are assumed to be approximately $30,000 for a PA and $140,000 for a primary care allopathic physician, the difference between the physician and the PA in total training costs in 2008 may be calculated as $140,000 minus $30,000, plus the protracted training ($140,000 – $30,000 + $325,000). The differential is nearly $435,000 per PA that society gains by having a PA trained instead of a physician. Put another way, the PA produces $435,000 worth of patient care before the physician begins practice.

If salary costs are used as a proxy for employment costs, the physician-PA differential is $74,000 (the differences between the average primary care salaries of $142,000 for physicians and $65,000 for PAs). This means the salary cost of a PA is 0.45 of a physician. If it requires 10% of a physician's time to supervise a PA, 10% of $142,000 should be added to the cost of employing a PA. The PA-doctor cost ratio as viewed by an employer would then become $65,000:$156,000, or 0.42. When Record and colleagues (1980) made the original calculations using 1977 data, they found the cost ratio of hiring a PA to be 0.38 based on a wider disparity between PA and physician salaries. Since that time both physician and PA salaries have steadily climbed, and in 2008 are closer to 0.50.

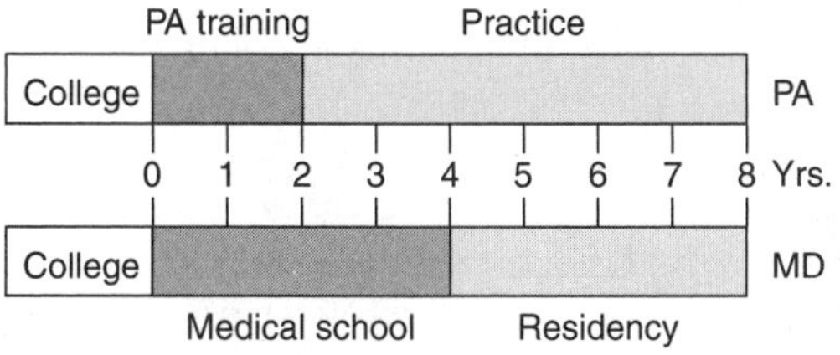

COSTS OF PRACTICING PHYSICIAN ASSISTANTS

Cost implications of the use of PAs can be viewed from three perspectives. The first is that of the entrepreneurial doctor or medical practice: Will revenue resulting from hiring a PA exceed the additional costs of compensating the provider? Second, if market conditions warrant, the focus is whether it is more desirable to hire a doctor or a PA. The third is the societal concern: How to deliver high-quality care at minimal cost? For many economists, the social economic view is all that counts; no matter where costs come from. In the end, all costs are ultimately borne by society.

Employment Costs of Physician Assistants

A number of direct and indirect costs must be considered when a PA is employed. These costs include salary, benefits, malpractice insurance, office space, equipment, support staff, supplies, and other direct and indirect expenses. Data on this subject are sparse, although there is little to suggest that costs other than compensation are different from those associated with employing a physician. Only one outcome study has been undertaken demonstrating that a PA uses no more laboratory and imaging orders and drugs for an episode of care than a physician (Exhibit 11-20) (Hooker, 2002). Aside from anecdotal reports suggesting that malpractice insurance may be substantially less for the PA because the litigation rate is less than it is for physicians, there

EXHIBIT 11-19

Cost Comparison of Physician Assistant and Physician Training Programs in 2008 Dollars

	PA student	MD student
Cost/year	$15,000	$35,000
Years of training	2	4
Total	$30,000	$140,000

EXHIBIT 11-20
Multivariate Regression Cost Model Holding Different Valuables Constant While Examining for Differences Between Types of Providers

Provider	N	Total Cost	Visit Cost	Med Cost	Image Cost	Lab Cost
BRONCHITIS EPISODE COST						
Physician	1,336	$234.74	$133.63*	$96.42**	$3.31	$1.37
PA	411	$224.13	$92.23*	$125.74	$4.65	$1.50
TENDINITIS EPISODE COSTS						
Physician	264	$183.33**	$144.77*	$30.14	$7.50	$0.93
PA	90	$149.80**	$98.77*	$40.65	$9.53	$0.84
OTITIS MEDIA EPISODE COSTS						
Physician	6,264	$188.39*	$140.07*	$47.77	$0.0	$0.54
PA	2,008	$136.60*	$83.29*	$52.99	$0.0	$0.32
URINARY TRACT INFECTION EPISODE COSTS						
Physician	1,633	$262.17*	$142.73	$83.91	$17.67*	$17.86**
PA	878	$210.50*	$97.70*	$91.50	$5.80*	$15.48**
TOTAL	12,866					

*Significant at $p < 0.001$.
**Significant at $p < 0.01$.

Data from Hooker, R.S. (2002). A cost analysis of physician assistants in primary care. Journal of the American Academy of Physician Assistants, 15(11), 39–42, 45, 48 passim.

seems to be little to suggest that PAs lose any of their cost-effectiveness by the way they practice medicine.

In contrast to other costs, the income differential for PAs and physicians is clearly quite large. Most PAs are employees and therefore are salaried, whereas self-employed physicians receive not only a stream of revenue for their own services but also entrepreneurial benefit from employing a revenue-generating provider.

Salary Data

Based on U.S. Bureau of Labor Statistics data collected in 2008, $74,270 was the median salary estimate for an experienced family medicine PA in that year. The figure for a primary care physician in the same year was approximately $149,850 (U.S. Department of Labor, Bureau of Labor Statistics, 2008). Therefore, the PA was at 0.50 of the salary of the physician in primary care. This ratio has fluctuated between 40% and 50% for 30 years. The ratio is higher when using American Medical Association (AMA) and AAPA data

and lower when using Bureau of Labor Statistics data. Differences between the the Bureau of Labor Statistics data and AAPA (or AMA) data may be due to bias selection; professional society members (such as doctors and PAs with high salaries) are more likely to join than those with low salaries. In 2009, the AAPA estimates that the average annual salary for a PA was $89,898.

What is more difficult to calculate is the benefits associated with each type of employment (doctor vs. PA). The doctor may be a partner of a medical group, may have bonuses at the end of the year, and different time-off arrangements. The PA tends to be salaried and not a partner in the practice. As information emerges from various countries where salary and income are more standardized and can be more accurately accounted for, the differences may be a more reliable gauge of worth of a career.

Perquisites (Fringe Benefits)

Although the *compensation* package (which includes salary and benefits) of a PA may differ monetarily from that of a physician colleague in the same work organization, there are some parallels in the types of perquisites offered. For example, in 2006 60% of doctors reported receiving a signing bonus that averaged $20,480 (Merritt et al, 2006). For PAs a signing bonus is between $5,000 and $10,000. Relocation allowances are another $5,000 to $10,000.

Other perquisites include health insurance, malpractice insurance, a retirement plan, allowances for journals and continuing education, and paid time off to take coursework. Retirement benefits run between $4,500 and $4,800 for PAs compared to $14,225 for internists and $12,529 for family practitioners who do not deliver babies.

Financials are another fringe benefit that are folded into PA and doctor compensation. In 2006, 24% of PAs reported receiving a bonus based on their individual performance, with revenue generated being the most common yardstick. Extra pay was also received for overtime, assisting on surgeries, administrative duties, and on-call availability and services. In all, 68% of PAs reported some form of additional pay besides their base salary (AAPA, 2007a).

Compensation-Production Ratio

One of the better ways to examine the net value of a PA is the income generated to the employer in private practice. Compensation, which includes salary and benefits collectively, is usually examined. The most useful ratio is the amount of compensation the employer forgoes to retain the PA divided by the amount of revenue the PA returns to the employer. Basically, the smaller the ratio the more economical the provider is to the practice. The Medical Group Management Association (MGMA) collects these data annually (Exhibit 11-21). In 2004, the compensation-production ratio for PAs was 0.27. For comparison, the compensation-production ratio for family practice physicians was 0.57; for pediatricians, 0.49; for NPs, 0.42; and for psychologists 0.79. These findings suggest that PAs are relatively more economical to employ since they return more revenue for their salary than other providers (MGMA, 2005).

Substitution Ratios

Substitution is the degree of labor one worker can assume for another. Primarily the level of delegation and comparative productivity of

EXHIBIT 11-21

Compensation to Gross Charges Ratio for Physician Assistants and Other Types of Providers, 2004

Provider Type	No. of Providers	Medical Practices	Mean
Overall for primary care PAs	259	73	0.267
ORGANIZATION TYPE			
Single specialty	36	17	0.252
Multispecialty	223	256	0.239
OTHER PROVIDERS			
Family practice physician (without obstetrician)	1,621	232	0.527
Internal medicine physician	1,289	187	0.541
Pediatric physician	941	147	0.485
Nurse practitioner	392	138	0.420
Midwife (outpatient and inpatient)	51	24	0.658
Optometrist	91	35	0.494
Psychologist	68	26	0.793
Podiatrist	60	37	0.485

Data from Medical Group Management Association. (2005). Physician Compensation and Production Survey: 2005 Report Based on 2004 Survey. Englewood, CO: Medical Group Management Association.

physicians and PAs for the delegated services determine the physician-PA substitution ratio. A substitution ratio of 1.0 implies unity and is achieved when one PA completely substitutes for one doctor. PAs in rural and isolated clinics commonly function at very high levels, often replacing the physician who was previously occupying that role (DeBarth, 1996). These accounts are largely anecdotal, however, and little is known about the types and numbers of patients seen by physicians versus PAs in comparable settings. The best studies occur in large managed care settings in which some of the variables can be controlled and physicians and PAs work alongside each other, seeing similar patients at the same time and under the same circumstances.

Using an urban healthcare center as a paradigm, one study constructed production functions that would best exploit the possibilities of substituting PAs for physicians. It was estimated that one PA could replace one-half of a full-time physician. From data developed in a national survey of physicians, Scheffler (1979) estimated that a 10% increase in the medical office visits output of a practice would require, on average, an increase of 3.5% in physician hours or 5.4% in PA hours. These percentages suggest a marginal substitution ratio of 0.63, as compared with the overall 0.50 ratio estimated by Zeckhauser and Eliastom (1974).

Another mathematic model tested with data from seven HMOs to demonstrate the potential impact of PAs and NPs on physician requirements found that in adult medicine, the addition of 12.7 PAs and/or NPs would permit physician numbers to drop from 16.4 to 9.7. Thus, the 12.7 PAs and/or NPs could replace 4.6 physicians (Schneider & Foley, 1977). The respective substitution ratio is calculated as 0.53.

Record (1981a) estimated that if enough PAs were hired to perform all of the services for which they were considered competent by physicians in the Department of Internal Medicine at Kaiser Permanente, and if the PA and physician work weeks were equal, the substitution ratio would be 0.76. Steinwachs and colleagues (1986) studied ambulatory care in another HMO and found the substitution

ratio to be .38 in adult care and .48 in pediatrics. The ratios might have been higher if the base had been primary care, as it was in the Record study (1981a), with outpatient specialty services excluded. Hooker (1993) developed data that suggest the ratio was 0.90, and Page's work (1975) in the military was close to unity (0.99).

Most of the estimates of substitution ratios fall in the range of 0.65 to 0.95, suggesting it would take, on average, approximately one PA to substitute for three-fourths of a primary care doctor. For managers, this suggests that four PAs could replace three physicians.

REIMBURSEMENT

There are four major ways a physician is reimbursed for his or labor: fee for service, fee per case, per capita, and lump-sum payment (salary). As employees of doctors, PAs must be cost-effective to allow the reimbursement rate to adequately compensate for their labors and the cost to the physician employer for his or her risk in employing the PA. Reimbursement of PAs directly also occurs, depending on various scenarios. The three major methods of reimbursing American PAs for services is Medicare, Medicaid, and third-party reimbursement from private insurance companies.

Medicare Coverage for Physician Assistants

The first Medicare coverage of medical services provided by PAs was authorized by the Rural Health Clinic Services Act in 1977. In the two decades following this act, Congress incrementally expanded Medicare Part B payment for services provided by PAs authorizing coverage in hospitals, nursing facilities, rural federally designated health professional shortage areas (HPSAs), and for first assisting with surgery. In 1997, the Balanced Budget Act extended coverage to all practice settings at one uniform rate (85% of the prevailing reimbursement rate for doctors).

Since 1998, Medicare pays the PAs' employers for medical services provided by PAs in all settings at 85% of the physician's fee schedule

(Exhibit 11-22). This payment includes work performed in hospitals (inpatient, outpatient, and emergency departments), nursing facilities, homes, offices and clinics, as well as first assisting with surgery. Assignment of fees is mandatory and state law determines supervision and scope of practice. Hospitals that bill Part B for services provided by PAs may not at the same time include PA salaries in the hospital's cost reports.

Outpatient services provided in offices and clinics may still be billed under Medicare's "incident-to" provisions if Medicare's restrictive billing guidelines are met. This form of billing allows payment at 100% of the fee schedule if: (1) the physician is physically on site when the PA provides care, (2) the physician treats all new Medicare patients (PAs may provide the subsequent care), and (3) established Medicare patients with new

medical problems are personally treated by the physician (PAs may provide the subsequent care).

According to the Balanced Budget Act, PAs (using the 85% reimbursement benefit) may be either W-2, leased employees, or independent contractors. The employer would still bill Medicare for the services provided by the PA. All PAs who treat Medicare patients must have a provider identification number (PIN). In 2002, the Centers for Medicare and Medicaid Services issued new instructions that permitted PAs to have an ownership interest in an approved corporate entity (e.g., professional medical corporation) that bills the Medicare program if that corporation qualifies as a provider or supplier of Medicare services. The new policy also removed a provision that prohibited ambulatory surgical centers from employing PAs.

EXHIBIT 11-22
Medicare Policy for Physician Assistants

Setting	Supervision Requirement	Reimbursement Rate	Services
Office/clinic when physician is not on site	State law	85% of physician's fee schedule	All services PA is legally authorized to provide that would have been covered if provided personally by a physician
Office/clinic when physician is on site	Physician must be in the suite of offices	100% of physician's fee schedule*	Same as above
Home visit/house call	State law	85% of physician's fee schedule	Same as above
Skilled nursing facility and nursing facility	State law	85% of physician's fee schedule	Same as above
Office or home visit if rural Health Professional Shortage Area	State law	85% of physician's fee schedule	Same as above
Hospital	State law	85% of physician's fee schedule	Same as above
First assisting at surgery in all settings	State law	85% of physician's first assist fee schedule**	Same as above
Federally certified rural health clinics	State law	85% of physician's fee schedule	Same as above
HMO†	State law	85% of physician's fee schedule	Same as above

*Using carrier guidelines for "incident to" services.

**For example, 85% × 16% = 13.6% of surgeon's fee.

†Some Medicare/HMO risk contracts may exclude nonphysician providers.

Medicaid Coverage

All 50 states and the federal district cover medical services provided by PAs under their state-based Medicaid programs. The rate of reimbursement, which is paid to the employing practice and not directly to the PA, is either the same as or slightly lower than that paid to physicians.

Private Insurance

There are more than 100 health insurance companies in the United States. Private insurers generally cover medical services provided by PAs when they are included as part of the physician's bill or as part of a global fee for surgery. A long-standing American Medical Association (AMA) policy (April 1978) recommends that:

> ... reimbursement for services of a physician['s] assistant be made directly to the employing physician. In instances where the PA is providing services in the physician's office and in conjunction with the physician, the cost of such services would appropriately be a part of the physician's charge as is now the case with other personnel he employs. When the PA provides physician-like services to a patient under the direction of, but in a location physically remote from the employing physician, AMA has recommended that the physician bill for such services on the basis of the usual, customary and reasonable charges concept.

Although insurance companies have discretion regarding what rate they may reimburse a

PA for services, the standard rate that emerged after the Balanced Budget Act of 1997 is at 85% of the prevailing rate for the doctor in the same setting. Over the past two decades, a number of actions by state insurance regulators and a few litigations against companies such as Blue Cross of Georgia in the early 2000s resulted in most companies honoring the medical services of PAs and NPs.

ISSUES REGARDING THE EFFECTIVENESS OF PHYSICIAN ASSISTANTS

How cost-effective is a PA? The answer, though not known exactly, is contained in the difference between the physician-PA substitution ratio (0.75) and the PA-physician cost ratio (0.45). The meaning of these two numbers is that a PA can substitute for *at least* 75% of primary care physician services. This service is undertaken at approximately 45% of the physician's salary. If the physician's time to see patients is reduced because of supervision, then the ratio is 50%. The social cost figures are even more impressive because the PA-physician ratio, including training costs, is smaller than the employment cost ratio. Finally, the employment of a primary care PA is fairly economical because the compensation-production ratio at 27% is more efficient than most other types of providers (including family medicine doctors at 53%, and NPs at 38%). Exhibit 11-23 presents a summary of the

EXHIBIT 11-23
Cost-Effectiveness of Primary Care Physician Assistants*

Issue Examined	Range	Average or Best Study
Delegation	0.40:1.0	0.83
Supervision	0.10:0.60	0.10
Physician-PA substitution ratio	0.40:1.0	0.75
PA-physician cost ratio (salary)	0.40:0.50	0.43
PA-physician cost ratio (with supervision)		0.52
Compensation-production ratio	0.25:0.52	0.38
Societal cost training a PA (compared with a physician)		0.20
Average no. of outpatients seen	18:35	21.7
PA-physician cost-benefit ratio	Unknown	Unknown

*Based on a review of the literature, using conservative estimates, and extrapolating to 2005 costs.

economic exercises in this chapter. These figures, however, must be viewed with caution since they are based on the "best studies" (those studies considered the most rigorous in investigation), or the average of different studies, using fairly conservative figures.

Prescribing Authority

All states, the District of Columbia, and Guam authorize prescribing privileges for PAs and most of those allow some limited prescribing of controlled substances. The first state statute to authorize prescribing privileges for PAs was passed in Colorado in 1969. It stipulated that graduates of the University of Colorado child health associate program (i.e., pediatric PAs) could prescribe medications without immediate consultation from supervising physicians provided that the latter subsequently approved the script. New York authorized prescribing privilege to PAs in 1972; Maine, New Mexico, and North Carolina followed in 1973. By 1979, 11 states had passed laws allowing PA prescribing privileges. Over the next three decades, states gradually authorized PA prescribing either by statute or by regulation. The argument in most instances was in recognition that prescribing medication is part of the PA's clinical role and the supervising physician has the authority to delegate such tasks to qualified health professionals. By 2008, all states sanctioned PA prescribing.

Prescribing authority generally applies to the outpatient or ambulatory setting. Medications for patients in the hospital are considered medical orders and usually fall under the purview of institutional medical staff bylaws. States typically place certain stipulations on PA prescribing activities. These may include (1) requiring physician cosignature for a PA prescription, (2) limiting the drugs that a PA may prescribe (e.g., those listed in a specific formulary), (3) excluding selected schedules of drugs, usually schedule II agents (i.e., those defined by the Controlled Substances Act as having the potential for abuse), (4) prescribing using drug treatment protocols, and (5) limiting the quantities of certain drugs that PAs may prescribe.

Hooker and Cipher (2005) examined the national trends in PA and NP prescribing and found that over a 6-year period, on average, doctors, PAs, and NPs wrote prescriptions for 60% to 70% of the visits. The mean number of prescriptions was 1.3 to 1.5 per visit depending on the provider. PAs were more likely to prescribe a controlled substance than were physicians or NPs (19.5%, 12.4%, and 10.9%, respectively). Overall, PAs and NPs are prescribing in a manner similar to doctors.

Prescribing Behavior

Although all 50 states permit PAs to prescribe, full understanding of the implications of this policy are yet to be determined. In 2008, the AAPA Research Division estimated that PAs practicing in family medicine and general internal medicine wrote 1.5 prescriptions, and emergency medicine PAs 1.4. These three specialties wrote the most prescriptions (AAPA, 2008a). In an analysis of 5 years of National Ambulatory Medical Care Survey (NAMCS) data, Hooker and Cipher (2005) analyzed the likelihood of prescribing by type of provider: PA, NP, and doctor. The likelihood of prescribing was similar among the three types of prescribers.

BARRIERS TO PRACTICE EFFECTIVENESS

On a public policy level, the phrase *barriers to practice* refers to factors known to have a significant limiting effect on the practice effectiveness of PAs and other nonphysician healthcare practitioners. Barriers to practice are commonly used within discussions of the utilization of PAs to denote the multiple health system factors that limit the full capabilities of PAs to provide healthcare services. These factors involve medical, legal, and economic elements and prevent PAs from discharging the full range of authorized medical tasks for which they are educated and certified to perform (Office of Technology Assessment, 1986; Emelio, 1994; Office of Inspector General, 2001).

PAs are often constrained in their capabilities to augment medical practices because of restrictions imposed by states. Barriers to the full practice effectiveness of PAs may reduce or eliminate the cost benefits that accrue from their use and deter them from serving populations in need of medical care services or from practicing in certain areas. Uneven state medical practice acts, the lack of authorization to prescribe medications in some states, and the absence of private third-party reimbursement that exists in many rural ambulatory practice settings have been shown to have restrictive effects on PA use (Willis, 1993).

While conventionally defined barriers to practice (i.e., state government regulatory policies for supervision requirements and prescribing authority) clearly work to affect levels of PA clinical productivity in a broad sense, on the day-to-day practice level, findings suggest that differences in the delegatory styles of individual employing physicians are also important determinants of PA effectiveness. On a fundamental level, barriers to practice (i.e., practice laws and regulations) represent the parameters drawn for PAs and advance practice nurses, usually by physicians. At the margins, because clinical activities between physicians and PAs overlap considerably, scope of practice and professional domain issues arise among these health professionals. Physicians now share a great deal of their medical diagnostic and therapeutic responsibilities with PAs. This willingness to share medical functions is a result of forces affecting the evolution of the division of medical labor in the U.S. health system.

States and their licensing boards have considerable control over the practice activities of PAs and NPs through their authority to license and regulate the healthcare occupations. Restrictions to the full practice effectiveness of PAs and similar healthcare providers historically reduced or eliminated the cost benefits that accrue from using these professionals because they were prevented from serving populations in greatest need of medical care services or from practicing at all. This set of barriers has gradually been reduced and, for all intents and purposes, has been minimal since 2008.

PA practice favorability scores ranged from a high (maximum attainable) of 100 points in three states (Washington, Iowa, and Montana) to a low of 0 (lowest attainable) in Mississippi, with a mean score of 73.1. Twenty-one states had practice favorability scores of 90 or greater, and 14 had scores less than 5. Lower scores generally correlated with the lack of PA prescriptive authority. A significant relationship ($P < 0.001$) was observed between practice favorability scores and a state's PA-population ratio. States tended to cluster into three groups, reflecting the association between favorability scores and PA-population ratios: states with high favorability scores and high PA-population ratios, states with midrange scores and midrange ratios, and states with low scores and consequently low ratios. These findings confirm the widely held view that scope of practice regulations, the existence of prescribing authority, and eligibility for reimbursement all affect PA use. If these factors are unfavorable, they serve as barriers to PA practice effectiveness. This policy analysis is believed to have played a significant influential role in states improving their enabling legislation for nonphysician clinicians in the 1990s. The work of Wing and colleagues (2004) showed that substantial changes took place over a 10-year period preceding the year 2000. These changes were entirely on the state level and almost all states improved enabling legislation, prescribing authorization, and insurance reimbursement. Now that all states have more or less similar legislation, reimbursement, and prescribing, the significant barriers seem like remote history.

JOB SATISFACTION OF PHYSICIAN ASSISTANTS

Job satisfaction is not usually thought of as an economic issue. However, a high rate of turnover of professional personnel in a clinic is disruptive to patient care and organizational stability, as well as to the individual clinician. When employment attrition occurs, productivity and the efficiency of the healthcare service are negatively affected. At one time the major reason PAs, NPs, and physicians left an organization was because of management (Pantell, Reilly, & Liang, 1980).

Research on PAs and job satisfaction is fairly extensive and PAs seem to be reasonably satisfied with their work experience and practice conditions. PAs express an overall level of satisfaction that compares favorably with that of other professionals such as lawyers, accountants, and engineers (Perry, 1978). Holmes and Fasser (1993) found PAs reporting less stress and lower turnover rates than nurses and many other healthcare workers. PAs also are more satisfied than NPs, who sometimes regard themselves as better-trained and more effective alternative practitioners.

The major determinants of job satisfaction among PAs seem to be the professional and personal support provided by the PA's supervising physician, the amount of responsibility for patient care, income, and opportunities for career advancement (Baker et al, 1989). Two studies suggest the strongest correlates of both job performance and job satisfaction are the degree of physician supervisory support and amount of responsibility for patient care (Freeborn, Hooker, & Pope, 2002). Location in smaller communities is also associated with greater satisfaction (Sells & Herdnener, 1975), although a more recent study found that satisfaction levels were equally high for PAs practicing in both urban and rural settings (Larson, Hart, & Hummel, 1994). Lack of opportunities for career advancement has been frequently cited as a major concern and the main cause of attrition from the PA profession (Osterweis & Garfinkel, 1993; Willis, 1993). Inadequate financial compensation and control over income are other reported sources of dissatisfaction (Willis, 1993). Acceptance by patients and by other healthcare workers has not been found to be a significant problem (Nelson, Jacobs, & Johnson, 1974; Record et al, 1980; Record & Schweitzer, 1981a, 1981b).

Clinical responsibility and professional autonomy among PAs is highly correlated with the level of job satisfaction, the extent of professional and personal support provided by the supervising physicians, and the opportunities for career advancement. The majority of studies addressing the job/career satisfaction of PAs

reveal that they are largely satisfied in their professional roles and are quite happy with their career choice—a set of findings that are a bit surprising in view of the status of PAs as dependent practitioners.

Holmes and Fasser (1993) reported findings of occupational stress and professional retention in a survey conducted of 1,360 randomly selected practicing PAs responding to a mailed questionnaire. The typical respondent was male (53%), white (88%), age 37 years (mean), and devoted most work time to patient care activities. Job satisfaction was high overall, and it was correlated positively with independence, challenge, and job security. Issues of salary, perceived opportunities for advancement, and the management style of the employer were associated with the highest levels of job dissatisfaction and role stress.

When Freeborn, Hooker, and Pope (2002) compared perceptions about the practice environment and job satisfaction of PAs, NPs, and physicians in primary care, they identified that autonomy was not so much a problem. This finding may have been due to progressive human resource aspects of practice in a managed care organization. However, the common areas of dissatisfaction included patient load and the limited amount of time with patients. PAs and NPs were more likely than the physicians to experience stress on a daily basis and indicated they were less likely than physicians to choose the practice setting again (Exhibit 11-24). In the HMO where this study took place, PAs/NPs were significantly less satisfied than physicians with their incomes and fringe benefits.

Researchers at the AAPA identified that by 1999 only 15% of all PAs who have ever graduated from a formal PA program had left the profession. The AAPA surveyed the profession and with a 74% return identified that by all measures PAs were satisfied with their work environment, satisfied with clinical practice, satisfied with their job, and had a favorable outlook on the profession (Marvelle & Kraditor, 1999).

In one of the few career satisfaction studies that compared PAs with other occupations that have similar levels of responsibility, Freeborn and Hooker (1995) examined PAs in

EXHIBIT 11-24
Kaiser Permanente Primary Care Provider's Attitudes About Selected Aspects of Practice

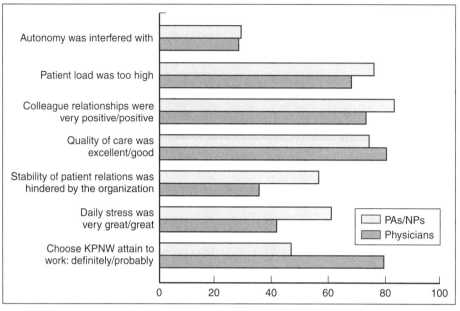

Data from Freeborn, D. K., Hooker, R. S., & Pope, C. R. (2002). Satisfaction and well-being of primary care providers in managed care. Evaluation & The Health Professions, 25(2), 239–254.

an HMO with NPs, optometrists, mental health workers, and chemical dependency counselors. PAs expressed the most satisfaction with the amount of responsibility, support from coworkers, job security, working hours, supervision, and task variety. They were less satisfied with workload, control over the pace of work, and opportunities for advancement. Chemical dependency counselors expressed the highest levels of satisfaction across various dimensions of work; optometrists expressed the lowest level of satisfaction (Exhibit 11-25). NPs also tended to be satisfied with most aspects of practice in this setting. In a number of instances they were more satisfied than the PAs. Most PAs were also satisfied with pay and fringe benefits (Freeborn & Hooker, 1995).

These findings, along with those of other studies, suggest that institutions, group practices, and HMOs are favorable settings for PAs. The organization of health care in an HMO model may be consistent with how the PA views himself or herself as a member of a healthcare team.

Perry and Redmond (1984) noted the following:

> Little is known about why PAs leave their careers. Clearly some do so to raise families and some may return to resume at least part-time. We estimate that the attrition rate is approximately two percent a year. Background may play a role since men, former military medical corpsmen, and graduates of military PA programs exhibited the lowest attrition in one study.

As of 2007, the annual annulment (death, disability, retirement) rate for PAs in the United States was estimated at 7%. This estimate is still considered very low for any occupation. How long PAs remain in their careers as clinicians remains for further analysis. Clear evidence exists that PA employment results in the production of more revenue than the costs of their employment in almost all settings. Yet for various reasons, PAs also tend to be underused in some clinical practice settings. For example, PAs are not highly represented in pediatrics, geriatrics, and psychiatry. Understanding this deselection for

EXHIBIT 11-25
Comparison of Job Satisfaction Between Nonphysician Providers

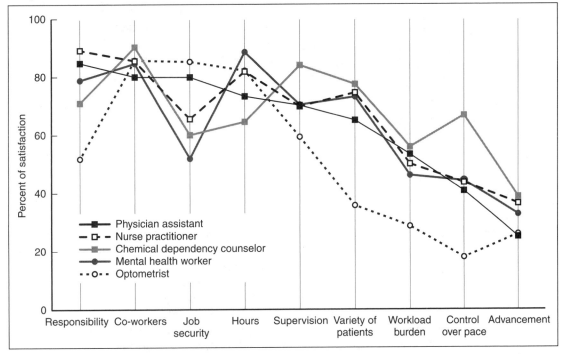

Data from Freeborn, D. K., & Hooker, R. S. (1995). Satisfaction of physician assistants and other nonphysician providers in a managed care setting. Public Health Reports, 110(6), 714–719.

certain roles in high demand is an area of research that bears exploring.

Research on Physician Assistant Economics

The literature about the economics of PA education and employment is modest. It is also somewhat outdated in the sense that national productivity has not been evaluated. Because this literature reveals large areas missing and many questions unanswered, a brief list of economic questions is presented.

■ **Case reports:** Writing about PAs in clinical roles and comparing their value to that of a doctor in the same role provides an opportunity to see how a PA can be used in common situations. Diagnostic codes, procedure codes, patient characteristics, and revenue generated should be compared.

■ **Cost benefit:** What is the cost benefit of a PA to an organization? Do PAs negate any of

their cost-effectiveness by managing patients differently? What are some of the differences between clinics with and without PAs?

■ **Cost utility:** What is the cost utility of a PA and does the chronic disease management of a patient by a PA have any different utility than with a doctor?

■ **Team use:** Does the incorporation of a PA on a team of doctors and nurses change the productivity and output? Does a doctor-PA team improve care when compared with a doctor-doctor team?

■ **Economy of scale:** Is there some optimal level when the addition of one more PA to an organization changes the output?

■ **Education:** What is the opportunity cost of a PA education? How does this differ by type of institution and by size of PA program? What are the differences between public and private tuition PA programs? Do these differences in cost of education have any predictive value on the role the PA selects?

- **Rate of return:** What is the rate of return to a PA education for the individual, institution, and society?

- **Cost of PA programs:** What is the cost of starting a PA program and maintaining a PA program? What is the cost per student per month and is this changing compared to inflation?

- **Patient benefit from PA education:** What does a patient receive in turn for being a patient attended by a PA in training?

- **Role satisfaction:** Are PAs satisfied with their roles? Are there PA roles that are more satisfying than others?

- **Productivity over time:** What is the lifetime productivity of a PA under given circumstances?

SUMMARY

Knowledge about performance and the potential contribution of PAs continues to be a significant source of scrutiny. Virtually all studies demonstrate an advantage to systems, whether they are large or small, when a PA is added to the staff. Clearly a large portion of primary care services can be safely delegated to PAs. In settings where PAs provide these services, they perform at levels of productivity that compare favorably with physicians. When the difference between substitution ratios and cost ratios are compared (even when the ratios are conservatively estimated) the differences are so large as to ensure cost savings for employers. Prepaid group practice studies and research from other large institutions suggest that physician comfort levels and practice styles in delegating medical tasks

to the PAs with whom they work have a significant influence on PA use and effectiveness in clinical practices. In studies of performance and patterns of utilization of PAs and NPs, scholars have noted a marked difference in the observed versus normative rates of delegation of medical tasks by HMO physicians when working with both PAs and NPs.

Measures of the clinical practice activities and professional characteristics of these healthcare providers continue to be observed in inpatient and outpatient settings. Results suggest that PAs and NPs are underused in many healthcare systems. The factor most critical in determining the effective use of PAs is the medical task delegation style of the supervising physicians. We offer that staffing efficiency in many organizations could be increased if physicians were more aware of the clinical roles and practice capabilities of these PAs and were better equipped to delegate tasks appropriately.

The societal cost benefits of PAs in the form of education suggest that a great deal is gained when PAs are trained because they provide care at substantial savings for 5 years longer than physicians. Many of the barriers in the form of restrictive legislation and reimbursement policies that at one time interfered with full use of PAs have largely been removed.

Finally, the cost advantages of employing PAs instead of physicians remains strong after four decades of observation. The cost difference between the income of doctors in primary care and PAs in primary care has been hovering around 50% salary ratio since the early 1990s. However, this employment investment could diminish if the gap between physician and PA earnings significantly narrows.

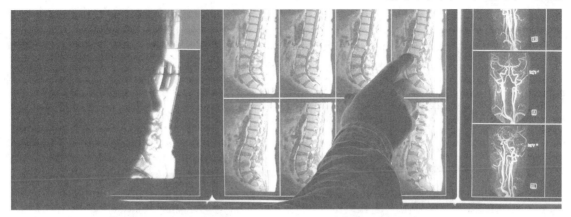

CHAPTER 12

PHYSICIAN ASSISTANT PROFESSIONAL RELATIONSHIPS

JAMES F. CAWLEY ■ RODERICK S. HOOKER ■ DAVID P. ASPREY

The ultimate test of a relationship is to disagree but hold hands.

—*Alexander Penney*

ABSTRACT

Physician assistants (PAs) have forged relationships with physicians, nurses, managed care, the federal and state governments, and patients as they have sought recognition. All are integral members of healthcare delivery in the United States and a strong relationship is needed with each entity. Issues about international medical graduates are germane as Canada and other countries are alert to a need to take advantage of the available trained stock of medical practitioners. Because of the need to communicate, a rich legacy of PA journalism emerges and provides both a forum for advances in PA information and a means of promulgating achievements.

INTRODUCTION

The U.S. Department of Labor estimates that more than 100 occupations deal with patients in some aspect of the healthcare workforce. This number is a dramatic contrast to the way medicine was originally organized. In the colonial period of America up through the 1930s, all medical services were under the purview of the physician. The patient's family provided assistance informally. Formal nursing arose from a need to assist the physician in treatments, tend to the sick, and develop public health roles. Since the 1860s there has been a constant genesis of new healthcare occupations. Most healthcare occupations have taken a common path—an assistant to the physician or nurse. Because the origin of the American physician assistant (PA) movement is no different, it is not surprising that the profession should try to foster a relationship with medicine, nursing, and other players in the healthcare workforce for support and survival.

PHYSICIANS

Doctors of the 20th century were unique in that their authority was generally unquestioned. Even when they were employees of a hospital and a board oversaw the granting of privileges they essentially reported to no one. Only later, after 1975, did peer review and oversight begin to take shape. This sovereign profession of doctors was a force to reckon with and individual power had been consolidated with the American Medical Association (AMA). The doctor dominated the hierarchy of medicine, law, and religion, and the basis for this is embedded in sociology, which identifies that the influence of the profession resides in knowledge and competence (Goode, 1960; Freidson, 1970; Fuchs, 1974): "In some cases, [the dependence we have on doctors as a society] may be entirely subjective, but no matter: Psychological dependence is as real in its consequences as any other" (Starr, 1982).

PAs originated from a concept developed by physicians—that they had a need for an assistant who could assume medical responsibility and extend their usefulness. As a result of this endeavor, a close working relationship with physicians has held PAs in good stead. Therefore, it is not surprising that PAs and their employers agree about the degree of supervision and autonomy, and physicians report that the quality of their lives has improved as a result of hiring a PA.

Attitudes Toward Physician Assistants

Autonomy in medicine is typically regarded as possible only when a monopoly exists in that occupation. Yet, as Starr (1982) points out, physicians did not set out to gain a "monopoly of competence," rather, they wanted to use facilities and work with technical assistants while maintaining control of the division of labor. Thus, one might expect that the emergence of the PA and nurse practitioner (NP) would be generally acceptable and perhaps desirable to physicians as long as their professional autonomy is not jeopardized.

Abbott and colleagues (2007) add that American physicians are a very heterogeneous social category with varying levels of intraprofessional competition and influence. In other words, although physicians generally enjoy a powerful and prestigious position relative to other medical workers, they vary considerably in how they perceive this power and prestige. The power difference between physicians and other occupations is often described

as physician dominance, but this authority is on a very large continuum. Some physicians seek out PAs as colleagues engaged in a team effort to provide care to the needful of society. Other physicians object to any role that may threaten their position in medicine.

The theoretic basis of the relationship between physicians and PAs is best understood when viewed as part of a larger system of stratification of medical care occupations. Although there are more than 100 healthcare occupations, physicians have established hierarchical dominance relative to all the other occupations. The physician is considered more powerful in terms of influence and prestige than nurses, aides, and auxiliaries (Shortell, 1974; Larson, 1977).

Unfortunately, the literature on physician attitudes toward PAs is sparse and may be outdated. Appropriate roles for PAs were not well defined in the minds of most physicians who have responded to surveys and inquiries in the last century. The empirical research on physicians' receptiveness to PAs varies by scope, purpose, geographic location, and method. Of the few studies available, several have asked physicians:

- whether PAs should practice independently or with a physician,
- whether they approve of the concept of a PA,
- whether they would hire a PA for their practice, and/or
- what types of tasks PAs might handle.

Sometimes these studies were specifically about PAs, and other times they queried physicians about a hypothetical assistant. For example, a survey of Wisconsin physicians in the 1960s examined physicians' receptivity to hypothetical "doctors' assistants" or "clinical associates." Approximately 40% said they would employ such a person (Coye & Hansen, 1969). In another study undertaken at the same time, mothers of small children were asked whether they would feel comfortable having a PA handle specific tasks. Having a pediatric PA care for their children was acceptable to 94% of the mothers. However, when the same question about specific task delegation was presented to the pediatrician—patients' willingness to accept the patient care services of PAs—the pediatrician's willingness to delegate these tasks fell far below (Patterson, 1969).

Spanning the 1970s and 1980s, several surveys about attitudes of physicians regarding PAs examined the hypothetical duties and the actual activities of PAs. Physicians who employed PAs and those who had no contact with PAs were surveyed. Some of the questions centered on taking histories, taking blood pressure readings, casting, and suturing. All concluded that routine activities were most appropriate for PAs, and regardless of specialty, type of practice, or community need, most thought it practical to employ a PA (Borland, Williams, & Taylor 1972; Legler, 1983). Sometimes the surveys concluded that physicians felt PAs could provide appropriate care, but legal and liability questions often arose, suggesting there might be some reluctance in employing a PA (Yanni, Backman, & Potash, 1972).

Other times the surveys showed a generally favorable attitude toward PAs, but only a few physicians saw PAs as a solution to the primary care doctor shortage (Haug Associates, 1973). A mail survey of Army physicians stationed worldwide found that a majority (74%) of physicians would welcome a PA to relieve them of seeing routine or minor problems, and 81% believed that the quality of care would be improved or at least not changed by PA use. Most Army physicians approved the assignment of PAs to remote locations, even when they would have an independent role in the care of active-duty personnel (Stuart & Blair, 1974). In the rural South, a very high percentage of physicians expressed a favorable attitude toward PAs, even though many had never worked with them (Joiner & Harris, 1974; Fenn 1987).

In a study of physicians' attitudes toward the effect PAs have on quality of care, risk of malpractice, role threat, and gender bias in a large health maintenance organization (HMO), internists and pediatricians had favorable attitudes toward NPs and PAs. Obstetricians and gynecologists had somewhat less favorable attitudes (Exhibit 12-1).

Several questions were asked to determine whether these physicians—who at the time of this study in 1977 were predominantly men—might have had gender bias, because most of the PAs were men and the NPs were predominantly women. Physician responses indicated that PAs more than NPs should be awarded certain privileges and participation, suggesting the existence of some gender bias at the time (Johnson & Freeborn, 1986).

In Minnesota, rural family physicians were surveyed about their confidence in the various abilities of PAs. There was a high degree of confidence in the areas of preventive medicine and routine care. Some concern was expressed about the proficiency of PAs taking calls, covering the emergency department, and making hospital rounds—activities that involve a broader base of clinical knowledge and diagnostic skills. Other concerns were an increased workload for physicians resulting from their assumed supervisory role; an increased number of complex cases seen by physicians; increased physician liability; job competition among PAs, NPs, and physicians; and supervisory guidelines for physicians regarding collaborative relationships (Bergeson et al, 1997). These attitudes may be different in group and staff model HMOs, in which the role and responsibilities of PAs may be broader and more institutionalized. In an HMO, the doctor and the PA are both salaried, meaning they are closer to being "peer clinicians" than in a private office-based setting. Higher levels of acceptance and collaboration are likely. By the late 1990s, within HMOs such as Kaiser Permanente, Group Health Cooperative, and Harvard Pilgrim Health Plan, the majority of physicians did not know what it was like to work *without* PAs (Jacobson, Parker, & Coulter, 1998).

Responsibilities and Privileges

At one time doctors were asked whether it was a good idea to be on a first-name basis with PAs and NPs. In general, these HMO physicians (almost all men) were less inclined to be on a first-name basis with NPs than with PAs. The doctors were also asked about certain privileges such as (1) wearing the same clinical coats except for the identification tag,

EXHIBIT 12-1
Physician Attitudes Toward Physician Assistants

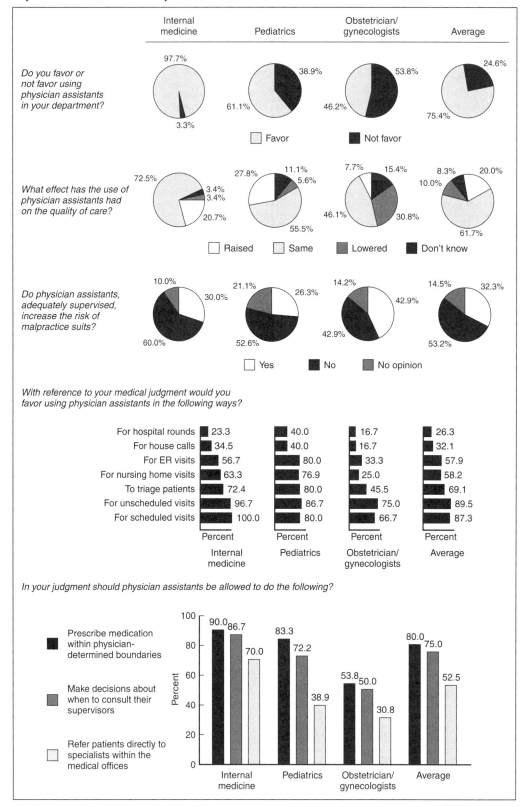

Data from Johnson, R. E., & Freeborn, D. K. (1986). Comparing HMO physicians' attitudes towards NPs and PAs. Nurse Practitioner, 11(1), 39–49.

(2) having access to areas reserved for physicians, (3) participating in decisions about how outpatient care was to be delivered, and (4) sitting on various clinical committees. Although physicians were generally accepting of PAs, no consistent pattern in their acceptance or attitudes toward PAs emerged in this study (Johnson & Freeborn, 1986).

Prescribing

Prescribing is considered the last domain of physician autonomy and has been described as "the most common and overt expression of the physician's power" (Pelligrino, 1976). That prescriptive authority has come slowly for PAs may be a result of physicians being reluctant to share this power. The physician's level of confidence in PAs prescribing tends to be more attitudinal than experiential. In Montana, supervising physicians were surveyed about authorizing PAs to prescribe specific agents. Minnesota physicians were asked a similar set of questions. In both instances the physicians strongly supported proposed legislation (Willis & Reid, 1990; Zellmer, 1992).

Objections to Physician Assistants

No matter how overwhelming the acceptance of PAs by physicians may appear, all physicians do not share this view. In fact, some doctors object to PAs. Shortly after the introduction of PAs, some notable health policy observers expressed the notion that the creation of PAs and similar providers was an abdication by physicians of their social responsibilities (Roemer, 1977). Roemer believed that physicians should have been required to spend time in community service practice.

Medicine was and still is criticized for its unwillingness to serve in rural and other undesirable settings. By establishing PAs as doctor-dependent providers who would serve in undesirable settings, one can argue that medicine was attempting to address their critics while maintaining physician dominance of medical practice. For some physicians professional dominance is jeopardized by PAs and other nonphysician clinicians (e.g., NPs, clinical nurse specialists [CNSs], nurse anesthetists,

and nurse-midwives). One argument advanced by Lichter (1995) is that profit motives and faulty patient satisfaction surveys have contributed to the rise of nonphysician clinician demands for an expanded scope of practice (Lichter, 1995). However, several arguments can be made to counter this view. First, most policy analysts, economists, and medical sociologists, whose views are endorsed at very high levels, assert that the use of PAs is an important component in improving healthcare access and efficiency. The U.S. healthcare delivery system and its personnel are perceived by the public to have a number of problems, prompting the need for major reform measures. Many of these problems relate to the composition of its healthcare workforce and the impact of provider specialty and geographic distribution (White, 1992; Pew Health Professions Commission, 1993). In its third report, the Council on Graduate Medical Education (COGME) found that:

> The rising physician/population ratio will do little to improve the public's health or increase access to services; moreover, it will hinder cost-containment efforts. There is an imbalance of physician specialty distribution, with too few primary care physicians and too many specialist physicians. America's medical educational system is disarticulated between its undergraduate and graduate (GME) components and should be more responsive to regional and national workforce needs. Shortages in the number of primary care physicians contribute to continuing problems in health services access. There continues to be a decline in interest in generalist training among recent medical graduates; only 16% of medical graduates selected residencies in primary care areas and a 57% match rate in internal medicine residency programs in 1993. The preparation of physicians for roles in primary care is often inadequate for future practice responsibilities, particularly in managed care systems. There is a need for better health workforce planning and to restructure financing and reimbursement systems to attain the appropriate specialty mix, racial/ethnic composition, and geographic distribution of physicians. (COGME, 1994)

Strategies aimed at strengthening the ability of the U.S. healthcare workforce to deliver primary care and improve effectiveness in reducing costs and increasing access will require many years to attain if physicians are the only professionals assumed to deliver medical care services. If overall policy goals for the workforce put forth by the COGME and others are to be achieved, it seems likely that such efforts will require the participation of nonphysicians such as PAs and NPs. Future healthcare delivery systems have been envisioned in which the bulk of primary care services are delivered by PAs and NPs, as physicians assume an increased amount of staff management and administrative and clinical consulting duties. Such changes in healthcare professional roles would likely be economically more efficient for medical practices and be a more rational way to use medical training and talent (Meikle, 1992).

Another counter-argument is that medicine is being practiced differently and more efficiently now than in the past. We have discarded scalpels that need resharpening and needles that need sterilization and have replaced them with disposable instruments of better quality because of the cost-effectiveness of these innovations. Likewise, we have replaced many traditional physician services with alternatives that are more economical than those provided by physicians and in some instances are superior to them. Optometrists have taken over the refraction component of ophthalmology care, not because they wanted to, but because physicians were willing to share this role to free their time for other eye services such as surgery. Midwives have been providing birthing services long before there were competent physicians interested enough in assuming this role. The use of PAs is a natural evolution in the healthcare workforce.

Lichter (1995) claimed that, "antiintellectualism contributed to the rise of PA/NP expanded scope of practice, often achieved legislatively." There may be some truth to this statement because PAs make no claim to be elite providers, and instead may be more like nurses that are comfortable allying themselves to the needs of consumers. As Starr (1982) pointed out, "[Medicine], by its nature, is an inegalitarian institution; it claims to enjoy a dignity not shared by ordinary occupations and a right to set its own rules and standards. These claims go against the democratic grain. They are also exceptionally hard to establish and enforce in a fluid, rapidly expanding society." The PA role seems more like a blend between the skills of a physician and the patient-oriented role of the nurse. These attributes appear to be attractive to the consumer.

Other arguments contend that the advent of medical boards guaranteed educational training of practitioners and any movement away from education as the basis of licensure is a step away from medical standards that will have negative long-term consequences (Lichter, 1995). What is not accounted for in this view is the superior educational development that has come out of collaboration between PA training programs and physician training programs. As Estes (1993) stated, "The educational system producing physician assistants is more advanced, efficient, and cost-effective than that producing physicians."

Organized Medicine

A relationship between the American Academy of Physician Assistants (AAPA) and the American Medical Association (AMA) has waxed and waned over the years. In 1994, the AMA granted observer status for the AAPA to sit in on the AMA House of Delegates. In 1995, the AMA House of Delegates adopted a set of guidelines for the working relationship between physicians and PAs (see Chapter 14). The guidelines recognize that PAs practice with physician supervision and the PA and physician together should determine the PA's role in patient care. They suggest that there is no role for PAs to be in competition with physicians or to practice medicine independently from physicians. This recognition came in deference to the practice advocated by NPs. The AMA Board of Trustees wrote:

> [NPs] use terms like "collaboration" and "interdependent" whereas PAs use "delegation" and

"supervision." PAs regard themselves as "agents" of the physicians, legally and practically, and view delegated medical acts and understanding the delegatory style of physicians with whom they work as their particular responsibilities. They define "collaboration" as synonymous with physician supervision. In contrast, NPs work towards "independent" practice and decision making under the nurse practice acts. (Gara, 1995)

A similar relationship with organized medicine exists between the AAPA and the American Academy of Family Physicians. The goal of this partnership is to work on issues affecting continuing medical education. So it appears, for now, that the relationship between organized medicine and the PA profession is secure, providing it remains as physicians want it.

Physician Assistants as Professionals

The question of whether PAs are true professionals has arisen on a number of occasions and is relevant when discussing the professional relationships PAs must maintain with physicians. Some would argue that PAs do not qualify as professionals because they do not possess their own body of knowledge and lack total autonomy in their work. Rather, they share a body of knowledge with physicians, who are recognized as the ultimate profession, and are granted a substantial degree of work autonomy within their defined practice. Yet, the standard of what constitutes a professional appears to be changing. PAs have made great progress in regulating and legislating their field as well as establishing title definition and protection, rules for entry into the profession, accreditation of educational programs, and certification of graduates. Whereas this progress has been incremental, it is based on the increasingly accepted concept of delegated or negotiated autonomy via the supervising physician.

There is a need for more research about PAs and healthcare delivery and a description of the unique aspects that PAs bring to medical practice. PAs have thus far not generated a large body of knowledge about themselves or

their practice aspects, but they have resisted the temptation to create an arcane language and "science" in an attempt to bestow professional status on themselves. They remain true to their calling as competency-based providers of health care, with the majority in primary care and many caring for the medically underserved. The PA profession should continue to strive for status as professionals in the altruistic sense, just as physicians ponder returning to their roots in service to society.

Evolution of the Physician–Physician Assistant Relationship

The ideal relationship between a physician and PA has not been fully articulated in spite of the rhetoric coming from the professional societies of physicians and PAs. In an interview with a group of physicians on this subject it was expressed that, "the role of the PA has to change because integrative models will provide the kind of preventive medicine that managed care demands. The PA is frequently thought of as a substitute, whereas he or she should be complementary to the physician. Physicians will soon begin to lose this. When they do, the relationship between physicians and PAs will be greatly enhanced." Another physician expressed that there is "an abysmal lack of knowledge about PAs." Still another wished that "PAs programs that are tightly integrated with medical school programs should serve as role models and sources of information for 'unintegrated' programs" (Blessing & Davis, 1988).

Some physicians offer that the establishment of a collegial role with a PA comes with familiarity. Given time, the attitude of physicians toward PAs will improve. The relationship between physicians and PAs should begin with medical students being exposed to PAs and learning more about "how a team approach facilitates good medical care" (Blessing et al, 1998).

Ongoing PA utilization is dependent on the physician's readiness to hire, work closely with, or otherwise promote the activities of PAs and other nonphysician providers (Glenn & Hofmeister, 1976). Clearly there is a wide range of opinions; however, since early studies were undertaken the visibility of PAs in healthcare systems has steadily improved. Physician attitudes toward an expanded role for the PA in the future are quite favorable (Lapius, 1983; Legler, 1983). Future attitudes toward acceptance of PAs will depend on the practice patterns of PAs, whether they are viewed as colleagues or competitors and if the economics of PA employment does not infringe on physician income. Contemporary and well-structured research on PA roles may be necessary to adequately address the spectrum of physician attitudes.

NURSES

In their first decade of existence PAs struggled to distinguish themselves from nurses. When assigned to hospital roles PAs were sometimes placed in nursing departments. In outpatient settings sometimes PAs were linked with a registered nurse (RN), believing this relationship would strengthen the PA's role (Lairson, Record, & James, 1974). Early in the development of the profession, some believed the logical place for PAs was within the nursing profession (Bergman, 1971).

Conceptual Models of Nursing

Nurses have formulated a number of conceptual models that constitute formal explanations of what nursing is. As Fawcett (1994) has noted, four concepts are central to models of nursing: person, environment, health, and patient care. The various nursing models define these concepts differently, link them in diverse ways, and give different emphasis to the relationships among them. Moreover, different models emphasize different processes as being central to nursing. For example, Roy's Adaptation Model identifies adaptation of patients as a critical factor in nursing (Roy & Andrews, 1998). In this model, human beings are biopsychosocial adaptive systems who cope with environmental change through the process of adaptation. Within the human system, there are four subsystems or response modes: physiological needs, self-concept, role function, and interdependence. These subsystems constitute adaptive modes that provide mechanisms for coping with environmental stimuli and change. The goal of nursing, according to this model, is to promote patient adaptation during health and illness.

Martha Rogers, by contrast, emphasizes the centrality of the individual as a unified whole. Her model views nursing as a process in which individuals are aided in achieving maximum well-being within their potential (Rogers, 1994). Nurse researchers increasingly are turning toward these conceptual models for their inspiration in formulating research questions and hypotheses. Other conceptual models of nursing that have been used in nursing studies include King's Open System Model (Johnson, 1998), Neuman's Health Care Systems Model (1989), Orem's Model of Self-Care (1995), and Parse's Theory of Human Becoming (1992). Exhibit 12-2 lists eight conceptual models of nursing, together with a study for each that claimed the model as its framework.

In addition to conceptual models that describe and characterize the entire nursing process, nurses have developed other models and theories that focus on specific phenomena of interest to nurses. An important example is Nola Pender's Health Promotion Model, a conceptual map (Pender & Pender, 1996). Another example is Mishel's Uncertainty in Illness Theory (1998), which focuses on the concept of uncertainty—the inability of a person to determine the meaning of illness-related events. According to this theory a situation appraised as uncertain will mobilize individuals to use their resources to adapt to the situation. Mishel's conceptualization of uncertainty has been used as a framework for qualitative and quantitative studies.

These theories, separately and in the aggregate, establish the theoretical basis of nursing and the contributions they bring to medicine. The body of nursing is theory-based and differs conceptually from allopathic medicine, in which there is no unifying theory other than science as a whole. Thus, medicine lacks a theoretical basis but instead is composed of biology, chemistry, and physics. Only psychiatry is a separate and distinct theory.

EXHIBIT 12-2
Examples of Studies Linked to Conceptual Models of Nursing

King's Open System Model	What is the effect of a nurse-client transactional female adolescents' oral contraceptive intervention on adherence? (Hanna, 1993)
Levine's Conservation Model	What are the dimensions of fatigue as experienced by patients with congestive heart failure? (Schaefer & Potylycki, 1993)
Neuman's Health Care Systems Model	What is the relationship between mood symptoms and daytime ambulatory blood pressure during a 12-hour period in black female caregivers and noncaregivers? (Picot et al, 1999)
Parse's Theory of Human Becoming	What are the factors that influence young women's perceptions of risk for sexually transmitted diseases? (Parse, 1992)
Orem's Model of Self-Care	What is the relationship between self-care agency and abuse on the one hand and physical and emotional health on the other among women in intimate relationships? (Campbell & Soeken, 1999)
Roger's Science of Unitary Human Beings	What is the efficacy of a Rogerian-based intervention of therapeutic touch on anxiety, pain, and plasma T-lymphocyte concentration in burn patients? (Turner et al, 1998)
Roy's Adaptation Model	Do formal cancer support groups help women adapt to the physiological and psychosocial sequelae of breast cancer? (Samarel et al, 1998)

Advanced Practice Nurses

Evolution of patterns in the division of medical labor in U.S. medicine reveals that several types of nonphysician health professionals make important contributions and expand the services available to patients. As part of this evolution of health professional roles, PAs and various levels of nurses have been increasingly incorporated into medical practices and health institutions' staffing.

Advanced practice nurse (APN), or advanced practice registered nurse (APRN), is the overarching term that encompasses the following four roles in nursing:

- Certified nurse-midwife (CNM)
- Certified registered nurse anesthetist (CRNA)
- Clinical nurse specialist (CNS)
- Certified nurse practitioner (CNP)

APNs complete graduate-level education programs and acquire specialized clinical knowledge and skills, preparing them to provide direct care to patients as a component of their practice. The APN level of nursing builds on the competencies of RNs. As a result, APNs demonstrate increased depth and breadth of knowledge, increased synthesis of data, increased complexity of skills and interventions, and significant role autonomy. The APN is educationally prepared to assume responsibility and accountability for health promotion and the assessment, diagnosis, and management of patient problems, which includes the use and prescription of pharmacological and nonpharmacological interventions.

Nurse Practitioners

NPs are typically graduate-prepared nurses with additional advanced nursing education beyond the RN preparation. NPs are educated to meet core competencies as well as to serve specific patient populations, such as in pediatric, adult, family, women's health, or geriatric care. The NP curriculum is based on theoretical constructs from many health disciplines and includes course work in pharmacology, physiology, pathophysiology, epidemiology, health assessment, diagnosis, clinical decision-making, and management. As part of their education, NP students receive intensive clinical experiences with typically more than 600 supervised clinical hours in their practice area (Berlin et al, 2002). Although NPs are more visible in the United States, their presence is gaining worldwide.

Nurse practitioners work in many settings, including family practice offices, urgent care centers, nursing homes, home care, community clinics, schools, and rural health clinics. Although NPs stand on their nursing credentials as being independent, almost all maintain collaborative working relationships with physicians. In the United States, NPs are licensed by the state in which they practice and have board certification in their area of practice (usually through the American Nurses Credentialing Center [ANCC] or National Certification Corporation [NCC]).

An NP can serve as a patient's "point of entry" healthcare provider. The core philosophy of the field is individualized care. NPs focus on patients' conditions as well as the effects of illness on the lives of the patients and their families. Informing patients about their health and encouraging them to participate in decisions are central to the care provided by NPs.

Most NPs treat acute and chronic conditions through prescribing medications, physical therapy, tests, and therapies for patients. Many NPs have a DEA registration number that allows them to write prescriptions for federally defined controlled medications. Similar to PAs, they may bill Medicare, Medicaid, and private insurance for services performed.

In 1965—the same year as the inception of PAs—the first NP demonstration project, funded by the Commonwealth Foundation, was initiated at the University of Colorado Medical Center. Henry Silver, MD, and Loretta Ford, RN, were the developers of this program in pediatrics. The intent was to extend the nurse's role in pediatric medicine. As a 5-year project it was designed to prepare nurses to provide comprehensive well-child care in noninstitutional settings and to study the program outcomes for their applicability for curriculum changes in collegiate nursing programs (Ford, 1979). This course of study was 4 months, followed by 20 months of field experience with a pediatrician. At completion of this program these nurses were granted a certificate. Graduates of this program were called pediatric NPs.

Programs soon spread across the United States. As of 2008, about 125,000 NPs were estimated to be in active clinical practice, representing 51% of all APNS. Of all NPs, about 4,500 are CNMs. There are approximately 337 institutions (predominantly schools of nursing), containing approximately 1,488 accredited educational programs or separate tracks for NPs. The trend in annual graduations of NPs has been declining since 2000, with a drop from 7,100 graduates in 2000 to 6,000 graduates in 2008 (Exhibit 12-3).

NPs can practice either independently or with limited supervision from doctors in all but seven states. In all states except Georgia they can prescribe medications with some level of authority, although some states do prohibit them from prescribing narcotics. This number is a bit contentious because as of 2004 there were 141,209 nurses who held NP credentials but only 65.7 were employed with the position title of "nurse practitioner" (U.S. Department of Health & Human Services/Health Resources Services Administration [US DHHS/HRSA], 2006).

The NP profession has expanded to an international level (Exhibit 12-4). The National Organization of Nurse Practitioner Faculties (NONPF) is the organization that promotes NP education at the national and international levels. Starting in 1974 as a small group of educators meeting to develop the first NP curriculum guidelines, NONPF has evolved as the leading organization for NP faculty sharing the commitment of excellence in NP educations. Today, the organization represents a global network of over 1,200 educators.

The International Council of Nurses (ICN) Network was launched in 2000 to do the following:

- Serve as a forum for exchange of knowledge
- Serve as a resource for the development of APN/NP roles and the appropriate educational underpinning
- Serve as a vehicle for ICN to harness specialist expertise
- Help ICN more effectively meet its mandate as the global voice of the profession
- Provide a mechanism to promote and disseminate information from any of the network members and ICN

EXHIBIT 12-3
Nurse Practitioner Enrollment and Graduation of Master's Level, 2005

Clinical Track/National Certification Examination	No. of Schools	Students								
		Full Time		Part Time		Total		Graduations		
		Number	%	Number	%	Number	%	Number	%	
Family	268	4,927	58.3	6,621	53.0	11,548	55.4	3,144	53.3	
Adult	137	959	11.4	2,440	19.5	3,399	16.3	872	14.8	
Pediatric	93	671	7.9	875	7.0	1,546	7.4	552	9.4	
Pediatric acute care	7	48	0.6	5	> 0.1	53	0.3	0		
Gerontological	54	124	1.5	194	1.6	318	1.5	98	1.7	
Women's health	48	315	3.7	441	3.5	756	3.6	286	4.8	
Neonatal	54	224	2.7	267	2.1	491	2.4	191	3.2	
Adult acute care	60	535	6.3	926	7.4	1,461	7.0	3,970	6.7	
Adult psychiatric and mental health	44	124	1.5	346	2.8	470	2.3	162	2.7	
Family psychiatric and mental health	15	116	1.4	49	0.4	165	0.8	22	0.4	
NP dual tracks	65	316	3.7	263	2.1	579	2.8	167	2.8	
Undeclared	2	78	0.9	11	0.1					
Not specified	4	7	0.1	45	0.4	52	0.2	9	0.2	
TOTAL	851	8,444		12,483		20,838		5,900		

Data from Fang, D., Wilsey-Wisniewski, S., & Bednash, G. D. (2006). 2005–2006 Enrollment and Graduations in Baccalaureate and Graduate Programs in Nursing. Annual Report. Washington, DC: American Association of Colleges of Nursing.

■ Act as the base for future international collaboration around advanced practice and the NP role, including international conferences

Clinical Nurse Specialist

CNSs are RNs who are experts in the diagnosis and treatment of illness and the promotion of wellness in the presence or absence of disease. They are considered independent practitioners who function in a collaborative role with the physician. In fact, many demographic studies on NPs and APNs classify the CNS as an NP.

Most CNSs (93%) receive their education through a master's program; 3% are prepared through a post-master's certificate. The CNS curriculum concentrates heavily on advanced skills in assessment, intervention, health promotion, illness prevention, and critical thinking. In addition, the educational preparation is theoretically grounded in multiple theories of nursing and theories from other disciplines (Huch, 1992).

CNSs use theory and research to guide their care. They work in communities, hospitals, home care settings, and across healthcare delivery systems. They develop and manage population-based programs of care and collaborate with other providers and multidisciplinary teams to ensure that patients receive the range of healthcare services needed to restore wellness. In 2004 there were 72,521 CNSs, representing 24% of all APNs (US DHHS/HRSA, 2006).

Certified Registered Nurse Anesthetist

Established in 1956, the CRNA credential refers to an APN who provides anesthetics to patients in collaboration with surgeons, anesthesiologists, dentists, podiatrists, and other qualified healthcare professionals. When anesthesia is administered by a CRNA, it is recognized as the practice of nursing; when administered by an anesthesiologist, it is recognized as the practice of medicine. CRNAs practice in every setting in which anesthesia is delivered: traditional hospital surgical

EXHIBIT 12-4
Nurse Practitioners Globally

Nurse practitioners (NPs) are formally recognized in Canada, Australia, Great Britain, and New Zealand. Although their role is not as well defined as in the United States and their numbers are small, the profession is growing on a global level.

AUSTRALIA
The government of New South Wales enacted the Nurses Amendment (Nurse Practitioner) Act in 1998. This provision allows for recognition and accreditation of NPs and authorizes NPs to perform diagnostic services and limited prescribing. Since the enactment of this provision, NPs have established themselves in South Australia, Northern Territory, Queensland, and Western Australia. There are approximately 200 NPs and a dozen NP programs in Australia.

CANADA
Canada is struggling with meeting demand for healthcare services and a number of initiatives are underway, including importing doctors, PAs, and NPs and expanding NP services. A 2005 report by the Canadian Institute for Health Information (CIHI) and the Canadian Nurses Association showed that the number of NPs in Canada increased by more than 20% from 2003 to 2004. This was an increase of 153, from 725 in 2003 to 878 in 2004. The number of provinces and territories licensing NPs increased from seven in 2003 (Newfoundland and Labrador, Nova Scotia, New Brunswick, Ontario, Alberta, the Northwest Territories, and Nunavut) to eight in 2004 (with the addition of Saskatchewan) (CIHI, 2005). However, because the number of NPs in Canada is not considered adequate to meet current demands, much less future demands, some emphasis is beginning to shift to educating and employing PAs.

UNITED KINGDOM
The first group of NPs were qualified in the United Kingdom in 1991. They were then invited to attend the Nurse Practitioner Conference in Colorado in 1992. At this conference these NPs met with representatives of the American Academy of Nurse Practitioners and the University of Colorado. It was agreed that NPs in the United States and the United Kingdom would work together to improve communication and share knowledge and experiences.

suites and obstetrical delivery rooms; critical access hospitals; ambulatory surgical centers; the offices of dentists, podiatrists, ophthalmologists, plastic surgeons, and pain management specialists; and the U.S. Military, Public Health Services, and Department of Veterans Affairs healthcare facilities.

Nurses were the first professional group to provide anesthesia services in the United States and have been doing so for more than 125 years. Established in the late 1800s, anesthesia has since become recognized as the first clinical nursing specialty. The discipline of nurse anesthesia developed in response to requests of surgeons seeking a solution to the high morbidity and mortality attributed to anesthesia at that time. Surgeons saw nurses as a cadre of professionals who could give their undivided attention to patient care during surgical procedures. Serving as pioneers in anesthesia, nurse anesthetists became involved in the full range of specialty surgical procedures, as well as in the refinement of anesthesia techniques and equipment.

CRNAs practice with a high degree of autonomy and professional respect. In regard to education, 37% of CRNAs have attended a master's program; 58% received their preparation through a post-RN certificate. In 2004, there were 32,523 CRNAs, representing 13% of all APNs (US DHHS/HRSA, 2006).

Certified Nurse-Midwife
CNMs are registered nurses who receive additional training to provide primary health care to women. This care includes evaluation, assessment, treatment, and referral to a specialist, if required. CNMs have been recognized for their contributions to reducing the rates of infant and maternal mortality, premature births, and low-birth-weight neonates. Their skills as primary care providers are also evidenced by low rates of cesarean birth, episiotomies, and epidural anesthesia use and their high rates of success in vaginal birth after cesarean. Seventy percent of women who receive care from nurse-midwives are considered vulnerable to poor health outcomes by virtue of age, socioeconomic status, education, ethnicity, or location of residence. Whereas 56% of CNMs received their educational preparation in this specialty through a master's program, 5% obtained a post-master's certificate; 36% were estimated to have received their nurse-midwife preparation through a certificate program.

The practice of nurse-midwifery was established in the United States in the 1920s by such early leaders as Mary Breckinridge and Hattie Hemschemeyer. Desirous of promoting child health, the midwives provided prenatal care for pregnant women and assisted physicians. They also supported women during labor and birth at home. By the early 1930s, there were only two sites for the practice of nurse-midwifery in the United States: Frontier Nursing Service and Maternity Center Association. Over the next 20 years, nurse-midwifery expanded in response to physician shortages, the emergence of a childbirth education movement, and women's demands for participation in birth. In the 1940s, the greatest expansion occurred in the South and Southwest. Midwives were providing care in home births, birthing centers, and, occasionally, in community hospitals (Dawley, 2003).

In development since the 1940s, a national organization to represent midwives was established in 1955 in Kansas City, Missouri, with the founding meeting of the American College of Nurse-Midwifery. A series of conflicts within organized nursing about the place and role of nurse-midwives in the newly reorganized American Nurses Association and the National League for Nursing took place during this time (Dawley & Burst, 2005). Ultimately, the American College of Nurse-Midwifery merged with another organization, the American Association of Nurse-Midwives, to create the American College of Nurse-Midwives (Dawley, 2005). As of 2004, there were 32,523 CNMs, which constitutes 4% of all APNs (USDHHS/HRSA, 2006).

Legal Recognition

The board of nursing in each state, under the authority of the state's nursing practice act, establishes statutory authority for licensure of RNs, which includes the use of a title, authorization for a scope of practice, standards of practice, and disciplinary grounds. When an RN engages in practice that is determined to be beyond the identified scope of nursing practice, as in advanced practice nursing, legal authorization for that practice must exist in state law. Any title, even if issued by a national certification body, only carries legal status if

that title is recognized or authorized in statute or regulation. Some jurisdictions require certification by a national professional body as one prerequisite for state authorization to practice as an APN. Licensure or legal recognition is based on congruence between education, practice, and a competence assessment method that is psychometrically sound and legally defensible.

Comparing Physician Assistants and Nurse Practitioners

The origins of PAs and NPs are similar in time and concept. Whereas the ideologies of the two professions may remain distinct to some, enough analysis exists to suggest that NP service in the United States and elsewhere is remarkably similar to the service provided by PAs (Hooker & McCaig, 1996; McCaig et al, 1998). Approximately one-third of U.S. PAs and somewhere over one-half of NPs are in primary care (Hooker, 2006). Primary care in this case is defined as family practice, general internal medicine, pediatrics, and obstetrics and gynecology. NPs are five times more likely to be in pediatrics or women's health than PAs. However, when other subspecialties are included, such as geriatrics, urgent care, corrections medicine, and occupation and environmental medicine, the percent of PAs in primary care approaches parity.

Despite their divergent training (and sometimes acrimonious debate), PAs and NPs are commonly thought of as similar types of healthcare providers. In a number of clinical settings, such as managed care health systems and ambulatory clinics, the roles of PAs and NPs are regarded as interchangeable, and open positions are often advertised as being able to be filled by either provider. Major research reports and policy analyses that have examined both of these health professions consider PAs and NPs to be equivalent when used in ambulatory practice roles (Office of Technology Assessment, 1986). Even on the clinical level, PAs and NPs have similar views about their roles (Freeborn & Hooker, 1995; Freeborn, Hooker, & Pope, 2002) (Exhibits 12-5 and 12-6).

EXHIBIT 12-5
Venn Diagram of Doctors, Nurses, and Physician Assistants

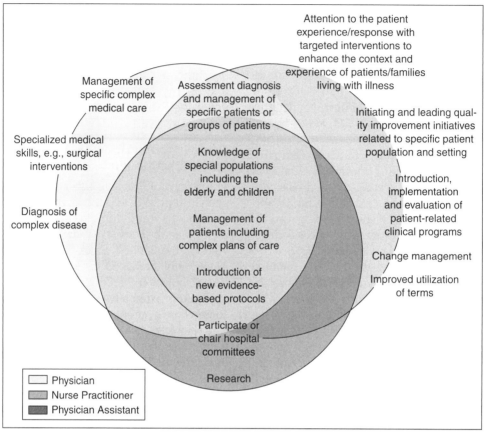

Yet, important differences between PAs and NPs persist (Exhibit 12-7). As healthcare professionals, NPs and PAs possess distinctive professional orientations and educational backgrounds, have different state regulatory systems, and show practice characteristics that appear to be moving in different directions. NPs believe that as nurses they are empowered to act independently, with the authority to prescribe drugs without physician oversight. They want nurse reimbursement rates to be brought up to physician rates for a "like service" (Safriet, 1994). In the early introduction of new health practitioners, patients viewed NPs and PAs differently (Conant et al, 1971). These differences were thought to have important implications for the future roles of both professions in a reformed healthcare system, but as of 2009 very little has emerged to identify what these differences are.

Physician Supervision

The NP profession has long maintained that its scope of practice is "collaborative" and does not require the supervision of a physician, but most NPs have some form of legal and practice connection to physicians. The developing prospect of a clinically based doctorate in nursing practice (DNP) for NPs and other APNs provides evidence that NPs are increasingly likely to establish themselves as independent practitioners and share with physicians the domain of medical practice. A document drafted by the National Council of State Boards of Nursing titled, "The Future Regulation of Advanced Practice Nursing," states, "Fully licensed APNs will be independent practitioners. After licensure, there will be no regulatory requirements for supervision" (National Council of State Boards of Nursing, 2006). The document outlines how DNP

EXHIBIT 12-6
Percentage of Kaiser Permanente Providers Satisfied or Very Satisfied With Specific Aspects of Their Employment

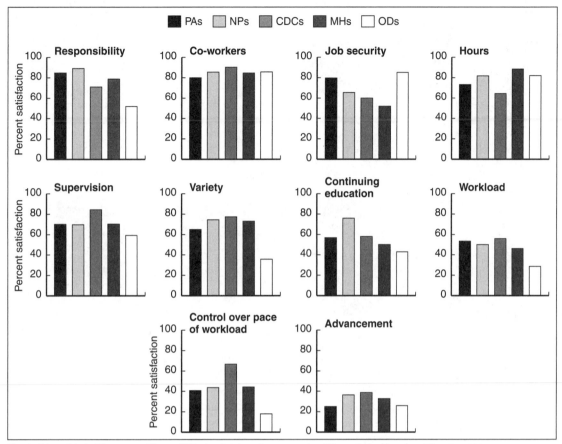

PAs, physician assistants; NPs, nurse practitioners; CDCs, chemical dependence counselors; MHs, mental health workers; ODs, optometrists.

Data from Freeborn, D. K., & Hooker, R. S. (1995). Satisfaction of physician assistants and other nonphysician providers in a managed care setting. Public Health Reports (Washington, DC 1974), 110(6), 714–719.

graduates would become licensed as independent providers by state boards of nursing. It is tantamount to a formal declaration of independent medical practice by the NP profession. As of 2008 there are 67 DNP programs in the United States.

This movement is not entirely unexpected. However, what is of interest is physicians' malaise in response to these aggressive moves that likely will place NPs in direct competition with primary care physicians. The rationale for this malaise is the ongoing need for additional primary care providers. Physicians are unlikely to be able to meet the anticipated demand for medical care services in the future, and APNs, armed with the DNP degrees, are likely to seek to deliver medical

care services independent of physicians. One physician states that, "it seems virtually certain that the [APN] graduates will provide a number of services that have traditionally been viewed as being solely within the domain of physicians, and will do so in independent practice settings" (Whitcomb, 2006).

This rise in autonomy represents an interesting shift in physician attitudes toward NPs and PAs. With many workforce experts calling attention to a crisis in primary care, and with declining interest in primary care among recent medical graduates, it appears to be a wide open field for nonphysicians. Yet, PAs also are exhibiting less interest in primary care, with 65% of the profession now working in specialties. The door would appear to be

EXHIBIT 12-7
Characteristics of Nurse Practitioners and Physician Assistants, 2008

Characteristic	Nurse Practitioner	Physician Assistant
Average age	43.6	41.5
Female (%)	92	78
Average years in practice	9.0	9.5
Number employed	115,000	65,000
Background	Registered nurse	Nurse, emergency medical services, medic, respiratory therapist, physical therapist, other
Number of U.S. degree-granting institutions with programs	202	141
Number of program tracks	381	145
Curriculum focus	Health assessment, diagnosis, treatment	Primary care
Length of education	21–43 months; mean, 22 months	18–39 months; mean, 27 months
Master's degree granted at graduation (2007)	84%	78%
Number of annual graduates (2008)	5,500	5,800
Average salary (2007)	$73,600	$86,430
Certificate requirements	Certification required before practice as of 2006 (NCC, AANP, ANCC, NCBPNP)	Certification required before practice (PANCE)
Recertification	Every 5 years	Every 6 years
Practice autonomy	Autonomous in 43 states	Physician supervision requried in all states
Primary care clinicians	85%	44%
Full time	50%	85%

Sources: *Curran, 2007; Buppert, 2004; Hooker, 2006; U.S. Department of Labor, 2007; AAPA, 2008b; Christian, Dower, & O'Neil, 2007; AACN, 2008.*

open for NPs with doctoral degrees to enter and perhaps dominate primary care delivery. The recent utilization of NPs in for-profit medical clinics set in large retail chains is but further evidence of this trend.

A move by NPs to independent practice in primary care may evoke opposition among some physician groups, but one observer downplays such opposition: "I am aware that some state medical societies are actively opposing the development of DNP programs by colleges and universities and the granting of an expanded scope of practice to APNs by state officials . . . I believe it is wrong for the (medical) profession to block the APN movement" (Whitcomb, 2006).

PAs believe themselves to be a segment of the health workforce that could continue to augment physicians in meeting future demands for medical care services and are not seeking independent practice. Rather than advocating meekly handing over a segment of medical practice to NPs, a group that has been at times overtly hostile to physicians and sometimes militant in their assertion of independent practice, it seems reasonable workforce policy to consider those nonphysicians who are trained in the medical model, who have sought a practice relationship that is not threatening to physician groups, and who are equally effective in providing quality and cost-effective medical care.

Patient Outcomes

Little has been undertaken to compare outcomes of care between NPs and PAs. One study assessed the quality of diabetes care among 46 family medicine practices employing either an NP or a PA (but not both). Compared with practices employing PAs, practices employing

NPs were more likely to measure hemoglobin A_{1c} (HgbA1c) levels (66% vs. 33%), lipid levels (80% vs. 58%), and urinary microalbumin levels (32% vs. 6%); to have treated high lipid levels (77% vs. 56%); and to have patients attain lipid targets (54% vs. 37%). Practices with NPs were more likely than physician-only practice to assess HgbA1c levels (66% vs. 49%) and lipid levels (80% vs. 68%). These effects could not be attributed to use of diabetes registries, health risk assessments, nurses for counseling, or patient reminder systems (Exhibit 12-8). Practices with either PAs or NPs were perceived as busier and had larger total staff than physician-only practices (Ohman-Strickland et al, 2008).

EXHIBIT 12-8
Adjusted Probabilities of Appropriate Assessment, Treatment, and Target Attainment Among Diabetic Patients by Practice Type

Measure Assessed (all patients)	Total Number of Patients	Percent (95% CI)			Pair-Wise Comparison, Rate Ratio (P Value)		
		Practices with NPs N = 9	Practices with PAs N = 9	Practices With Physicians Only N = 28	NP vs. PA	NP vs. Physician Only	PA vs. Physician Only
HbA1c in last 6 months	846	65.5 (57.7–72.5)	33.4 (17.9–53.4)	48.9 (36.8–61.2)	1.96 (0.005)	1.34 (less than 0.001)	0.68 (0.21)
Blood pressure (BP) at last three visits	846	80.1 (64.1–90.0)	75.0 (47.5–90.8)	83.2 (74.3–89.4)	1.06 (0.72)	0.96 (0.63)	0.90 (0.50)
Lipids in last 12 months	846	80.1 (72.6–86.0)	58.2 (45.4–69.9)	68.3 (55.3–78.9)	1.37 (0.004)	1.17 (0.007)	0.85 (0.29)
Microalbumin in last 12 months	846	31.9 (14.1–57.1)	6.1 (2.7–13.3)	18.6 (10.8–30.1)	5.26 (less than 0.001)	1.72 (0.10)	0.33 (0.2)
Treated or assessed and on target (all patients) HbA1c unadjusted	846	98.2	99.4	100.0	NA	NA	NA
BP	846	76.1 (61.4–86.5)	81.5 (72.7–87.9)	78.3 (69.5–85.2)	0.93 (0.48)	0.97 (0.72)	1.04 (0.58)
Lipids	846	76.6 (66.6–84.4)	55.9 (43.4–67.8)	65.7 (60.1–71.0)	1.37 (0.004)	1.17 (0.03)	0.85 (0.20)
Microalbumin	846	79.6 (61.7–90.5)	61.4 (34.7–82.6)	65.7 (53.5–76.1)	1.30 (0.26)	1.21 (0.11)	0.93 (0.79)
At target (only if assessed) HgbA1c	439	100.0	100.0	100.0	NA	NA	NA
BP	653	78.0 (63.9–87.7)	81.8 (72.3–88.5)	79.0 (71.1–85.3)	0.95 (0.63)	0.99 (0.86)	1.04 (0.64)
Lipids	566	77.2 (65.3–85.9)	64.7 (52.2–75.5)	72.0 (62.8–79.7)	1.19 (0.09)	1.07 (0.32)	0.90 (0.37)
Microalbumin	166	98.2 (92.8–99.6)	86.4 (45.4–98.0)	97.7 (87.5–99.6)	1.13 (0.07)	1.01 (0.71)	0.88 (0.9)

Data from Ohman-Strickland, P. A., et al. (2008). Quality of diabetes care in family medicine practices: Influence of nurse-practitioners and physician's assistants. Annals of Family Medicine, 6(1), 14–22.

Professional Enablers and Barriers

The attributes that facilitate or inhibit full expression of a profession are referred to as *enablers* and *barriers*. These attributes factor into the future roles of PAs and NPs in health care (Exhibit 12-9). For example, one attribute of PAs that is considered an enabler of the profession is the idea that they are unencumbered by "doctor-nurse" conflicts and traditional role perceptions. As a result, some analysts believe that PAs have somewhat clearer identities, greater mobility, and willingness—by role, definition, and name—to serve as physician associates than NPs. Their roles are more flexible because of this willing dependence on the physician. However, many of the barriers to full use for NPs, including institutional "job" dependence, limited power when compared with physicians, legal status less than optimal, partial reimbursement, and variance on qualifications and training, are also common to PAs.

Barriers unique to NPs include time-control needs and a relative lack of professional organization. PAs, on the other hand, may be limited by the social and/or political license afforded NPs because of a lack of a homogeneous professional base. PAs began their profession drawing initially on experience as corpsmen, but then quickly expanded to include applicants with diverse medical backgrounds. However, a nursing background is the common denominator for all NPs, and this background provides professional acceptance.

Unlike PAs, who have a single national academy that consolidates all PA efforts (the AAPA), no single organization represents all NPs. The American Academy of Nurse Practitioners, the American College of Nurse Practitioners, the American Nurses Association (ANA), and the National Alliance of Nurse Practitioners all claim some representation and have their advocates and critics. Other organizations represent different specialties of NPs nationally, such as the National Association of Pediatric Nurse Associates & Practitioners (NAPNAP); Association of Women's Health, Obstetrics, and Neonatal Nurses (AWHONN);

EXHIBIT 12-9

Physician Assistant and Nurse Practitioner Enablers and Barriers to Future Roles in Health Care

Enablers: NPs	Enablers: PAs
Professional base	Role flexibility
Independence from physicians	Willingness to assume dependent posture with physicians
Cost-savings potential	Cost-savings potential
Interchangeability with PAs	Interchangeability with NPs
Social appeal	Relatively greater mobility than NPs
Nursing numbers offer wide political potential to influence legislation	Professional organization
	Relatively clear identity
Large number of training programs granting graduate degrees	

Barriers: NPs	Barriers: PAs
Physician independence	Physician dependence
Limited relative power	Limited relative power
Limited (but growing) reimbursable functions	Limited (but growing) reimbursable functions
Limited power (absolute)	Limited power (absolute)
Limited mobility compared with PAs	Lack of homogeneous professional base such as nursing
Specialized training	Variable qualifications/training
Predominantly women with inherent time-control needs (i.e., need for part-time or day-shift work, child dependence)	Small number of training programs. Range from junior colleges to graduate programs in academic medical centers
Professional disorganization	

and the National Association of Nurse Practitioners in Reproductive Health. Four national NP certification boards exist for credentialing NPs, depending on specialty and preference, and many states have certification processes as well. The ANA, a powerful special-interest group, often acts on behalf of NPs. Although this splintering of NP factions has delayed the development of strong alliances between NPs and PAs (at least on the national level) efforts are underway to create a national alliance of clinicians (PAs and NPs). The American Academy of Nurse Practitioners seems to be emerging as one of the stronger organizations.

Although many people object to the tension between the two nonphysician groups, this tension can also be viewed as healthy, if society is considered best served when there is competition. When both providers strive to improve their image and demonstrate their ability to deliver quality care, patients must surely benefit in the end. Along with the public, the respective professions benefit when each is compared alongside the other, as well as with physicians. Delivering quality care at affordable cost and providing choice in types of providers can only enhance the image of U.S. medicine.

Even in the absence of far-reaching healthcare reform, it is anticipated that requirements for the use of NPs are expected to increase in an ever-expanding and demanding health system. If universal access for the United States were to occur, changes are envisioned for NPs, particularly in helping to meet primary care delivery needs (Harper & Johnson, 1998). Projections include requirements for higher numbers of NPs (along with PAs) to fulfill roles as primary care practitioners in private practices, in expanding managed care systems, and in institutional settings.

Attitudes Toward Physician Assistants

To evaluate nurses' attitudes toward PAs, a survey was conducted in two hospitals. Hospital X employed 19 PAs to work in adult and pediatric ambulatory clinics, the emergency department, the neonatal intensive care unit (NICU), and the newborn nursery. Hospital Y employed no PAs (Exhibit 12-10).

EXHIBIT 12-10
Nurse's Attitudes Toward Physician Assistants

1. *In general, do you believe the PAs with whom you have worked to be professionally competent?*

Hospital*	Yes	No
X	91.4%	8.6%
Y	74.2%	25.8%

2. *In general, do you object to performing functions at the request of a PA you believe to be professionally competent?*

Hospital	Yes	No
X	27.9%	72.1%
Y	36.5%	63.5%

3. *In general, are you or would you be comfortable working with a PA?*

Hospital	Yes	No
X	78.4%	21.6%
Y	56.2%	43.8%

4. *Of PAs and NPs, which do you personally prefer?*

Hospital	PA	NP	Both	Neither
X	8.1%	11.1%	58.6%	22.2%
Y	9.6%	35.6%	32.9%	21.9%

5. *How would you describe your overall attitude toward the PA profession?*

Hospital	Positive	Negative	Indifferent
X	52.3%	10.3%	37.4%
Y	35.4%	21.5%	43.1%

6. *I do not clearly understand the need for PAs in the healthcare system.*

Hospital	True	False
X	37.1%	69.2%
Y	47.9%	52.1%

7. *I do not clearly understand the need for PAs in the hospital.*

Hospital	True	False
X	64.1%	35.9%
Y	74.7%	25.3%

8. *My state Nurse Practice Act:*

	Hospital X	Hospital Y
Allows me to legally take orders from a PA	12.3%	6.0%
Legally requires me to take orders from a PA	2.8%	1.5%
Does not allow me to legally take orders from a PA	34.9%	16.4%
I do not know what the Nurse Practice Act says in regard to PAs	50.0%	76.1%

*Hospital X = 19 PAs; hospital Y = no PAs.
Data from Erkert, J. D. (1985). Nurses' attitudes toward PAs. *Physician Assistant, 9*(12), 41–44.

The results of this study indicated that nurses who have experience working with PAs or who have an understanding of the role of the PA in the healthcare system have more positive attitudes toward them than those who do not have such knowledge or experience (Erkert, 1985). Although some tension exists between PAs and nurses on the academic level, the roots of PAs go deeply into the nursing profession. Many PAs had their primary introduction to medicine through nursing. Approximately one-fourth of all PAs had some nursing experience. The early military corpsmen were typically trained in part by nurses and were often under nursing departments in field and stateside hospitals.

MANAGED CARE ORGANIZATIONS

PAs have been employees of managed care organizations since the late 1960s. Key healthcare reform policy goals are to lower medical care access barriers, contain cost, and incorporate largely new organizational structures ("managed competition") in health services delivery. In effect, this goal means a reliance on HMOs and other types of prepaid and managed care delivery systems. The clinical staffing mix of HMOs and other managed care organizations tends to be based in large part on the capabilities and efficiency of employed healthcare professionals. PAs and APNs are used to provide the required range, access, and quality of medical diagnostic, therapeutic, and preventive care services in a manner acceptable to enrollees.

Many believe these efforts result in improved levels of medical service access, promote greater effectiveness in medical care resource allocation, and place less emphasis on ability to pay as a criterion for people seeking health insurance coverage. As HMOs and other managed care plans become the principal locus of primary care services for many individuals, it is likely that there will be an increased demand for a full range of primary care providers (Crane 1995; Crane & Carpenter, 2006).

Analysts frequently use HMO staffing patterns to estimate national clinical workforce requirements (Weiner, 2002). This has occurred in some of the military branches and other federal systems. Based on a national survey of group and staff-model HMOs, researchers found that two-thirds of the HMOs employ a PA and/or an NP. A correlation analysis also found that HMOs with the lowest ratio of primary care physicians to members also had the highest percentage of PAs and NPs as employees (Dial et al, 1995). The authors concluded that PAs and NPs are being used in high ratios to substitute for physician services in these settings.

GOVERNMENT

As PAs have legally defined their role through legislation and policy, relationships with various federal and state government entities were (and are) necessary (see Chapter 13). Interaction with the federal government results from the need for funding of health profession education. For decades this has been through the federal grant system under Title VII, as well as reimbursement policies through Medicare and Medicaid.

Physicians receive a large share of the more than $5 billion Medicare subsidy of graduate medical education (GME) through direct medical education (DME) and indirect medical education assistance (IMEA) payments. These funds go to teaching hospitals to support the clinical education of physicians and include training assistance for a number of other healthcare professionals. However, this Medicare funding does not support PAs or APNs. In the past, federal dollars supporting PA and NP training have been administered through grant awards programs.

Federal support for PA education is authorized under Title VII Section 747 of the Public Health Service Act, whereas nursing education is funded by Title VIII. Federal support for nursing education focuses on student recruitment incentives and support to train additional numbers of nursing school faculty.

Current incentives and rewards for teaching hospitals sponsoring GME programs are driven more by institutional needs than by societal needs. Changing the structure and financing policies of Medicare to better emphasize the training of generalist physicians has not come to fruition. Making health profession educational programs receiving federal support more accountable to the public in terms of graduate outcomes (e.g., patterns of specialty and practice location) is now an increasingly accepted premise.

Medicare policy has been slow to respond to shifting patterns of physician education and practice. It has long been advocated that generalist physician numbers could be promoted by shifting the locus of GME training experiences to increase residents' time in outpatient and ambulatory care clinics, yet Medicare does not allow funding support in these settings. A policy change in the financing of health profession education is a key part of healthcare reform. The Clinton administration's proposed bill, the Health Security Act, contained an extensive array of changes affecting GME size and funding. Although this was not enacted, a major reform policy goal remains in place and is aimed to produce a 55% level of primary care physicians in the workforce. To help attain these goals, there has been the development of a new fund to support the cost of academic health center functions beyond the usual provision of patient healthcare services, establishment of an institute for healthcare workforce development, a series of initiatives to augment Title VII and VIII funding above the current level, and a GME funding pool of $200 million for advanced practice nursing. This later proposal should be modified to include PAs in the likelihood that they will be used at the same level as or higher than NPs and other advanced practice nurses in reform-restructured inpatient staffing. Incremental changes are anticipated in Congress that may eventually achieve this goal. Until then, PA education will have to rely on limited support through the Bureau of Health Professions.

PHARMACISTS

The last remaining barrier for full use of PAs was prescribing. On an individual level, in settings where a PA works with a pharmacist (usually within an institution), there is wide acceptance of PAs and the way they prescribe (Hooker, 1993). Although historically a few pharmacists opposed the ability of PAs to prescribe, these objections have largely disappeared, perhaps because of the increasing clinical role that pharmacists have been developing since the mid-1990s. For the most part, pharmacists do not seem concerned about PAs from a safety perspective.

One study that examined PA views of drug information sources showed that PAs rated pharmacists as the best sources of drug information. Next in descending order of drug information reliability were journal articles, physicians, detail persons, and other PAs. This study also found that PAs view pharmacists with increasing regard the more they come in contact with them (Fincham, 1985; Fincham, 1986).

PATIENTS

The patient's viewpoint is generally considered the most important element in the appraisal of PA acceptance in American society (Exhibit 12-11). Although relationships with physicians and nurses are placed high on the list of importance, the PA-patient relationship is the reason PAs have been able to thrive in such a competitive

EXHIBIT 12-11
How Patients View Physician Assistants Is Critical to Their Success

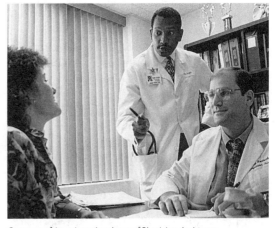

Courtesy of American Academy of Physician Assistants.

environment. The prioritization of the PA-patient relationship is important because if consumers are not satisfied with PAs, no alliance with organized medicine will ensure the PA profession's future. If patient acceptance and satisfaction with PAs was low, it is doubtful that PAs would still be in existence.

Attitudes Toward Physician Assistants

Patient attitudes and satisfaction with their providers is important because satisfied patients are more likely to follow through on recommendations made by the provider (Janis, 1980). Even before formal PA education had produced more than a few dozen PAs, researchers in the late 1960s were asking mothers of young children if they would feel comfortable with a theoretical "doctor's assistant" who could manage many of the common childhood illnesses. Ninety-four percent said such a "PA" would be acceptable (Patterson, 1969).

The first study on patient acceptance of clinically active PAs was conducted within a few years after PAs were beginning to be noticed. This study, anticipating that PAs would be dispersed throughout different socioeconomic classes, sought to determine in which social strata PA acceptance would be highest. The results showed that in 1970 the upper-middle-class community was more readily accepting of PAs (and NPs) than lower-middle-class communities (Conant et al, 1971).

In 1972, a study was undertaken in Los Angeles to assess patient acceptance of and attitudes toward the use of PAs in different roles. Acceptance was highest among unmarried, middle-class respondents who had some exposure to college. As the perceived complexity of procedures a PA might perform was increased, approval decreased; 91% of all respondents approved most procedures, such as injections, administered by PAs. This approval rating diminished to 34% in the case of first examination of a patient with a head injury by a PA (Strunk, 1973). In another 1972 study, patients rated PAs highly in terms of technical competence (89%), professional

manner (86%), and access to services (79%). Patients also reported improvement in the quality of care (71%) (Nelson, Jacobs, & Johnson, 1974). Other studies helped reinforce findings that PAs were generally well received by the patients they served regardless of rural or urban setting or social status (Oliver et al, 1986; Smith, 1981; Storms & Fox, 1979).

To address a charge by some that physicians treat patients of higher socioeconomic status and PAs treat those of lower status, Crandall, Haas, and Radelet (1986) undertook a study in three primary care centers in Florida. Data from this study showed no consistent or substantively significant relationships between the patients' social status and the type of provider. In another study using a random survey of all households in Kentucky, Mainous, Bertolino, and Harrell (1992) found that a substantial proportion of households came in contact with PAs and NPs and that satisfaction with PAs and NPs was quite high.

Elizondo and Blessing (1990) examined patient expectations of PAs in dealing with a series of personal, social, psychological, and health-related items. Results indicated that patients expect the PA to be involved with these problems but do not expect the PA to be an expert. In a follow-up survey a few years later the subject groups were PAs, supervising physicians, and PA educators. The results were compared with those of the previous study, and the findings indicated a higher level of confidence in the abilities of PAs.

Provider attitudes affect the outcome of select disorders and the level of patient satisfaction. The confidence and attitudes of three primary care PAs and 18 physicians were assessed 3 weeks after a clinic visit for low back pain in a large HMO. Patients of more confident providers were significantly more satisfied with the information they received than patients of less confident providers. Differences could not be explained by years in practice, length of visit, patient demographics, or the type of providers (Bush, Cherkin, & Barlow, 1993).

In another HMO study by Freeborn and Pope (1994), members in the Pacific Northwest region of Kaiser Permanente rated the "technical competence, skill, and ability" of physicians, PAs, and NPs as "satisfied or very satisfied" more than 75% of the time. Hooker (1993) analyzed the same population spanning an 18-month period in the early 1990s with regard to how members viewed physicians, PAs, and NPs. A 57-item questionnaire specifically asked about satisfaction with a particular medical office visit and a specific provider. Samples were drawn randomly from the automated appointment system and sent within 1 week after a patient's medical office visit. When health plan members were asked how satisfied they were with their latest encounter, adult practice PAs and NPs scored within 1% to 2% of physicians (between 88% and 90% favorable). The technical skill of PAs and NPs rated within 3% to 4% of physicians. As for overall satisfaction, members regarded adult medicine PAs and NPs almost the same and statistically indistinguishable from each other. In this study, pediatricians were viewed approximately 10% more favorably than pediatric PAs and NPs for reasons not clear in this study.

Hooker, Potts, and Ray (1997) compared the attitudes and satisfaction levels of patients with physicians, PAs, and NPs in the same HMO. Analyzing more than 40,000 returned questionnaires, they found neither statistical differences between PAs and NPs nor differences between PAs/NPs and physicians across five different departments (Exhibit 12-12).

Even when select variables were examined, such as length of experience, gender, and age of the provider, no differences emerged to show any statistical difference.

To assess the extent to which the experiences of older patients vary according to type of primary care provider, Hooker, Cipher, and Sekscenski (2005) undertook a national, cross-sectional survey of Medicare beneficiaries. Satisfaction data, patient sociodemographic characteristics, healthcare experience, types of care, and types of insurance were surveyed. A total of 146,880 completed surveys from 321,407 randomly sampled Medicare beneficiaries nationwide (45.7% of total surveyed) were analyzed. Approximately 3% identified a PA or an NP as their personal provider. For questions on satisfaction with their personal care clinician, results were similar across the the various providers (Exhibit 12-13). Patients who reported an NP as their primary care provider were significantly more likely to be Medicaid recipients as compared with patients who reported receiving care from a PA or physician. Patients who reported a physician as their primary care provider were more likely to have supplemental insurance as compared with patients who reported receiving care from a PA or NP. The authors concluded that Medicare beneficiaries are generally satisfied with their medical care and do not distinguish preferences based on type of provider. Overall primary care providers, be

EXHIBIT 12-12
Patient Satisfaction: Comparison of Average Scores for Physician Assistants/Nurse Practitioners and Physicians in an Internal Medicine Department, 1997 ($N = 41,000$)

Question	PAs/NPs	Physicians
How *courteous* and *respectful* was the clinician?	93	94
How well did the clinician *understand* your problem?	90	90
How well did the clinician *explain* to you what he or she was doing and why?	91	90
Did the clinician *use words* that were easy for you to understand?	93.5	94
How well did the clinicians *listen* to your concerns and questions?	88	91
Did the clinician spend *enough time* with you?	90	90
How much *confidence* do you have in the clinician's ability or competence?	90	91.5
Overall, how satisfied are you with the service that you receieved from the clinician?	90	91.5

* Italicized words identify the patient satisfaction characteristic surveyed. No statistical differences were found at $P < 0.001$.

Data from Hooker, R. S., Potts, R., & Ray, W. (1997). Patient satisfaction: Comparing physician assistants, nurse practitioners and physicians. Permanente Journal, 1(1), 38–42.

EXHIBIT 12-13

Comparison of Health and Provider Ratings by Medicare Recipients, 2000–2001

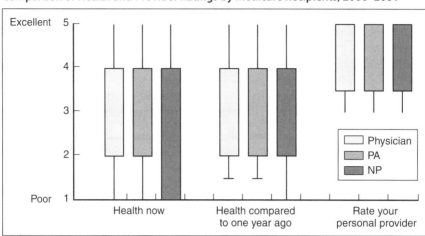

Data from Hooker, R. S., Cipher, D. J., & Sekscenski, E. (2005). Patient satisfaction with physician assistant, nurse practitioner, and physician care: A national survey of Medicare beneficiaries. Journal of Clinical Outcomes Management, 12(2), 88–92.

they PAs, NPs, or physicians, seemed to be viewed similarly favorably by the elderly.

In 2007, the AAPA undertook a national survey on patients' perceptions of PAs. The survey was managed by Fleishman-Hillard, an international communications company, and was conducted by Opinion Research Corporation. The questions were part of an omnibus poll using a nationally representative random sample. Just over 1,000 adults were interviewed by telephone. Two out of three adults responding to the nationwide poll said they are aware of the PA profession. Just over 80% of all respondents said they would be willing to be seen by a PA for a routine health visit in the event their primary medical doctor was not available. Of those previously treated by a PA, 90% said they would be willing to see a PA again. Of those who have never been treated by a PA, 76% said they would be willing to see a PA. The results seem to point that one way to increase patient willingness to be treated by a PA would be to increase contact between the public and PAs.

Even though there are approximately 65,000 clinically practicing PAs in a country of more than 281 million people, 51% of those surveyed said they had been treated by a PA.

(The percentage based off the weighted base would be 47 percent.) To test whether the respondents were confusing PAs with other healthcare professions, all were asked to describe the primary responsibilities of a PA and, for those previously treated by a PA, what condition they presented to the PA. The responses confirmed the public has a general understanding of what a PA does. Respondents mentioned that PAs "do everything a doctor does," provide patient care, write prescriptions, diagnose illness, and take the burden off the doctor. Conditions or procedures mentioned by those previously treated by a PA, such as colds, the flu, allergies, asthma, annual checkups, gynecological examinations, and general surgery, are common to PAs. Nine percent of those previously seen by a PA said they were treated by a PA because the physician was not available.

Roblin and colleagues (2004) undertook a retrospective observational study of 41,209 patient satisfaction surveys randomly sampled from visits provided by pediatric and adult medicine departments from 1997 to 2000. Adjusted for patient and visit characteristics, patients were significantly more likely to be satisfied with practitioner interaction on visits attended by PAs and/or NPs than visits attended by doctors in both the adult and pediatric practices (Exhibit 12-14). Patient satisfaction did not differ significantly by practitioner type for most conditions and presenting condition.

Parents

Parents of children are mentioned because of their reaction to the concept of pediatric PAs and child health associates (CHAs). In the mid-1960s, a few years preceding full deployment of CHAs, three separate studies reported favorable parent acceptance of pediatric-trained assistants on alternate pediatrician patient visits at approximately one-half the usual pediatric fee (Austin, Foster, & Richards, 1968; Skinner, 1968). In structured interviews in the homes of 145 mothers in the Seattle area, roughly one-half of the group had regular pediatric care from private pediatricians, one-third from an HMO, and the rest from public health clinics. Approximately 75% of the mothers approved of the pediatric assistant for well-child care, and 94% indicated they would be willing to use the assistant if the physician and assistant were well trained and capable (Patterson, 1969). A third study found that the pediatrician's time could be better spent delegating at least 50% of the workload to PAs (Anderson & Powers, 1970).

Silver and Ott (1973) reported that 94% of the parents expressed satisfaction with the joint services they received from a pediatrician and a CHA team and with their opportunity to maintain adequate communication with the physician. Half the parents of children seen in this setting thought that joint care was better than care they received from a physician alone.

Henry and Hooker (2008) examined the attitudes of rural communities in their regard to PAs staffing a clinic in town. This study compared PAs' perspectives of their role in rural health with the perspectives of the communities they serve in order to understand shared and differing views on access to health care. PAs and local residents in eight remote Texas communities were interviewed. Conversations with the PAs in these communities suggest that townspeople are not concerned that a PA is in the clinic instead of a physician—that it is irrelevant to the community. Their own patients and the positive feedback they receive reinforce their views. Conversations with community members (clinic patients and nonpatients) suggest otherwise.

In the aggregate, each community was clearly appreciative of the clinic's presence in the town. Residents understood that the PA was filling a role as clinician in the town and were glad for what he or she provided, but they perceived this role as mostly treating "little conditions." Yet most claimed that the level of health care "could be better." One important note is that discussion focused on the level of health care rather than on the specific PA. Many were quick to say that their concerns over health care had nothing to do with the PA personally—the PA was doing a good job—but the town needed *more* health care than the PA could provide. One community member, representing the majority of responses, said (referring to the PA), "[She's] very good and is lots of help. She helps everyone. I've been living here for 18 years and have been going to the clinic all that time." When the same respondent was asked what people think about not having a physician in town, she responded: "[It's] not really a good deal. We need a full-time doctor . . . it would be better." It is clear that residents understand the difference between a physician and a PA. They know their town does not have a physician

EXHIBIT 12-14
Satisfaction of Encounter When Attended by a Physician Assistant/Nurse Practitioner or a Doctor

	Difference in Satisfaction (0–100 scale) for Visits Attended by a PA/NP vs. a Doctor	
	Adult Medicine	*Pediatric Medicine*
Pace of care	1.33	1.14
Provider interaction	0.87	0.35
Overall experience	0.90	1.23

Data from Roblin, D.W., Becker, E. R., Adams, E. K., et al. (2004). Patient satisfaction with primary care: Does type of practitioner matter? Medical Care, 42(6), 579–590.

and they have thoughts, opinions, and concerns about the level of health care in their town.

Interestingly, the communities that were the most satisfied with having only a PA at the clinic were those towns that have had the same PA for the longest amount of time (6–10 years). This finding suggests that the relationships that are built between a PA and the community over years of working together make an impact on the community's trust and commitment to the clinic and the PA, as well as overall perception of health care. Anecdote aside, the aggregated results suggest that while PAs and community members agree that the level of the town's health care was at least moderately good, there are varying perspectives on the role of the autonomous PA in the town (Henry & Hooker, 2008).

One of the problems with evaluating patient acceptance and satisfaction with healthcare providers in general is the asymmetry of information. The healthcare consumer can neither choose the best treatment because of lack of time, nor judge whether the treatment is adequate unless he or she is a clinician. The patient may perceive the best care is related to the sense of comfort felt when the patient is seen by a certain provider, even though the best care is not being delivered. For many patients the "halo effect" predominates in their thinking, and the clinician (physician, PA, NP, or CNM) is often held above reproach when surveys are conducted.

From the literature, it appears that PAs are held in high regard by patients regardless of socioeconomic status, condition, and setting. These views may reflect confidence in the PA's ability to take care of their medical conditions. The most recent findings suggest patients like the provider as long as the provider is courteous, explains the care, uses terms they can understand, and listens to their complaints. Most likely, *satisfaction* represents the perception of patients whose healthcare need was largely met. Additional studies are needed to measure and compare both satisfaction and outcome of all types of providers in all types of settings. Some of the current literature is outdated and the few contemporary studies were undertaken in well-defined settings

in which PAs and NPs have long been established.

INTERNATIONAL MEDICAL GRADUATES

International medical graduates (IMGs) (formerly known as *foreign medical graduates*) have filled gaps in American medical services during most of the 20th century. Fully one-quarter of all U.S. licensed physicians are IMGs and close to 30% of all resident physicians are IMGs. The vast majority of IMGs in the United States are born and trained overseas. Not all IMGs in the United States are licensed or enrolled in U.S. GME programs. Recognizing this population as a potential source of medical providers, some state medical boards have explored various approaches to assist IMGs who have failed to meet requirements for licensure. This effort includes remedial activities to correct deficiencies in knowledge and skills or limited licensure that allows IMGs to practice as physicians in certain settings and/or under supervision. As barriers to medical licensure have increased, many have sought ways to enter health care in lieu of completing the lengthy and expensive medical licensure process.

Some IMGs have sought access to PA licensure as a permanent career change, and others as an interim step toward licensure as physicians. Unlicensed IMGs have organized to promote state laws to make it easier for them to train or practice as PAs. These attempts to recast IMGs as PAs have been criticized as creating a double standard for PA qualification, jeopardizing public safety, and creating a regulatory bureaucracy that would be prohibitively expensive (Fowkes et al, 1996; Stanhope, Fasser, & Cawley, 1992).

In the early 1990s, following the passage of a law in Florida that permitted IMGs to seek PA credentials, the AAPA Professional Practice Council issued an official position paper on the issue of IMGs attempting to become PAs. The paper asserts that entry to the PA profession should require graduation from an accredited PA educational program and passage of the national certifying examination.

Furthermore, "Passage of an examination by itself is inadequate to define the knowledge needed to practice as a PA."

This position paper is in part a result of observations that the socialization to the PA role and understanding of the physician-PA relationship is part of the knowledge base required of the PA. These aspects of the PA role are taught and experienced as a PA student. Additionally, having states develop or administer their own examinations as an alternative entry mechanism would compromise the uniformity of a national PA qualifying standard and possibly discourage reciprocity between states. Moreover, there is evidence that IMGs lack the knowledge and skills necessary to practice as PAs or to validate fast-track or abbreviated educational programs as appropriate solutions.

In California, surveys in 1980, 1993, and 1994 collected information about the interest and preparedness among IMGs seeking PA certification. These surveys revealed that few of the IMGs were interested in becoming PAs as a permanent career, and few could show a commitment to primary care of the underserved. Of the 50 IMGs accepted into California's PA programs in recent years, 62% had academic or personal difficulties. Only 34 IMGs became certified. The City University of New York/Harlem Hospital PA Program developed an accelerated program for IMGs in 1992. None of the IMGs who took the same clinical competency examination developed for PA students passed (Stanhope, Fasser, & Cawley, 1992).

Some states, including Maryland, Florida, Michigan, and Washington, have used different approaches to alternative pathways to PA licensure for IMGs (Bottom & Evans, 1994; Cawley, 1995). Additional preparatory programs in California that have assessed the readiness of unlicensed IMGs to enter PA programs have shown that the participants did not demonstrate knowledge or clinical skills equivalent to those expected of licensed PAs (Fowkes et al, 1996).

In 2007, the Ontario government launched a large health initiative that included recruiting PAs and converting IMGs into PAs. In total, 40 IMGs were given a course upgrade in general medicine and instructed that they could work as PAs but not consider themselves doctors. They are not referred to as anything but PAs and are eligible for membership in the Canadian Associaton of Physician Assistants. After 2 years working as PAs they are eligible to opt out of working as a PA and apply for a residency in family medicine or some other postgraduate training regimen. This experiment is observed under the *HealthForceOntario* initiative through 2012 (Kuttler, 2007c).

PEERS WITHIN THE PHYSICIAN ASSISTANT PROFESSION

Key professional relationships for PAs are those maintained among their peers. One method of fostering these relationships is through the growing number of publications written by and for PAs. How and what a profession says about itself is an evolving process, and the way it promotes itself in journalism and literature is a measurement of the profession's status and maturity. The increasing numbers of articles and books authored by PAs has allowed more than one publication to exist at the same time. As the profession expands into other countries, such publications will serve as a forum for global communication about the profession.

Ongoing challenges for PA publications include the following:

- Competitive and increasingly difficult business of print journals
- Use of the Web as an alternative source of medical education sources
- Challenge of recruiting sufficient manuscripts from PA clinicians
- Lack of a firm research infrastructure in the profession

However, these challenges have the potential to be overcome with the expansion of the profession outside of the United States.

Journals

The history of PA journals is rooted in the era of the profession's initial development. Although some have folded, others have endured with the support of professional societies (Exhibit 12-15).

PA Journal

Charles B. Slack, Inc., a publisher in New Jersey, launched the first official journal of the American Academy of Physician Assistants in 1970. Initially, the volumes were titled *Physician's Associate*. This name reflected the few years that the AAPA was the *American Academy of Physician's Associates*. Later, when the name changed to the AAPA, the name *PA Journal* was adopted.

The first PA professional journal listed a number of influential members of the profession, including Don Detmer, MD, who served as Editor; Ann Bliss, MSW; Carl Emil Fasser, PA; Bill Stanhope, PA; David Lawrence, MD, MPH; Steve Turnipseed, MX; John Ott, MD; and Bill De'Ak, MD. Later known as the "Green Journal" because of its distinctive cover, the *PA Journal* served "as a forum for the discussion and presentation of important issues related to the advancement of the physician's assistant and other health professional auxiliaries."

Physician Assistant

While the *PA Journal* was still in publication, a small independent publisher, United Business Publications, Inc., launched a magazine in 1976 called *Physician Assistant*. Both journals were competing for essentially the same audience and the same advertising revenue. Ultimately, neither journal proved particularly viable financially, and the first version of *Physician Assistant* folded a few years later.

Meanwhile, a new prospective publisher, F & F Publications, entered discussion with the AAPA concerning the possibility of a new journal for the profession. An agreement was reached whereby the AAPA granted a 1-year endorsement to *Health Practitioner*. (The initial plan was to distribute it to PAs and NPs.)

EXHIBIT 12-15
Timeline of Physician Assistant Journalism

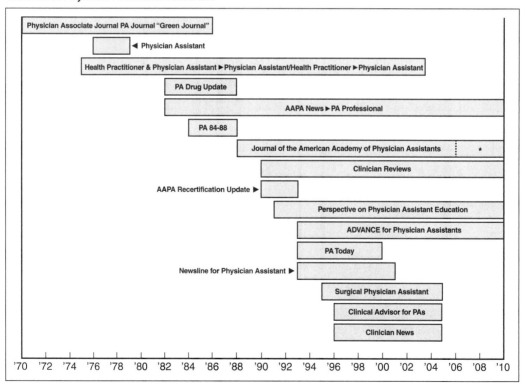

Journal of the Physician Assistant Education (formerly *PPAE*) '06–'10.

The first issue of *Health Practitioner* was distributed at the May 1977 AAPA Conference in Houston, Texas. By the end of the year the tag line "Magazine for Physician Assistants" was added to the title. Next, the title *Physician Assistant* was obtained from the original publisher, and that title took the place of the tag line for the March 1978 issue, which was called *Health Practitioner and Physician Assistant Magazine*. Starting with the next issue, the name was simplified to *Health Practitioner/Physician Assistant*. In August 1979 the order was reversed, and the name became *Physician Assistant/Health Practitioner* (reflecting the fact that the audience was primarily PAs). Meanwhile, PW Communications took over the publication from F & F Publications. In 1983, *Health Practitioner* was dropped from the title, and the publication became known as *Physician Assistant*.

Although the initial AAPA endorsement of what was originally called *Health Practitioner* expired after the March 1978 issue, in January 1983, after the *PA Journal* had finally folded, *Physician Assistant* again became the official publication of the AAPA; that relationship continued through June 1987, when the AAPA was ready to introduce its own new publication (Tiger, 1992). After being sold multiple times to various publishers, *Physician Assistant* folded in 2004.

Journal of the American Academy of Physician Assistants

In 1988, for the first time, the AAPA published a journal with editorial control in the hands of the academy: the *Journal of the American Academy of Physician Assistants (JAAPA)* has its own staff, editorial board, and PA editors. Initially published by Mosby and currently published by Haymarket Media. It is a scholarly peer-reviewed monthy publication that includes some coverage of the PA profession and AAPA updates. Leslie Kole, PA, was appointed the founding editor-in-chief in 1988 and served as full-time in-house editor based in the AAPA headquarters until 2003. At the time the AAPA retained Haymarket Media as publisher, it appointed Sarah

Zarbock, PA, as editor-in-chief. Tayna Gregory, PhD, serves as editor (Exhibit 12-16).

The AAPA Board of Directors approves the appointment of the 13-member Editorial Board of *JAAPA*. Members of the Editorial Board serve 3-year terms. Members include a representative of the AAPA Board, usually the immediate past president, the founding editor, and a variety of distinguished clinical and academic PAs. Typical *JAAPA* departments include "From the AAPA," CME articles, case reports, and "CAT Clinic." Articles on bioethics, evidence-based medicine, PA health services research, dermatology, new drug information, and surgical issues are also included, as well as editorials by guests and the editor-in-chief. As of 2008, *JAAPA* has published more than 8,000 pages of clinical articles, policy papers, surveys, scientific studies, editorials, debates, letters, and essays. More than 90% of the contributions have

EXHIBIT 12-16
Journal of the American Academy of Physician Assistants

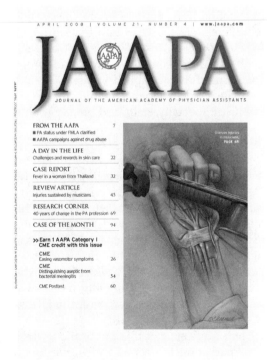

Courtesy Haymarket Media.

been authored by PAs. It competed side by side with *Physician Assistant* for readership and advertisement revenue until *Physician Assistant* folded.

In 2008, *JAAPA* won several awards from the Society of National Association Publications. These awards were for: (1) scholarly journal, most improved, for the April 2007 redesign of *JAAPA*; (2) peer-reviewed article in a scholarly journal for "Pandemic influenza: A brief history and primer" (January 2007); and (3) peer-reviewed article in a scholarly journal for "High-altitude illnesses: From the limited to the potentially lethal" (January 2007). *JAAPA* is a membership benefit of the AAPA and is distributed to all AAPA members.

ADVANCE for Physician Assistants

In 1993, *ADVANCE for Physician Assistants* was launched as a new publication "to provide timely and useful information about clinical and practice issues" (Exhibit 12-17). *ADVANCE for PAs* strives to reach the growing PA market as a major publication in the field. Over the past decade *ADVANCE* has excelled in two areas: being a source of useful clinical information and, perhaps more importantly, being a reliable source of information regarding the profession itself. The editor and staff comb the data from the AAPA and professional societies to publish statistics on new graduates and experienced clinicians as well as data by specialty, state, and other variables.

Clinician Reviews

Clinician Reviews was a breakaway publication of *Physician Assistant*. Formed in 1990 by two PAs, David Mittman and Tom Yakeren, the publication aimed to do what others had failed to do—appeal to a wider audience than just PAs. This publication started out as a high-quality, glossy monthly journal that was marketed to PAs and NP/CNMs. It published clinical articles and occasionally reported on issues that politically or economically affected PAs and NPs (Exhibit 12-18).

The significance of this publication was its joint marketing to PAs and NPs, reinforcing the developing perception that, in regard to staffing, PAs and NPs were interchangeable in

EXHIBIT 12-17
ADVANCE for Physician Assistants

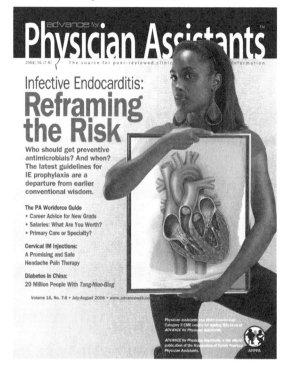

the healthcare industry. *Clinician Reviews* went through several format changes, but its audience always remained NPs and PAs. It currently is published in tabloid format and is co-edited by Randy D. Danielsen, PhD, Dean of the Arizona School of Health Sciences. *Clinician Reviews* claim a subscription distribution of more than 80,000.

Journal of Physician Assistant Education

Journal of Physician Assistant Education (JPAE) is the research-based journal of the Physician Assistant Education Association (PAEA). It is the only academically focused journal for PAs and the most scholarly. The journal originated as a newletter for PA educators called *Perspective on Physician Assistant Education* and was circulated by the PAEA. In 1998, with underwriting from the AAPA and Donald Pederson, PhD, PA, of the University of Utah PA Program as editor, it began as the quarterly journal *Perspective on Physician*

EXHIBIT 12-18
Clinician Reviews

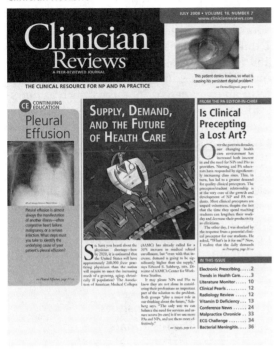

Courtesy of Clinicians Group, LLC, Clifton, NJ.

EXHIBIT 12-19
Journal of Physician Assistant Education

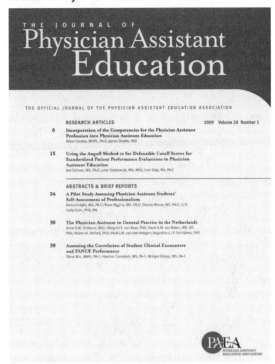

Courtesy of the Physician Assistant Education Association.

Assistant Education. In 2005, the PAEA assumed full management of the publication and appointed P. Eugene Jones, PhD, PA, as editor-in-chief. Ultimately, the journal evolved into the *JPAE* and serves primarily as a platform to disseminate research on the education and behavior of PAs. It receives international submissions as the rigor and quality of research continues to improve (Exhibit 12-19).

Specialty Journals

Surgical Physician Assistant was a small quarterly journal that started in 1995 and was focused on clinical literature of interest to surgical PAs. Although it was somewhat an official journal of surgical PAs, it was sent to all PAs (members and nonmembers of the AAPA). The journal folded due to lack of revenue in 2003. *Arthritis Practitioner* was a publication directed at PAs and NPs in rheumatology but ran out of funding in 2007.

The first official journal of a specialty PA society is the *Journal of the Dermatology Physician Assistants* published by the Society of Dermatology Physician Assistants (SDPA). The quarterly publication began in 2007 and hopes to build on the growing number of dermatology PAs. Its mission is to help improve dermatological patient care by publishing current practice-related educational information for the PA profession. The premier issue included articles on clinical dermatology, surgical dermatology, cosmetic dermatology, and professional development. The journal is free for SDPA members and costs $30 per year for nonmembers.

Constituent Chapter Newsletters

Since the development of constituent chapters of PA professional organizations, there has been an attempt to collect and redistribute information on the decentralized and local PA level. Usually this is by and for PAs in state chapters of the AAPA or affiliations. A giant boost in these publications came in the mid-1980s when the Leaderle Corporation made unrestricted grants to all 50 state-affiliated chapters of the AAPA to purchase personal computers and other equipment for the purposes of generating newsletters.

Magazines

Other publications in the history of the PA profession include non-peer-reviewed magazines (as opposed to journals). Peter Frishauf, founder of *Health Practitioner/Physician Assistant*, produced a series of publications that ran for 5 years—*PA 84* through *PA 88*. Another example is *PA Drug Update*, which was created in the 1980s as a magazine of continuing medical education for physician assistants. Underwritten by Pfizer Pharmaceuticals, it had a number of topics written by specialists in various fields and was distributed to PAs. *AAPA Recertification Update* began in 1990 as a special publication to prepare students and graduates for the recertification process. It ended after 4 years of publication. *PA Professional* was launched in 2009 as a monthly magazine targeting PAs. It replaced the *AAPA News*.

Books

PAs have authored more than 30 books (Exhibit 12-20). Topics range from certification review to clinical practice to studies of the PA profession itself.

Electronic Resources

Through support by Duke University, PAs have a number of online forums: the PA Forum, Student PA Forum, PA Faculty Forum, and PAs in Primary Care Forum. Known as lists, these forums are usually lively exchanges of opinions by PAs and address a wide range of subjects.

Additional online sources include the various websites of PA professional organizations. For example, the AAPA website provides information about the PA profession as a service to answer commonly asked questions about PAs and the Academy. Popular sections of the site include PA program information, position papers of the AAPA, current data on PA practitioners and students, legislative and legal information, and the contact information for the profession's leadership. Other online sources of information about PAs are shown in Exhibit 12-21. This is a partial list of more than 150 websites, most of which are managed by individual PA education programs.

In an era where print media, such as newspapers and print journals, face increasing competition from other sources, the future of PA publications is uncertain. However, there is a need for more media related to PAs. The existing publications intended for PAs struggle with declining advertising revenues and may require greater levels of subsidy from their organizational sponsors to sustain their operations. There is not as of yet a global journal intended for PAs, although that may be a desired goal.

Research on Relationships With Other Professionals

Much of the available information regarding relationships that PAs have with various other professionals is anecdotal or outdated. Relationships for PAs are a broad area of research and involve the disciplines of history, policy, sociology, anthropology, and organizational theories. A brief list of some research topics is presented here.

- **Case studies:** How PAs and doctors interact needs to be recorded using sociological investigation techniques.

- **Sociology:** Where does concordance and divergence of attitudes lie in views between PAs and doctors, nurses, and patients about how well they are perceived?

- **Economics and ethics:** Willingness to be seen is a concept that probes patient's trade-offs and inclinations in willing to be seen by a PA or wait longer to be seen by a doctor. How willing are patients to be seen by a PA, NP, or doctor if they have to make time trade-offs or economic trade-offs?

- **History:** What are the historical markers that identify where PAs gained acceptance by nursing and other professionals?

EXHIBIT 12-20
Selected Books for Physician Assistants

1972	*The Physician's Assistant: Today and Tomorrow,* by Alfred M. Sadler, Blair Sadler, and Ann Bliss; first book on the PA profession, published by Yale University Press.
1975	*The Physician Assistant: A National and Local Analysis,* by Ann Suter Ford, published by Praeger Publishers.
	The Physician's Assistant: Today and Tomorrow, 2nd edition, by Alfred M. Sadler, Blair Sadler, and Ann Bliss, published by Ballinger.
1977	*The New Health Professionals: Nurse Practitioners and Physician's Assistants,* by Ann Bliss and Eva Cohen, published by Lippincott Williams & Wilkins.
	The Physician's Assistant: A Baccalaureate Curriculum, by Hu Myers.
1978	*The Physician's Assistant: Innovation in the Medical Division of Labor,* by Eugene Schneller, published by Lexington Books.
1980	*Physician's Assistant Examination Review,* by Thomas D. Aschenbrener.
1981	*Staffing Primary Care in 1990: Physician Replacement and Cost Savings,* by Jane Cassels Record, published by Lippincott Williams & Wilkins.
	The Art of Teaching Primary Care, edited by Archie Golden, Dennis G. Carlson, and Jan L. Hagen, published by Springer.
	The Role of the Physician Assistants in Primary Care, by Judith Greenwood, published by CRC.
1982	*Physician Assistants: Their Contribution to Health Care,* by Henry Perry and Bena Breitner, published by Human Services Press.
1984	*Alternatives in Health Care Delivery: Emerging Roles of Physician Assistants,* by Reginal D. Carter, published by W. H. Green.
1986	*Physician Assistants: Present and Future Models of Utilization,* edited by Sarah F. Zarbock and Kenneth Harbert, published by Praeger.
1987	*The Physician Assistant in a Changing Health Care Environment,* by Gretchen E. Schafft and James F. Cawley, published by Aspen.
1993	*The Roles of the Physician Assistant and Nurse Practitioner in Primary Care,* edited by D. Kay Clawson and Marian Osterweis, published by the Association of Academic Health Centers.
	Selected Annotated Bibliography of the Physician Assistant Profession, 4th edition, by Susan M. Anderson, published by the AAPA.
1994	*Managing Risk Through Quality PA Practice: A Guide for Health Care Providers,* published by the AAPA.
1995	*Physician Assistant Career Planning Guide,* by Julie A. Edin, published by Betz.
1996	*The Physician Assistant Emergency Medicine Handbook,* by Steven W. Salyer, published by W. B. Saunders.
1997	*Don't Call Me Doctor,* by G. B. Randall, published by Morris Publications.
1998	*Physician Assistant Legal Handbook,* by Patricia A. Younger, published by Aspen.
	National Certifying Examination for Physician Assistant, by Jack Rudman, published by National Learning Corp.
	Primary Care for Physician Assistants: Pretest Self-Assessment and Review, edited by Rodney L. Moser, published by McGraw-Hill.
2000	*Physician Assistant's Clinical Companion,* published by Springhouse.
2001	*Physician Assistant's Guide to Research and Medical Literature,* by J. Dennis Blessing, published by F. A. Davis.
	Physician Assistant's Drug Handbook, by J. Dennis Blessing, published by F. A. Davis.
	Physician Assistant Review, by Patrick C. Auth and Morris D. Kerstein, published by Lippincott Williams & Wilkins.
2002	*Physician Assistant Secrets,* by David A. Tecchio and Donna Hall, published by Lippincott Williams & Wilkins.
	A Kernel in the Pod, by J. Michael Jones, published by Xlibris.
	Clinical Procedures for Physician Assistants, by Richard W. Dehn and David P. Asprey, published by Saunders.
	Opportunities in Physician Assistant Careers, revised edition, by Terence J. Sacks, published by McGraw-Hill.
2003	*Physician Assistants in American Medicine,* 2nd edition, by Roderick. S. Hooker and James. F. Cawley, Churchill Livingstone.
	Getting Into the Physician Assistant School of Your Choice, 2nd edition, by Andrew J. Rodican, published by McGraw-Hill Medical.
	A Comprehensive Review for the Certification and Recertification Examinations for Physician Assistants, edited by Claire Babcock O'Connell and Sarah F. Zarbock, published by Lippincott Williams & Wilkins.
2004	*The Physician Assistant Medical Handbook,* 2nd edition, by James B. Labus, published by Saunders.
2007	*The Physician Assistant's Business Practice and Legal Guide,* by Michelle Roth-Kauffman, published by Jones & Bartlett.
	Appleton & Lange's Review for the Physician Assistant, 5th edition, by Anthony Miller and Albert Simon, published by McGraw-Hill Medical.
2008	*Physician Assistant: A Guide to Clinical Practice,* 4th edition, edited by Ruth Ballweg, Edward Sullivan, Darwin Brown, and Daniel Vetrosky, published by Saunders.
	Ethics and Professionalism: A Guide for the Physician Assistant, by Barry A. Cassidy and J. Dennis Blessing, published by F. A. Davis.

EXHIBIT 12-21
Online Sources of Information About Physician Assistants

Source of Information	Website Address	Comment
Bureau of Labor Statistics, U.S. Department of Labor	http://www.stats.bls.gov/oco/ocos081.htm	Projects PA growth
American Academy of Physician Assistants home page	http://www.aapa.org	Continuously updated
American Academy of Physician Assistants list of PA programs	http://www.aapa.org/pgmlist.php3	Includes all U.S. PA programs
Physician Assistant Education Association	http://www.paeaonline.org/	Official organization of U.S. PA programs
Journal of the Physician Assistant Education Association	http://www.paeaonline.org/publications. html#JPAE	PA education journal website
Surgical Physician Assistant	http://www.surgicalpa.com/	Journal website
National Commission on Certification of Physician Assistants	http://www.nccpa.net/	Credentialing body for graduate PAs
Journal of the American Academy of Physician Assistants	http://www.jaapa.pdr.net/	Official journal of the AAPA
PA History Project	http://www.aapa.org/pahistorysociety/schol_ awards.htm	
Physician Assistant Jobs	http://www.physicianassistantjobs.com/	Job locator
Physician Assistant Career Center	http://www.paworld.net/postresume.htm	Employment and information blog
Veteran Affairs Physician Assistant Association	http://www.vapaa.org/	—
Internet Journal of Academic Physician Assistants	http://www.ispub.com/journals/ijapa.htm	—
U.S. News and World Report ranking of graduate PA programs as of 2009	http://grad-schools.usnews. rankingsandreviews.com/grad/pas/ search	—
Accreditation Review Commission on Education for the Physician Assistant	http://www.arc-pa.org/	Lists current accredited PA programs
Centralized Application Service for Physician Assistants	http://www.portal.caspaonline.org/	Application service
United Kingdom Academy of Physician Assistants	http://www.ukapa.co.uk/	Oficial site for PAs in the United Kingdom
Canadian Association of Physician Assistants	http://www.caopa.net/	Official site for PAs in Canada

- **Behavior:** What are the attitudes of various professions and public attitudes about doctoral degrees for PAs and NPs?

- **Organization:** Why do some institutions employ PAs exclusively and others employ NPs exclusively?

- **Gender and generation:** Do the attitudes of PAs and NPs about each other transcend generations and gender?

SUMMARY

No profession stands alone; all are built on relationships with other players in the same arena. From the beginning, the physician-PA relationship began as a strong one and continues today. The evidence is overwhelming that physicians accept PAs in their many and varied roles, and this attitude is not likely to change as long as PAs avoid seeking independent practice. Relationships with other populations such as nurses, NPs, pharmacists, organized medicine, and patients are stronger today than they have ever been. PA journalism, the richest form of communication, has emerged as a solid venue for PAs to evidence their contribution to society. This enterprise has expanded as the profession has grown and will likely continue, an acknowledgment that the PA profession has come of age and is an important group to observe.

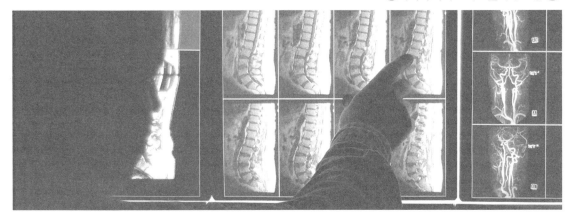

CHAPTER 13

LEGISLATION AND POLICY

JAMES F. CAWLEY ■ RODERICK S. HOOKER ■ DAVID P. ASPREY

The less people know about how sausages and laws are made, the better they'll sleep at night.
—*Otto von Bismarck*

ABSTRACT

Laws that address the conduct of doctors and other health professionals are evolutionary, and their historical roots are anchored over a period of 100 years. Collectively, this body of laws spells out what a doctor may do and to whom he or she may delegate medical authority. Since the first physician assistant (PA) graduate was employed, federal and state legislation has emerged as a fabric of laws stitched together. For Americans, the cloth is made up of the states, territories, the District of Columbia, and federal systems; together they provide a remarkable patchwork quilt. States are not uniform in how they enact laws, and PA legislation is no exception. However, all 50 states enable PAs to work, prescribe, and be reimbursed for their services. That accomplishment came about through legal activism, concern for public safety, coordinated political action, and professionalism.

INTRODUCTION

Legislation regarding the U.S. physician assistant (PA) profession is fixed in statutes enacted decades ago for physicians and subsequently for nurses and other health personnel. These medical practice statutes evolved over the course of the 20th century into their highly codified form today. A significant part of medical practice evolution has been the broadening of scopes of practice that now permits various personnel to perform heretofore restricted medical tasks. During the past half-century, this evolution has led to a significant proliferation of health professions and their respective licensing processes. Currently, there are more than 36 regulated health professions in the United States and more than 200 health vocations.

With the introduction of PAs and nurse practitioners (NPs) in 1965, state health occupation regulatory acts needed to be modified to allow these providers to perform tasks that were traditionally in the domain of the physician. In 2000, all states had enabling legislations; by 2007 all 50 states permitted prescribing authority for PAs and NPs. Legislative and regulatory changes in state medical practice acts to accommodate PA practice included defining the required qualifications for occupational licensure or certification, defining scope of practice, developing supervisory stipulations, establishing board representation and governance policies, creating professional disciplinary standards, and granting prescribing authority. Acts providing prescribing authority for PAs were the most difficult to obtain and tended to meet significant resistance. Evolving from a patchwork of laws among various jurisdictions, modern PA practice regulations are growing in their degree of similarity. The evidence to date demonstrates that PAs handle the delegated role, assuming a great deal of responsibility, and the result is improved healthcare access for U.S. citizens (Jonsson, Norden, & Hanson, 2007).

Medical licensure laws to regulate physicians were enacted in the United States during the late 19th and early 20th centuries as a matter of public necessity. Protection of the public against quackery, commercial exploitation, deception, and professional incompetence required legally enforceable standards for entrance into and continuing practice in the medical profession. Therefore, the state medical practices were developed to specify ethical and educational requirements for physicians relating to personal character, scientific education, and practical training or experience.

Unlike medical licensure laws, state licensure statutes for PAs, allied and auxiliary health personnel, and nurses were not enacted to correct abuses of independent entrepreneurial practice. Instead, the latter statutes have usually been "friendly" regulations enacted with the cooperation of the professions and occupations and designed to protect both the regulated personnel and the public from unqualified and unethical practitioners.

The forms of licensure, however, are generally similar to medical practice acts, except that in some states, PAs' licensure is permissive rather than mandatory. Accordingly, the statutes define the practice of the various professions and occupations and prescribe the personal, educational, and certification of professional competence qualifications required for such practice. The most significant and contemporary issues regarding licensure of PAs concern the effect of licensure provisions on the distribution of tasks and duties. For physicians, with unlimited licenses to perform all medical functions, the critical questions are what medical functions they

may delegate and under what conditions such delegations can be made. For PAs, the problems are more numerous and complex. Because their licenses are limited to a particular segment of health service, it is sometimes necessary to identify functions that they may not legally perform under ordinary circumstances. These determinations require interpretation of the scope of permissible practice as defined by the relevant licensure statute and the scope of exclusive practice as defined by the statute. For example, a PA in a urology practice may be violating his scope of practice if he removes a wart from the patient's foot. In Missouri, an early licensure statute stipulated that PAs could not refract and fit patients with prescription lenses. Other examples arose largely out of territorial imperative of some special interest group that felt their scope of practice was threatened.

Functions within the scope of practice for a PA may be either "independent of" or "dependent on" receiving orders, direction, or supervision from a physician. Many variables are involved in determining whether a given function is dependent, and if so, the nature and degree of supervision required for its performance. The same complexity characterizes another problem related to the PA scope of practice: the delegation of medical functions. Unlike some allied health personnel, such as physical therapists and occupational therapists who have unique skills not likely to be duplicated by a physician, the PA has the same skills more or less than those of a physician. Therefore, delegation is not an issue of authorizing personnel to use their exclusive professional skills, but one of authorizing PAs to perform medical functions that the physician would normally have to do through delegation of medical functions to the PA.

In general, scope-of-practice issues are the most uncertain area in the legal regulation of PAs, because the licensure statutes or related court decisions have not adequately addressed how PAs should be viewed—as providers with their own set of jurisdictions or as employees of physicians. After more than four decades of experience with delegation of physician tasks to PAs, that so few cases have come under the legal spotlight reflects some confidence that PAs are practicing within their legal scope of practice.

OVERVIEW OF STATE LEGISLATIVE PROCESSES

Each of the 50 states possesses a state-defined right to retain power to protect the public health. No state abrogates this right and each regulates the practice of various occupations, including physicians, nurses, physical therapists, and PAs. Each state writes its own laws and wide variations exist in the structure and content of the laws. For PAs to institute changes in policy or legislation is a lengthy, but worthwhile process, outlined as follows (Gara & Davis, 2008).

- First, PAs raise the question about whether changes in policy could be made. Individuals may band together and poll their colleagues in practice about problems and issues they may be experiencing or have in common, such as with insurance reimbursement, prescribing, or supervision.
- Second, the state PA professional society, usually a constituent chapter of the American Academy of Physician Assistants (AAPA), commonly seeks advice from the government affairs section of the AAPA. This consultation allows practice environments in other states to be compared. Summaries of PA state laws and regulations are reviewed. See Appendix III.
- Third, a group of PAs with legislative interest may seek the assistance of sympathetic representatives in the state legislature to see if they will sponsor a bill. Typically, this step requires some agreement between the state medical society and the individuals seeking the legislation regarding the terms of the policy change being requested. Bipartisan support is usually recommended because different political parties will have different levels of influence in the state house or state senate.
- Fourth, when the bill is introduced, it usually goes to a committee that will make a recommendation and then introduce it in the House and Senate with a recommendation. Regular contact with representatives or staff members as to when the bill will be discussed in committee is important. Being present to give testimony if needed is usually required.
- Fifth, after a committee approves a bill, it goes to the full chamber for vote. A bill that passes in one chamber needs to be introduced in the second chamber.
- Finally, once passed by both chambers (and sometimes changed to reach agreement), the bill must be signed by the governor to become law.

Exhibit 13-1 is an example of Wisconsin's legislative process.

PHYSICIAN ASSISTANT LEGISLATION HISTORY

Early medical licensure statutes reflected the recommendations of the Flexner report on medical education published in 1910, which initiated efforts to raise standards of medical school admission, instruction, and curriculum to place these schools under the jurisdiction of universities and to provide full-time faculty and adequate facilities for teaching and clinical experience (Starr, 1982). The incorporation in medical licensure laws of requirements that proprietary schools could not meet resulted in the closing of medical doctor diploma mills. Standards of ethics and competency provided in the early licensure laws for PAs were derived from the view of leaders of the medical profession that medicine should be based on an educational system that was responsive to the needs and the social and scientific status of the country at that time (see "AAPA Guidelines for Ethical Conduct" in Appendix IV).

Although vast changes have taken place in the social and scientific status of the country since the original enactment of the medical practice acts, no fundamental changes have been made in the statutory standards of professional

EXHIBIT 13-1
How a Bill Is Introduced Into the Wisconsin Legislature

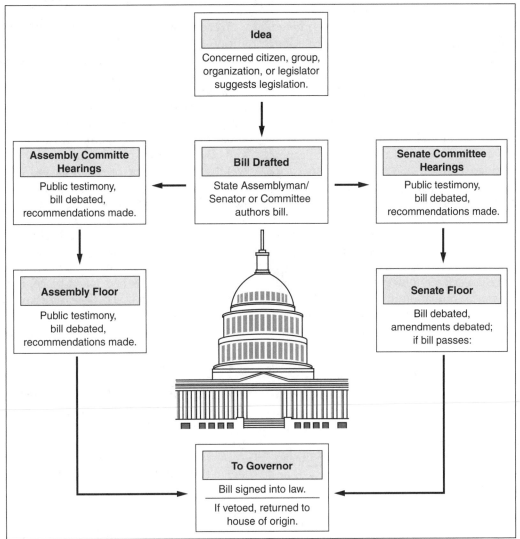

Idea

Concerned citizen, group, organization, or legislator suggests legislation.

Assembly Committee Hearings

Public testimony, bill debated, recommendations made.

Bill Drafted

State Assemblyman/ Senator or Committee authors bill.

Senate Committee Hearings

Public testimony, bill debated, recommendations made.

Assembly Floor

Public testimony, bill debated, recommendations made.

Senate Floor

Bill debated, amendments debated; if bill passes:

To Governor

Bill signed into law.

If vetoed, returned to house of origin.

competence and ethical behavior. In investigating the adequacy of current licensure laws to meet modern scientific and social conditions, the important question of authority for delegation of functions must be considered.

Initial PA statutes took either a broad, delegatory direction or a more restrictive, regulatory direction. Statutes based on a delegatory model affirmed the notion of task delegation by a doctor to an employee without any specific delineation of the performance of those tasks. Other states used the regulatory model by enacting laws that accepted the principle of physician task delegation as the basis of PA practice but placing specific stipulations on PA scope of practice and medical task performance.

The first state laws for PAs—passed in the 1970s—allowed broad delegatory authority for supervising physicians. Many were simple amendments to the medical practice act that allowed physicians to delegate patient care tasks within the physician's scope of practice to PAs who practiced with the physician's supervision.

Over time, a majority of states moved toward the regulatory model (Gara, 1990; Gara & Davis, 2008). For example, between 1971 and 1991, the law enabling PAs to practice in Connecticut (Public Health Act 171) stipulated that legal prohibition against the practice of medicine would not apply to PAs. An additional statement defining the PA according to necessary education and national certification was added in 1981. In 1991, the Connecticut legislature passed a new statute addressing PA licensure and prescriptive rights to replace the former delegatory law. The new law allows for the licensure of PAs and grants PAs the authority to prescribe, dispense, and administer controlled substances. Criteria for licensure, which includes an academic degree (the baccalaureate degree), graduation from an accredited PA program, passage of the National Commission on Certification of Physician Assistants (NCCPA) certification examination, maintenance of continuing education requirements, 60 hours of pharmacology instruction, and appropriate application and renewal fees, were also defined in the law. The law precludes individuals lacking minimal credentials from identifying themselves as PAs.

Currently, PAs are recognized as healthcare practitioners authorized to perform physician-delegated medical diagnostic and therapeutic tasks (diagnosis, testing, treating, and follow-up of patients) by professional licensing boards in all 50 states, Guam, and the District of Columbia. In 2000, Mississippi was the last state to formally recognize the PA practice. In 2007, Indiana was the last state to grant prescriptive authority. In fact, state regulatory agencies now tend to recognize prescribing activities by PAs within circumscribed boundaries as an essential component of their modern practice roles (Hansen, 1992; Wing et al, 2004).

Since the turn of the century, more than 150 pieces of legislation across most of the 50 states, have addressed some improvement in PA policy (A. Davis, personal communication, May 14, 2007). American territories such as Puerto Rico, the Virgin Islands, and American Samoa lag behind their state counterparts in enacting permissive legislation for PAs.

Trends among states adopting policies that allow PAs to practice are illustrated in Exhibits 13-2 and 13-3. Exhibit 13-2 details the professional practice indices for PAs from 1992 to 2000 (Wing et al, 2004). The original index, developed by Sekscenski and colleagues (1994), first identified the wide differences in enabling legislation in the 50 states and the District of Columbia. By using weighted values for prescribing and ease in insurance reimbursement and scope of practice, an assessment was calculated for each state for PAs and NPs. In 2002, Wing and colleagues recalculated the weights based on new research and compiled differences between the states over an 8-year span to show what changes had taken place. From a rank order of values, Washington state remains first with a perfect score of 100 and New Jersey the last, with a score of 42 (in 2002).

Exhibit 13-3 shows the states in terms of PA growth per capita. From 1992 through 1996 and into 2002, all states grew in PA presence and 15 states experienced a growth of over 100% of PAs. Four of the 15 had growth of over 200%, with Mississippi experiencing a 549 percent growth since legislation in 2000 permitting PAs to practice (Wing et al, 2004).

LICENSURE, REGISTRATION, AND CERTIFICATION

Before entering practice, a PA must meet specific requirements designated by the state. Like all of health occupations licensure, PA practice is regulated at the state level, and there are variations from state to state in terms of registration, certification, and licensure options.

Most states require licensure, which restricts practice to those who have met certain standards and qualifications and have been approved by a designated regulatory body. Under licensure, it is generally illegal for

EXHIBIT 13-2
Professional Practice Indices for Physician Assistants, 1992 and 2000

State	Original Index		Change	New Index
	1992	*2000*		*2000*
Alabama	39	89	50	61
Alaska	90	96.5	6.5	81.5
Arizona	99	99	0	82
Arkansas	54	98	44	59
California	58	97	39	83
Colorado	80	95	15	75
Connecticut	87	97	10	83
Delaware	55	68	13	82
District of Columbia	92	59	33	45
Florida	48	93	45	61
Georgia	59	96	37	77
Hawaii	38	99	0	87
Idaho	89	87.5	−1.5	72.5
Illinois	59	59	0	87
Indiana	37	77	40	50
Iowa	99	99	0	87
Kansas	87	96.5	9.5	75.5
Kentucky	42	75	33	54
Louisiana	37	60	23	54
Maine	94	94	0	83
Maryland	49	90	41	76
Massachusetts	83	92	9	82
Michigan	89	97	8	89
Minnesota	83	88	5	81
Mississippi	0	88	88	49
Missouri	39	97	58	61
Montana	98	99.5	1.5	91
Nebraska	93	94	1	79
Nevada	98	95.5	−2.5	64.5
New Hampshire	95	97	2	89
New Jersey	37	42	5	48
New Mexico	94	98	4	84
New York	98	99	1	84
North Carolina	92	94	2	94
North Dakota	87	88	1	69.5
Ohio	51	55	4	36.5
Oklahoma	46	96	50	77.5
Oregon	99	99	0	92
Pennsylvania	86	86	0	73
Rhode Island	93	97	4	88
South Carolina	37	80	43	52
South Dakota	94	97	3	81.5

(Continued)

EXHIBIT 13-2
Professional Practice Indices for Physician Assistants, 1992 and 2000—cont'd

State	Original Index		Change	New Index
	1992	*2000*		*2000*
Tennessee	42	99	57	86
Texas	77	93	16	67
Utah	93	98	5	85
Vermont	86	95	9	82
Virginia	42	67	25	47
Washington	100	100	0	82
West Virginia	95	99	3	84
Wisconsin	97	95	0	83
Wyoming	97	97	0	81

From Wing, P., et al. (2004). The changing professional practice of physician assistants: 1992 to 2000. Journal of the American Academy of Physician Assistants, 17(1), p. 39. Reprinted with permission of the publisher.

EXHIBIT 13-3
Practicing Physician Assistants per 100,000 Population by State, 1992, 1996, and 2000

State	Number			Percentage of Change
	1992	*1996*	*2000*	*1992–2000*
Alabama	2.7	4.6	5.3	98
Alaska	20.8	32.3	40.3	94
Arizona	8.9	9.4	12.5	40
Arkansas	1.2	2.3	1.9	59
California	5.1	8.6	10.3	101
Colorado	11.0	14.9	18.8	71
Connecticut	15.3	15.8	21.8	43
Delaware	7.7	9.1	10.9	42
District of Columbia	5.9	30.7	25.7	336
Florida	8.2	8.8	11.8	44
Georgia	9.0	12.2	15.0	66
Hawaii	4.6	7.9	6.9	61
Idaho	5.7	8.6	13.6	139
Illinois	2.1	3.4	6.4	204
Indiana	2.4	2.5	3.9	63
Iowa	9.3	11.1	16.4	76
Kansas	10.6	11.6	16.2	53
Kentucky	6.2	7.9	11.2	81
Louisiana	2.2	3.2	5.5	149
Maine	24.6	21.7	29.5	20
Maryland	13.9	16.4	20.0	44
Massachusetts	8.9	9.9	12.6	42
Michigan	10.4	10.6	15.3	47
Minnesota	7.1	6.7	10.9	53
Mississippi	0.2	1.2	1.3	549

EXHIBIT 13-3
Practicing Physician Assistants per 100,000 Population by State, 1992, 1996, and 2000—cont'd

State	Number			Percentage of Change
	1992	*1996*	*2000*	*1992–2000*
Missouri	2.0	3.9	4.6	128
Montana	7.3	12.0	17.7	143
Nebraska	13.0	18.6	24.2	86
Nevada	6.2	7.8	9.1	47
New Hampshire	12.7	11.3	14.4	14
New Jersey	2.3	2.2	5.2	126
New Mexico	10.4	17.4	19.3	86
New York	12.3	17.3	23.5	91
North Carolina	15.5	18.1	23.5	52
North Dakota	18.2	23.6	30.0	65
Ohio	4.5	6.9	9.4	109
Oklahoma	5.0	11.3	15.9	218
Oregon	6.3	7.1	9.3	75
Pennsylvania	11.5	12.4	16.1	40
Rhode Island	10.5	10.0	11.3	8
South Carolina	2.1	5.3	7.4	250
South Dakota	19.5	24.0	31.2	60
Tennessee	5.7	6.1	7.9	39
Texas	4.8	8.6	11.1	130
Utah	9.1	9.9	13.7	51
Vermont	12.7	13.8	20.3	60
Virginia	4.6	6.3	8.3	81
Washington	11.4	13.8	18.9	65
West Virginia	10.1	13.8	24.4	142
Wisconsin	12.3	10.2	13.8	13
Wyoming	12.5	13.7	20.0	60
United States	**7.4**	**9.6**	**12.8**	**73**

From Wing, P., et al. (2004). The changing professional practice of physician assistants: 1992 to 2000. Journal of the American Academy of Physician Assistants, *17(1), p. 45. Reprinted with permission of the publisher.*

someone to practice in an occupation without meeting the specified requirements. Only a few states require either registration or certification, and these requirements are less restrictive. Registration serves only as an official list of those practicing. Certification restricts the use of the title "Physician Assistant-Certified" and involves obtaining a valid certificate from the NCCPA. Certification is typically a voluntary process meant to designate a level of professional competence; however, individuals who are not certified may still practice in the occupation. In some states, certification is required to practice as a PA, and the term is used loosely to mean the traditional definition of licensure.

Of those states that require and regulate licensure, the specific requirements, fees, documents, and process needed to become licensed vary. The licensure process is administered by an agency or board, which develops specifications for licensure and determines which examination is accepted. The purpose of this process is to protect the health and safety of the public, helping to ensure that a person working under a PA title is appropriately trained and qualified.

The application process to obtain a license to work as a PA is determined by the state and is very involved. For example, Alaska—one of the most permissive states in regards to licensure—requires applicants to complete 11 documents. The process typically takes 3 months if all the necessary forms are available and requires several hundred dollars in fees.

Generally, state boards or agencies require individuals seeking a license to practice as a PA to:

- graduate from a PA educational program accredited by the Accreditation Review Commission for the Physician Assistant (ARC-PA);
- be certified by the NCCPA by passing the Physician Assistant National Certifying examination (PANCE), a 300-item, multiple-choice question examination; and
- complete a screening questionnaire about criminal malpractice history.

NCCPA certification is required for PA qualification in 49 states (and is recognized by Ontario and Manitoba). More than 92% of the 69,000 PAs in active clinical practice in 2007 hold NCCPA certification (AAPA, 2006b). When a state requires certification, the PA must document that he or she has a certificate from the NCCPA that has not expired. The laws generally do not refer to "recertified," they merely require "active" or "continuing certification." For licensure, some states require only initial NCCPA certification and do not require PAs to maintain active certification beyond the initial 2-year period. More than 30 states, however, require that PAs maintain an active NCCPA certification status in order to be licensed.

To some, the licensure concept for a PA may cause confusion because the term tends to imply autonomous function. That the majority of states license PAs and other health professions raises the possibility of confusion for the public as well as for legislation intended to apply to PAs. However, licensure is the most rigorous method of regulation. In a licensed profession, no individual may practice without permission granted by the state. This type of rigorous regulation of PA practice is already in place in every state, even though it is not universally termed "licensure." Licensing PAs holds the profession to rigorous standards and creates credential parity with other health professions. An additional rationale for using "licensure" as the regulatory term for PAs is to ensure that laws that should apply to PAs indeed do so. Many categories of health law refer to "licensed providers." These laws usually intend to include providers who have a specific state-authorized scope of practice. When a state uses a regulatory term other than "licensure" for PAs, they can be unintentionally excluded from provisions that apply to "licensed healthcare providers."

As states evolved and changed their regulatory laws to licensure, many used the occasion to modernize the law in other ways. Of the 32 states that changed to licensure since 1992, 14 also expanded prescriptive authority to include controlled substances. In examining supervision requirements, only one state changed during this time period to allow some form of off-site practice. All other states that changed to licensure already granted some form of off-site practice privilege to physician assistants. In addition, 6 states made the supervision requirements, as measured by the number of PAs a physician can supervise, more restrictive, while 10 lessened the restriction and 16 made no change. Gradually, states have enacted provisions dealing with the reimbursement of PAs by third parties. Of the states that changed to licensing PAs, three increased the reimbursement status of PAs by requiring their services be covered in some form.

REGULATING PHYSICIAN ASSISTANT PRACTICE

Recognition of PAs in state medical practice and PA practice acts typically involves the passage of a statute by the legislature that modifies the existing act to explicitly allow physicians to delegate medical tasks to qualified assistants. The statute normally contains language that defines the circumstances of physician task delegation, terms of physician supervision of the PA, and enumeration of who may qualify as a PA.

Next, the state health regulatory authority, that is, the Department of Health, writes and promulgates regulations based on the statute. Regulations are a more detailed delineation of the authority contained in the statute and contain the details of the processes of applying for and obtaining a license and stipulate the standards of qualification, expected conduct, and disciplinary consequences of inappropriate behavior. In most instances, the regulations specify that a governing body, either the medical board or a separate PA examining board, review and oversee the process of granting a license and monitoring and approving practice activities. In many states, the board of medicine appoints a subgroup to undertake the oversight functions of PA regulation, that is, a PA advisory committee. A separate PA board is in effect in almost one-quarter of states.

Although there is some variation, most state laws have abandoned the concept that a medical board or other regulatory agency should micromanage physician-PA teams. For example, the Wyoming Board of Medical Examiners does not recognize or bestow any level of competency upon a PA to carry out a specific task. Such recognition of skill is considered the responsibility of the supervising physician. However, a PA is expected to perform with similar skill and competency and to be evaluated by the same standards as the physician in the performance of assigned duties. Considerations for regulating PA practice include the specific state practice act, supervision required, scope of practice, scope of employment, and other factors.

State Practice Acts

State practice acts vary widely, both in regulatory approach and in the scope of practice they authorize. They may influence the formal prescriptive authority and the administrative protocols organizations develop. State practice acts are intended to ensure quality of care, but organizations ranging from small physician offices to large medical centers and institutions typically provide their own controls on quality in addition to or over and above state practice acts.

Although state practice acts may provide a weak mechanism for guiding actual practices within a state, they play an important role in defining professions and restricting what PAs can do. In some instances they can even define the amount of care a physician can delegate. For example, in Virginia the regulations about PA management state that the supervising physician shall see and evaluate any patient who presents with the same complaint twice in a single episode of care who has failed to improve significantly.

Because these acts may present a threat of litigation for PAs and physicians when practicing within a state, they cannot be simply ignored. The development of model state legislation, such as the model developed by the AAPA's government affairs department (shown in Appendix III), can provide a foundation for achieving national consensus regarding state legislation for PAs (Physician Payment Review Commission, 1994).

Supervision

Various state statutes require that a physician supervise a PA. *Supervision,* as defined by law, is considered "responsible control." *Control* implies the establishment of the overall limits of and the policies to be followed by the supervised professional and the day-to-day supervision of care. Direct supervision requires the physician be in the facility and occasionally in the same room as the individual performing the duty. Direct supervision further implies that the physician will be immediately available if the need arises.

More often, supervision is indirect and may be implied or explicitly stated, but usually requires the availability of the physician for consultation. *Availability* need not necessarily be the physical presence of the doctor. Carrying a beeper or a cellular telephone that provides a means of availability may be appropriate, depending on the circumstances of the practice site and the rules imposed by the state boards responsible for licensure. A typical way this type of supervision is defined is provided in a New York state statute:

> Supervision shall be continuous but shall not be construed as necessarily requiring the physical presence of the supervising physician at the time and place where such services are performed. (N.Y. [Educ.] Law 6542[3])

The degree of supervision and availability usually depends on the complexity of the task, risk to the patient, training of the PA, setting in which care is rendered, necessity for immediate medical attention, and the number of other professionals the physician supervises. Generally, the more complex the task and the greater the potential risk to the patient, the more direct and explicit are the expectations for the supervision. Backup physician supervision must be made available if for some reason the usual methods of contact fail or the supervising physician is out of town.

Review implies the physician will regularly read the notes and examine the work the PA is undertaking. This process may consist of a review of medical record progress notes made by the PA or some other predetermined means of ensuring supervision. Generally, the doctor should be able to demonstrate that the supervised PA is performing at the expected skill level and is compliant with any protocols and procedures that may be in place to ensure quality of care. This should be done with some regularity (Harty-Golder, 1995; Moses & Feld, 2007). The specific mechanism by which this is accomplished and with what frequency is generally left to the discretion of the supervising physician and the PA.

Delegation of Functions

The delegation of functions, or delegation agreement, outlines the broad duties and specific patient problems and procedures that the physician delegates to the PA. A delegation of functions may be as broad or as specific as the physician/PA team determines is necessary. Ideally, it would be reviewed and revised frequently. Such agreements are becoming a commonplace element of the process of state licensure. For example, the Alaska state licensure application includes a section in which the supervising physician and PA outline a collaborative plan regarding the PA's practice, authority, liability, and ongoing assessment of work performance.

The delegation of functions by physicians to PAs is the cornerstone of licensure for the practice of medicine. Because the statutory definitions of medical practice give physicians an unlimited license to perform all functions of health service, even those for which other healthcare personnel may also be licensed (or even better suited), the doctor can determine what can and should be done by his or her employees. However, the concomitant licensing of other healthcare personnel indicates that the statutes do not contemplate all healthcare service to be conducted by physicians.

Scope of Practice

Scope of practice refers to the specific regulations of practice set by the individual state licensing boards in a PA practice act. In essence, each state outlines what a PA is authorized to do. Scope of practice may differ from state to state. When revising practice regulations, boards generally reflect what constitutes the "usual and customary" practice in a specific area. PA scope of practice is generally defined by the following four elements:

- Education and experience
- State law
- Facility policy
- Physician delegation

The scope of practice of PAs is constantly evolving as they gain additional skill and experience and as medicine evolves and new practices become routine. However, PA scope of practice should be limited to those tasks for which they are adequately prepared as a result of their education and training and experience working with physicians in clinical practice.

Scope of Employment

In traditional legal theory, an employer is responsible for the acts of the "servant" during the period the servant performs on behalf of the employer. The thinking is that the employer derives benefit (generally profit) from having the servant (employee) and therefore should pay for any damages the servant might cause (Grumbach & Coffman, 1998). For example, in an early English case, the court held that a master is not responsible for the acts of a servant when the servant is "going on a frolic of his own." In *Joel v. Morrsion* (1834,

6C & P, 501, 172 Eng. Rep. 1338) the court determined that if the servant steps beyond the bounds of "his master's business," then the master should not be held liable.

What generally determines the "scope of employment" in health care, as in many other businesses, is the employment contract (job description) and the delegation agreement (written guidelines or policies). These documents are the basis for determining whether the employee has truly been doing the "master's business."

If a hospital emergency department has hired a PA for a specific emergency medicine role and the PA begins administering cancer therapy without checking with the supervising physician, then the PA is out of the scope of his or her employment, especially if the PA has no prior experience in providing cancer therapy. In this instance, the PA is clearly going beyond the duties the emergency department had hired the PA to perform.

Scope-of-employment violations can subject the employee to dismissal or can make the PA responsible for all damages in a negligence action. In the case of a negligence claim, if the hospital can prove that it did not know about the employee's activities and had no reasonable way of obtaining that information, it can escape liability and place the entire burden on the "frolicking" employee's shoulders.

Protocols

Protocols are procedures for carrying out a set of processes in the course of medical treatment. Written clinical protocols are sometimes mentioned with regard to the regulation of PA practice, but are generally considered an undesirable means to do so. Protocols may be useful for dealing with very specific clinical entities (e.g., anaphylaxis) but they are by nature rigid, unable to anticipate all variations of a situation, and rapidly become outdated. Clinical protocols also may impair the clinical judgment exercised by PAs and are ineffective in improving the diagnosis and treatment of disease (AAPA, 2006b). There is no evidence that requiring extensive clinical protocols at the state regulatory level protects public

safety. This requirement may actually hinder care, as it decreases the ability to utilize clinical judgment and individualize treatment for a specific patient.

American Medical Association (AMA) guidelines for physician/physician assistant practice do not recommend protocols in delineating physician and PA practice. Instead, the AMA policy calls for "mutually agreed upon guidelines that are developed by the physician and the physician assistant" (AMA, 2001).

Sometimes an employer or regulatory body, in discussing protocols, actually wants a description of how the PA and physician will practice together. For the sake of clarity, the terms *practice description* and *job description* are defined here.

Practice Description

A *practice description* is a broad explanation of the practice and how the physician and PA will relate within the practice. Various items can be described in a practice description, such as the patient population of the practice and types of services provided (e.g., family practice, general surgery, obstetrics and gynecology). Sometimes the practice description spells out the physician supervision mechanism and may include case conferences, chart review, or availability of the physician on site or by telecommunication; and the hospital, nursing home, and call responsibilities in the practice.

Job Description

A *job description* outlines the PA's duties in the practice and is not necessarily regulated. It may describe the activities of the PA, along with the relationship of the PA to patients and other personnel (such as supervision of clerks or laboratory personnel). A job description might include the types of patients the PA will see, hours the PA will work, call responsibilities, and settings in which the PA is expected to provide care.

Credentialing

Credentialing is the process utilized by licensed healthcare facilities (hospitals, nursing homes, surgical centers, and others) to validate the background and assess the qualifications of healthcare professionals to provide patient care services. Determination of credentials is based on an objective evaluation of a person's current licensure, training or experience, competence, and ability to perform the privileges (authorizations granted by the governing body of an institution to provide specific care services within defined limits) requested.

In general, PAs are credentialed by the medical staff and authorized through privileges in a manner parallel to that used for physicians. Privileges are generally granted in accordance with community need and norms. Any privileges granted by a facility must conform to state law. The primary purpose for credentialing providers is to protect healthcare organizations and institutions from the legal liability that could result from the actions of unqualified providers. Evaluation of an organization's credentialing program features prominently in surveys by the Joint Commission and the National Committee for Quality Assurance (NCQA). By ensuring that providers are qualified, credentialing also promotes quality care.

The process for credentialing PAs in outpatient settings is evolving, but it is also regulated by state laws, by the standards of accrediting agencies, and by an institution's governing board. It is usually not as extensive as the process of obtaining inpatient credentialing. Typically, individual physician practices do not conduct formal credentialing processes. They may, however, confirm licensure and certification when hiring a PA (Calabrese, Crane, & Legler, 1997).

Federation of State Boards

The Federation of State Boards of Medical Examiners (FSBME) is a national nonprofit organization representing the 70 medical boards of the United States and its territories and 14 state boards of osteopathic medicine. The FSBME, which has a PA serving as a member of its governing board of directors, insures public safety through effective systems of medical licensing and discipline and addresses issues such as Internet prescribing, defining

sexual boundaries between providers and patients, measuring the quality of international medical education, physician mobility, and emergency preparedness. The FSBME also provides a credentialing service for PAs. All state and federal boards recognize this credentialing service, which permits quicker credentialing for PAs who move. The official journal of the FSBME is the *Journal of Medical Licensure and Discipline*. More information about the organization is available on their website at http://www.fsmb.org.

ORGANIZED MEDICINE AND PHYSICIAN ASSISTANTS

In many states, the state medical society is regarded as the voice of medicine. As state legislators considered bills that modified PA regulation and delegated scope of practice, they commonly asked, "What's the medical society's position on this bill?" During the past decade, state medical societies have shown an increased willingness to work as colleagues with PA state societies on health law issues. Today, most state PA organizations have sustained relationships with their respective state medical societies (Gara & Davis, 2008). This increased level of communication has had a positive impact on the development of state laws and regulations governing PA practice (Exhibit 13-4).

EXHIBIT 13-4
Ann Davis, PA, AAPA Director of State Governmental Affairs and Ed Freidman, PA, Past AAPA President

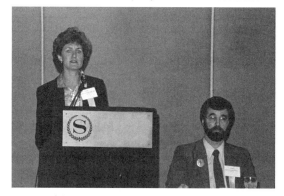

Courtesy of the American Academy of Physician Assistants.

The policies of organized medicine on the national level have also played a significant role in state regulation of PA practice over the past 10 years, the result of stable and productive relationships with physician leaders. In 1995, the AMA issued guidelines that offered a framework for physician-PA practice; these were adopted as policy by many state medical societies and used as a default position by others (Davis, 2002).

PRESCRIPTIVE AUTHORITY

Prescribing authority for PAs was obtained through legal and political negotiating on a state-by-state basis over four decades. It was a long but successful process that at its heart increasingly recognized the skills and contributions of the PA role to society.

The first statute authorizing prescribing privileges for PAs was passed in Colorado in 1969. That statute stipulated that graduates of the University of Colorado Child Health Associate Program (one of the first three PA programs and one specific to pediatrics) could prescribe medications without immediate consultation from a supervising physician, provided that the latter subsequently approved the prescription. New York authorized PA prescribing privileges in 1972; Maine, New Mexico, North Carolina, Oklahoma, and Kansas followed. By 1979, PA prescribing privileges existed in 11 states (Weston, 1980). The preponderance of states passed PA prescribing authority in the 1980s and 1990s. In 2006, Indiana became the last state to authorize PA prescribing.

Currently, all states, as well as Guam and the District of Columbia, authorize the supervising physician to delegate prescriptive responsibility to PAs, and 46 states include controlled substances in that authorization (Exhibits 13-5 and 13-6). In fact, most states permit PA prescribing privileges for Schedule II through Schedule IV drugs. (Schedule I drugs are not relevant to this discussion because it is illegal for licensed practitioners, including physicians, in the United States to prescribe these drugs.) The prescribing privilege for Schedule II drugs is limited in about six states. In the other states, the prescribing privilege applies to Schedule III through Schedule V drugs, including prescription legend drugs, with some restrictions on prescribing Schedule II and III drugs. PAs may also prescribe over-the-counter medications or drug preparations that do not, by law, require the written order of a licensed prescriber.

In general, PAs are authorized to sign prescriptions using their own names and prescription pads bearing the names of themselves and the supervising physician. States that allow PA prescribing of controlled substances require PAs to obtain their own Drug Enforcement Administration (DEA) registration number.

Initial Resistance

Approval of PA prescribing authority has been controversial at times, depending on the state. In a comparative analysis of state regulatory experiences and policy approaches authorizing PA prescribing, Cohen (1996) found that experiences and policy varied widely. Prescribing was a particularly troublesome barrier to PA practice effectiveness in states such as Maryland and Ohio until their laws were changed in the mid 2000s.

Why were state regulatory agencies initially reluctant to allow prescribing privilege to PAs? One reason was the perception that PAs were not sufficiently trained in pharmacological modalities to be competent prescribers. Further, because the agencies regulating PA practice have historically been largely composed of physicians, a second reason was the perception of increased legal liability of supervising physicians. The belief was that PAs lacked prescribing competence.

Physician reluctance may have also resulted from cultural factors that the medical profession may not wish to share the act of prescribing. This cultural factor is that the act of prescribing had at one point been described as "the most common and overt expression of the physicians' power" (Pelligrino, 1976). Throughout history the ingestion of substances has been associated with magical, mystical, and religious elements that transcend any

EXHIBIT 13-5
Types of Prescriptive Privileges for Physician Assistants by State, 2009

Jurisdiction	Restrictions	Controlled Substances
Alabama	Formulary	
Alaska		Schedules III through V
Arizona		Schedules II through III limited to a 14-day supply with board prescribing certification (72 hours without)
		Schedules IV through V, not more than five times in 6-month period per patient
Arkansas		Schedules III through V
California	PAs may write "drug orders" which, for the purposes of DEA registration, meet the federal definition of a prescription	Schedules II through V
Colorado		Schedules II through V
Connecticut		Schedules II through V
Delaware		Schedules II through V
District of Columbia		
Florida	Formulary of prohibited drugs	
Georgia	Formulary	Schedules III through V
Guam		Schedules III through V
Hawaii		Schedules III through V
Idaho		Schedules II through V
Illinois		Schedules III through V
Indiana		Schedules III through V
Iowa		Schedules III through V and Schedule II (except depressants)
Kansas		Schedules II through V
Kentucky		
Louisiana		Schedules III through V
Maine		Schedules III through V
		Board may approve Schedule II for individual PAs
Maryland		Schedules II through V
Massachusetts		Schedules II through V
Michigan		Schedules III through V
		Schedule II (7-day supply) as discharge medication
Minnesota	Formulary	Schedules II through V
Mississippi		Schedules II through V
Missouri		
Montana		Schedules II through V (schedule II limited to 34-day supply)
Nebraska		Schedules II through V
Nevada		Schedules II through V
New Hampshire		Schedules II through V
New Jersey		Schedules II through V (certain conditions apply)
New Mexico	Formulary	Schedules II through V
New York		Schedules III through V
North Carolina		Schedules II through V (schedules II–III limited to 30-day supply)
North Dakota		Schedules III through V

EXHIBIT 13-5
Types of Prescriptive Privileges for Physician Assistants by State—cont'd

Jurisdiction	Restrictions	Controlled Substances
Ohio		Schedules III through V
Oklahoma	Formulary	Schedules III through V
Oregon		Schedules II through V
Pennsylvania	Formulary	Schedules III through V (limited to 30-day supply unless for chronic condition)
Rhode Island		Schedules II through V
South Carolina	Formulary	Schedules III through V
South Dakota		Schedules II through V (schedule II limited to 30-day supply)
Tennessee		Schedules II through V
Texas	In specified practice sites	Schedules III through V (limited to 30-day supply)
Utah		Schedules II through V
Vermont	Formulary	Schedules II through V
Virginia		Schedules III through V
Washington		Schedules II through V
West Virginia	Formulary	Schedules III through V (schedule III limited to 72-hour supply)
Wisconsin		Schedules II through V
Wyoming		Schedules II through V

pharmacological effects. When coupled with the ingrained urge to "take something" for an illness, this historical association gave extraordinary power to the person (in recent years, the doctor) who had the exclusive right to provide the "something" (Pelligrino, 1976).

Physicians may have been reluctant to share the act of prescribing because it gave the physician the authority to define the clinical situation as medical, it established the patient as "truly ill," and it implicitly reinforced the physician's ability to handle the illness. The act of prescribing maintained the physician's power by providing the physician time for the illness to unfold when a diagnosis is uncertain or a condition is obscure, even though scientific observation may indicate no medication is needed (Pelligrino, 1976). Sharing prescribing privileges with PAs removed physicians as the only source of such power.

The symbolic weight of prescribing had other practical implications for the doctor. For one thing, prescribing a drug indicates to the patient that the doctor is concerned and is trying to help. Prescribing a drug can take the place of communicating with the patient. Finally, prescribing can be used to both guide and end the office visit, as well as to provide a link with the patient for continuing visits (Pelligrino, 1976). Thus, delegating prescribing authority to PAs may have been perceived as reducing this power of the physician.

Economic factors may have also contributed to the debate over prescriptive authority for PAs. The initial purpose of the creation of PAs was to alleviate a shortage of physician services. More recently, however, given the more abundant supply of physician services, the distinction of whether PAs complement physician services or are alternatives for physician services is less clear. The latter situation implies that PAs are currently in competition with physicians for patients.

Opposition to prescribing privileges for PAs from other healthcare professions, such as pharmacists, was another possible reason. The opposition, however, was basically confined to attempting to influence regulatory agencies

EXHIBIT 13-6
Controlled Substance Act

> **Schedule I** drugs have no accepted medical use in the United States and have a high abuse potential. Some examples are heroin, marijuana, LSD, peyote, mescaline, and psilocybin.
>
> **Schedule II** drugs have a high abuse potential with severe psychic or physical dependence liability. Controlled substances consist of certain narcotic, stimulant, and depressant drugs. Examples of the narcotics are opium, morphine, codeine, methadone, and meperidine. Examples of the stimulants are amphetamine and methamphetamine. Examples of the depressants are amobarbital, pentobarbital, secobarbital, and methaqualone.
>
> **Schedule III** drugs have an abuse potential less than those in Schedules I and II and include compounds containing limited quantities of certain narcotic drugs and non-narcotic drugs such as paregoric and barbituric acid derivatives not included in another schedule.
>
> **Schedule IV** drugs have an abuse potential less than those listed in Schedule III and include such drugs as phenobarbital, chloral hydrate, meprobamate, chlordiazepoxide, diazepam, and dextropropoxyphene.
>
> **Schedule V** drugs have an abuse potential less than those listed in Schedule IV and consist of preparations containing limited amounts of certain narcotic drugs generally for antitussive and antidiarrheal purposes.

and state legislatures through testimony and lobbying efforts. Such efforts may have delayed the granting of prescribing privileges in some states but were not sufficient to prevent them.

A key determinant in the outcome of whether prescriptive authority would be granted was the position of the involved stakeholder groups, such as medical societies and nursing groups. At one time, a number of medical and nursing groups asserted that PAs were not qualified to prescribe because of the short duration of their training (2 years). PA proponents asserted that the PA act of prescribing was always under the supervision of the employing physician and that their training program required them to have formal instruction in pharmacology.

Legal Basis for Prescriptive Authority

Statutes authorizing state medical and health occupation boards to regulate medical practitioners constituted the legal basis of PA prescribing activities. Typical state regulatory acts establish PAs as the agents of their supervising physicians, predicated on the legal doctrine of *respondeat superior* (the employer is considered responsible for the actions of the employee), and PAs maintain direct liability for the services they render to patients. Supervising physicians define the broad parameters of PA practice activities and the standard to which PA services are held and are vicariously liable for services performed by their PAs.

Preparation for Prescribing

Concerns about patient safety and physician liability have some historical validity given the substantial amount of variation that has characterized the evolution of PA training and educational programs. The pharmacology and therapeutics component of the PAs' educational experience had been singled out as a major area of concern (Camp, 1984). However, because knowledge of pharmacology is a required component of practice for a PA, ARC-PA accredited PA programs must include formal course instruction in basic and clinical pharmacology. ARC-PA standards mandate that PA programs teach "the principles of clinical pharmacology and medical therapeutics appropriate to the medical therapy for common problems in clinical practice" (ARC-PA, 2006).

During the clinical year, PA students obtain clinical training and experience by rotating through inpatient and outpatient settings. The contents of these clinical rotations and preceptorships stress the appropriate use of drugs and medications as part of patient care management. Pharmacology and medical therapeutics are also part of the core requirements of every PA program. A national survey of PA educational programs in 2007 revealed that the typical PA student received an average of 75.4 hours of instruction in pharmacology, with a range of 32 to 160 hours (PAEA, 2007).

The University of Utah has developed a model clinical therapeutics curriculum, which is used by a number of PA programs.

Additionally, testing knowledge about prescriptions is part of the PANCE. On the PANCE, 18% of the examination items relate to pharmaceutical aspects of patient care management (Arbett, Lathrop, & Hooker, 2009). Specifically, the exam assesses knowledge of pharmaceutical therapeutics defined as: mechanism of action, indications for use, contraindications, side effects, adverse reactions, follow-up and monitoring of pharmacological regimens, risks for drug interactions, clinical presentation of drug interactions, treatment of drug interactions, drug toxicity, methods to reduce medication errors, cross-reactivity of similar medications, and recognition and treatment of allergic reactions.

To meet requirements for continuing certification, the NCCPA requires PAs to obtain 100 hours of continuing medical education (CME) hours annually and to recertify by formal examination (the Physician Assistant National Recertifying Examination [PANRE]) every 6 years. Nineteen states require PAs to maintain ongoing NCCPA certification, and a number of states have similar CME requirements for PAs to maintain state licensure. Some states require PAs to obtain specific CME in pharmacological patient management prior to being granted prescribing authority.

Drug Enforcement Administration Registration

Every provider who administers, prescribes, or dispenses any controlled substance, other than as a direct agent of another registrant, must be registered with the DEA. A PA who is required to register must submit a completed Form DEA-224 to the DEA. Before 1994, PAs, NPs, and certified nurse-midwives (CNMs) were registered similar to physicians with a registration number beginning with the letter A or B, followed by a letter corresponding to the first letter of their last name. In 1994, the DEA chose to reclassify nonphysician providers under the term *midlevel practitioners* and required new registration numbers beginning with the M

(for *midlevel*) and the first letter of the prescriber's last name, followed by a computer-generated sequence of seven numbers. For more information, or to obtain a registration application, contact the DEA registration unit at 800-882-9539.

The DEA will register a PA to prescribe controlled substances only if the particular state allows PAs to prescribe controlled substances and only after the PA has completed all of the requirements imposed by state law. Some states require controlled substance registration with a state agency, for which PAs should apply before applying for a DEA registration. If the PA fails to obtain a state PA practice license or controlled substance registration (if applicable), or has the license revoked or rescinded, then the DEA cannot issue a registration. If an existing DEA registrant loses his or her state privileges, then the DEA must also rescind or revoke the federal controlled substance registration.

PAs may use the same DEA registration number when practicing in different locations within the same state. However, effective 2007, a separate DEA registration is required for each state in which the PA practices. In addition, the privileges associated with registration will change based on state law. If, for instance, a PA moves from a state that allows PAs to prescribe Schedule II drugs to one that does not, the PA's DEA registration will no longer allow Schedule II prescriptions.

DEA registration must be renewed every 3 years. The certificate of registration must be maintained at the registered location and kept available for official inspection. Every prescriber registered with the DEA receives a re-registration application approximately 60 days before the expiration date of his or her registration. If more than one practice location is used from which he or she dispenses controlled substances from personal supplies, then each location must be independently registered. A move to a new location requires a request for modification of registration in writing to the DEA office.

There are some exceptions to this process, such as being in the Armed Forces or working for other government agencies, such as the

Public Health Service and the Veterans Administration. Other administrative details such as record-keeping requirements, inventory, prescription orders, control and reporting of substance theft or loss, and guidelines for prescribers of controlled substances can be found in the *1993 Mid-Level Practitioner's Manual: An Informational Outline of the Controlled Substances Act of 1970.*

Dispensing of Medication

The authority to dispense medications is regulated by the state; however, pharmacists have strongly defended their rights in terms of dispensing and insist that prescribing and dispensing activities be separately regulated. Despite this concern, physicians in one-half of the United States have the authority to delegate dispensing privileges to PAs. PAs dispense medications from office supplies in some practices—most commonly those set in rural clinics or practices in states that do not specifically prohibit dispensing (Henry & Hooker, 2007). Note that in most jurisdictions, giving patients drug samples that have been supplied by a drug company is not considered the same as dispensing (Gara & Davis, 2008).

Physician Assistant Prescribing Trends

PAs prescribe in a wide variety of settings, and studies of patient expectations and satisfaction levels affirm the notion that PAs are expected to perform prescribing activities as part of their roles in patient management. Nationwide, PAs are estimated to have over 221 million patient visits and to write or recommend more than 300 million prescriptions in 2008. This amounts to nearly 10% of all prescriptions written annually (AAPA, 2008a).

Among the medications most commonly prescribed by PAs were antihypertensives, cholesterol-lowering agents, bronchodilators/respiratory therapy agents, agents to treat diabetes, gastrointestinal medications, and oral contraceptives. Sixty percent or more of the PAs reported prescribing urinary or vaginal agents, upper respiratory medications, gastrointestinal agents, anti-arthritic anti-gout agents, and analgesics. The mean number of prescriptions written by each PA was 50 per week (AAPA, 2006c).

Safety, Efficacy, and Acceptance of Physician Assistant Prescriptive Authority

Although the data to assess the safety and effectiveness of PA prescribing are sparse, research specifically focused on PA prescribing activity is largely positive in terms of safety and efficacy. (*Safety,* in this context, refers to the prescribing that minimizes the risk of an adverse consequence from the drug prescribed, and *effectiveness* refers to the contribution of the drug to the outcome of treatment.) A low proportion of suits involve PA misconduct related to prescribing (Cawley, Rohrs, & Hooker, 1998).

In the Kaiser Permanente HMO system, episodes of care were tracked when the care was exclusively by physicians or PAs. Four specific primary care morbidities were evaluated from the onset to resolution: otitis media, urinary tract infections, shoulder bursitis, and acute bronchitis. One outcome criterion was safety, as measured by the rate of adverse effects from antibiotics and other drugs provided in the treatment of upper respiratory infection. No differences in rates were observed between PA and physician clinical measures. In some instances, the choice of medication by the PA was less expensive than that of the physician, resulting in an improved cost benefit (Hooker, 2002).

An Iowa study reported that 95% of physicians and 93% of PAs believed that practicing PAs were qualified to prescribe medication with little or no supervision by the physician (Ekwo et al, 1979). Similarly, all 29 Montana physicians responding to a 1989 survey expressed confidence in the ability of the PAs they were supervising to prescribe therapeutic agents, with 40% having no reservations regarding PAs prescribing any agent (Willis & Reid, 1990).

A consistent finding is that when PAs are delegated the prescribing decision or provided protocols to guide them in specified clinical situations, they do at least as well as physicians in writing prescriptions, ordering drug treatment, and producing "good" processes of care. Although the evidence is not sufficient to generalize to all PA prescribing, it does appear sufficient to predict adequate performance of PAs when they are delegated the handling, including the drug treatment, of acute episodes of illness in office-based primary care. Liability insurance premiums have not increased appreciably, and the remarkably few malpractice claims have not centered on prescribing as an issue of safety.

Other Research

Analyzed data from the National Ambulatory Medical Care Survey (NAMCS) from 1997 through 2003 revealed that prescribing patterns among PAs, NPs, and primary care physicians were similar (Exhibits 13-7 and 13-8). The characteristics of all the patients seen were similar for geographical region of visit, age, and gender, but differed by ethnicity and race. An NP or a PA was the provider of record for 5% of the primary care visits in the NAMCS database. The three clinician types were likely to write at least one prescription for 70% of all visits, and the mean number of prescriptions was 1.3 to 1.5 per visit (range 0 to 5) depending on the provider. PAs were more likely to prescribe a controlled substance for a visit than a physician or an NP (19.5%, 12.4%, and 10.9%, respectively). Only

EXHIBIT 13-7
Likelihood of Prescribing at a Visit by Type of Prescriber (% of visits)

Number of Prescriptions	Doctor	PA	NP
0	38.9	39.8	32.7
1	27.1	25.6	27.5
2	15.2	16.3	15.2
3	8.0	7.6	7.6
4	3.8	6.8	—
5	6.8	6.8	10.1

Data from Hooker, R. S., & Cipher, D. J. (2005). Physician assistant and nurse practitioner prescribing: 1997–2002. Journal of Rural Health: Official Journal of the American Rural Health Association and the National Rural Health Care Association, 21(4), 355–360.

EXHIBIT 13-8
Mean Number of Prescriptions Written by Type of Prescriber, 1997–2002

	PA	NP	Doctor	Total
NONCONTROLLED SUBSTANCE				
Urban	1.5	1.5	1.4	1.4
Rural	0.9	1.8	1.6	1.6
CONTROLLED SUBSTANCE				
Urban	0.2	0.1	0.1	0.1
Rural	0.1	0.2	0.2	0.2
Total for all prescriptions	1.4	1.7	1.4	1.4

Data from Hooker, R. S., & Cipher, D. J. (2005). Physician assistant and nurse practitioner prescribing: 1997–2002. Journal of Rural Health: Official Journal of the American Rural Health Association and the National Rural Health Care Association, 21(4), 355–360.

in nonmetropolitan settings did differences emerge. NPs who worked in rural areas wrote significantly more prescriptions than physicians and PAs (Hooker & Cipher, 2005).

The presence of prescribing authority has been shown to have a profound effect on the number and utilization of PAs, particularly in rural states. This finding is illustrated by experiences observed in several western states (Willis & Reid, 1990). For example, the Montana legislature amended the state's medical practice act to permit PA prescribing within specific but typical parameters. In 1988, there were 26 PAs practicing in Montana; in 1991, 43; and in 1995, 130 (Willis & Reid, 1990).

Another example of the impact of PA prescribing authority was observed in Texas in the early 1990s following the passage of a PA prescribing bill. At that time, Texas had 26 federally certified rural health clinics. Less than 5% of the state's PA clinicians were in practice in small rural communities (less than 10,000 population). Texas PA practice regulations permitted neither prescribing of medications nor off-site practice supervision, despite the fact that the state had more than 70 counties either partially or fully designated as provider shortage areas. Shortly after the passage of PA prescribing regulations in 1991, there was a marked increase in the number of PAs employed in rural health clinics (Henry & Hooker, 2007).

In 1992, the number of PAs had nearly quadrupled to 99, and the percentage practicing in rural communities had tripled from 5% to 15% (Hooker & Cawley, 2003). In 2006, about one-third of all PAs worked in communities of less than 50,000 population (AAPA, 2006a).

A consistent finding of most research studies on the prescriptive practices of PAs appears to be that when PAs are given prescriptive authority, through either delegated power or protocols to guide them in specified clinical situations, they do at least as well as physicians in writing prescriptions, ordering drug treatment, and producing "good" processes of care. Although the evidence is not sufficient to generalize to all PA prescribing, it does appear that PA performance is generally adequate for all aspects of acute episodes of illness in office-based primary care.

LOBBYING

In modern Washington DC, it is a necessity for health professions organizations to engage in lobbying, the attempt to influence or sway a public official toward desired legislation. In the healthcare field, lobbying typically involves clinicians meeting with their government representatives to have a brief, meaningful conversation in an effort to influence policy direction with the representatives' votes. Representation is critical on Capitol Hill if health professions groups are to maintain their practice prerogatives and, importantly, to be reimbursed for their services through Medicare. Some health professions groups appear omnipresent in conducting lobbying activities. For example, the pharmaceutical industry, among the most prominent and powerful groups in Washington DC, employed 675 lobbyists and spent more than $91 million in 2002 (Angel, 2004). The PA profession, appropriately and similar to virtually all other major health professions, maintains a regular presence on Capitol Hill.

Lobbying got its name from a practice that developed in the 1860s, when citizens would gather in the lobby of the Willard Hotel in Washington, one block from the White House. Lore has it that when persons sought to petition President Ulysses S. Grant, they would intercept Grant in the Willard Lobby to make their requests. The practice of lobbying thus grew.

Clinicians typically share the attitude that involvement in political affairs, particularly lobbying, is a messy set of activities best left to others. They commonly feel that there is no need for them to pay attention to the political side of the profession and regard politics as an activity that is a bit unsavory and that diverts attention from patient care. Whereas this thinking is perhaps convenient, it is shortsighted and ignores the modern realities of medical politics. In the contemporary world of the health professions and health policy, politics require interest and involvement from health professionals.

Research on Physician Assistant Legislation and Policy

The literature about PA legislation and policy provides a number of lessons about how a new profession is introduced into society and how it is securitized. However, many research questions remain unanswered. Some areas of policy-focused research are listed here.

- **State laws:** What has been the timeline of policy development that permitted or restricted the full deployment of PAs? What were the enablers and barriers erected and who were the principals involved?

- **Policy:** What are the trends and policy changes that occurred as the profession moved from largely unrestricted PA use to highly codified laws and policies? Did legislative experiments allowing PAs to practice in some states stimulate similar legislation in other states?

- **Licensure:** In which states is it easiest to obtain a PA license and in which states is it the most difficult? How do these states compare? Does the ease or difficulty of the PA licensure process reflect the ease of practice in the state?

■ **Scope of practice:** How do practice descriptions compare among PAs in various disciplines across states and within states?

■ **Prescribing:** What are the characteristics of PA practices in which prescribing is formulary-restricted? What are the characteristics of practices that are not formulary-restricted?

■ **Model state law:** How close are states in fitting into the AAPA model state law for PAs? What are the characteristics of states that fit "tightly" within the AAPA model and those that fit "loosely"?

■ **Lobbying:** How does the AAPA lobby Congress and what has been the result of this lobbying in terms of legislation and policy reimbursement?

SUMMARY

Establishing and standardizing the regulation of PAs has been an evolutionary journey from a simple attitude that a doctor can delegate anything to an assistant to highly regulated laws and policies transcending all jurisdictions. All states, the District of Columbia, and the majority of U.S. territories have enacted statutes and regulations that define PAs, describe their scope of practice, discuss supervision, designate the agency that will administer the law, set application and renewal criteria, and establish disciplinary measures for violations of the law. Although each state writes its own laws, there has been an effort to standardize the structure and content of most laws. Because occupational regulation changes with the times, state chapters and the AAPA are required to closely monitor legislative and regulatory affairs. It is necessary for the clinically active PA to be familiar with the regulations of each state and jurisdiction in which they practice. PAs also need to be aware of modern practice standards and the disciplinary consequences of not meeting such standards (Exhibit 13-9).

EXHIBIT 13-9
References for Legislation Issues Available From the American Academy of Physician Assistants

The Legislative Action Center
http://members.aapa.org/vocus/index.htm
Provides information on state and federal legislation affecting PAs and information for PAs preparing to lobby their representatives

AAPA's Legislative Agenda for the 110th Congress
http://www.aapa.org/gandp/agenda_110congress.html
Physician Assistants: State Laws & Regulations,
10th edition, http://www.aapa.org/aapastore
Comprehensive summary of state laws and regulations authorizing PA practice; includes the AAPA policy, "Guidelines for State Regulation of Physician Assistants," model state legislation for PAs, chart of practice requirements, and a listing of PA state regulatory authorities

Model State Legislation for PAs
http://www.aapa.org/gandp/modelaw.html
A model state legislation to be used as a template for PA practice regulations

Guidelines for State Regulation of Physician Assistants
http://www.aapa.org/manual/
06-GuideforStateRegs.pdf
Proposed guidelines for state regulation of PA practice

Physician Assistant Scope of Practice
http://www.aapa.org/gandp/issuebrief/pascope.pdf
An explanation of what elements factor into the duties a PA can perform: education/experience, state law, facility policy, and delegatory decisions made by supervising physicians

Taking Charge: State Government Affairs Handbook
http://www.aapa.org/members/cor-pubs/takecharge.pdf
(a "members-only" section of the website)
A resource guide for state chapters concerning all aspects of the state legislative process

Team Building: Developing Effective Organizational Relationships
http://www.aapa.org/members/cor-pubs/teambldg.pdf
(a "members-only" section of the website)
Provides strategies and suggestions for developing partnerships with other state organizations
    Another useful reference is the article "Lessons learned from service to the state licensing board" by N. Genova, 2002, in *Journal of the American Academy of Physician Assistants, 15*(12), 8–11 available at http://www.jaapa.com. This article provides insights from working with medical board officials on issues affecting PAs.

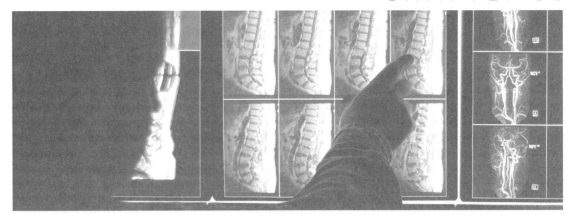

CHAPTER 14

LEGAL ISSUES OF PHYSICIAN ASSISTANT PRACTICE

RODERICK S. HOOKER ■ DAVID P. ASPREY ■ JAMES F. CAWLEY

Law and order are the medicine of the body politic and when the body politic gets sick, medicine must be administered.
—B. R. Ambedkar, Indian Nationalist
(1891–1956)

ABSTRACT

All states have laws governing physician assistants (PAs) that are enabling and restrictive. The laws, in turn, permit certain activity but at the same time create liability for the PA's employing or supervising doctor. Legal doctrine guides doctors, agencies, and the courts in how to address liability when it occurs. In the United States, Canada, and Australia legal doctrine is largely the responsibility of the state/province. In Great Britain and the Netherlands such doctrine falls under the central government. Medical boards are responsible for licensing services and administering systems to monitor provider behavior, ensure public safety, and provide appropriate medical discipline. The National Practitioner Data Bank collects this information. The results are that PAs present a very low level of liability for malpractice
when compared to doctors and advanced practice nurses.

INTRODUCTION

Physician assistants (PAs) were created in response to a changing healthcare system. As a result, the U.S. legal system has needed to address the PA phenomenon. One of the primary aspects of using PAs is supervision. State, provincial, and federal systems have put into place regulatory and contractual arrangements in which a doctor is obligated to properly supervise the PA. Lack of proper supervision not only results in potential tort liability of the practice but also may affect reimbursement for services provided.

The scope of services that a PA is permitted to perform can be quite broad, ranging from routine examinations and diagnostic maneuvers, prescribing medications, and performing minor surgery. Procedures permitted to be performed by PAs can be explicit or implicit, depending on state law, the reviewing medical board, and the arrangement between the supervising doctor and the PA.

LIABILITY OF PHYSICIANS WHO SUPERVISE PHYSICIAN ASSISTANTS

One of the most discussed topics regarding employment of a PA is the set of legal doctrines that binds the doctor to the action of the PA. Doctrines are principles of government and tend to have a legal connotation. Legal doctrines commonly used to assess a physician's liability for mistakes of a PA include the following:

- *Respondeat superior* (from the Latin "let the master answer"), in which the employer is considered responsible for the actions of the employee
- *Negligent supervision,* in which an employer fails to reasonably monitor and control an employee's actions
- *Negligent hiring,* in which an employer can be considered negligent if an employee had an easily discoverable record of misconduct or was aware of an employee's past misconduct
- The *"captain-of-the-ship" doctrine,* in which a physician is considered liable for the negligent acts of other employees
- The *"borrowed-servant rule,"* in which an employing physician is considered liable for the actions of a borrowed servant PA because the physician is considered the person in control of the PA's actions

Since the mid-1980s statutory regulations have emerged from various states suggesting a legislative trend to reduce and limit the liability for physicians who supervise PAs. Generally, the standard of care applicable to PAs is the same as the standard of care for a physician. The tendency is for the elements of each cause of action to reflect the mistakes of PAs and not to hold supervising physicians liable (Gore, 2000).

However, physicians striving to reduce liability from PAs working under them should focus on three main areas: (1) selection, (2) supervision, and (3) standard of conduct.

PAs learn most from the habits of the physicians who supervise them, irrespective of whether the habits are good or bad.

The American Medical Association (AMA) recognized these concepts when its 1995 House of Delegates adopted the following guidelines for physician/PA practice:

- The physician is responsible for managing the health care of patients in all practice settings.
- Health care services delivered by physicians and PAs must be within the scope of each practitioner's authorized practice as defined by state law.
- The physician is ultimately responsible for coordinating and managing the care of patients and, with the appropriate input of the PA, ensuring the quality of health care provided to patients.
- The physician is responsible for the supervision of the PA in all settings.
- The role of PAs in the delivery of care should be defined through mutually agreed upon guidelines that are developed by the physician and the PA and based on the physician's delegatory style.
- The physician must be available for consultation with the PA at all times either in person or through telecommunication systems or other means.
- The extent of the involvement by the PA in the assessment and implementation of treatment will depend on the complexity and acuity of the patient's condition and the training and experience and preparation of the PA as adjudged by the physician.
- Patients should be made clearly aware at all times whether they are being cared for by a physician or a PA.
- The physician and PA together should review all delegated patient services on a regular basis, as well as the mutually agreed upon guidelines for practice.
- The physician is responsible for clarifying and familiarizing the PA with his or her supervising methods and style of delegating patient care. (AMA, 2001)

PHYSICIAN ASSISTANT LIABILITY

In general, each state-licensed practitioner is directly liable for his or her own actions in tort and negligence; therefore, physicians, nurses, PAs, and others are independently liable for their malpractice. Licensed practitioners are also separately liable to their individual licensing and registration boards for any professional misconduct. Hospitals and physician professional groups may also be responsible for the malpractice of any employed licensed practitioner that occurs within the scope of employment (Cawley, 2005).

Agency

In the eyes of the law, the PA serves as the agent of the physician. *Agency* refers to a legal relationship whereby one party (the agent— the PA) is authorized to represent another (the principal—the physician) in dealings with third parties (patients). Agents owe their principals three duties: loyalty, obedience as to reasonable directions, and care (which includes the duty to notify).

Agency authority may be *contractual, apparent,* or *inherent.* When contractual, the scope of authority is clearly communicated to the agent; when apparent, the authority is communicated to the third party; under inherent, the principal is liable even when the agent acts in violation of the principal's orders or exceeds the scope of authority. Authority also may either be *expressed,* in which the orders from the principal are clearly defined, or *implied,* in which authority is based on a reasonable belief by the agent. The circumstances under which the authority is granted may result from contract, custom, circumstance, or be judicially defined in the event that litigation occurs.

Under the theory of *apparent agency,* a principal (an employing physician or hospital) "holds out" an agent (a PA) to the community as one who possesses certain authority, inducing the formation of a belief on the part of the third party that the agent may provide certain services. Principals that employ PAs have a legal duty to their prospective patients to provide non-negligent care. This is called *vicarious liability.*

Agency, or more precisely, apparent agency, assumes that caregivers do not misrepresent themselves. Plaintiffs have claimed that they assumed that a provider was a physician simply because the provider wore a stethoscope and lab coat. Therefore, most state PA practice laws require PAs to clearly identify themselves as PAs. For example, statutes in Texas, Maryland, and other states—in addition to imposing legal responsibility on the employing physician for the PA's acts or omissions— expressly require a PA to wear a name tag identifying himself or herself as a PA while engaging in professional activities. The distinction between the PA and the physician must always be clear and obvious to patients and the PA must never be misrepresented to patients as a medical student, student in training, or any other inaccurate typing. Misrepresenting the status of a PA or failing to disclose that status has resulted in administrative sanctions and can form liability under the theory of misrepresentation.

The *Whittaker* Case

What is the legal basis for the expansion of PA activity? For example, does a state's medical practice act or PA practice act permit a PA to insert a pacemaker in a patient suffering severe bradycardia? For most jurisdictions, legal authorities have not had to deal with the underlying issues associated with these questions. In a few states, however, the answers have begun to emerge from court decisions, opinions of attorneys general, or legislative enactment. As a practical matter, delegation of health service functions is predominantly governed by prevailing custom and practice. In the few relevant court decisions, however, it has been held that professional custom is no defense for a contravention of licensure laws.

One case in particular is important to illustrate, not only because of the court's handling of elements of licensure, custom, and supervision in deciding the delegation question, but because of its influence on the development of the PA profession. The case *People v. Whittaker*

(No. 35307, Justice Court of Redding Judicial District, Shasta County, Calif. [December 1966]) involved the right of a neurosurgeon to use a trained surgical assistant to assist in brain surgery. For various reasons the case became a pivotal event affecting the fledgling PA profession.

Roger G. Whittaker was a former Navy corpsman and engineering technology student at the University of California. He had attended the Navy's Hospital Corps School and Operating Technician School. A Vietnam veteran, he was attending college with veterans' benefits and took a job as an assistant with neurosurgeon George C. Stevenson. Stevenson was the only practicing neurosurgeon within 275 miles of Redding, California. Whittaker and Stevenson were reported to the California State Board of Medical Examiners.

Whittaker was charged with practicing medicine without a license because he operated a cranial drill and Giegle saw, positioned by the surgeon, to bore holes and excise skull flaps during neurosurgical operations. The surgeon was charged with aiding and abetting an unlicensed person to practice medicine. Despite the testimony of the chairman of the board of Redding Memorial Hospital that said the defendant was a "better neurosurgical assistant than I am," Whittaker was found guilty in one of three cases before the jury, and his employer was found guilty of having aided and abetted him. However, Whittaker and Stevenson were found not guilty on the other two charges because the jury felt that their services were beneficial. The court imposed nominal penalties. Both received suspended sentences of 30 days in jail; Whittaker was fined $50, and his employer $200. A jury empanelled before a justice of the Peace Court found both parties guilty of the charge in which the surgeon had sufficient time to call another physician to assist him but did not try to do so. As a standard for judging the physician's use of an unlicensed trained assistant, working under direct supervision, the following instruction was given to the jury:

In determining whether acts in this case, if any, performed under the direct supervision and control of a duly licensed physician, were legal or illegal, you may consider evidence of custom and usage of the medical practice in California as shown by the evidence in this case.

The *Whittaker* judgment was successfully appealed because of its importance as a test of the right of a physician or surgeon to use an extra pair of hands under conditions not constituting a medical emergency. This particular case was significant for its allowance of prevailing "custom and usage of the medical practice" in the state to determine the propriety of a physician's delegation and supervision of patently medical, but essentially mechanical, functions.

An interesting footnote to this case is that Dr. Eugene Stead, the founder of the PA program at Duke University, was called to serve as an expert witness. Stead testified that Whittaker provided a much-needed medical service and put forth the concept of the delegation of medical tasks to assistants. In the course of the legal proceedings, Stead had the opportunity to meet Whittaker and told him about the new educational program that had been inaugurated at Duke. Whittaker became a member of the third PA class at Duke and later, president of the AAPA (Condit, 1993; Carter, Thompson, & Stanhope, 2008) (Exhibit 14-1).

EXHIBIT 14-1
Roger Whittaker, PA-C (left) Passing the AAPA Presidential Gavel to Daniel Fox, PA-C, 1977

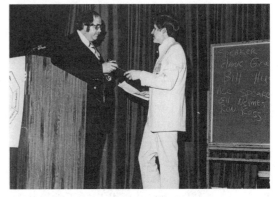

Courtesy of the American Academy of Physician Assistants.

The key issue in the licensure of PAs is the scope of functions that may be delegated to them and the educational and certification qualifications to permit such delegation safely. A shortage of PAs and other skilled healthcare personnel, new scientific and technological developments, and new methods of organizing health services have made the question of delegation all the more important. Across the states, licensure laws are being amended to authorize broader scope of functions for qualified PAs.

MALPRACTICE LITIGATION

In addition to being responsible for licensing services, medical boards are responsible for administering systems to monitor provider behavior, ensure public safety, and provide appropriate medical discipline. Each state board has investigative units responsible for the identification of medical misconduct. Examples of medical misconduct include (but are not limited to) the following:

- Practicing fraudulently
- Practicing with gross incompetence or gross negligence
- Practicing while impaired by alcohol, drugs, physical disability, or mental disability
- Being convicted of a crime
- Filing a false report
- Guaranteeing that treatment will result in a cure
- Refusing to provide services because of race, creed, color, or ethnicity
- Performing services not authorized by the patient
- Harassing, abusing, or intimidating a patient
- Ordering excessive tests
- Abandoning or neglecting a patient in need of immediate care

As the number of PAs in practice increases, the number of reported cases of malpractice lawsuits involving allegations of negligence by PAs has increased. Legal precedents have been set.

Negligence

A claimant who brings a medical negligence action against any healthcare provider must prove that four elements existed in the situation in question: duty, breach of duty, proximate cause, and damages.

Duty

A claimant first must show that the healthcare provider had a *duty* to provide medical care. For example, in all states but Vermont, healthcare providers are not required to stop and render care in a roadside emergency (Vt. Stat. Ann. tit. 12 519). Therefore, they cannot be found negligent for failure to provide care in such a situation. On the other hand, some courts have ruled that a physician on call in an emergency department has a duty to render medical assistance to any emergency patient whether or not the person is eligible for treatment at that facility (*Guerrero v. Copper Queen Hospital*, 537 P2d 1329). In most circumstances, the duty to treat is activated when medical treatment is begun and continues until the patient has recovered from the condition or has released the healthcare provider from the continuing duty to treat.

Breach of Duty

Breach of duty is predicated on provision of the standard of care of a reasonably prudent physician practicing under the same or similar circumstances. This is an objective standard, and an expert witness in a medical negligence trial is not asked what he or she personally would have done in the situation. Rather, the determination of breach of duty is based on what an average, reasonably prudent healthcare provider in the community would have done. Of the four requisite elements in negligence cases, breach of duty is the most difficult to prove.

A precedent for standard of care for physicians was spelled out in 1988 (*Pike v. Honsinger*, 155 NYS2d 201, 49 NE2d 760 [1988]). In this case, a PA and the employing physician differed in terms of the PA's capacity to handle a specific surgery. The physician (and a surgeon), by taking charge of the case, implied that he had a reasonable degree of learning and skill that is ordinarily possessed by physicians and surgeons in the locality in which he practices, and which is ordinarily regarded by those conversant with the employment as necessary to qualify him to engage in the business of practicing medicine and surgery. For the PA, upon consenting to treat a patient, it becomes his duty to use reasonable care and diligence in the exercise of his skill and the application of his learning to accomplish the purpose for which he was employed. There must be a want of ordinary and reasonable care, leading to a bad result if either is at fault. As applied here breach of duty necessitates a lack of reasonable care under the circumstances.

Proximate Cause

In addition to the duty to treat and a breach of that duty, negligence involves proving that the breach of duty was the cause of the claimant's injury. For example, a healthcare provider may have been negligent in a case of wrongful death. However, if the healthcare provider can show that the patient would have died regardless of the treatment rendered, the negligence cannot be held to be the *proximate cause* of death.

Damages

The fourth criterion for a negligence suit is that a claimant must have sustained some form of *damage*. For example, medication errors frequently are made in hospitals; too much, too little, or the wrong type of medication is given, or it is administered via the wrong route. Although many of these errors can be blamed on negligence, the vast majority of them result in little or no damage. Medical negligence suits routinely cost more than $20,000 to prosecute, and it is unlikely that an experienced malpractice attorney would accept a case with estimated damages less than $50,000.

Standard of Care

As mentioned previously, in a medical negligence action involving a physician, the duty is breached only when the physician has not performed as a reasonable and prudent physician would have performed under the same or similar circumstances. But to what standard of care should a PA or other healthcare extender be held: to that of a reasonably prudent PA or that of a reasonably prudent physician? Two federal court opinions involving a technician and a PA illustrate the confusion in this area.

In the case of *Haire v. United States* (No. 75-55-ORL-CIV-R, 1976), the mother of a 23-month-old girl took her child to the pediatric clinic at a military medical center in Florida. The child was seen by a medical technician. This technician had worked as a medic in Vietnam for 2 years and had received in-service training, which primarily involved observing the supervising pediatrician, before being assigned to the clinic. The medical technician examined the child and recorded that she had a runny nose as a result of an upper respiratory infection. He prescribed a decongestant and discharged her. Over the next 10 days, the child's appetite diminished and her runny nose persisted. On the tenth day, her temperature was noticeably elevated. The next day, her mother brought her back to the clinic, and the medical technician saw the child again. He examined the child's ears and throat and listened to her chest. He then told the mother that the patient's tonsils were causing her distress and discharged the child without referring her to a physician. The next day the patient's mother noted "twitching" of her daughter's hands and a temperature of 103°F. She rushed the child to a local emergency department, where a physician performed a lumbar puncture and diagnosed *Haemophilus influenzae* meningitis. Despite the rapid institution of appropriate treatment the child died 3 days later.

The child's family sued the medical center, claiming that the "physician extender" failed to diagnose or test for meningitis and that the child should have been referred to a physician on her second clinic visit. At the trial, a board-certified pediatrician testified on behalf of the family that if a pediatrician had seen the child on the second visit, the physician would have suspected meningitis and conducted ophthalmic and neurological examinations to confirm the diagnosis. The court held the technician to the standard of care of a board-certified pediatrician, and because he had not performed the neurological and ophthalmic examinations that a board-certified pediatrician would have performed, the court found him negligent. In 1976 the parents were awarded $15,000 each for emotional suffering.

In the case of *Polischeck v. United States* (535 F Supp 1261 [ED Pa. 1982]), another federal court took a different approach. A 44-year-old woman experienced a headache associated with nausea, vomiting, and fever. She complained to her husband of pressure behind her eyes and the feeling that the "top of her head was blowing off." The next day she went to the emergency department of a government medical center and was evaluated by a PA. Her temperature was 100.4°F and her blood pressure was 144/90 mm Hg. The PA questioned the patient about her illness and recorded that she had experienced "sudden onset of headache 4 days ago with malaise, nausea, and ocular myalgia." A brief neurological examination revealed photophobia but no nuchal rigidity. A complete blood count demonstrated a slightly elevated white blood cell count. The PA diagnosed flu syndrome, prescribed an analgesic/anxiolytic/muscle relaxant, and instructed the patient to return to the emergency department if her symptoms became worse. This medical center allowed PAs to use their discretion in deciding whether to consult a physician and did not require supervising physicians to review the charts of patients seen by PAs, so the patient was not seen by a physician and her chart was not reviewed or countersigned by a physician.

Two days later, on a Friday, the patient returned to the emergency department when her condition had not improved. The same PA saw her and referred her to the emergency department physician. The physician examined the patient, diagnosed "headaches, etiology unknown," and advised the patient to go to the internal medicine clinic the following Monday if her headaches persisted, or sooner if they became worse. That evening the patient's husband could not rouse her. He took her

back to the emergency department, where the same physician examined her and diagnosed intracerebral hemorrhage. Because the medical center was not equipped to handle this type of patient, she was transferred to another hospital, where an arteriogram demonstrated a large subdural hematoma and a right posterior communicating artery aneurysm. A frontoparietal craniotomy was performed. However, the patient never regained consciousness and she died 3 days later.

The patient's husband filed suit in federal court, claiming that the medical center was negligent in not having his wife seen by a physician on her first visit. He also claimed that the physician was negligent in treating the patient on her second visit. At the trial the plaintiff's expert medical witnesses testified that the standard of care in the community required that patients not be discharged from emergency departments until they had been seen or at least their charts had been reviewed by a licensed physician. However, the court reasoned that the PA himself was not negligent in failing to diagnose the patient's subarachnoid hemorrhage on her first visit. Indeed, it hardly seems reasonable to expect a person with only 2 years of general medical training to be able to recognize a medical condition when it is presented in a patient possessing only some of the condition's textbook symptoms.

Therefore, the court held the PA to the same standard of care as other PAs in the community with similar training and, compared with these peers, he was not negligent. However, the court found the medical center negligent for failure either to have the patient seen or to have her records reviewed by a physician on her first visit, as was standard in the community.

These two decisions disagree about the standard of practice that a PA must meet. Decisions in other cases involving healthcare extenders may be helpful in clarifying this issue.

- *Thompson v. Brent* (245 S2d 751 [La. 1971]): In removing a cast from a patient's leg with a Stryker saw, a nurse accidentally cut the patient's leg, leaving a scar. The court held her to the standard of care of a physician and ruled that she had been negligent.

■ *Barber v. Reinking* (411 P2d 861 [Wash. 1966]): A practical nurse administered an injection that caused injury to a patient. In that state only registered nurses were authorized by law to administer injections. The court held the practical nurse to the standard of care of a registered nurse and ruled that she had been negligent.

Evidence of Standard of Care

How is the standard of care proved in a medical negligence suit? In addition to hiring an expert witness, the plaintiff's attorneys most likely will subpoena all hospital or clinic manuals, regulations, and protocols referring to PAs. These usually are admissible evidence of the applicable standard of care. If a PA has failed to follow a hospital's protocol or other applicable regulation, there will be strong, though not necessarily conclusive, evidence that the standard of care was not met. Violation of a state law regarding the duties of PAs also is strong evidence of a breach of the standard of care (Exhibit 14-2).

In addition to hospital or clinic protocols and regulations, the courts may consult guidelines

EXHIBIT 14-2
Physician Assistant Legal References

Vt. Stat. Ann. tit. 12 519

Guerrero v. Copper Queen Hospital, 537 P2d 1329

Pike v. Honsinger, 155 NYS2d 201, 49 NE2d 760 (1988)

Haire v. United States, No. 75-55-ORL-CIV-R, 1976

Polischeck v. United States, 535 F Supp 1261 (ED Pa. 1982)

Thompson v. Brent, 245 S2d 751 (La. 1971)

Barber v. Reinking, 411 P2d 861 (Wash. 1966)

Thompson v. United States, 368 F Supp 466 (WD La. 1973)

Whitney v. Day, 300 NW2d 380 (1980)

This is an incomplete list and does not represent the range of legal cases or literature on litigation involving PAs. The reader is referred to the legal literature for recent cases.

issued by professional organizations, including standards used by the Joint Commission. Therefore, it is important that PAs also be aware of the guidelines issued by these organizations.

There is controversy, however, with regard to the precise definition of what constitutes the PA standard of care. Although data are limited, current evidence indicates that the increase in the number of malpractice claims, the size of awards, and rate increases physicians have been undergoing in the 1980s has not been the PA experience.

NATIONAL PRACTITIONER DATA BANK

Are PAs safe to employ? Can they provide competent care? For more than four decades policymakers and opponents of PAs have questioned whether it is in society's best interest to sanction PAs. The one predominant question that arises is whether PAs increase liability. Unlike doctors, nurses, dentists, and some other health occupations, PAs have a relatively short history and their scrutiny for quality of care has not been as lengthy. Because scrutiny of PAs has been relatively brief since they were first legislated under the 1966 Allied Health Professions Act (PL-751) and legislation fully extended to all 50 states in 2000, a full assessment of their safety has not been undertaken. With that said, some attempts have been made to address the question of safety. Two studies (Brock, 1998; Cawley, Rohrs, & Hooker, 1998) examined a few years of federal data in the 1990s. Both studies concluded there was little evidence that patient care was being compromised by PAs.

In 2008, a research team set out to answer the fundamental question of whether PAs provide care safely or less safely than doctors. The intent was to address this question more systematically than it had been before using a federal source of data: the National Practitioner Data Bank (NPDB). The NPDB is a unique repository of all state board actions or malpractice actions against physicians, dentists, PAs, NPs, and other licensed healthcare professionals. It was originally established in 1990 to restrict the ability of incompetent practitioners to move from state to state without discovery of previous substandard performance or unprofessional conduct. Since then, it has expanded to serve as a registry for the following:

- Medical malpractice payers
- Medical and dental state licensing boards
- Hospital and other healthcare entities
- Professional societies with formal peer review
- Department of Health and Human Services Office of the Inspector General
- U.S. Drug Enforcement Administration
- Federal and state government agencies
- Health insurance plans

All PAs (as well as doctors, nurses, dentists, chiropractors, and others) applying for privileges to a hospital or medical center must submit information that is then forwarded to the NPDB for clearance. From 1990 through 2008, the NPDB produced information on more than 414,000 reported actions, malpractice payments, and Medicare/Medicaid exclusions that involved 18 different types of providers. The variables in the NPDB are large, inclusive, and comprehensive. A list of those pertinent to this report is presented in Exhibit 14-3.

To provide annual information on how three different types of providers were reported to the NPDB for adverse outcomes, fraud, misappropriation of professional role, and other actions, 17 years of data (January 1, 1991 to January 1, 2008) regarding physicians, PAs, and advanced practice nurses (APNs) were analyzed. (APNs in this case refer to NPs, certified nurse specialists [CNSs], CNMs, and certified registered nurse anesthetists [CRNAs]). This analysis involved 324,285 entries (Exhibit 14-4). The chi-square test showed a statistically significant difference in malpractice payments and adverse actions between provider types ($\chi^2 = 576.67$; $p < 0.0001$).

Exhibit 14-5 displays the average age of the provider at time of event leading to the report. A comparison on means among three types of healthcare providers reveals statistically significant differences in mean age at the time of the event leading to report between physicians and PAs, physicians and APNs, as well as PAs and APNs (F = 280.19 and $p < 0.0001$). There are significant differences in mean age at the time of the adverse action leading to report between physicians and PAs, physicians and APNs (F = 65.44 and $p < 0.0001$). PAs and APNs were younger than physicians for malpractice reports but not between themselves.

EXHIBIT 14-3
Variables Examining Physician Assistants in the National Practitioner Data Bank

Independent Variables	Dependent Variables
Physician assistants	Total number of malpractice payments
Advance practice nurses (NPs, CRNAs, CNSs, CNMs)	Average amount of malpractice payments
Doctors (MD, DO, MBBS)	Average years of practice
	Total number of adverse events/actions
	State medical board licensing actions
	Clinical privileges actions
	Professional society membership actions
	Practitioner exclusions from Medicare and Medicaid programs
	U.S. Drug Enforcement Administration actions
	Year of adverse action
	Basis of action
	State of license

EXHIBIT 14-4
National Practitioner Data Bank Entries by Provider Type, 1991–2007

Type of Provider	Total Entries	Malpractice Reports		
		Malpractice Payments	*Adverse Actions*	*Number of Involved Providers*
Physician	320,034	245,267	74,767	268,919
PA	1,536	1,222	314	1,509
APN	2,715	2,608	107	3,265
TOTAL	324,285	249,097	75,188	273,693

Total entries $\chi^2 = 576.7$; $p < 0.0001$.

Malpractice Payment field RECTYPE M AND P $\chi^2 = 181.4$; $p < 0.0001$.

Adverse Action field RECTYPE A AND C $\chi^2 = 565.7$; $p < 0.0001$.

Number of Involved Providers $\chi^2 = 1395.8$; $p < 0.0001$.

Data compiled from the National Practitioner Data Bank.

Exhibit 14-6 reports medical malpractice payments by reason for payment and provider type. This table is useful in demonstrating the main reasons for malpractice payments. The chi-square test shows a significant association between reasons of malpractice payment and type of healthcare provider ($\chi^2 = 11,525.38$ and $p < 0.0001$).

Physicians totaled 104,353 medical malpractice payments spanning 17 years, and PAs had 252 payments during the same reporting period. The leading category of reason for medical practice payment for both physicians (34,021 of 104,353) and PAs (129 of 252) was diagnosis error (Exhibit 14-7).

Exhibit 14-8 displays the unadjusted mean, median, and total malpractice payments for the three provider types over the 17-year study period. The total malpractice payments for the 17 years for all providers exceeded $58 billion (in 2007 dollars). PA payments comprised 0.3% of the total and APN payments comprised 1.2% of the total. The average APN payment was the highest at $282,083. The average physician payment was $236,720, while the average PA payment was $164,988. The average physician payment was 1.4 times higher than the average PA payment.

EXHIBIT 14-5
Characteristics of Providers in the National Practitioner Data Bank, 1991–2008

Provider	Reports by Provider			Age (average in years) at Time of Event Leading to Report	
	Number of Reports	*Average Number of Reports per Provider*	*Number of Providers*	*Adverse Action**	*Malpractice†*
Physician	320,034	1.19	268,919	48 (±11)	43 (±11)
PA	1,536	1.02	1,509	41 (± 9)	37 (± 9)
APN	2,715	0.83	3,265	43 (± 9)	41 (± 9)

*$F = 65.44$ and $p < 0.0001$.

†$F = 280.19$ and $p < 0.0001$.

± standard deviation.

Data compiled from the National Practitioner Data Bank.

EXHIBIT 14-6
Medical Malpractice Payments by Reason for Payment and Provider Type, 2004–2008

Reason for Payment	Total	Physician	PA	APN
Diagnosis	84,193	83,130	678	385
Surgery	66,605	66,451	56	98
Treatment	44,603	44,028	301	274
Obstetrics	21,700	21,114	8	578
Medication	13,676	13,446	104	126
Anesthesia	8,611	7,592	10	1,009
Monitoring	3,859	3,757	22	80
Miscellaneous	3,663	3,600	38	25
Equipment/product	980	966	2	12
IV and blood products	858	839	3	16
Behavioral health	235	230	0	5
TOTAL	248,983	245,153	1,222	2,608

Data from Hooker, R. S., Nicholson, J., & Le, T. (2009). Does the employment of physician assistants and nurse practitioners increase liability? Journal of Medical Licensure and Discipline, 95(2), 6–16.

EXHIBIT 14-7
Mean Malpractice Payment by Year, 1991–2008

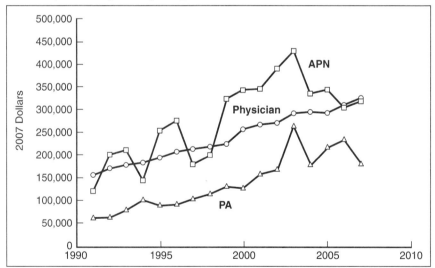

Data from Hooker, R. S., Nicholson, J., & Le, T. (2009). Does the employment of physician assistants and nurse practitioners increase liability? Journal of Medical Licensure and Discipline, 95(2), 6–16.

EXHIBIT 14-8
Malpractice Payment (Unadjusted) Amount for the Period Jan. 1, 1991–Dec. 31, 2007

Type of Provider	Number of Entries	Mean (000)	Median (000)	Sum (000)
Physicians	245,267	$236,720	$115,000	$58,053.59
PAs	1,222	$164,988	$72,500	$201.62
APNs	2,608	$282,083	$125,000	$735.67
TOTAL	249,097			$58,990.88

Data from Hooker, R. S., Nicholson, J., & Le, T. (2009). Does the employment of physician assistants and nurse practitioners increase liability? Journal of Medical Licensure and Discipline, 95(2), 6–16.

The NPDB data suggest the rate and amount of malpractice payments for PAs is relatively low compared with that for physicians. In fact, the NPDB data reveal one claim per eight practicing physicians versus one claim per 107 PAs over the same time period. These findings support perceptions that PAs pose a low risk of malpractice liability to the public in general and to employing practices in particular. One reason postulated for this observed low risk is the communication skills that PAs may have in patient encounters (Brock, 1998). Whether PAs have communication skills that limit liability remains to be researched. Another explanation is that they may avoid risky encounters with patients and avoid procedures that have high liability profiles, such as births and anesthesia.

Work is needed to further understand the rate of litigation and malpractice by number of visits and types of visits that are managed by physicians, PAs, APNs, and other types of providers. Although the NPDB has some flaws in its collection methodology, these flaws should not be discounted completely because the criteria for data bank entry affect all providers equally. This analysis of the existing data should offer some reassurance that the delegated responsibility of patient care from the physician to the PA is a relatively safe one (Hooker, Nicholson, & Le, 2009).

TORT REFORM

Tort reform refers to measures that would modify the current medical liability system to limit the number of legal claims and amounts awarded in cases prosecuted by personal injury lawyers that are perceived to unfairly burden insurance policyholders with high premiums. At times, tort reform has become a politicized matter with medical groups, particularly the AMA, labeling tort reform a "crisis" issue. The AMA has spent considerable sums lobbying for legislation favorable to their hoped-for objectives to change the present medical malpractice liability law.

Tort law is traditionally a matter of state "common law" and legislation. A number of states have addressed this issue in the past by passing various types of measures that modify the tort liability and resolution system. In some states, legislation has passed attempting to deal with alleged abuses of the tort system by placing caps on the amount of money that juries can award for "pain and suffering." Bills of this sort cap awards for noneconomic damages at a certain level (e.g., $250,000) and place limits on attorney's fees and other damages that plaintiffs can collect in medical malpractice suits.

Some proposals go beyond simply applying liability caps to physicians and hospitals, and extend such limits on liability to any entity providing healthcare products or services. Under such legislation, civil suits against drug makers, insurance companies, and medical device manufacturers would be subject to the same caps on noneconomic and punitive damages as suits against physicians (Dowling & Glendinning, 2005).

Tort reform adherents advocate the idea of capping malpractice awards and this notion has found some degree of legislative acceptance. Caps exist in 16 states and have been in place in California since 1975. Typically, such laws limit awards that a plaintiff may receive for pain and suffering at $250,000 to $500,000. However, there is no conclusive evidence that caps save much money. One study of verdicts in 22 states concluded that caps have no effect on the size of the overall compensation awarded by juries, and that what seemed to influence outcomes were factors such as the severity of injury, the requirement for medical expert screening of cases, and the election experiences of the judge (Baker, 2005). A RAND Corporation study concluded that the California law had reduced net recoveries for plaintiffs by 15% and had cut attorneys' fees by 60%; defendant liabilities were trimmed by 30% (Lohr, 2005). There is also doubt that caps will work to limit overall compensation awarded to plaintiffs because lawyers may shift the damage awards to categories of compensation that are not capped (Baker, 2005).

One perceived change resulting from these caps has been reluctance on the part of lawyers to take medical malpractice cases, thus reducing the opportunity for victims of medical negligence to have access to the court system. Others feel that such caps are futile and unfairly penalize less-fortunate groups, such as the poor and the elderly, who have less economic capacity than the average citizen (Liptak, 2005).

On the other side of the argument is convincing data that show there is no such thing as an "epidemic" of medical malpractice. Reviews of existing evidence of the rates of serious injuries and malpractice suits cite data from studies done over the past 30 years in Utah, Colorado, and California by researchers. Rates have not risen steeply in the past 10 years; the rates show that there are 6 to 25 serious injuries from medical malpractice for every lawsuit filed. In the states for which there is the best recent information—Texas, Florida, and Mississippi—reports show that the rate of claims has been steady or even declined in relation to population and economic growth over the past 15 years (Baker, 2005).

Another issue is the question of the necessity for a federal remedy to the matter of medical malpractice liability, as has been proposed in the past decade. Is this the most appropriate way to deal with an issue that is primarily in the purview of the states because they license and regulate the practice of medicine? Most would agree that the overall goals for the reform of medical malpractice liability include limiting overall health system costs, adequately compensating the victims of medical mistakes, and providing incentives for health providers and facilities to avoid errors. Many believe that more needs to be done within the medical care system to reduce the number of errors. States commonly deal with these matters and may be in the best position to solve them rather than a federally imposed ruling.

Tort reform has been front and center in a number of states where legislatures have struggled with the competing interests of the medical profession versus the trial lawyers. For example, in 2004 Maryland's medical malpractice carrier announced that premiums would raise by 33%. This led to considerable wrangling between the governor and the legislature, who differed on remedies to deal with the malpractice issue. Following considerable politization of the issue the final legislative solution, in addition to limitations of awards on noneconomic damages, was for the state to essentially levy a health maintenance organization (HMO) user's fee to subsidize physician malpractice insurance premiums. Several years later, a large amount of this subsidization was shown not to be utilized by the state's malpractice carrier and was subsequently refunded to the state treasury. In confrontations of this sort, consumers seem to be caught in the crossfire. One comment of interest throughout this discussion in Maryland was the bewilderment of the public who, in the words of one person, saw this issue as "rich doctors fighting with rich lawyers" (Cawley, 2005).

A view commonly held by advocates of tort reformers is that the tort system is responsible for rising medical insurance premiums. Baker (2005) identifies cyclical economics of the insurance industry and states that tort reform would have little impact on malpractice insurance premiums. He explains why there is little connection between the rates or amounts of medical malpractice awards and insurance premiums. The main observation is that the combination of the stock market bubble bursting in 2001, coupled with a downturn in interest rates and the September 11, 2001 attacks, led insurance companies to be at the bottom of the cycle. The result was that premiums rose steeply thereafter not only in the medical malpractice area but also in the entire property and casualty insurance business.

In the overall picture of health policy, the cost of medical malpractice is small—less than 1% of total healthcare costs. The automobile liability and workers' compensation businesses total amounts are higher than medical malpractice, and overall numbers and premium rates in these areas are proportionately higher than the premiums paid by physicians.

For the PA profession, the tort reform issue presents some difficult choices. On one hand, there is seemingly natural temptation to side with physicians on this issue because most PAs are employees of physician practices. PAs are sometimes the targets of lawsuits when physicians and healthcare facilities are sued and share their frustrations with the current system. On the other hand, PAs view themselves as advocates for their patients and espouse the values of the rights of citizens to seek appropriate redress of alleged medical negligence (Cawley, 2005).

The AAPA developed a policy statement on this issue that was approved by the 2004 AAPA House of Delegates. This position holds that:

> It is critical to assure that any medical liability insurance reform in the United States treats patients fairly . . . tort reform alone is not the answer. Caps on noneconomic damages may perhaps be appropriate if they are part of comprehensive medical liability insurance reform whose impact is borne equitably by attorneys, insurers, providers, and patients.

On the matter of liability caps, the AAPA believes that "a $250,000 cap on noneconomic damages paid for medical malpractice is too low and that fair and comprehensive reform of the medical liability insurance system is needed. Appropriate goals of a fair medical liability insurance system include compensating injured patients, deterring poor quality medical care, and assuring affordable medical liability insurance" (AAPA House of Delegates, 2005).

Medical errors can be a difficult episode in a provider's professional career. For the individual PA, the best approach, if one has made a medical error, is to bear in mind the bioethical value of truth telling. In the past several years, there has also been a movement to admit to error and to offer an apology (Banja, 2005). In a number of states, laws have passed allowing providers to offer apologies to injured patients and families and exempting such apologies from admission in courts.

Research and Legal Issues

While liability is one of the reasons used to not employ a PA there is little research to identify what the safety and efficacy of PAs are. A number of questions arise as to what is the liability of PA employment.

- **Case studies:** Describe cases in which a PA was found liable or incompetent, convicted of fraud, or exonerated for skill and duty.

- **Federation of State Boards of Medical Examiners:** What is the rate of various disciplinary issues brought before state boards of medical examiners by population and type of provider?

- **State comparisons:** How do the various states compare in their laws of liability?

- **Liability rate:** What is the rate of liability per 10,000 visits in primary care comparing a PA, an NP, and a doctor? How do these rates compare per medical specialty?

- **Adverse event:** What changes and trends are occurring in adverse events regarding PAs?

- **Supervision liability:** When does physician supervision become an issue in liability involving a PA and when is the PA alone held accountable for his or her actions without involving the doctor?

SUMMARY

Although state laws governing PAs continue to emerge, the one constant held is that the PA is bound to the supervising doctor. Legal doctrines are the theories of behavior that guide doctors, agencies, and the courts in how the laws concerning PAs should be interpreted. Medical boards are responsible for licensing services, administering systems to monitor provider behavior, ensuring public safety, and providing appropriate medical discipline if liability or malpractice issues are raised.

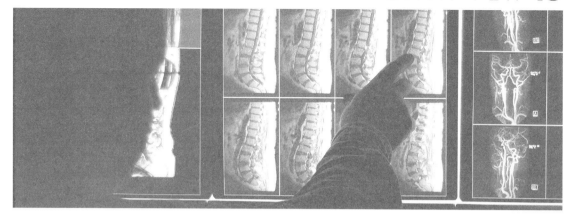

CHAPTER 15

PROFESSIONAL AND WORKFORCE ISSUES

JAMES F. CAWLEY ■ RODERICK S. HOOKER ■ DAVID P. ASPREY

The reward for work well done is the opportunity to do more.

—Jonas Salk

ABSTRACT

Issues related to the professional practice of medicine as a physician assistant (PA) and the practice dynamics associated with the workforce tend to shape policy and governance. Factors that impact the culture and environment of the PA's practice have the potential to influence core issues such as job satisfaction, scope of practice, and role delineation. Although these profession and workforce issues may be viewed as peripheral to the clinical practice of medicine, they do influence the behavior of PAs.

INTRODUCTION

Professional issues influence the behavior of physician assistants (PAs) in various ways. They may be organizationally based or political in nature; many issues draw lines as to which side of the healthcare environment PAs are placed when viewed by physicians. The issues under discussion in this chapter represent contemporary changes in healthcare delivery and review traditional views of caregivers and services. As new patterns of service delivery evolve, the boundaries between and within some professions tend to blur.

Health workforce issues, defined as the interaction among the various health professions as they relate to supply and demand in the medical marketplace, have become increasingly important for policymakers and providers alike. A key characteristic that has made PAs valuable in the U.S. health workforce is their adaptability. PAs like stem cells, begin with all the basic ingredients for development. Both are able to grow and change to meet the environment where they come to rest. These include changing demands in the health care system.

PROFESSIONAL ISSUES

Issues relating to or connected with a profession are considered professional issues. They may arise at any time and almost under any circumstance. Throughout their history, PAs have faced such professional issues as enabling legislation, prescriptive authority, and insurance reimbursement. Today, PAs are confronted with issues related to their professional growth.

Physician Assistant Unions

Efforts to organize PAs have met with acceptance and resistance since the first PAs were incorporated into a healthcare worker's union around 1975 with Kaiser Permanente in Colorado. In 2000, New York led the nation in the number of unionized PAs through their affiliation with the Service Employees International Union (SEIU), Local 1199, in New York City. The union began incorporating PAs in 1988, and in 1997 the local union created a PA division, which represents PAs exclusively. Local 1199 is the first and closest thing to a PA-only union in the country. As of 2000 it had unionized more than 500 PAs, including 75 at the Catholic Medical Center in New York City and 157 at the Riker's Island correctional facility. About half are located in hospitals within New York State (Herrick, 2000).

To be a union member or member of a collective bargaining unit, one has to be a *nonmanagement employee*. Most physicians are independent contractors and are not eligible to join a union. Likewise, PAs who are self-employed cannot join a union.

The Quality Health-Care Coalition Act, HR 1304, introduced in the Congressional sessions of 1999 and 2000, proposed dramatic revisions to federal antitrust laws to allow self-employed physicians to organize and collectively bargain with managed care organizations. This legislation met with major opposition from the insurance and hospital industries, the Department of Justice, and the Federal Trade Commission. The bill passed the House amidst a flurry of hostile wrangling, but no bill was ever introduced in the Senate. Similar bills have been enacted into law in some states. Their impact remains to be seen.

Can supervising physicians who are employees join collective bargaining units?

Neither the National Labor Relations Board (NLRB) nor the courts has provided definitive guidance on this issue. It depends on the facts in each case. The NLRB distinguishes between "authority arising from professional knowledge and authority encompassing front-line management prerogatives." In 1994, the Supreme Court disagreed with this distinction in its decision *NLRB v. Health Care and Retirement Corp.* This case involved charge nurses and the question of whether or not they were management. Despite a court ruling that found the charge nurses to be members of management, the NLRB continues to find that most nurses and healthcare professionals who direct other employees are employees and not supervisors (AAPA, 2006b).

Conversely, the majority of courts and the NLRB generally see physicians as supervisors. However, the NLRB has recognized physician bargaining units and considered only department heads to be management in a few cases. In some instances, physicians who clinically supervise PAs might be considered nonmanagement if they did not exercise control over the PA hours, hiring, firing, salaries, and performance evaluations.

The 1999 AAPA census found nationwide that 3.9% of all PAs were members of a union. These figures may not reflect part-time and per diem PAs, who are also covered by union contracts but may only have a quasi-membership status within the union (AAPA, 2000). Whereas the New York unionization rate is almost triple that of any other state, the vast majority of PAs are not in unions. Not all efforts to unionize PAs have been successful. Although little is known about union successes, much less failures, the authors know of unionization efforts within Kaiser Permanente in Portland, Oregon. In 1988 and 1999 a movement to organize PAs and advanced practice nurses (APNs), 230 full-time employees, into a collective bargaining union met with defeat. A Kaiser Permanente strike of 1,000 PAs, nurses, pharmacists, optometrists, physical therapists, and other healthcare workers in Colorado lasted 20 days in 2000. All but a few PAs joined the strike (Hughes, 2000). However, in 2002 the PAs and APNs agreed to be represented by the union and have been part of a union to date.

Unionized PAs report that collective bargaining has allowed them to influence how care is delivered and to increase stipends in continuing medical education (CME), work ratios, shift times, and the formation of professional practice committees that decide work and care issues (Herrick, 2000).

Pharmaceutical Industry Representatives

Interactions between pharmaceutical representatives and healthcare providers have long been examined. Although initial attention was almost exclusively focused on physicians, expanded prescribing privileges for PAs and other nonphysician providers has resulted in greater interactions with pharmaceutical representatives. PAs and nurse practitioners (NPs) are responsible for a growing number of prescriptions and pharmaceutical companies increasingly have been promoting their role in health care. For example, one company specializes in hiring PAs and NPs as pharmaceutical representatives and another company targets PAs as prescribers of interest.

As the focus of the pharmaceutical industry has moved toward NPs and PAs as prescribers, retail prescriptions from these providers increased 22% in the first 8 months of 2006 compared to the same time period in 2005. Physician retail prescriptions increased at a significantly slower rate during this time period—only 2%. Within these 12 months, detailing by pharmaceutical sales representatives to PAs and NPs increased 9% compared to the same time period the previous year, while detailing to office- and hospital-based physicians continued to decrease: 6% and 16%, respectively. Of the top products detailed to NPs and PAs during this time, details for Nexium increased 28%, followed by details for Singulair, which increased 24%. According to Verispan's Pharmaceutical Company Image study, the majority of PAs (86%) see at least one sales representative each week, with an average of 6.8 representatives seen per week. Eighty-five percent of NPs reported seeing sales representatives each week, with an average of 5.9 seen per week (Anonymous, 2006).

A professional issue associated with the presence of pharmaceutical company representatives involves gifts distributed to physicians, PAs, and NPs by pharmaceutical representatives. The intent of such gifts is to influence favorable prescribing. More than one-half of the $11 billion spent in promotions in 1996 was funneled through company sales representatives. As a result of concern regarding prescribing influence, ethical guidelines on gifts that doctors receive have been developed. Basically, a prescribing doctor may accept only from drug representatives that which would benefit patients or the practice. Similar guidelines have been developed for PAs and NPs.

Certain jurisdictions have considered banning pharmaceutical representatives from medical settings (Massachusetts) or requiring them to have a license (the District of Columbia). The ethical issues in this area relate to the degree to which the pharmaceutical representatives influence important medical decisions such as prescribing. Some have called for a complete prohibition of the receipt of money or favors of any sort provided by pharmaceutical companies involving medical education (Angel, 2004). This approach would mean that pharmaceutical companies would be forbidden from conducting marketing activities that involved medical students, residents, fellows, and faculty in medical education settings and supporting continuing medical education sessions conducted by professional organizations.

In a 2008 report, a task force from the Association of American Medical Colleges (AAMC) called for a complete disengagement of drug company activities in undergraduate as well as graduate medical education. The report urges medical schools and teaching hospitals to adopt policies that prohibit drug industry gifts and services to physicians, faculty, residents, and students, and to curtail the involvement of industry in continuing medical education activities. Under these guidelines, companies could not engage in activities such as providing lunches for conferences and seminars, providing gifts (pens, mugs, etc.), and other enticements to influence medical students. The policy directions discussed in the report have been implemented in many medical schools and teaching hospitals. It urges all academic medical centers to accelerate their adoption of policies that better manage, and when necessary, prohibit, academic-industry interactions that can inherently create conflicts of interest and undermine standards of professionalism. Some believe that industry will also voluntarily discontinue those practices that compromise professionalism as well as public trust. It is of interest to note that the task force included three CEOs of major drug companies as well as prominent medical educators and clinicians (AAMC, 2008).

The professional difficulty with such reform will not be so much in the areas of medical education, but in the involvement of industry in support of professional organizational meetings. Many professional organizations, such as the AAPA, depend heavily on the revenue derived from their annual conferences, which in turn are dependent on drug company support and involvement in their exhibit hall displays and CME sessions.

Physician Assistant Participation in Execution

Of the 37 states with the death penalty, most use lethal injection. In 2000, the AAPA refined an existing policy on executions in its code of conduct. Although PAs can certify death (after the prisoner is officially pronounced dead), witness an execution, and relieve the acute suffering of a condemned person before the execution, they should not participate in a legally authorized execution. As a policy of statement there are no formal consequences.

Assisted Suicide

Assisted suicide has been a topic of debate among healthcare professionals for decades, and PAs are no exception. In 1997, Oregon became the first and only state to legalize provider-assisted suicide and, in 1998, 16 patients used provider-assisted suicide; an additional 27 patients did the same the following year. These numbers represents nine provider-assisted suicide deaths per 10,000 total Oregon deaths. From 1998 to 2007 there

have been a little over 300 assisted suicides reported.

Barbara Coombs Lee, the executive director of the Death with Dignity advocacy group, which helped create the Oregon law, is an attorney and former PA. However, no known case of assisted suicide involving a PA has been reported. Attitudes about this act are likely to change with time and along with it will be the more open involvement of patients, their caregivers, physicians, nurses, pharmacists, and PAs.

In a Michigan survey conducted in 1994, 48% of responding PAs tended to support provider-assisted suicide and 40% were opposed (Hayden et al, 1995). No survey has been published since this surfaced as a professional issue in the 1990s, and the issue has largely been ignored.

Impairment

Impairment of professional performance by alcohol, other drugs, or mental illness is a common professional issue for all health professionals. An estimated 12% to 14% of physicians experience such problems at some time during their lives, mostly due to chemical dependence. In 1985 the North Carolina Academy of Physician Assistants created a standing committee to address impaired PAs, modeled after a similar program for physicians in the state. Over the first 11 years 29 PAs were referred for assessment and treatment by the impaired physician program in the state (Exhibits 15-1 and 15-2) (Mattingly & Curtis, 1996).

In work published by Ganley and colleagues (2005), a 6-year retroactive chart review was undertaken to compare outcomes between chemically dependent physicians and PAs under contract with the North Carolina Physicians Health Program (NCPHP). Of 233 physicians, 212 (91%) had a good outcome, compared to only 20 of 34 PAs (59%) in this sample. Fifteen percent of physicians and 37% of PAs were female with basically the same outcome. Alcohol was the predominant substance used by both groups. Most subjects in both groups were between the ages of 30 and

EXHIBIT 15-1
Problems/Diagnoses of Impaired Physician Assistants (North Carolina)

Diagnosis	No. of PAs	%
Opioids	7	24
Alcohol	5	17
Polysubstances	5	17
Dual diagnosis	3	10
Psychiatric disorder	3	10
Sexual misconduct	2	7
Other	2	7
Marijuana	1	3
Unsubstantiated	1	3
TOTAL	N = 29	

Data from Mattingly, D. E., & Curtis, L. G. (1996). Physician assistant impairment. A peer review program for North Carolina. North Carolina Medical Journal, 57, 233–235.

EXHIBIT 15-2
Status of Physician Assistant Impairment Cases in North Carolina

	No. of PAs	%
Contract agreements	13	45
Assessed and released	9	31
Not currently licensed in NC	—	10
Not currently in NC	3	10
Other	1	3

Data from Mattingly, D. E., & Curtis, L. G. (1996). Physician assistant impairment. A peer review program for North Carolina. North Carolina Medical Journal, 57, 233–235.

55, with best outcomes between the ages of 25 and 29, and the worst in those older than 55. With paucity of data on PAs in the literature, the present study may be one of the first to single out this group and compare their recovery rates with those of physicians while receiving similar services (Ganley et al, 2005).

Other states have modeled their PA impairment programs after either the North Carolina model or the individual state's existing program for physicians. A support program within the AAPA, called the Caduceus Caucus, assists AAPA members with alcohol and drug addiction (Exhibit 15-3). Suggested readings on the topic of impairment are shown in Exhibit 15-4.

EXHIBIT 15-3
Caduceus Caucus Program for Physician Assistants

Purpose: To provide a resource for information and advocacy for physician assistants involved with issues of impairment.

ACTIVITIES:

- Provide continuing education on various impairment issues at AAPA Annual Conferences
- Conduct refresher seminars for constituent chapter impairment committee members
- Encourage AA/ACOA/NA Al-Anon type meetings at various AAPA functions
- Act as a resource for chapter CME committee members for potential speakers on impairment issues
- Establish a telephone network of concerned colleagues to provide information and guidance to PAs facing problems rooted in impairment issues
- Issue periodic newsletters to provide updated information on programs, lectures, books, articles, etc., of benefit to members
- Explore means of raising funds to continue providing services to AAPA members

Liability Insurance

As the role of the PA expanded, the need for professional liability insurance developed. No matter how careful and competent PAs are, mistakes are made and sometimes judgments on those mistakes are rendered. The future of PA practice can be dependent on whether PAs are properly protected in the event they are sued. Usually, a PA is the employee of a physician, group, or institution, in which case there may be adequate coverage under the employer's plan or a group rate. However, the AAPA offers these rationales for PAs having personal professional liability coverage:

- Even though PAs are dependent practitioners and the supervising physician is responsible for their actions, each health provider is responsible for his or her own negligent acts.
- As more patients, their friends, and malpractice lawyers become aware of PAs, they see a potential malpractice target if they believe they've received a poor standard of care.

EXHIBIT 15-4
Suggested Reading for Impairment Issues

Drunk Driving, the Legal Criteria (AAPA position paper, adopted 1991) http://www.aapa.org/policy/drunk-driving.html

A brief discussion of the AAPA's position on drunk driving and recommendations for blood alcohol levels

Physician Assistant Impairment (AAPA position paper, adopted 1990, amended 1992, reaffirmed 2004) http://www.aapa.org/manual/13-Impairment.pdf

Discusses a range of issues concerning impairment and PAs

Developing an Impairment Committee: A Guide for AAPA Constituent Chapters, available from AAPA staff, ext. 3207

A guide on how to implement an impairment committee within the state chapter

Mott, J. S., & Borden S. L. (1994). The impaired PA. *Journal of the American Academy of Physician Assistants, 7*(9), 682–684, http://www.jaapa.com and available from AAPA staff, ext. 3207

A discussion on issues of impairment and physician assistants and the current status of the AAPA and state chapters in dealing with impaired providers

Paine, S. J. (1996). Legal issues surrounding professional impairment. *Journal of the American Academy of Physician Assistants, 9*(12), 16–19, http://www.aapa.org/gandp/impair.html.

Review of the signs and events that might lead a PA to suspect impairment and approaches to addressing the problem of the impaired colleague

previous employer paid the premiums for coverage. However, the previous employer may request reimbursement. (AAPA, 2007f)

Professional liability insurance coverage generally depends on the duties that are performed, the geographic area of practice, and the limits of liability chosen (Exhibits 15-5 and 15-6). The American Continental Insurance Company has classified PAs by the type of activities in which they participate. Class I PAs tend to be in the cognitive disciplines

EXHIBIT 15-5
Classification of Physician Assistants for Liability Insurance

Class A: A PA who performs tasks ordinarily reserved for a physician and who works under the direction and supervision of a qualified licensed physician to assist in the diagnostic management of patients.

Class B: A PA who does one of more of the following:

- Assists in surgery (any exposure to an operating room other than for observation with a general practitioner/family practice or general surgeon)
- Is exposed to trauma/emergency room procedures or responsibilities thereof (10 hours or less per week)
- Is exposed to obstetric (OB) care limited to prenatal or postnatal care
- Assists in anesthesiology

Class C: A PA who is involved in one or more of the following:

- Assists in surgery (any exposure to an operating room other than for observation with orthopedic surgeon, OB/GYN surgeon, cardiovascular surgeon, thoracic surgeon, neurosurgeon, and/or plastic surgeon)
- Is exposed to trauma/emergency room procedures or responsibilities thereof (more than 10 hours per week)
- Is exposed to OB care, including delivery room responsibilities
- Is exposed to cardiac catheterization laboratory

Class D: Students currently attending an AAPA-approved PA program.

Source: CM&F Group, Inc. Retrieved September 4, 2008, from http://www.cmfgroup.com/mal/pa.

- A personal policy provides separate limits of liability to meet the needs of a PA's specific type of practice.
- The policy is owned by the individual PA, which means there is no conflict of interest between a PA and his or her employer in the event a claim is filed.
- A personal defense attorney is provided in the event of a claim.
- An individual policy can be written to cover duties in more than one position, such as in situations in which a PA chooses to moonlight.
- Individual coverage can follow a PA from position to position, even if a

EXHIBIT 15-6
Examples of Full-Time Physician Assistant Annual Liability Insurance Rates for Different Classes of Physician Assistant Activities by Geographic Regions, 2008*

Location	Physician Assistant Type			
	Class A ($)	Class B ($)	Class C ($)	Class D ($)
New York City	1,932	2,415	2,898	150
New York State	1,610	2,013	2,416	150
Houston, Texas	1,932	2,415	2,898	150
Texas (most areas)	1,610	2,013	2,416	150
Tennessee	1,610	2,013	2,416	150
Oregon	1,610	2,013	2,416	150
California	1,640	2050	2,460	150
District of Columbia	1,610	2,013	2,416	150
Florida, Dade County	1,932	2,415	2,898	150
Florida State	1,610	2,013	2,416	150
Louisiana	1,932	2,415	2,898	150

*Values are based on $1,000,000/$6,000,000 professional liability protection, including deposition fees/expense, Good Samaritan Coverage, assault coverage, first aid expense, medical payments, conformance to statute, and consent to settle.

Data from CM&F Group, Inc. Retrieved September 4, 2008, from http://www.cmfgroup.com/mal/pa.

(e.g., psychiatry, pediatrics, family medicine), whereas Class III PAs are in the surgical specialties. Generally speaking, Class II PAs carry twice as much liability as Class I PAs, and Class III PAs carry three times as much liability insurance as Class I PAs. PA students (Class IV) are approximately one-tenth as much as a Class I PA for liability purposes.

Abortion

Legislation on PAs involved with abortions varies by state. Because of the shortage of qualified providers, attention has been directed to the idea that PAs, NPs, and certified nurse-midwives can expand access to abortion services, which is estimated to average around 4,000 per day. After the U.S. Supreme Court declared in *Roe v. Wade* that women had a fundamental right to terminate a pregnancy, most states enacted laws decriminalizing abortion when performed by a physician. Six states (Arizona, Kansas, New Hampshire, Oregon, Vermont, and West Virginia) do not specify that a physician must perform this procedure. At the same time, most states define the scope of practice of PAs as the practice of medicine by trained and licensed professionals under the supervision of physicians. Inconsistencies between physician-only abortion laws and PA statutes have generated some confusion in the medical community over whether PAs working under the supervision of physicians can legally perform abortions. Three attorneys examined some of the case studies surrounding abortions and wrote that "any perceived conflict between physicians-only and PA statutes should not preclude PAs from performing this common surgical procedure" (Lieberman & Lawlani, 1994).

With the introduction of mifepristone, an abortifacient that is distributed directly from the manufacturer to medical practitioners rather than pharmacies, a number of laws came into effect. Missouri and Michigan law prohibits PAs from performing abortions, and a regulation in Tennessee says that PAs may not accept the delegated authority to issue a prescription or dispense any drug or medication whose sole purpose is to cause or perform abortion. In 1991, California's attorney general ruled that the state's physicians-only law precludes PAs from performing abortions; however, in New York the health department reached the opposite conclusion. The Rhode Island Department of Health lifted the physicians-only restriction on medical, but not surgical, abortion. The Montana State Supreme Court overturned a law prohibiting PAs from performing abortions in Montana.

Emergency Medical Treatment

Legal regulations of PA practice at times apply to special settings such as the emergency department. EMTALA is the Emergency Medical Treatment and Labor Act (42 USC §1867, Ch. 7), a law that took effect in 1986 to ensure that all individuals have access to appropriate emergency care and that they are not inappropriately transferred to another facility. Sometimes referred to as the "COBRA" or "anti-dumping law," the EMTALA provisions were passed by Congress within a larger bill called the Consolidated Omnibus Budget Reconciliation Act of 1985. The legislative language is found in section 1867(a) of the Social Security Act, codified at 42 USC §1395cc and §1395dd. The regulations are found primarily at 42 CFR §489.24, et seq.

The EMTALA law requires that a hospital provide an appropriate medical screening examination to any individual presenting to the hospital requesting emergency care. One purpose of the medical screening examination is to determine whether an emergency medical condition exists. If the clinical staff determines that an emergency medical condition does exist, they must either provide the treatment necessary to stabilize the individual or, if the facility and staff are unable to provide the care needed, the individual may be transferred. The law includes specific criteria that must be met regarding transfers.

The EMTALA law and regulations allow for PAs to conduct medical screening examinations as long as written hospital policy specifies that PAs be among the providers the hospital deems qualified to conduct them. Individual PAs must be granted authority, through privileges or some other mechanism, to be authorized to conduct the examinations. The regulations state:

> "In the case of a hospital that has an emergency department, if an individual (whether or not eligible for Medicare benefits and regardless of ability to pay) comes by himself or herself or with another person to the emergency department and a request is made on the individual's behalf for examination or treatment of a medical condition by qualified medical personnel (as determined by the hospital in its rules and regulations), the hospital must provide for an appropriate medical screening examination within the capability of the hospital's emergency department, to determine whether or not an emergency medical condition exists." (AAPA, 2006b)

Signing a Death Certificate

Ruling on a death allows families and others involved to start the process of closure. The need to sign a death certificate is not a topic that involves most PAs, but it may be necessary in certain circumstances, especially in rural areas. Policies regarding PA signatures on death certificates are decided on the state level, and they are slowly moving toward uniformity.

In Washington state, a funeral director or other person in charge of internment may accept a PA signature on a death certificate if the PA was the last person in attendance of the deceased. Washington state law permits PAs to sign death certificates. However, at one time, coroners would not accept a death certificate signed by a PA.

In New York, PAs may not sign a death certificate; only a licensed physician, duly designated coroner, or medical examiner can sign a death certificate. However, a PA may make a death pronouncement in lieu of the supervising physician.

Idaho law regarding certifying death is somewhere in between New York and Washington State. The law reads:

> A certificate of each death which occurs in this state shall be filed with the local registrar of the district in which the death occurs, or as otherwise directed by the state registrar,

within five (5) days after the occurrence. However, the board shall, by rule and upon such conditions as it may prescribe to assure compliance with the purposes of the vital statistics act, provide for the filing of death certificates without medical certifications of cause of death in cases in which compliance with the applicable prescribed period would result in undue hardship; but provided, however, that medical certifications of cause of death shall be provided by the certifying physician, physician assistant, advanced practice professional nurse or coroner to the vital statistics unit within fifteen (15) days from the filing of the death certificate.

Common Errors in Practice

For the PA the opportunity to practice medicine is a limited license (in most states) and governed by a set of rules and policies. The state board of medical examiners usually oversees these rules. Although a fair amount is known about the activity and conduct of PAs in certain states, little has been aggregated and compared across states.

Through discussion with representatives of state boards of medical examiners or attorneys who either work for the boards or defend PAs, a list of common errors has emerged (Exhibit 15-7). These are offered as the accumulation of wisdom of many people who regulate the activity of PAs and not promulgated as evidence of fact.

Other Professional Issues

The AAPA, through its Councils and House of Delegates, identifies and addresses various professional issues that arise. A summary of professional issues that have been addressed in policy by the AAPA is provided in Exhibit 15-8. Additional professional issues are considered by the AAPA each year. A partial list of these topics is presented in Exhibit 15-9.

WORKFORCE ISSUES

A key characteristic that has made PAs valuable in the U.S. health workforce is their adaptability. The pleuropotency of PAs is their capability to work with physicians in almost any clinical practice setting. Over time they have been able to adjust to the changing demands in the healthcare system and fill niches in the medical workforce. Physicians are beginning to appreciate this capability. After a period in which PAs were somewhat invisible on the health workforce policy scene, influential leaders in medicine have recently taken note of their current roles and potential.

Health workforce issues—the interplay among the various health professions as they relate to supply and demand in the medical marketplace—have become increasingly important as to improving access to care. A shortage of physicians, which has led to an expansion of medical school enrollment and output (Iglehart, 2008). The prevailing wisdom in health workforce policy circles is that medical schools must expand their capacity in order to meet the anticipated demand for physician services expected in the next 10 to 20 years. This projected demand is based on the assumptions of an expanding and aging population, decreased physician productivity, and an increasing gross domestic product (Salzberg & Grover, 2006).

The expansion of medical education to meet anticipated demand brings direct challenges to the PA profession and to PA education, suggesting that changes are needed in the profession's educational direction, structure, and output. One belief is that PAs and NPs are likely to assume a greater role in medical care in the future. In part, this view holds that the physician workforce will not be able to meet the anticipated future demand for medical care services, and that "PAs will assume an expanded scope of practice in which they take on new responsibilities for patient care" (Whitcomb, 2007b). This view has led to suggestions to lengthen the period of PA education, which currently averages 26 months. Given the increasing complexities of modern medicine and the difficulties faced by primary care providers in patient management, it is easy to understand how individuals outside of the PA profession may feel that

EXHIBIT 15-7
Issues Likely to Jeopardize the Career of a Physician Assistant

1. Failure to pay attention to the whole person
   a. Complaint A was addressed, but B was ignored.
   b. The appropriate questions were not asked of the patient.
   c. The patient and the PA each understood the relationship to be different than it was.
   d. The PA terminated the relationship, but the patient did not have any alternative for care.
   e. A romantic or inappropriate relationship developed between the PA and the patient.
2. Inappropriate or inadequate supervision
   a. A formal relationship with the physician was not maintained.
   b. The physician supervised more PAs than the law allows.
   c. The change of supervising physicians was not formally made or documented.
   d. The board of medical examiners was not informed that the previous supervising physician relationship was terminated.
3. Inappropriate prescribing
   a. Appropriate forms were not completed allowing authorization for the prescriptive privilege.
   b. The PA prescribed a drug that is not considered appropriate for the scope of practice or the clinical basis of the practice.
   c. The PA prescribed for self or for family.
   d. The medical record entry was not made or did not reflect the prescription that was written.
4. Failure to adequately and accurately document in the medical record
   a. The medical record failed to document the care that was given.
   b. The sloppiness of handwriting suggested an indifference to organization and care of the patient to some reviewers (and juries).
   c. The medical record entry was subject to a loose interpretation.
5. Failure to communicate
   a. The perception of the patient or the patient's family was that the provider was rude, impertinent, arrogant, indifferent, or callous.
   b. The PA lied to the patient or family, and it is then discovered that he or she lied intentionally.
   c. The patient or patient's family's concerns or complaints were not acknowledged and documented.
6. Misrepresenting self
   a. The PA did not disclose that he or she is a PA and/or explain what a PA is, if asked.
   b. The PA failed to wear a name tag that distinguishes him or her as a PA.
   c. The PA misrepresented himself or herself as a physician (by calling himself or herself a doctor even if he or she has a doctorate degree).
7. Becoming visible to the board of medical examiners
   a. The PA failed to register an address change or name change.
   b. The PA failed to renew his or her license.
   c. The PA misrepresented (lied) on a state or federal government form.
   d. The PA failed to file paperwork in the required timeframe.
8. Failing to stay current with administrative or legislative changes
   a. Legislation can change the law.
   b. The board of medical examiners can change the rules.
   c. The standards of care can change in the community, the state, or even nationally.
9. Failure to know the state laws and rules
   a. The PA must understand the PA licensing act in his or her state.
   b. The PA must understand the PA rules that the board of medical examiners oversees.
   c. The PA must understand the letter and intent of the pharmacy laws, rules, and policies for both prescribers and pharmacists.
10. Boundary violations
    a. The PA mishandled prescriptions, samples, and medication dispensing.
    b. The PA documented interactions with patients that seem seductive or solicitous.
    c. The PA committed alcohol or substance abuse violations.

EXHIBIT 15-8

American Academy of Physician Assistants Policy Statements

Guidelines for Amending Medical Staff Bylaws (Adopted 1987, amended 1993, 2003, and 2007)

PAs and their supervising physicians must seek delineation of their clinical privileges in hospitals and managed care systems. The criteria and process for granting clinical privileges to PAs is similar to the process for physicians and is outlined in the medical staff bylaws. In most hospitals, the medical staff credentialing process involves simultaneous consideration of applications for medical staff membership and for clinical privileges. These guidelines are intended to assist medical staff in making appropriate changes to the bylaws that authorize the granting of membership and clinical privileges to PAs.

Clinical Practice Guidelines (Adopted 1997; reaffirmed 2004)

Mandatory clinical practice guidelines are standard fare for many medical providers as managed care and corporate interests transform the U.S. healthcare system. Along with guidelines come corporate mandates for efficient use of resources, assessment of provider productivity, and measurement of clinical outcomes. This document provides an analysis and commentary on the trend of standardized medical care in the name of more efficient use of resources. When predicated on sound medical and scientific data, guidelines can lessen provider variability in treatment and diagnosis.

End-of-Life Decision-Making (Adopted 1997; reaffirmed 2004)

The AAPA does not advocate assisted suicide; however, the AAPA feels that the ethical, compassionate, well-intentioned provider who discusses voluntary self-termination of life by competent, informed terminally ill patients should not be subject to prosecution. PAs are frontline caregivers for the dying. They should take a leadership role in educating the public, policymakers, other health professionals, and their patients regarding the need for enlightened and progressive policies in this area. The AAPA believes that the most effective way to minimize the issue of assisted suicide is to optimize care and maximize quality of life for patients at the end of life.

Guidelines for the Ethical Conduct for the PA (Adopted in 2000; amended in 2004, 2006, 2007)

Essentially, this policy is the AAPA's code of ethics. The full text of this policy appears in Appendix IV.

Genetic Testing in Clinical Practice (Adopted 2001; amended 2006)

Primary care providers are typically the providers who screen patients for genetic disorders and provide access to counseling and testing. PAs need to know which genetic disorders they themselves can diagnose and manage and those that require referral to a genetic specialist. PAs should be aware of the advantages and disadvantages of the currently available types of genetic tests: carrier screening, diagnostic testing, presymptomatic testing, and predictive testing.

Guidelines for the PA Serving as an Expert Witness (Adopted 1977; amended 1987, 1991, 2001; reaffirmed 2004)

A PA may serve as a witness in a legal proceeding in several capacities. These guidelines discuss serving as an expert witness and giving opinions in professional liability (medical malpractice) cases. Accompanying notes and references outline other roles a PA may have as a witness or consultant, preparation for testifying, legal terms, strategies and tactics that may be encountered.

Managed Care in Rural America (Adopted 1997; amended 2004)

PAs are a key component in any system that serves the healthcare needs of rural America. The AAPA makes the following recommendations regarding use of PAs in rural areas:

- PAs are qualified to be primary care providers in managed care systems. Including PAs on the list of primary care providers allows patients the option of seeking care from a PA who is an integral part of the physician-PA team.

- As managed care plans are implemented in rural areas, state and federal agencies and other stakeholders need to recognize the importance of exceptions, modifications, and alternatives to certain regulatory and practice requirements. This flexibility can help preserve and expand the availability of needed healthcare services.

- States, communities, and managed care organizations need to actively develop solutions to problems in education, recruitment, and retention of healthcare providers in rural areas.

PAs as Medicaid Managed Care Providers (Adopted 1996; amended 1997; reaffirmed 2004)

PAs are a critical part of the health workforce providing care for Medicaid patients. To facilitate the continued delivery of services, the AAPA believes that states should include the following provisions in Medicaid managed care plans:

- PAs should be recognized as primary care providers, either by naming them specifically with their supervising physicians, or by naming them within a group.

EXHIBIT 15-8
American Academy of Physician Assistants Policy Statements—cont'd

- PAs should be included on the list of providers in order to allow Medicaid beneficiaries the option of seeking care from a physician-PA team that may in fact already be serving as their current providers.
- States should assign a maximum patient panel that recognizes the proven productivity of PAs and physicians and does not provide a disincentive for utilizing PAs on the healthcare team. This can be achieved by increasing a supervising physician's panel size by an appropriate number or by directly paneling the PA.

PAs as Medical Review Officers (Adopted 1991; amended 2004)

The federal government requires mandatory drug and alcohol testing as a safety precaution for more than 7 million transportation workers, such as bus drivers, railroad workers, airline mechanics, and flight crews. The U.S. Department of Transportation (DOT) issued extensive rules

governing alcohol and drug tests in 2001. The role of a Medical Review Officer (MRO) is mandated through federal regulations. According to the regulations, a medical review officer is "a person who is a licensed physician and who is responsible for receiving and reviewing laboratory results generated by an employer's drug testing program and evaluating medical explanations for certain drug test results." To qualify as an MRO, the individual must be licensed as a physician (doctor of medicine or osteopathy). The AAPA believes that the medical knowledge and training necessary to ensure competence as an MRO are not limited to licensed physicians. As practitioners trained in the medical model to provide physician services, PAs have the background necessary to perform successfully the duties of an MRO.

For more information regarding the AAPA's stance on various issues, visit http://www.aapa.org/gandp/pro-issues.html.

EXHIBIT 15-9
Selected Professional Issues of the Physician Assistant Profession

- Reauthorization of State Child Health Insurance Program legislation
- Title VII funding for PA education
- The Doctor of Nursing Practice (DNP) degree for NPs
- License portability for healthcare professionals
- Medicare fraud and coding
- Telemedicine
- PAs as independent contractors
- Measuring continuing competency and re-entry to practice
- Doctoral degrees for PAs
- International medical graduates and entry into the PA profession
- Accreditation of postgraduate PA programs
- Supervision and delegation of supervision
- Specialty recognition/certification

2 years is a relatively short time in which to prepare for encountering the wide range of clinical problems faced by modern clinicians. Moreover, the discussion of PA specialty recognition and certification has called attention to additional realities, such as younger and less experienced PA graduates, increasing rates of specialization, an increase in PA postgraduate programs, and greater scrutiny of credentialing and regulatory agencies. Collectively, these factors raise legitimate questions regarding the adequacy and depth of current PA education (Kohlhepp, 2006).

Richard Cooper (2007), a leading advocate for the expansion of the health workforce, believes the United States is facing a substantial physician shortage and that U.S. workforce policy should call for an increase in the output of medical school graduates, NPs, and PAs. In speaking about both PAs and NPs, Cooper unequivocally asserts that "neither discipline has expanded its training capacity to the degree that will be required, and, like physicians, neither will have a supply of practitioners that will meet future demand."

Is there any consensus on the expansion of PA graduates and, if so, how should that consensus be expressed? In an attempt to answer the first part of that question, the Physician Assistant Education Association (PAEA) conducted a survey in 2006 to assess the degree of PA program expansion. Nearly one-half of existing programs stated that they either "possibly" or "probably" would increase their class size (or already had done so). This is roughly the same proportion seen among medical schools. However, there were also concerns expressed by respondents related to the limited clinical sites and the lack of qualified faculty (Glicken & Lane, 2007). Yet, academic medicine has unequivocally called for an expansion of medical school graduates. Should PA education consider a similar policy?

Leaders in medicine are essentially saying that they are counting on PAs to pick up a proportion of the slack in the workforce and that raising the output of educational programs should be considered. In an attempt to determine the dimensions of current program expansion, surveys have been conducted but little has been done in terms of policy direction with the information in response to calls for a greater supply of PA graduates. This raises the question of who determines PA educational policy: Is it the professional organizations or is it left to individual institutions?

Recent history suggests that it is market forces in higher education, rather than a concerted effort by the professions' organizations, that tends to set the course of PA education. This was certainly the case in the second phase of PA program expansion in the late 1990s, when the number of programs more than doubled. In this instance, the professions' organizations refrained from taking any public positions on program expansion. Generally, since its development, the PAEA has traditionally shied away from taking official positions on workforce policy issues. In view of the recent challenges presented to PA education by prominent leaders in medicine, it may be time for a more assertive organizational approach to addressing PA workforce policy issues to shape the direction for the profession.

Federal Involvement in Workforce Issues

For decades, the federal government has been extensively involved in helping to shape workforce policy in the United States. The federal role in health workforce policy was prominent and included the funding of workforce study groups, such as the Graduate Medical Education National Advisory Committee and the Council on Graduate Medical Education, as well as programs that offered direct support to schools for training health professionals. However, the federal government is now perceived to be withdrawing from involvement in health workforce activities (Iglehart, 2008).

The present expansion of medical education is occurring more as a private-sector activity than with the traditional federal subsidy it enjoyed for almost a century. If PA programs were to expand their enrollment, it would likely occur as a private-sector activity as well. What this trend means is uncertain. Federal support of health workforce training typically took into consideration perceived problematic areas that affected society and the health sector, such as insufficient numbers of providers in primary care and in rural and underserved areas, and imbalances in racial or ethnic composition. Consequently, in recent years the federal training grants for PA education have integrated these identified priorities as preferences. In doing so, they have selected proposals for grant support that has attainable goals consistent with these priorities.

Research and Professional and Workforce Issues

The literature about PA professional and workforce issues is limited. Following are suggestions for areas of further research.

- **Professionalism:** What are issues for PAs in the 21st century with regard to professionalism?

- **Unions:** Do PAs who belong to unions have any work, salary, or benefit characteristics that differ from those working in similar settings without union representation?

- **Attitudes:** What are the attitudes of PAs compared to NPs and doctors regarding various social issues, such as assisted suicide, abortion, impairment, and autonomy?

■ **Prescribing:** What are the trends in the pharmaceutical industry in targeting PAs and NPs compared with those of doctors?

■ **Health workforce policy:** Will private sector expansion in the workforce address issues of shortages? Can Americans attain the workforce needed without federal policy direction or subsidies?

■ **International PAs:** What are the political and professional issues for PAs by country?

SUMMARY

Professional issues for PAs vary depending on the era, prior accomplishments, comparisons with other professionals, experience, and policy climates. Some of these issues relate to unions, interactions with pharmaceutical representatives, provider-assisted suicide, impairment issues, liability insurance, abortion, emergency medical treatment, and signing death certificates. Although some of these issues are uniquely specific to PAs, many are shared in common with other health professionals.

Similarly, workforce issues have become increasingly influenced by PAs. As the total number of PAs in the workforce increases, the PA profession appears to have reached a critical mass that has caused national organizations and individual investigators to increasingly include PAs when examining the national healthcare workforce. The PA profession would benefit from additional original research on many workforce-related questions in order to be prepared to assist policymakers in developing programs to address our nation's needs for healthcare providers.

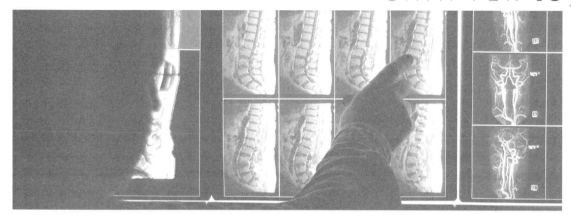

CHAPTER 16

PHYSICIAN ASSISTANT
PROFESSIONAL ORGANIZATIONS

JAMES F. CAWLEY ■ DAVID P. ASPREY ■ RODERICK S. HOOKER

My own business always bores me to death;
I prefer other people's.
— *Oscar Wilde (1854–1900),*
Lady Windermere's Fan, *1892*

ABSTRACT

How physician assistants (PAs) are represented and remain a viable part of their country's healthcare mission and goals is complex. Within the U.S. healthcare environment lies a set of organizations that represent the profession: the American Academy of Physician Assistants (AAPA), the Physician Assistant Education Association (PAEA), the National Commission on the Certification of Physician Assistants (NCCPA), and the Accreditation Review Commission on Education for the Physician Assistant (ARC-PA). Organizations affecting PAs outside of the United States are now emerging and include the Canadian Association of Physician Assistants, the Netherlands Association of Physician Assistants, and the United Kingdom Academy of Physician Assistants.

INTRODUCTION

Organizations are social arrangements usually with rules of conduct and a hierarchy. A doctor's office, a group of retired nurses, or a professional group developed to promote a specialized interest constitute an organization. Physician assistants (PAs), like other special groups, are represented and remain a viable part of their country's healthcare mission and goals via organizations. Within the United States a number of organizations have been established to assume vital functions for the PA profession:

■ The American Academy of Physician Assistants (AAPA)
■ The Physician Assistant Education Association (PAEA)
■ The National Commission on the Certification of Physician Assistants (NCCPA)
■ The Accreditation Review Commission on Education for the Physician Assistant (ARC-PA)

These organizations are influential bodies comprised of members, officers, and staff devoted to the specific mission of their agency. The AAPA looks after members' interests in federal and state legislative activities. The PAEA speaks for PA educators and sponsoring institutions to ensure there is dialogue between educators, government agencies, and practicing PAs. The NCCPA assures the public and health regulatory agencies that PAs meet a standard level of knowledge and have skills necessary for safe and effective clinical practice. Finally, The ARC-PA ensures that PA educational programs meet established standards for accreditation (Exhibit 16-1). Similar counterparts are found in England, the Netherlands, and Canada.

The creators of these organizations planned these structures after existing medical organizations but also to be different in certain respects than previous professional societies and organizations. The foundations for these organizations were laid early in PA development and all have evolved and matured into institutions respected within and external to the profession.

THE AMERICAN ACADEMY OF PHYSICIAN ASSISTANTS

Shortly after the second PA class graduated in 1968, it became apparent that some form of communication among all PAs was needed and that it was necessary for the fledgling profession to have some form of representation on the national level. The early graduates of Duke University decided that an organization was necessary to reach out to all PAs, both students and graduates (Stanhope, Fasser, & Cawley, 1992). Out of this effort, the AAPA was born in April 1968, and the first newsletter representing the nascent profession was sent to all graduates in 1969. At the time, the Medex program was developing in Seattle, Alderson-Broaddus was launching its program in West Virginia, and the

EXHIBIT 16-1
Physician Assistant Professional Organizations

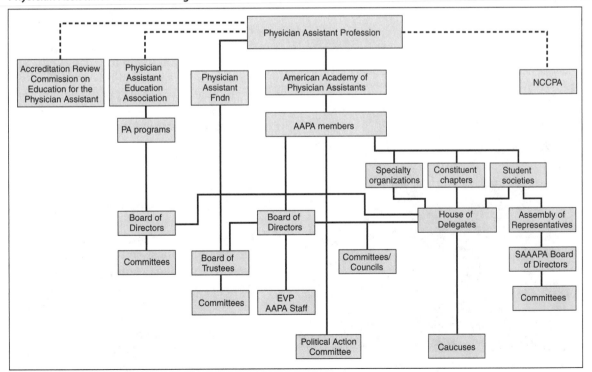

Colorado Child Health Associate (CHA) program was producing graduates. From a group of 15 PAs gathered together in a rented trailer in Durham, North Carolina, the AAPA organization has grown (Exhibit 16-2) to a membership that represents a substantial number of PA graduates of U.S. educational programs.

The effort to establish the first professional organization was not a direct lineage; there was competition for an institution that could represent all PAs. After the founding of the AAPA, other organizations emerged, aiming to represent and provide services to the new profession. These were proprietary membership associations:

- The American Association of Physician Assistants (a group of U.S. Public Health Service PAs at Staten Island Public Health Hospital)
- The National Association of Physician Assistants
- The American College of Physician Assistants (which originated from the Cincinnati Technical College PA program) (Ballweg & Wick, 1999)

In the early 1970s, the AAPA, along with other now-defunct organizations, vied for the

EXHIBIT 16-2
Early Leadership of the American Academy of Physician Assistants [From left, Paul Moson, PA; Carl Fasser, PA-C; Robert Jewitt, MD; Donald Fisher, PhD; J. Rhodes Havarty, MD; and Thomas Piemme, MD.]

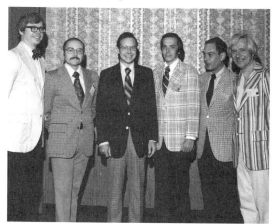

Courtesy of the American Academy of Physician Assistants.

opportunity to represent all PAs. Newly graduated PAs were asked to join or support one or another organization. Eventually, most PAs selected the AAPA, and today it is the national professional society representing all PAs. The AAPA survived this initial period and prospered in part because of its strong leadership. This leadership came with the newly hired Executive Director Donald Fisher, PhD, the support of a number of prominent physicians (Alfred Sadler, Tom Pimme, Joseph Hamberg, and Hu Myers), and the national prominence of its early presidents, including Thomas R. Godkins, PA, Carl E. Fasser, PA, and Paul Moson, PA.

Initally incorporated in North Carolina and later headquartered in Alexandria, Virginia, today the AAPA has grown into a prominent national health professions organization (Exhibit 16-3).

Purposes and Objectives

The AAPA's mission is to promote quality, cost-effective, and accessible health care and to promote the professional and personal development of PAs. As part of this mission, the AAPA works to do the following:

- Enhance the role and utilization of PAs
- Promote the PA profession to the public
- Establish and maintain moral and ethical guidelines for the assurance of continuity in the quality of healthcare delivery by its members
- Ensure the competency of PAs through active involvement in continuing education and certification processes
- Promote and conduct research on the PA profession
- Encourage its membership to render quality service to the public
- Develop, sponsor, and evaluate continuing medical education (CME) or medical-related educational programs for the PA
- Assist in defining the role of the PA
- Participate in the development of criteria leading to certification
- Develop, coordinate, and participate in studies having an impact directly or indirectly on the PA profession

EXHIBIT 16-3
American Academy of Physician Assistants Building in Alexandria, Virginia

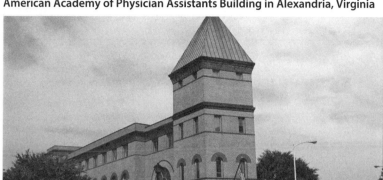

Courtesy of the American Academy of Physician Assistants.

- Serve as a public information center for its membership, health professions, and the public
- Participate in certification of PAs

Organizational Structure

The AAPA is a federated structure of 57 chartered constituent chapters representing the interests of PAs in 50 states, the District of Columbia, Guam, the Air Force, the Navy, the Army, Public Health Service/Coast Guard, and the Department of Veterans Affairs. PA educational programs have formed student societies that make up the Student Academy of the American Academy of Physician Assistants (SAAAPA).

Governing Bodies

The leadership of the AAPA consists of a president, a vice president who is also speaker of the House of Delegates, a secretary, a treasurer, first and second vice-speakers, and a board of directors. The president and speaker of the house are the most visible of the elected executive board. The House members elect the speaker of the house and vice-speakers. The chair of the board of directors is elected by board members. The board also includes individuals elected by fellow AAPA members.

The AAPA House of Delegates was formed in 1977 as part of governance restructuring that took place to meet an expanding membership. The House meets annually to adopt legislation and devlop policy. As a policymaking organ of the profession, the House considers resolutions put forth by the AAPA's standing committees, Councils, constituent chapters, and board of directors; the SAAPA; the PAEA; the Surgical Congress; and the Medical Congress. Other affiliates of the AAPA include the Physician Assistant Foundation, which grants scholarships to deserving PA students, and a Political Action Committee, which supports federal candidates supportive of the PA profession.

The development of the PA profession and the AAPA were virtually synonymous for the first two decades. PAs were elected as leaders and served in various roles (Exhibits 16-4 and 16-5).

Staff

The permanent staff of the AAPA is led by an executive vice president, a chief operating officer, a vice president for member programs, a

EXHIBIT 16-4
Leadership of the American Academy of Physician Assistants

Years	President	Speaker of the House
2010–2011	Patrick Killeen	Bill Fenn
2009–2010	Steven Hanson	Bill Fenn
2008–2009	Cynthia Lord	Bill Fenn
2007–2008	Gregor Bennett	Paul S. Robinson
2006–2007	Mary Ettari	Paul S. Robinson
2005–2006	Rick Rohrs	Paul S. Robinson
2004–2005	Julie A. Theriault	Steven Hanson
2003–2004	Pam Scott	Steven Hanson
2002–2003	Ina Cushman	Steven Hanson
2001–2002	Edward Friedman	Thomas Lemley
2000–2001	Glen E. Combs	Thomas Lemley
1999–2000	William Kohlhepp	Ina Cushman
1998–1999	Ron L. Nelson	Ina Cushman
1997–1998	Elizabeth Coyte	William C. Kolhepp
1996–1997	Sherrie L. Borden	William C. Kolhepp
1995–1996	Lynn E. Caton	William C. Kolhepp
1994–1995	Debi Atherton Gerbert	M. Randolph Bundschu
1993–1994	Ann L. Elderkin	M. Randolph Bundschu
1992–1993	William H. Marquardt	Debi Atherton Gerbert
1991–1992	Sherri L. Stuart	Debi Atherton Gerbert
1990–1991	Bruce C. Fichandler	Suzanne Reich
1989–1990	Paul Lombardo	Sherri L. Stuart
1988–1989	Marshall R. Sinback, Jr.	Sherri L. Stuart
1987–1988	Ron L. Nelson	Bruce C. Fichandler
1986–1987	R. Scott Chavez	Bruce C. Fichandler
1985–1986	Glen E. Combs	Bruce C. Fichandler
1984–1985	Judith B. Willis	Bruce C. Fichandler
1983–1984	Charles G. Huntington	Burdeen M. Camp
1982–1983	Ron L. Fisher	R. Scott Chavez
1981–1982	Jarrett M. Wise	Charles G. Huntington
1980–1981	C. Emil Fasser	Charles G. Huntington
1979–1980	Ron Rosenberg	John Weed
1978–1979	James E. Konopa	Elaine E. Grant
1977–1978	Dan P. Fox	William Hughes
1976–1977	Roger G. Whittaker	*
1975–1976	Thomas R. Godkins	*
1974–1975	C. Emil Fasser	*
1973–1974	Paul F. Moson	*
1972–1973	John A. Braun	*
1971–1972	Thomas R. Godkins	*
1970–1971	John J. McQueary	*
1969–1970	William D. Stanhope	*
1968–1969	William D. Stanhope	*

*House of Delegates not established until 1977.

EXHIBIT 16-5
Past Leaders of the American Academy of Physician Assistants [From left, Steven Crain, PhD, Former EVP; Lynn Caton, PA-C; Sherrie Borden, PA-C; Bill Kohlhepp, PA-C (all past presidents; circa 1993)]

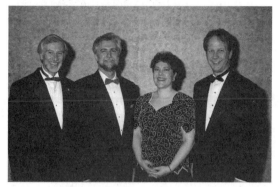

Courtesy of the American Academy of Physician Assistants.

EXHIBIT 16-7
Bill Leinweber, Executive Vice President of the American Academy of Physician Assistants

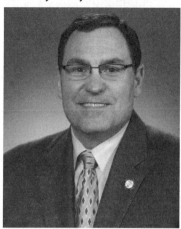

Courtesy of the American Academy of Physician Assistants.

vice president for governmental and professional affairs, a vice president for information and research services, a vice president for clinical affairs and education, and a vice president for finance and administrative services. Within this framework are a wide variety of technical and professional staff members who deliver an assortment of services for the membership and inquiries (Exhibits 16-6 and 16-7).

Governmental and Professional Affairs

The AAPA is the primary voice in Washington working with public and private policymakers to represent the interest of PAs. Consequently, the AAPA acts as the profession's advocate before federal regulators and policymakers, including the U.S. Congress. In

EXHIBIT 16-6
AAPA Executive Vice President and Professional Staff

Name	Tenure	Number of Employees
Bill Leinweber	2008–present	85
Stephen Crane	1993–2007	80
Harry A. Bradley	1992–1993	46
F. Lynn May	1984–1992	19
Peter D. Rosenstein	1981–1984	5
Donald W. Fisher	1973–1981	3

this role, the AAPA provides assistance for policymakers about professional affairs and interprets and comments on proposed or enacted laws or regulations, such as Medicare and Medicaid. For example, as a response to the prodding of the AAPA's Government and Professional Affairs Department, the *Medicare Carriers Manual* was revised to expand the scope of medical services that PAs can provide. In 1994, a significant advance was gained when the Senate Finance Committee voted for an amendment expanding Medicare coverage for PA services to all outpatient settings at 85% of the physician's reimbursement rate. The 1997 Balanced Budget Act finalized the terms of reimbursement for PA services at 85% of the physician rate in all practice settings.

The AAPA has also worked aggressively to improve the regulations of PAs at the state level. The AAPA's State Government Affairs Program assists local chapters that need help with projects seeking to improve PAs' scope of practice through changes in laws or regulations. This responsibility requires constant monitoring of state legislative activities, the District of Columbia, and half a dozen territories. In this capacity, the AAPA sends representatives to the meetings of the Federation of

State Medical Boards and promotes communication among PAs who are members of state PA regulatory agencies and boards.

In 1998, reflecting the wishes of the House of Delegates to have a group devoted to broad national legislative and payment issues, the AAPA formed the Governmental and Reimbursement Committee (GARC). GARC monitors health-related policy issues and trends and makes recommendations to the House with regard to governmental affairs. The Committee is composed of appointed members and members of the AAPA's governmental affairs staff. Other governmental and professional services of the AAPA include providing consultations and grants for chapters struggling with improving legislation and a handbook on reimbursement policies and rationales of private insurers and Medicare.

Although it is impossible to list all of the accomplishments of the AAPA, a few examples may suffice. As the healthcare reform debate was in the spotlight for much of 1993, the AAPA played an important role in providing timely information to committees about the role PAs play on the healthcare team. The AAPA provided information to policymakers involved in the healthcare reform debate. Members of the AAPA were invited to the White House for briefings on health care, and then First Lady Hillary Rodham Clinton confirmed the rising importance of PAs in her address to the AAPA's annual conference that year. That healthcare reform effort is being continued today with substantial input by the AAPA on how well PAs can deliver health services.

In another instance of legislative information at the state-level, PAs can prescribe in all states, as well as in Guam and the District of Columbia. That PAs are commissioned officers in all the branches of the services and the U.S. Public Health Service is a direct result of the AAPA working in Washington.

Workshops and Regional Meetings

The Constituent Chapter Officers Workshop was an event organized by the AAPA and held in Washington, DC every fall. This event helped AAPA chapter leaders develop leadership skills, chapter organization, and programming. Leaders were given the chance to meet with their U.S. representatives, senators, and national health leaders. Additionally, five regional meetings were held nationwide throughout the year to provide chapter leaders opportunities to network and to meet with leaders of the AAPA.

A new biannual event, Adventures in Lobbying (AIL), has replaced the Contituent Chapter Officers Workshop. The event was started in 2006 in response to the ongoing need to orient new PA members and leaders to national-level legislative efforts and to maintain visibility for the AAPA and its issues on Capitol Hill. Held in February, AIL brings together state chapter leaders, SAAAPA leaders, representatives from the education sector, and AAPA leaders and staff to focus for 2 days on lobbying Congress for a series of PA legislative issues.

Research Division

The AAPA's research division involves projects ranging from internally initiated data collection and analyses to sponsored projects (Exhibit 16-8). The demand for data from members, leaders, vendors, and government

EXHIBIT 16-8
AAPA Research Division Activities

- Internally sponsored or initiated data collection, analysis, and reporting projects
- Member census
- Census of PA students
- Survey of conference preregistrants
- Survey of PA programs about applicants
- Annual conference evaluation
- Market research
- Breast and cervical cancer study
- Prospective survey of PA students' specialty decision
- Survey of demand for advance trauma life support
- Pathway II evaluation
- Survey to determine number of practicing PAs
- Survey of employment benefits
- Surveys regarding member wants, needs, and preferences
- Activities to promote and facilitate research by PAs
- Data book (historical data on AAPA members)

policy analysts is high because of the reliable and remarkably complete databases.

Some of the more important annual surveys conducted by the research division are the PA census, membership census, the student census, and the conference survey. Individual salary profiles are available to show the compensation range and average salaries of PAs in different areas and different specialties. Outcomes from these studies have improved management capability for the AAPA, improved revenue, helped promote the profession, helped form strategic alliances, and improved benefit negotiations for PAs.

Publications

The AAPA produces several publications, many of which are available electronically. The *Journal of the American Academy of Physician Assistants (JAAPA)* is the official clinical journal of the organization. Published monthly by Haymarket Inc., it provides news reports, clinical review articles, research reports, a review of research on the PA profession, and other subjects of general interest for the profession. It is sent to all PA graduates, regardless of membership. *JAAPA* has a full-time editor employed by the publisher, a part-time PA editor, and a 10-member editorial board that is appointed by the AAPA Board.

PA Professional (formerly AAPA News) is published monthly. It is intended to keep members up-to-date on issues affecting PAs. The publication includes updates on legislative and professional affairs, employment listings, educational program listings, and data and survey results.

Legislative Watch is a monthly summary of state PA legislative activities written by Governmental Affairs staffer Ann Davis, PA. It provides updates of changes in PA state practice acts and chapter activities related to legislation and regulation.

Education

The AAPA recognizes the importance of the scientific basis for the clinical practice of PAs and the need to provide more emphasis on activities in this area. To accomplish this goal the academy utilizes the Department of

Clinical Affairs and Education, a staff-driven unit, and a Clinical and Scientific Affairs Council. The council identifies and monitors clinical practice and scientific developments related to the practice of medicine as it concerns PAs. Responsibilities include developing reports, issuing papers, and selecting educational documents for the AAPA.

Continuing Medical Education

The AAPA's Education Council monitors trends in CME, assesses PA continuing education needs, develops methods to address those needs, develops reports and issues papers regarding educational concerns, and works with the AAPA on educational issues.

Public Education

The Public Education Program distributes information about PAs. Articles about PAs have appeared in major newspapers and on national television networks. On National PA Day, celebrated each year on October 6, public education activities are spotlighted. Some of these activities include blood drives, food collection and medical education for the homeless, helping people living with AIDS or HIV infection, and fundraising for local charities. The AAPA also produces *Fitting in the Pieces*, a public education how-to handbook that is distributed to all constituent chapters.

Annual Conference

The first AAPA conference was held in 1973 at Sheppard Air Force Base in San Antonio, Texas. Since then, annual attendance has continued to climb (Exhibit 16-9). Today, the AAPA's annual conference is attended by thousands of PAs from the United States and overseas. For many PAs, this is the one major conference they attend each year. Although the main focus of the conference is CME, other events include workshops, technical exhibits, and general sessions featuring nationally renowned speakers and academy leaders. Professional exchange draws most participants. Since 2000, research has become a subject of increased interest to attendees. In 2009, there were more than 60 research posters on display (Exhibit 16-10).

Traditionally, the conference spans Memorial Day. Time is set aside during the conference to

EXHIBIT 16-9
American Academy of Physician Assistants Conference

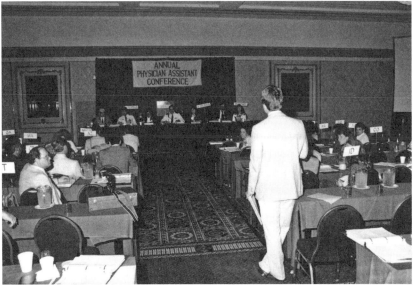

Courtesy of the American Academy of Physician Assistants.

honor those serving and who have served in the uniformed services.

Professional Recognition

The AAPA Academy Awards are the profession's top honors. Awards are given annually to PAs in recognition of the following categories:

- National Humanitarian
- International Humanitarian
- Rural PA of the Year
- Inner-city PA of the Year
- Outstanding PA of the Year
- Public Education Achievement Award
- Educator of the Year

Additionally, the Eugene Stead Award of Achievement honors an individual for his or her lifetime work that has had a broad and significant impact on the PA profession as a whole. The Distinguished Fellow Program of the AAPA recognizes members who have distinguished themselves among their colleagues and in their communities by their service to the PA profession, their commitment to advancing health care for all people, and

their exemplary personal and professional development. Other awards recognize excellence in publishing, public education, and a special honorary membership for those who have made important contributions to the profession.

Professional Practice Council

The Professional Practice Council (PPC) monitors health policy developments in the public and private sectors and writes papers on issues that affect the PA professional practice. The PPC has evaluated and written about the following:

- Stem cell research
- Needle/syringe exchange programs for the prevention of HIV transmission
- Immunization in children and adults
- Hospital privileges and credentialing
- Unlicensed medical graduates
- End-of-life decision-making
- Rural health care
- Telemedicine
- Substance abuse disorders
- PAs as Medicaid managed care providers

EXHIBIT 16-10
American Academy of Physician Assistants National Conferences and Attendance

Year	Location	Attendance	AAPA CME Lectures	Number of Posters	Number of Exhibits
2011	Toronto, ON				
2010	Atlanta, GA				
2009	San Diego, CA	6,414	400	60	363
2008	San Antonio, TX	7,349	400	73	505
2007	Philadelphia, PA.	7,848	400	75	522
2006	San Francisco, CA	9,500	375	56	485
2005	Orlando, FL	8,300	426	45	541
2004	Las Vegas, NV	10,800	380	57	537
2003	New Orleans, LA	9,198	418	52	472
2002	Boston, MA	9,120	299	88	656
2001	Anaheim, CA	7,346	380	50	678
2000	Chicago, IL	8,238	303	28	673
1999	Atlanta, GA	8,193	257	39	652
1998	Salt Lake City, UT	6,200	202	14	547
1997	Minneapolis, MN	6,676	304		504
1996	New York, NY	6,471	309		342
1995	Las Vegas, NV	6,817	269		442
1994	San Antonio, TX	5,349	212		396
1993	Miami, FL	4,346	201		349
1992	Nashville, TN	4,086	219		308
1991	San Francisco, CA	3,881	187		294
1990	New Orleans, LA	4,447	172		248
1989	Washington, DC	4,513	161		226
1988	Los Angeles, CA	3,490	159		158
1987	Cincinnati, OH	2,814	155		208
1986	Boston, MA	3,813	110		184
1985	San Antonio, TX	2,864	105		176
1984	Denver, CO	2,680	115		176
1983	St. Louis, MO	2,179	75		122
1982	Washington, DC	2,802	32		145
1981	San Diego, CA	1,877	29		96
1980	New Orleans, LA	2,205	28		103
1979	Hollywood, FL	1,955	32		88
1978	Las Vegas, NV	1,940	13		72
1977	Houston, TX	1,525	21		42
1976	Atlanta, GA	1,465	5		24
1975	St. Louis, MO	765	12		18
1974	New Orleans, LA	525	6		5
1973	Sheppard Air Force Base, TX	235	8		1

Data from the American Academy of Physician Assistants.

Generally, there is wide agreement among PAs that the AAPA has done a credible job of facilitating and promoting the profession. The PA profession enjoys a relationship with other professional medical organizations that is envied and continues to grow. It has succeeded in winning commission status in all the uniformed services. Medicare reimbursement for PAs has been achieved and continues to improve. The PA profession now enjoys Medicaid reimbursement as fairly standardized in most states. Legislation authorizing prescribing in most states continues to improve. These efforts have been driven by a sense of what is good for the public and what is good for the profession.

Some believe that with these accomplishments the AAPA should place more emphasis on the first part of the mission statement, ". . . to promote quality, cost-effective, and accessible health care . . . ." The AAPA has been in the forefront of many public health initiatives, including the promotion of *Healthy People 2010* (http://www.health.gov/healthypeople/), promulgated by the surgeon general. At the heart of this document is the goal of access for all people. As the AAPA expands its role, it may need to reassess its mission from time to time.

International Affairs

As a result of the increase in interest of PAs to work internationally and the interest among other countries in the PA profession, the AAPA devotes organizational resources to this area. The International Affairs Committee serves as a clearinghouse for information on international PA matters. *Guidelines for PAs Working Internationally,* provides the following guidance for PAs in the international arena:

■ PAs should establish and maintain the appropriate physician-PA team.
■ PAs should accurately represent their skills, training, professional credentials, and identity or service both directly and indirectly.
■ PAs should provide only those services for which they are qualified via their education and/or experiences, and in

accordance with all pertinent legal and regulatory processes.
■ PAs should respect the culture, values, beliefs, and expectations of the patients, local healthcare providers, and the local healthcare systems.
■ PAs should take responsibility for being familiar with and adhering to the customs, laws, and regulations of the country where they will be providing services.
■ When applicable, PAs should identify and train local personnel who can assume the role of providing care and continuing the education process.

The Physician Assistant Foundation

The PA Foundation seeks to foster the goals and objectives of the AAPA by supporting the educational and research needs of the profession (Exhibit 16-11). Founded in 1980 as the Education and Research Foundation, and later changed to its present name, it is the philanthropic arm of the AAPA. Most of its activity is focused on scholarships, such as the Breitman-Dorn Endowment, an unrestricted grant to assist doctoral students studying the activity of PAs. However, the foundation does help to support public health services for which PAs are part of the support staff, such as free clinics and homeless shelters.

Society for the Preservation of Physician Assistant History

The Society for the Preservation of Physician Assistant History (SPPAHx) is a component of the AAPA, serving as its historic arm, much like the PA Foundation serves as its philanthropic arm. Its mission is to preserve, study, and present PA history. Items related to ongoing development and importance of the PA profession are documented and made readily accessible to national PA organizations, educational programs, newsletter and journal publishers, and the general public. The archives maintain an integrated online, searchable database that identifies the existence and location of key documents, articles, books, films, oral history audio or videotapes, and other artifacts that detail the development, evolution, and benefits of the PA profession.

EXHIBIT 16-11
Physician Assistant Foundation Presidents

Years	President
2009–2010	Agnes Compagnone
2008–2009	Kent Wallace
2007–2008	Kent Wallace
2006–2007	Don Pedersen
2005–2006	Don Pedersen
2004–2005	Mary Ettari
2003–2004	Mary Ettari
2002–2003	John Byrnes
2001–2002	John Byrnes
2000–2001	Robin Hunter Busky
1999–2000	Robin Hunter Busky
1998–1999	Ann L. Elderkin
1997–1998	Ann L. Elderkin
1996–1997	Paul Lombardo
1995–1996	Paul Lombardo
1994–1995	Lorraine S. Atkinson
1993–1994	Lorraine S. Atkinson
1992–1993	Lorraine S. Atkinson
1991–1992	Lorraine S. Atkinson
1990–1991	J. Jeffrey Heinrich
1989–1990	J. Jeffrey Heinrich
1988–1989	J. Jeffrey Heinrich
1987–1988	James F. Cawley
1986–1987	James F. Cawley
1985–1986	James E. Konopa
1984–1985	Jarrett M. Wise
1983–1984	Jarrett M. Wise
1982–1983	James E. Konopa
1981–1982	James E. Konopa
1980–1981	Noel McFarlane
1979–1980	Donald W. Fisher

EXHIBIT 16-12
Presidents of the Society for the Preservation of Physician History

Year	President
2009	Carl Toney
2008	Richard Dehn
2007	Ruth Ballweg
2006	Pam Scott
2005	J. Dennis Blessing
2004	Ron Nelson
2003	J. Jeffrey Heinrich

PHYSICIAN ASSISTANT EDUCATION ASSOCIATION

The PAEA is the national organization representing PA educational programs. Originally known as the Association of Physician Assistant Programs (APAP), the organization was formed by a group of physicians and concerned PA program faculty in 1972 to facilitate communication and cooperation among PA programs. Initial concerns included accreditation of educational programs, certification, CME requirements of PAs, and the role delineation of PAs. The name change to PAEA came about in 2005 and coincided with a move from the headquarters of the AAPA to its own headquarters in Alexandria, Virginia.

The PAEA is the only national organization in the United States representing PA educational programs. Its mission is to pursue excellence, foster faculty development, advance the body of knowledge that defines quality education and patient-centered care, and promote diversity in all aspects of PA education. To accomplish its mission, the PAEA:

- Encourages and assists programs to educate competent and compassionate PAs
- Enhances programs' capability to recruit, select, and retain well-qualified PA students
- Supports programs in the recruitment, selection, development, and retention of well-qualified faculty
- Facilitates the pursuit and dissemination of research and scholarly work

The SPPAHx staff members have developed and maintained a website presenting the virtual history and benefits to the public of the PA profession. Other activities include liaison relationships with other PA, medical, and historical organizations. A professional archivist supports the collection by housing and preserving media, documents, artifacts, and other related materials that are not currently maintained in a suitable academic or physical environment. Other staff efforts include identifying areas needing more documentation and fostering studies and dialogue about the PA profession (Exhibit 16-12).

- Educates PAs who will practice evidence-based, patient-centered medicine
- Serves as the definitive voice on matters related to entry-level PA education, nationally and internationally
- Fosters professionalism and innovation in health professions education
- Promotes interprofessional education and practice
- Forges linkages with other organizations to advance its mission

The PAEA serves as a resource for individuals and organizations from various professional sectors interested in the educational aspects of the PA profession. Critical activities have included the collecting, publishing, and disseminating of information on member programs and their trends and characteristics. The *Annual Report on Physician Assistant Educational Programs in the United States* survey, now in its 24th edition, compiles the activities of PA programs annually. Another role of the PAEA is to provide effective representation to affiliated organizations involved in health education, healthcare policy, and the national certification of PA graduates.

Governance

The PAEA is governed by a board of directors elected by the membership. The Board consists of a president, president elect, past president, secretary treasurer, two directors-at-large, and student president (Exhibits 16-13 and 16-14).

Responsibility for all of the PAEA activities lies with the board of directors. The Board administers the PAEA's financial affairs, appoints standing and ad hoc committees, and conducts all association business between membership meetings. Board members are elected by the PAEA member programs. Only accredited programs can be full voting members.

Staff

The PAEA's day-to-day activities are handled by its professional staff, which includes an executive director, an associate executive director, a director of education and meeting

EXHIBIT 16-13
Presidents of the Physician Assistant Education Association (Formerly Association of Physician Assistant Programs)

Years	President
2009–2010	Ted Ruback, PA, MS
2009–2010	Justine Strand, MPH, PA-C
2008–2009	Dana Sayler-Stanhope, EdD, PA-C
2007–2008	Anita D. Glicken, MSW
2006–2007	Dawn Morton-Rias, EdD, PA-C
2005–2006	Patrick Knott, PhD, PA-C
2004–2005	Paul Lombardo, MPA, PA-C
2003–2004	James F. Cawley, MPH, PA-C
2002–2003	David Asprey, PA-C, PhD
2001–2002	Gloria Stewart, PA-C, EdD
2000–2001	P. Eugene Jones, PA-C, PhD
1999–2000	Donald Pedersen, PA-C, PhD
1998–1999	Walter Stein, PA, MHCA
1997–1998	Donald Pedersen, PA-C, PhD
1996–1997	Dennis Blessing, PA, PhD
1995–1996	James Hammond, MA, PA-C
1994–1995	Ronald D. Garcia, PhD
1993–1994	Richard R. Rahr, EdD, PA-C
1992–1993	Anthony A. Miller, MEd, PA-C
1991–1992	Albert Simon, DHSc, MEd, PA
1990–1991	Ruth Ballweg, PA, MPA
1989–1990	Steven Shelton, MBA, PA
1988–1989	Suzanne Greenberg, MS
1987–1988	Jesse Edwards, MS
1986–1987	Jack Liskin, MA, PA
1985–1986	Carl Fasser, PA, MS
1984–1985	Denis Oliver, PhD
1983–1984	Robert Curry, MD, MPH
1982–1983	Stephen Gladhart, EdD
1981–1982	Reginald Carter, PhD, PA
1980–1981	David Lewis, EdD
1979–1980	Thomas Godkins, PA, MPH
1978–1979	Archie Golden, MD, MPH
1977–1978	Frances Horvath, MD
1976–1977	C. Hilmon Castle, MD
1975–1976	Robert Jewett, MD
1974–1975	Thomas Piemme, MD
1973–1974	Alfred Sadler, Jr., MD

EXHIBIT 16-14
Leaders of the Physician Assistant Education Association [From left: Patricia Dieter, Ruth Ballweg, Anthony Miller, Albert F. Simon, and Sherrie Stolberg (circa 1993)].

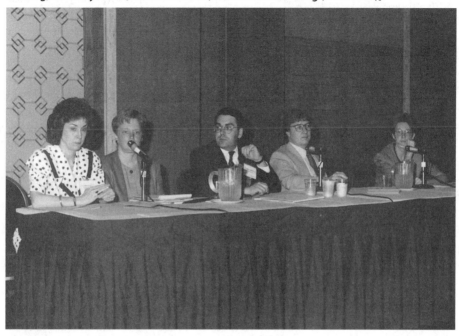

Courtesy of the American Academy of Physician Assistants.

services, an assistant director for data and research, an assistant director of marketing and communications, a manager of member communications, and a coordinator of meeting and membership services. Within this framework are various technical and professional staff members who provide services for the PAEA members (Exhibit 16-15).

Member Programs

As of 2009, the PAEA has 145 member PA educational programs located at various institutions across the United States. All currently accredited programs have elected to join the association. Only PA programs accredited by the ARC-PA, or its predecessor or successor organizations, are eligible for full program membership. Several yet-to-be accredited programs have chosen to affiliate with the association as "colleagues of the PAEA."

EXHIBIT16-15
Timi Agwar-Barwick, PAEA Executive Director

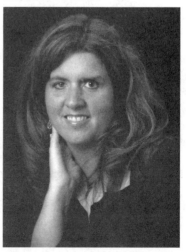

Courtesy of the Physician Assistant Education Association.

Services and Activities

The PAEA services include two national meetings of PA programs each year: the semiannual meeting in May and the education forum in October. It also provides publications, newsletters, consultation services, faculty development and leadership education programs, the systematic collection of pertinent PA program data, and tools to assess and improve the quality of PA education for individuals as well as for programs.

The organization has also formed special institutes to support activities particularly vital to the typical activities of PA program faculty. The Research Institute was established in 1996 as an organizational means to promote and fund research proposals that aim to explore topics pertaining to the conduct and process of PA education. It oversees all of the research activities, including the research grant programs and the production of the peer-reviewed *Journal of Physician Assistant Education*. The Faculty Development Institute, which was founded in 1997, oversees all of the PAEA's faculty development initiatives and workshops to expand and enrich the skills of PA educators. The Centralized Application Service for PA Applicants (CASPA) was instituted in 2001 and is an important revenue source for the PAEA. This service offers applicants a convenient web-based application service that allows applicants to apply to any number of participating PA educational programs by completing a single application.

ASSOCIATION OF POSTGRADUATE PHYSICIAN ASSISTANT PROGRAMS

Although not one of the four major organizations of the PA profession, one component of PA education involves the Association of Postgraduate Physician Assistant Programs (APPAP). This organization was formed in 1998 by a small group of postgraduate PA programs to further specialty education for PAs. Since 2007, the group contracts with the PAEA to provide some administrative services.

Since its founding, the APPAP has gained the support of the AAPA and the PAEA. A liaison representative of the APPAP now sits on the PAEA Board of Directors, and APPAP members work with the AAPA and PAEA on mutual goals designed to expand the PA profession. Member programs of the APPAP include those formal postgraduate PA programs designed to educate NCCPA-eligible or NCCPA-certified PAs for a defined period (usually 12 months) in a medical specialty. The APPAP member programs follow several models, including fellowships, master's degree programs, and residency programs. All APPAP member programs must award a certificate or degree or provide graduate academic credit. The APPAP's educational, professional, and informational purposes include the following:

- Assisting in the development and organization of postgraduate educational curricula and programs for PAs
- Assisting in defining the role of the PA, particularly in the specialties
- Assisting in the development of evaluation methodologies for postgraduate educational curricula and programs
- Serving as an information center for PAs, programs training PAs at the entry level, other medical and healthcare disciplines, and to the public with respect to postgraduate educational curricula and programs for PAs

NATIONAL COMMISSION ON CERTIFICATION OF PHYSICIAN ASSISTANTS

After formal education and training in an accredited program, the final stage in the professional preparation of a PA involves the national certification process. The PA certification process represents a distinct aspect of the evolution of PA profession systems and represents one different from most patterns observed in other nonphysician health professions. The development of a single respected system of national certification and recertification for PAs is considered an asset of the profession.

The NCCPA, founded in 1975, is a public organization that is the only credentialing organization for PAs in the United States. As of 2008, the NCCPA has certified more than 75,000 PAs. The mission of the NCCPA is to ensure the public and others that PAs credentialed by the NCCPA meet established standards of knowledge and clinical skills upon entry into practice and throughout their careers.

The NCCPA administers two national examinations used by state medical licensing boards: the Physician Assistant National Certification Examination (PANCE) and the Physician Assistant National Recertification Examination (PANRE). These examinations are developed by the National Board of Medical Examiners (NBME) under contract from the NCCPA. Other NCCPA functions include the following:

■ Establishing eligibility requirements for the PANCE and PANRE
■ Establishing standards for the examinations
■ Issuing and verifying certificates
■ Reregistering and recertifying PAs who meet CME and reexamination requirements

Initial certification through the PANCE is required for PA licensure in all states and U.S. medical jurisdictions, including the District of Columbia and U.S. territories. Most states require an NCCPA certificate in order for a PA to be licensed or to prescribe; more than one-half of the states require a current NCCPA certificate for license renewal.

History

The NCCPA arose as a result of the need for an independent agency to certify the level of preparation of the PA graduate for clinical practice. It was acknowledged that because program accreditation is not an infallible science, an additional mechanism to ensure a minimal level of clinical competence should be established. In 1971, the Division of Associated Health Professions of the U.S. Department of Health, Education, and Welfare (DAHP/DHEW), along with the Kellogg Foundation, set out to develop a certifying examination. This activity was later funded through the NBME. Initially called the National Certifying Examination for the Assistant to the Primary Care Physician, the examination was first administered in December 1973.

Parallel to the development of a national examination for PAs, key physicians within the American Medical Association (AMA) led the effort to develop an independent certifying agency. Thus, with the participation and support of the profession's then-young representative organizations (the AAPA and the APAP), the backing of the federal government, and funding from the Kellogg Foundation, the NCCPA was founded. Established in 1973, the organization worked to ensure employers, state boards, and patients that a standard related for the competency of PAs was in place. In 1975, the NCCPA was chartered with headquarters in Atlanta, Georgia. The first executive director of the NCCPA, David Glazer (1973 to 1996), and Thomas Piemme, MD, the first president of the NCCPA (1974), played pivotal roles in establishing the legitimacy of the NCCPA and its certifying examinations among state medical licensing boards.

At the time, various nurse practitioner, nurse clinician, and CHA programs were gaining momentum, as were Medex, physician associate, and PA programs. Graduates of most of these programs were eligible to take the Certifying Examination for the Assistant to the Primary Care Physician. Additionally, from 1974 through 1985, the NCCPA entry-level certifying examination was open to informally trained PAs who met certain eligibility criteria such as prior clinical experience working in a PA-like role. Only a few hundred took the examination.

Leadership

The NCCPA is led by a board of directors comprised of doctors, lawyers, PAs, and other elected representatives from the PA professional organizations (the AAPA and the PAEA) and other major medical organizations, such as the American College of Physicians-American

Society of Internal Medicine, American Academy of Family Physicians, the AMA, the American Academy of Pediatrics, the American College of Emergency Medicine, the American College of Surgeons, and the American Osteopathic Association (Exhibit 16-16). The Federation of State Medical Boards; major employers of PAs, such as the Department of Defense, the Department of Veterans Affairs, and the American Hospital Association; and members of the public are also included as representatives. The NCCPA maintains an observer status at the AAPA House of Delegates. The president of the NCCPA is the chief executive director and oversees staff members who work to assure that PAs meet professional standards of knowledge and skills (Exhibits 16-17 and 16-18).

Physician Assistant National Certification Examination and Other Examinations

The PANCE, the PANRE (a recertification examination), and the Pathway II (an alternative recertification examination) are administered by the NCCPA. These examinations assess essential knowledge and skills of PAs in conducting a variety of healthcare functions normally encountered in practice. The PANCE, developed by the NBME, consists of

300 standardized questions and is taken by nearly all PA educational program graduates. As of 2000, the test is administered via computer at special testing centers.

Content specifications for NCCPA examinations were developed and validated, in part, through use of role delineation studies. The first study was conducted by the NBME in the early 1970s. Subsequently, these studies were performed by the AAPA in 1979 and 1985. Several test-writing committees generate test questions for the PANCE, Pathway II, and the PANRE; test-writing committee members are appointed by the NCCPA and staffed by the NBME. The test-writing committee includes physicians and PAs who are employed in academic and clinical settings, including the primary care and clinical specialties. The test committee meets regularly to develop the content for each examination. The committee reviews the previous year's examination performance, finalizes the current examination blueprint, and makes assignments for and prepares new test items. In 1995, the number of certifying examinations administered totaled 2,913, with 2,272 attaining certification. The failure rate was 22%, with 641 candidates unsuccessful in reaching the pass/fail score level. In 2001, there were 4,267 first-time

EXHIBIT 16-16
National Commission on the Certification of Physician Assistants Board, 1997

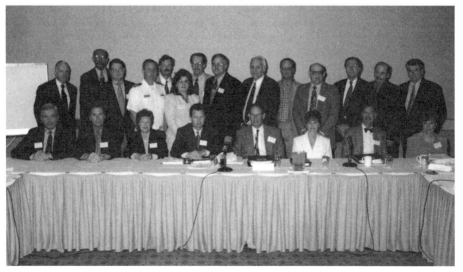

Courtesy of the American Academy of Physician Assistants.

EXHIBIT 16-17
**Presidents of the National Commission
on the Certification of Physician Assistants**

Year	President
2009	Edward J. Dunn, MBA, SPHR
2008	Lee B. Smith, MD, JD
2007	Randy D. Danielsen, PhD, PA-C
2006	William Kohlhepp, MHA, PA-C
2005	Dorothy "Disty" Pearson, PA-C
2004	John W. Ogle, MD
2003	Gary Winchester, MD
2002	Katherine J. Adamson, MMS, MA, PA-C
2001	Elaine Grant, MPH, PA-C
2000	Dewayne Andrews, MD, FACP
1999	John Hayden, MA
1998	Marshall Sinback, PA-C
1997	Marshall Sinback, PA-C
1996	Richard Rohrs, PA-C
1995	Richard Rohrs, PA-C
1994	Richard Gemming, PA-C
1993	Richard Gemming, PA-C
1992	Herschel L. Douglas, MD
1991	Herschel L. Douglas, MD
1990	Stanley R. Shane, MD
1989	Stanley R. Shane, MD
1988	Paul S. Goldstein, MD
1987	Paul S. Goldstein, MD
1986	Michael B. Sheldon, PA-C
1985	Michael B. Sheldon, PA-C
1984	Edmund C. Casey, MD
1983	Edmund C. Casey, MD
1982	Robert B. Bruner
1981	Robert B. Bruner
1980	Raymond H. Murray, MD
1979	Raymond H. Murray, MD
1978	J. Rhodes Haverty, MD
1977	J. Rhodes Haverty, MD
1976	Thomas Piemme, MD
1975	Thomas Piemme, MD
1974	Thomas Piemme, MD

EXHIBIT 16-18
**Janet Lathrop, MBA, President and
CEO of National Commission on
the Certification of Physician
Assistants, Inc.**

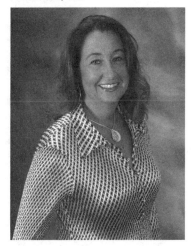

*Courtesy of the National Commission on
Certification of Physician Assistants.*

This blueprint is reflected in the PANCE, Pathway II, and PANRE. It was compiled using various sources, including data from the National Ambulatory Medical Care Survey and the National Hospital Discharge Survey (Exhibit 16-20).

To further establish the validity of the three NCCPA examinations, the organization periodically conducts an occupational analysis. The 1998 PA Practice Analysis project provided the fundamental basis of the content blueprint used in current NCCPA certifying and recertifying examinations (Cawley et al, 2001). Practice analyses of this sort are conducted periodically by national testing agencies as a means to verify the appropriateness of the content blueprint as well as the examination itself. The practice analysis lists the tasks and essential knowledge and skills that are representative of the actual abilities required of PAs in clinical practice. The results of this study identified the following knowledge and skills that rated most highly by practicing PAs:

- Skill in identifying pertinent physical findings
- Knowledge of signs and symptoms of medical conditions

PANCE takers who had a 91.5% pass rate (Exhibit 16-19). In 2007, 5,709 persons sat for the PANCE.

The NCCPA content blueprint identifies the clinical problems the PA should be prepared to encounter in a typical primary care practice.

EXHIBIT 16-19
Physician Assistant National Certification Examination Annual Scores

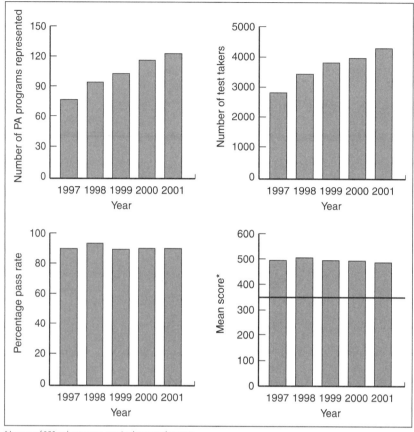

*A score of 350 or better was required to pass the exam.

Data from Hooker, R. S., Hess, B., & Cipher, D. (2002). A comparison of physician assistant programs by national certification examination scores. Perspective on Physician Assistant Education, 13(2), 81–86.

- Skill in recognizing conditions that constitute medical emergencies
- Skill in performing physical examinations
- Skill in conducting a patient interview
- Skill in associating current complaints with presenting history and identifying pertinent factors
- Knowledge of physical examination directed to a specific condition
- Skill in effective communication

The practice analysis study by Cawley and colleagues (2001) found few differences in the tasks performed by PAs based on the length of time worked in the profession. Some response patterns differed across specialties, particularly in the areas of cardiovascular/thoracic surgery, general surgery, and orthopedic surgery. However, consistently high ratings were observed in the domains considered being the essential functions of PA clinicians: history taking and physical diagnosis. PAs place great value on additional skills required in the practice of clinical medicine: diagnostic acumen, judgment, and knowledge in the development of an effective management plan. The consistency and high ratings of these findings suggest that the a central core of medical knowledge, tasks, and skills is valued and that the elements of this core are performed often and consistently by practicing PAs in virtually all specialties and settings (Exhibit 16-21). These domains of clinical knowledge deemed

EXHIBIT 16-20
**Examination Content for Physician Assistant National Certification Examination
and Physician Assistant National Recertification Examination**

% of Examination Content	Diseases, Disorders, and Medical Assessment
16	Cardiovascular system
12	Pulmonary system
10	Gastrointestinal/nutritional system
10	Musculoskeletal system
9	Eye, ear, nose, and throat
8	Reproductive system
6	Endocrine system
6	Neurological system
6	Psychiatric/behavioral system
6	Renal/urinary system
5	Dermatological
3	Hematological system
3	Infectious diseases
100%	

% of Examination Content	Knowledge and Skill Areas
18	Clinical therapeutics
18	Formulating most likely diagnosis
16	History taking and performing physical examinations
14	Clinical intervention
14	Using laboratory and diagnostic studies
10	Applying scientific concepts
10	Health maintenance
100%	

Data from National Commission on Certification of Physician Assistants. (2002). NCCPA Examination Content Blueprint, *Atlanta, GA: Author.*

important by practicing PAs are considered by the test-writing committees when developing the blueprint for the certification and recertifiation examinations. This practice analysis was redone and updated in 2004 (Arbett, Lathrop, & Hooker 2009).

Physician Assistant National Recertification Examination

In an effort to ensure career-long accountability for PAs, the NCCPA developed a recertification and reexamination process. Every 2 years, all certified PAs must reregister and submit documentation demonstrating that they participated in 100 hours of CME. This practice ensures the ongoing acquisition of new medical knowledge by PAs. Additionally, PAs are

EXHIBIT 16-21
Domains of Knowledge Deemed Most Important by Physician Assistants, Rank Ordered

1. Subjective data gathering
2. Assessment
3. Objective data gathering
4. Formulate and implement a plan
5. Clinical intervention procedures
6. Health promotion and disease prevention
7. Ancillary professional responsibilities

Data from Cawley J. F., Andrews, M. D., Barnhill, G. C., Webb, L., & Hill, K. (2001). What makes the day: An analysis of the content of physician assistant's practice. *Journal of the American Academy of Physician Assistants, 14*(5), 41, 42, 44, 47–50, 55–56 (passim).

required to be retested on their basic medical knowledge every 6 years. The intent of this reexamination process is to ensure the public that PAs are keeping abreast of the core knowledge to practice medicine.

In 1980, the NCCPA administered the entry-level examination for the purposes of recertification. This recertification was in part designed to identify any content areas that penalize individuals working in specialty practices and help identify the "core" area to be tested by a separate recertification examination. The PANRE was developed as a separate examination in 1984 and has been administered ever since. The PANRE consists of 300 multiple-choice questions. In 2007, a total of 7,438 examinees took the examination; 96% of examinees passed. NCCPA policy dictates that individuals who fail the PANRE once retake the examination; only 50 persons have failed the PANRE twice.

Some regard the NCCPA requirements for certificate maintenance and periodic recertification as a frustrating and time-consuming requirement. PAs must be mindful of the legitimacy derived from the profession's willingness to have a recertification by examination system. The intensity of the debate over recertification has quieted during the past decade as more PAs accomodate themselves to the reality of recertification by examination, a practice now common in most health professions.

Pathway II

In 1997, an alternative mechanism for meeting NCCPA recertification requirements grew out of the AAPA-NCCPA partnership that emerged in 1992. The Pathway II was a recertification examination developed in response to the needs of PAs who specialize in a particular medical field. The examination consisted of a take-home examination plus an elective component. However, this examination started to be phased out in 2006 and will be eliminated by 2010.

Controversies

The NCCPA, and in particular the PANRE, was the subject of criticism from the PA profession during the late 1980s and early 1990s. Such criticism was expressed in statements and resolutions from the AAPA House of Delegates. In particular, the NCCPA policy related to those PAs who fail the PANRE twice has been a topic of intense debate within the profession. The implications of this policy for those PAs practicing in the states requiring valid certification as a condition of licensure are significant. This NCCPA policy was known as "endpointing" because it defined the final consequences for those PAs who failed the PANRE twice. Under endpointing, such PAs lose their certification and must take and pass one of the three NCCPA examinations to regain certification status.

Another controversy involves predictors of success on the PANCE. PA educators are curious about candidate performance on the NCCPA examinations and the implications of these findings on adult learners for the recertification process. For example, is there a correlation between the academic degree received in PA education and the likelihood of passing the PANCE?

One study suggested that the NCCPA examination may need reevaluation because students without academic degrees and those with associate degrees who completed a PA program passed the NCCPA examination at a higher percentage than those with baccalaureate and graduate degrees. The study sample was nonrepresentative, but it was suggested that the discrepancy observed could indicate a cultural bias in the NCCPA examination (Hooker, Carter, & Cawley, 2004). Hooker, Hess, and Cipher (2002) looked at the correlation between PA training at the graduate level and performance on the PANCE and found that students who have graduated from a master's degree program on average do slightly better on the PANCE than those in a certificate or baccalaureate degree program. Nor could they find any other characteristics of programs (size, private, medical school association, duration) or characteristics of students (age, gender) that correlated with pass rates. On the other hand, Asprey and colleagues (2004), examining data over a longer time frame, found a correlation between PANCE test scores and academic degree awarded (Asprey, Dehn, & Kreiter, 2004a; Asprey, Dehn, & Kreiter, 2004b).

One reason for these discrepancies may have to do with the timing of the Hooker,

Hess, and Cawley survey, which was taken during a time of transition in PA education when the entry-level degree was becoming the master's degree; the data collected may only reflect the circumstances during those transition years (Cawley, 2003).

Specialty testing is a broad issue facing the profession, its representative organizations, and the NCCPA. Because specialization is a natural evolution in most healthcare professions, greater numbers of PAs are working in specialty practices. PAs representing specialty and subspecialty groups have spoken openly of the desire to have some form of recognition. The NCCPA is considering the development of specialty-specific examinations for practicing PAs. The NCCPA is the only national organization that has experience and expertise in PA testing, and has held a public forum on this topic. Representatives from many PA specialty organizations weighed in on the topic of specialty certification or some alternative, such as specialty recognition.

As part of the debate over specialty certification, the AAPA has expressed concern that a pathway of specialty certification would ultimately result in a narrowing of the career entry opportunities currently enjoyed by PAs. Specialty certification, particularly if determined by examination, could serve to place barriers to PAs seeking entry into particular specialties, thus adversely altering a long-cherished component of the PA profession and its employment pathways.

This issue has led to distinguishing between *specialty certification*, which is the term currently used by the NCCPA, and *specialty recognition*, which is a term that is preferred by the AAPA. Specialty certification connotes the establishment of a formal, nationally standardized examination administered to all PAs in a given clinical specialty through a process that would be expensive to develop and administer. The use of specialty-specific examinations would also require that there be a critical mass of persons in a particular specialty—that is, a minimum number of individuals eligible and willing to take the examination in order to make it economically feasible. Specialty recognition, on the other hand, is a concept that defines a process or series of achievements whereby a PA

who has worked for some period in a given specialty and fulfills a series of qualifying steps (e.g., has membership and fellow status in an AAPA-affiliated PA specialty group, provides documentation from a supervising physician of clinical proficiency in that specialty, attains other designated professional accomplishments in that clinical specialty) would then qualify for a privileged status in the AAPA. That status, known as *diplomate status* in some medical professional organizations, would then in turn be recognized by the national certifying agency, the NCCPA, and on that basis—and possibly other qualifiers (perhaps some form of take-home examination)—would award the PA specialty recognition as a PA with expertise in the relevant clinical specialty area.

Specialty recognition may be a middle-ground approach, one that would avoid the cost and intensity of administering specialty certifying examinations. The recognition process would offer those PAs who seek particular designation in a given specialty the public distinction that they seek for their accomplishments, but would avoid the costly pressurized approach of formal examination. Whether or not the recognition process would be sufficient in their minds or in the minds of employing physicians, hospitals, or regulatory agencies is an unknown at this point. In the summer of 2009, the NCCPA announced its intention to create a system of specialty certification examinations for five specialties and to have them in place by 2011.

THE ACCREDITATION REVIEW COMMISSION ON EDUCATION FOR THE PHYSICIAN ASSISTANT

The ARC-PA is the recognized accrediting agency that protects the interests of the public and the PA profession by defining the standards for PA education and evaluating PA educational programs within the territorial United States to ensure their compliance with those standards. It was initially formed as a component of the AMA's Committee on Allied Health Education and Accreditation (CAHEA), a national allied health professions accrediting entity. Later, the CAHEA was transformed into a more independent agency, the Commission on Accreditation of Allied Health Education Programs (CAAHEP), which was separate from the AMA. In 2001, the ARC-PA became a freestanding accrediting agency.

In accomplishing its mission to set standards for PA educational programs, the ARC-PA comprises a number of representatives. These representatives include the American Academy of Family Physicians, the AAPA, the American College of Physicians, the American Society of Internal Medicine, the American College of Surgeons, the AMA, the PAEA, and members of the public. The ARC-PA appoints site visitors, reviews applications for accreditation, and determines accreditation actions. As an agency to ensure public trust, the ARC-PA encourages excellence in PA education through its accreditation process by establishing and maintaining minimum standards of quality for educational programs. It awards accreditation to programs through a peer-review process that includes documentation and periodic site visit evaluation to substantiate compliance with the Accreditation Standards for Physician Assistant Education. The accreditation process is designed to encourage sound educational experimentation and innovation and to stimulate continuous self-study and improvement.

In addition to establishing educational standards and fostering excellence in PA programs, the ARC-PA provides information and guidance to individuals and organizations regarding PA program accreditation and makes public its accreditation actions (Exhibit 16-22).

Governance and Staff

The ARC-PA is overseen by a commission of 17 individuals that includes a chair, secretary, and treasurer. Commissioners are elected by the ARC-PA from a slate of nominees submitted by the ARC-PA collaborating organizations. Commissioners initially serve a 3-year term and are eligible for reappointment for a second term. The ARC-PA staff comprises an executive director, an associate director, and an administrative assistant (Exhibit 16-23).

Competencies for the Physician Assistant Profession

In 2005, the governing bodies of the AAPA, the ARC-PA, the NCCPA, and the PAEA jointly endorsed the "Competencies for the Physician Assistant Profession." The organizations collaborated to define the competencies that should be demonstrated by PAs in the domains of medical knowledge, interpersonal and communication skills, patient care, professionalism, practice-based learning and improvement, and systems-based practice. These competencies were defined in response to increased public interest in patient safety and an outcry to licensed healthcare providers to periodically demonstrate competence (Kohlhepp, Rohrs, & Robinson, 2005; Guerra, 2007).

The "Competencies" represent a desire and will to work together in the best interest of the people whom PAs serve—the public. They are organizational dynamics at their best that require high levels of communication and skill to maneuver among different but overlapping territory. They bring together interests in identifying measures to work together on the leadership and professional staff level to define gaps in knowledge and how to rectify them for the greater good.

GLOBAL PHYSICIAN ASSISTANT ORGANIZATIONS

As the PA profession grows in countries outside of the United States, so do the organizations that represent them. Examples of PA organizations from around the world are described in the following paragraphs.

Canadian Association of Physician Assistants

In 1997, Warrant Officer Thomas Ashman, bivouaced at Canadian Forces Station Alert Bay in Northern Canada as a PA, conceived the idea of a National Academy of Canadian PAs. In October 1999, the Canadian Academy of Physician Assistants (now the Canadian Association of Physician Assistants—CAPA)

EXHIBIT 16-22
History of the Accreditation Review Commission on Education for Physician Assistants

1973	The American College of Surgeons (ACS) adopts the *Essentials for an Educational Program for the Surgeon's Assistant.* The ACS Committee on Allied Health Personnel reviews applicant programs' compliance with these *Essentials.* In April, the Joint Review Committee for Educational Programs for the Assistant to the Primary Care Physician (JRC-PA) adds three graduate PAs as members-at-large for 1-year terms.
1974	The sponsors of the JRC-PA and the AMA recognize the AAPA as the fifth sponsor of the JRC-PA.
1975	The ACS becomes a sponsor of the JRC-PA.
1976	The review committees for primary care PAs and for surgeon's assistants are merged into the JRC-PA.
1976	The AMA House of Delegates votes to delegate its responsibility for adoption of proposed educational standards (also known as *Essentials*) to the AMA Council on Medical Education and authorizes the transfer of responsibility for accreditation from the AMA Council on Medical Education to its Committee on Allied Education and Accreditation (CAHEA).
	The new committee is a modification of the Council's former advisory Committee on Allied Health Education. These changes are instituted to achieve complete compliance with the U.S. Office of Education's criteria for national accrediting agencies. CAHEA is designed to represent communities of interest for which accreditation actions are taken. CAHEA is composed of representatives of allied health professions, medicine, the Council on Medical Education, and the public.
1978	The JRC-PA sponsors recognize the Association of Physician Assistant Program (APAP) as the seventh sponsor of the JRC-PA.
1981	The American Society of Internal Medicine (ASIM) withdraws its sponsorship of the JRC-PA.
1982	The sponsoring organizations reduce their representation from three to two members each, except for the AAPA, which continues to have three representatives.
1988	The JRC-PA is renamed the Accreditation Review Committee on Education for the Physician Assistant (ARC-PA).
1991	The AMA requests that administrative responsibility for the ARC-PA be undertaken by another sponsoring organization.
1991	The AAPA accepts administrative responsibility for the JRC-PA. The corporate offices of the ARC-PA are established in Marshfield, Wisconsin.
1994	The CAHEA is dissolved and accreditation activities are transferred to a new, independent agency, the Commission on Accreditation of Allied Health Education Programs (CAAHEP). The AMA beomes a sponsoring organization of the ARC-PA.
1995	The ARC-PA approves the addition of a third representative from APAP.
1995	The ARC-PA is incorporated.
1996	A study is initiated to determine the feasibility of the ARC-PA withdrawing from the CAAHEP system and establishing itself as a freestanding accrediting agency.
1998	ASIM returns as a sponsor of the ARC-PA when the association merges with the American College of Physicians.
2000	The members of the ARC-PA vote to become a freestanding accrediting agency for the PA profession as of January 1, 2001.
2001	ARC-PA begins operations as a freestanding accrediting agency.
2001	ARC-PA awards its first program accreditation as a new agency and becomes a member of the Association of Specialized and Professional Accreditors (ASPA).
2004	ARC-PA is awarded recognition by the Council for Higher Education Accreditation (CHEA).
2004	ARC-PA moves its corporate offices to Duluth, Georgia.
2006	ARC-PA enacts *Revision of Standards,* third edition.
2007	ARC-PA promulgates new *Standards* for the accreditation of PA postgraduate programs.
2009	There were 145 accredited entry-level PA programs and 3 accredited postgraduate PA programs.

was formed, and Ashman was elected founding president. CAPA's goal was to be a national professional organization that advocated for PAs across Canada. The organization's development was funded by the Canadian Forces with the intent that CAPA would become self-sufficient and expand to include a civilian component. In September 2001, CAPA, with assistance from the Canadian Forces Medical Services School, developed the Occupational Competency Profile (OCP) for the Civilian PA in Canada; this OCP was then adopted by the

John McCarty, Executive Director of the Accreditation Review Commission on Education for the Physician Assistant

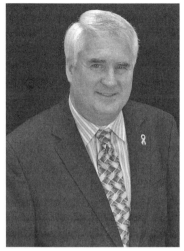

Courtesy of the ARC-PA.

Canadian Forces. In September 2002, the Canadian Forces inaugurated a redesigned PA program to align with requirements for accreditation by the Canadian Medical Association (CMA). The CAPA website is: http://www.caopa.net/.

CAPA's leadership includes an executive director, an elected president and officers, and five regional chapters. CAPA meets annually to provide leadership and medical education. A strong alliance between CAPA and the AAPA has existed since 2001.

Physician Assistant's Certification Council

The Physician Assistant's Certification Council (PACC) is an independent section of CAPA that administers and maintains the Canadian PA certification process. Certification includes an entry-to-practice examination, which is taken upon successful completion of a CMA-accredited PA program. The certification examination is administered independently of any training facility to ensure that the PA meets the standards set out in the OCP for the PA profession. CAPA aims to reassure the public that there is a national standard of care from PA providers who successfully complete this certification examination. Another priority of the PACC is to define continuing professional education (CPE) requirements for PAs to foster an ongoing professional learning process for all PAs.

The PACC's body of professionals includes a physician, an allied health professional, an educator, a consumer, a regulator, and two PAs. It also has two committees: the test-writing committee and the appeals committee. The test-writing committee's function is to ensure the utmost security of all testing material and to update the question bank used to formulate the certification examinations. The appeals committee is formed to deal strictly with matters that pertain to grievances, policy interpretation, and issues with examination process.

Conjoint Accreditation Service

The CMA Conjoint Accrediation Service (CMA CAS) was established in 1938 to provide accreditation services to various health-care educational entities. The CMA plays a central role in this process and believes that a collaborative approach among medical specialties and related health science professions is critical to providing safe and effective patient care. Since 1938, the CMA has played a leadership role to ensure national standards for the education of about 40,000 healthcare practitioners represented by 39 professional societies and 14 distinct health professions who perform diagnostic and therapeutic services to support physicians in the clinical setting. The CAS model:

- Brings health professions together under one umbrella for the benefit of the patient
- Promotes collaborative practices among physicians and other health professionals
- Brings the perspectives of physicians, employers, educators, and practitioners to deliberations concerning the education and competence of health professionals
- Establishes a reliable measure of educational quality for health professions

In June 2003, the CMA recognized the PA as a health professional. This act paved the way for a PA program accreditation process to begin. In June 2004, CMA/ARC-PA surveyed the Canadian Forces PA program for accreditation as a certificate-awarding program. Thus far, the CMA CAS has been involved in one accreditation process: the Canadian Forces Physician Assistant Program at Base Borden, Ontario. In 2007, the program was granted full 6-year accreditation status.

Netherlands Association of Physician Assistants

In the final decade of the last century, the Netherlands found itself faced with an increased number of patients, an aging population with multisystem illnesses, and rising costs of health care. The Ministry of Health chose to begin by developing a PA program. The following series of initiatives were undertaken:

- 2001: First PA program began at the Health Academy of Utrecht
- 2003: Second PA program established at the University Arnhem/Nijmegen
- 2003: Programs accredited by the Dutch Flemish Organization with one national curriculum
- 2004: Recognition of the profession by the Department of Education and Science
- 2006: Netherlands Association of Physician Assistants established

By 2009, five academic PA programs were actively educating PAs. A total of 200 PAs had graduated and were employed. The Netherlands has also established their own national organization and governing body for PAs, the Netherlands Association of Physician Assistants (NAPA).

United Kingdom Association of Physician Assistants, Ltd.

American-trained PAs have been able to practice in England under the general delegatory clause of the British Medical Act. Additionally, in 2006, 20 U.S. PAs were employed to work in Scotland as part of a 2-year demonstration project. Meanwhile, the Modernisation Agency of the National Health Service (NHS) worked extensively to develop the PA model in the United Kingdom. In 2005, NHS released *The Competence and Curriculum Framework for the Medical Care Practioner*. This document provided the groundwork for a large group of academics and policy people to examine the PA concept in more detail. A more concise and detailed follow-up document was released in 2006: *The Competence and Curriculum Framework for the Physician Assistant*. This document replaced the working title "medical care practitioner" in response to suggestions received through the public consultation process that the term "medical care practitioner" was confusing and that they did not mind the term "physician assistant."

The United Kingdom Association of Physician Assistants, Ltd. (UKAPA) is the official organization of PAs in the United Kingdom. Formed in 2006, the UKAPA suggested that the assessment of educational programs should work with the PA credential regulating body as part of an assessment team. In addition to the National Examination Board, other members forming the assessing body should include a member of the Royal College of General Practitioners (RCGP), Health Professions Council (HPC), and a delegate from the organization representing medical care practitioners (currently UKAPA, Ltd.). This work is under development and until such a body is formed, the steering committee will serve in this role to certify educational programs.

In response to the NHS *Competence and Curriculum Framework for the Physician Assistant*, UKAPA, declared that ". . . there should be some formal mechanism to include American PAs. The American PAs now have a body of experience in both systems and are well placed to provide much needed counseling in the critical transition phase." Registration of PAs with the General Medical Council began in 2007, with PAs practicing under Article 46, the Delegation and Referral clause of the General Medical Council's Handbook for Good Medical Practice. All principals agree this is a work in progress; a body of education accreditation, certification, and professional activity are the goals in the development of PAs in Great Britian.

Society of European Physician Assistants, Ltd.

A group of PAs stationed at military bases throughout Europe have created an informal group that put on meetings for medical education. This group has caught the attention of some who would like to see it grow.

The Austroasian Association of Physician Assistants, Ltd.

A group of Australian based PAs have tentatively created a name by which they hope to hold meetings.

Research and Physician Assistant Organizations

The organizations that represent PAs are not discussed in depth in the literature. Many research questions arise from the mere presence of these institutions. Following is a brief review of research areas in need of attention.

- **Case reports:** How did these organizations arise and what were the driving forces for the creation of these organizations?

- **Data:** What are the characteristics of individuals in the databases within each organization and do the variables compare and contrast with each other? What is the main purpose of the data and how are they used?

- **Organization:** How does the AAPA compare with the AMA, AOA, AAFP, AANP, and other organizations in terms of structure, influence, staffing ratios, policy development, and leadership?

- **Education:** Compare and contrast the PAEA with the AAMC and how it influences medical education.

- **Certification:** Compare and contrast the certification process of PAs in various countries. Does a certification process embedded in a professional society have an advantage over a process administered by a stand-alone organization?

- **Accreditation:** What is the evidence that an accreditation process for PA educational institutions provides a social good?

- **History:** What are the similarities and differences in how various PA professional organizations developed? Is there a one-person catalyst phenomenon or are such organizations a function of social organization?

- **Membership:** What does a PA receive for belonging to a professional society? Why do PAs belong or not belong to a professional society?

- **Global PA development:** What are the political issues for PAs by country and would an international PA congress be of any use to the profession?

- **Future:** What are issues for PAs in the 21st century in regard to organization?

SUMMARY

As the PA profession grew and matured, organizations arose to represent the various components of the profession. Each of these organizations, in turn, underwent their own maturation process. As of the new millennium, several U.S. organizations representing PAs or PA education are well established, have a defined domain, and well-defined constituencies. In turn, each of the organizations has a relationship with the other organizations and contributes to the efficiency of the profession as a whole. Each organization strives to achieve its own goals and, in turn, looks to its adjacent organizations for assistance. For many, the cooperation of these organizations represents a model of how to work toward a common goal: the promotion of improved health for citizens. This framework of professional organization is now spreading globally, with PA organizations now appearing in Canada, the United Kingdom, and the Netherlands.

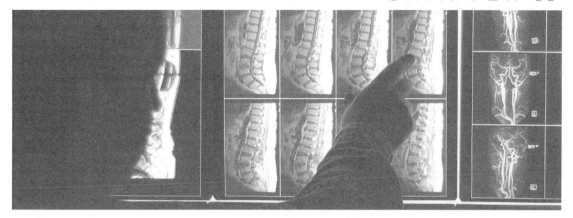

CHAPTER 17

PHYSICIAN ASSISTANTS IN THE FEDERAL WORKFORCE

RODERICK S. HOOKER ■ JAMES F. CAWLEY ■ DAVID P. ASPREY

It was once said that the moral test of Government is how that Government treats those who are in the dawn of life, the children; those who are in the twilight of life, the elderly; and those who are in the shadows of life, the sick, the needy and the handicapped.

—Hubert H. Humphrey (1911–1978)

ABSTRACT

The U.S. federal government is the largest single employer of physician assistants (PAs), employing approximately 5% of PAs. They are dispersed in all branches and agencies of the government that provide healthcare services, including the Departments of Defense, Veterans Affairs, Health and Human Services, Justice, and Homeland Security. The majority of these PAs are civil servants or hold a commission in the uniformed services. Many are also employed in contract roles for various agencies of the federal government domestically and on foreign shores. Most agencies that employ PAs are actively recruiting and have expanding needs for medical services.

INTRODUCTION

No two healthcare systems in the world are the same. Yet, the majority of developed countries are employers directly or indirectly of doctors, nurses, and other health providers. The exception is the U.S. government, where a very small group of doctors and nurses are federal employees. In spite of this, the U.S. federal government is the largest employer of physician assistants (PAs). As of 2009, approximately 5% of all employed PAs receive their earnings directly from the governmnt. They serve in the U.S. Armed Forces, Department of Veterans Affairs (VA), Bureau of Prisons (BOP), U.S. Department of Health and Human Services (HHS), and other federal agencies. The majority of federally employed PAs provide primary care services, and many work in positions previously occupied by physicians. Exact numbers of PAs are difficult to determine because many agencies and branches of the federal government, including the military, are constantly adding to the number of PAs delivering healthcare services among uniform, civilian, and contract jobs. However, the relevance of PAs in the federal workforce is evident by the qualifications standards for PAs set by the U.S. Office of Personnel Management (Exhibit 17-1).

The two largest federal agencies are the Department of Defense (DOD), which includes most military branches, and the Department of VA. In 2008, more than 1,300 uniformed PAs were on active duty, and over 1,600 civilian PAs were in the VA (Exhibit 17-2). Because a federal registry of healthcare workers is not available, these figures are based on communication with senior leaders in different departments and branches of the federal government. This chapter addresses PAs in the U.S. federal workforce. Canada has PAs in uniform and their role is addressed in Chapter 18.

EXHIBIT 17-1
Qualification Standards for Physician Assistants Positions Within the Federal Government (Series 0603)

The U.S. Office of Personnel Management defines the PA as someone who does the following:

- Assists a physician by providing diagnostic and therapeutic medical care and services under the guidance of the physician
- Assists in the examination and observation of patients by performing such duties as taking case histories, conducting physical examinations, and ordering laboratory studies during hospital rounds and clinic visits
- Carries out special procedures as directed by the physician; for example, giving injections or other medications, applying or changing dressings, performing lumbar punctures, or suturing minor lacerations

Basic requirements for a position in this series are as follows:

- Being a graduate of a physician assistant educational program, accredited by the Accreditation Review Committee on Education for the Physician Assistant or its predecessors, at a college, university, or educational institution that is accredited by an accrediting body or organization recognized by the Secretary, U.S. Department of Education
- Successfully completing the National Commission on Certification of Physician Assistants examination
- Maintaining certification, including completion of all requirements for continuing medical education and recertification

Applicants who meet these basic requirements may qualify for the following grade levels within the federal government if they meet the associated educational and/or specialized experience requirements described.

GS-07 (or equivalent)

- Completion of an accredited PA educational program (certificate of completion, associate degree, or bachelor's degree) **or**
- Completion of a bachelor's degree in a related healthcare or health-related science **and** graduation from an accredited PA educational program.

GS-09 (or equivalent)

- A minimum of 1 full year of work experience as a certified PA equivalent to the GS-07 grade level **and** graduation from an accredited physician assistant educational program as described previously
- Completion of the Master of Physician Assistant Studies **or**
- Completion of a master's degree in a related healthcare or health-related science **and** completion of an accredited PA educational program.

GS-11 (or equivalent)

- A minimum of 1 full year of work experience as a certified PA equivalent to the GS-09 grade level **and** completion of an accredited PA educational program as described previously **or**
- PhD or equivalent doctoral degree in a related health field **and** completion of an accredited PA educational program.

GS-12 and above (or equivalent)

A minimum of 1 full year of work experience as a certified PA equivalent to the next lower grade level **and** completion of an accredited physician assistant educational program.

Source: U.S. Office of Personnel Management.

EXHIBIT 17-2
U.S. Federally Employed Physician Assistants, 2008*

Branch	Active Duty	Billets†	Branch	Active Duty	Billets†
DEPARTMENT OF DEFENSE			**DEPARTMENT OF JUSTICE**		
U.S. Air Force			Bureau of Prisons	60	NA
Active Duty	270	298	Federal Bureau of Investigation	8	NA
Reserves	30	60			
Air National Guard	24	20	**DEPARTMENT OF HEALTH AND HUMAN SERVICES**		
			U.S. Public Health Service	140	NA
U.S. Army			Indian Health Service	25	NA
Active Duty	610	754	Food and Drug Administration	2	NA
Reserves	180	286	Centers for Disease Control		
National Guard	350	831	and Prevention	1	NA
U.S. Navy (including Marines)			Federal Occupational Health	4	NA
Active Duty	235	275	National Institutes of Health	6	NA
Reserves	44	80	Health Resources and Services		
			Administration	2	NA
DEPARTMENT OF HOMELAND SECURITY			National Health Service Corps	36	40
U.S. Coast Guard					
Active Duty	42	60	**DEPARTMENT OF STATE**		
Reserves	10	18	Peace Corps	30	NA
Immigration and Naturalization Service			**DEPARTMENT OF VETERANS AFFAIRS**		
Immigration Health Service	30	40	Veterans Health Administration	1,680	1,700
DEPARTMENT OF TRANSPORTATION			**OTHER AGENCIES**		
Federal Aviation Administration	2	2	Smithsonian Institution	2	NA
National Oceanic and			Central Intelligence Agency	4	NA
Atmospheric Administration	3	3			

*Data derived from various personal sources in the different agencies and branches, 2008. The numbers are likely to be different at the time of printing.
†A billet means an available position, although all are fluid and subject to change.
NA = data not available or does not exist.

MILITARY

The military of the United States, officially known as the U.S. Armed Forces, has five branches:

- Army
- Navy
- Marine Corps
- Air Force
- Coast Guard

The U.S. Public Health Service (USPHS), which is under the Department of HHS, and the National Oceanic and Atmospheric Administration (NOAA), which is under the Department of Commerce, also have active duty uniformed officers, known as the Commissioned Corps (discussed later in this chapter). These officers are considered uniformed services, not armed forces, because they do not carry weapons, but come under

the same rank, pay, and benefits systems as U.S. military agencies. The USPHS and NOAA can be militarized by the president during declared times of war.

All branches of the armed forces are part of the U.S. uniformed services and are under civilian control with the president of the United States serving as commander-in-chief. Except for the Coast Guard, all branches of the armed forces are part of the DOD. The Coast Guard falls under the authority of the Department of Homeland Security, but may be placed under the DOD in times of need, acting as a service to the Navy.

Approximately 1,500,000 personnel are currently on active duty in the military with an additional 1,260,000 personnel in the seven reserve/national guard components. As it is currently a volunteer military, there is no conscription. Although women are not usually assigned to serve in most combat assignments, they do serve in many noncombat specialties. Due to the realities of war, some of these non-combat positions see combat regularly.

As of 2008, approximately 1,300 PAs were on active duty in the military worldwide (Exhibit 17-3). They serve on land, sea, or in the air. Some serve in special hardship situations, such as isolated outposts, foreign lands, submarines, and the polar regions. In addition, approximately 500 PAs were employed in civilian practices that also serve in the Ready Reserves and National Guard in 50 states and four territories (Salyer, 2002).

Outside these figures are the many nonuniform (civilian) PAs on contract with military branches and federal agencies. A special group known as quasi-government employees work for companies such as Blackwater Security and Haliburton, Inc. These contract companies employ many PAs, some are former special forces, typically in direct support of military operations, such as in Iraq and Afghanistan.

Unlike most civilian PAs, the majority of military PAs have been medics and hospital corpsmen and received their training in the military. At one time, the typical military PA was a male, trained at an older age than his civilian counterparts that were assigned a

EXHIBIT 17-3
Army Physician Assistants in Sadr City, Iraq, August 2008

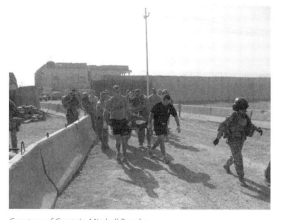

Courtesy of Captain Mitchell Brooks.

primary care role. Over the past decade that has changed; the ratio of female to male PAs is closer to 1:5. Job characteristics tend to differ as well. Level of responsibility is slightly higher, whereas closeness of supervision is lower for the military PA than for the civilian PA.

The history of the PA movement is anchored in the medic and corpsman. Many of the first PAs were returning Vietnam veterans who attended the early PA programs in the 1960s and 1970s (Hooker, 1991b). Although most of these PAs remained in civilian attire, a few donned the uniform again and returned to military service. All PAs in the uniformed services are commissioned officers.

The PA medical officer was initiated in the Army, Navy, and Air Force in 1971, and in the Coast Guard in 1975 (Stuart, Robinson, & Reed, 1973; Hooker, 1991a; Hooker, 1991b; Gwinn & Keller, 1999). Initially, all were non-commissioned officers, usually with senior enlisted rank. Their ranks swelled throughout the 1970s (Chitwood, 2008). The primary reason PAs took hold in the military was largely in response to the termination of the draft for physicians (Gaudry, 1977). When obligated service was removed for doctors (after the abolishment of the draft for military duty for men), those with little time invested in the military as a career tended to leave. In fact, the unplanned departure of more junior physicians from the military created a medical staffing vacuum of general medical officers. Not surprisingly, the services found it difficult to recruit physicians, especially given the expanding fee-for-service marketplace and substantial economic opportunities in the civilian sector. With a peacetime military and a need for medical officers, the military turned to PAs as a logical alternative (Hooker, 1989). Wanting to remain in their current roles, many PAs filled the medical officer gap and remain at high levels of visibility today.

One of the more interesting historical footnotes concerns the commissioning of PAs. Although it has not always been the case, all PAs currently in the U.S. uniformed services hold commissions as officers. The first PAs were in the enlisted ranks; they were the medics, corpsmen, or allied health personnel who matriculated through a formal PA training program (Amann, 1973). In the early 1970s, their rank status was changed from enlisted to warrant officer to reflect their technical skills and to avoid conflicts when directing services that involved officers (Hooker, 1989). In April 1978, the U.S. Air Force promoted enlisted PAs to commissioned officer status. This accession was considered consistent with the skills and responsibilities of an officer. It also took place because the Air Force warrant officer program had been discontinued in 1958, so the Air Force warrant officer structure was no longer an option. This left the Army, Navy, and Coast Guard PAs as warrant officers, in contrast to the commissioned officers in the Air Force.

As a consequence, discrepancies in rank, status, and career earnings for military pay emerged. These discrepancies were in stark contrast to the uniformity of rank, pay, and hierarchy of physicians, nurses, dentists, pharmacists, and physical therapists in the military that was present for more than 30 years. During a 20-year career beginning in 1970, the Air Force PA was making 25% more than his or her professional peer in the Army. This disparity became more apparent after econometric studies revealed that significant improvements in recruitment and retention could be achieved by commissioning PAs (Hooker, 1989). After intense lobbying by the AAPA, legislative representatives, PA leaders in the AAPA, and PAs in and out of uniform, and with some Congressional help, the surgeon generals of the different services eventually agreed to commission all military PAs (the Navy and Coast Guard in 1990; the Army in 1992). Military PA activists achieved their utmost goal in 1992 when the Coast Guard Reserve PA was commissioned. Seen as the close of an important chapter in PA professional development, the AAPA could move on to other professional issues, such as enabling legislation in states that lacked laws for PA practice, reimbursement standards, and prescribing rights.

The military and the PA profession maintain a strong kinship because it was the enlisted allied health professional in Vietnam and previous wars that gave rise to today's PA. As Assistant Surgeon General Moritsugu said to a group of Army PAs in 1994, "You are the germ plasm of all PAs" (Condit, 1993). The Medex PA program at the University of Washington was also composed of all former military servicemen. The founder, Dick Smith, reflected that although the Medex concept may have been controversial and resisted by some doctors, by choosing medics and corpsmen, he was recruiting war heroes to return to their homes and work with their communities. He believed it was this image that made them unassailable (R. E. Smith, personal communication, July 2006). Subsequent classes at Duke, Medex, and other programs were partially composed of veterans, many with Vietnam experience (Hooker, 1991). In fact, for the first 10 years, the majority of PA graduates were predominantly male veterans.

Today's military PA comprises former medics, technicians, and corpsmen who came up through the ranks, as well as some civilian PAs who entered the military. Although the number of civilian-trained PAs on active duty is not large, the number fluctuates from year to year depending on the various needs of each organization and their ability to recruit PAs. Incentives of rank and signing bonuses are enticements for recruitment of experienced PAs in times of need.

Education

At one time all of the armed services developed and maintained their own military PA schools. To meet demand at different times, some military branches contracted with civilian schools to train military PAs outside of their own programs. This took place with the Army and Air Force at the St. Francis University Master of Medical Science PA Program, the Coast Guard and Navy at the University of Nebraska and Duke University, and the Navy at the George Washington University in Washington, DC. In 1996, Congressional mandates to avoid government waste and combine training wherever possible under the auspices of the Interservice Training Review Organization allowed the

DOD to consolidate its military training programs. Mixed classes of PA students from the Army, Navy, Air Force, and Coast Guard, and at one time a few from the Federal BOP, were joined into an interservice PA training program at Ft. Sam Houston in San Antonio, Texas—the site of the former Army PA program. The student selection process remains the responsibility of each individual service.

Military Physician Assistant Role

The role of the PA in the military has been enhanced in a number of ways, beginning with deployment during international engagements such as in Vietnam, Panama, the Gulf War, Somalia, Haiti, Bosnia, Afghanistan, and Operation Enduring/Iraqi Freedom (Exhibit 17-4). PAs have been an integral part of combat-ready troops in the Army, Navy, Air Force, Marines, and Coast Guard. They also serve in the White House, the Pentagon, the Office of the Surgeon General, and in a number of policy development positions. Currently, the highest-ranking military PAs are colonels in the Air Force and Army and a captain in the Navy. Rear Admiral Michael Milner, the first of two PA flag officers, is in the U.S. Public Health Service. (The generic title of flag officer is used in the modern Navy to denote those who hold the rank of commodore, rear admiral or its equivalent, and above.)

EXHIBIT 17-4
Major Military Campaigns That Deployed Physician Assistants

Grenada (Operation Urgent Fury)
Panama (Operation Just Cause)
Gulf War: Iraq and Kuwait (Operation Desert Storm/ Desert Shield)
Northern Iraq for relief to Kurdish refugees (Operation Provide Comfort)
Balkans: Bosnia, Kosovo (Operation Joint Guard)
Somalia
Macedonia
Afghanistan
Iraq

Reserves

The military has a number of domestic options for PAs, including Reserve and National Guard units. Sometimes these units are called up in times of disasters such as floods, tornadoes, hurricanes, and wildfires, as well as combat and combat support in Iraq. For example, many reservists, including PAs, were called up after the September 11, 2001, terrorist attack on the World Trade Center in New York City and after the Hurricane Katrina disaster in New Orleans in 2005. PAs in Reserve and National Guard units take on special duties in medical units, prisoner of war units, harbor defense, port security, and training.

Historically, the military has always provided an opportunity for enlisted members to expand their medical training and skills while moving up the career ladder. Since the turn of the century, the military need for PAs has more than doubled because their ability to adapt to many roles is increasingly appreciated. Broad-based missions on diverse fronts require more medical services than when they are concentrated stateside. To expand the applicant pool for PA programs from within the military, the services allow officers and the enlisted from other career tracks to apply to become PAs. They apply through their respective services and then are screened and forwarded to the Interservice Physician Assistant Program (IPAP) for a starting date assignment.

Air Force

The Air Force has approximately 270 PAs on active duty, serving principally in primary care and family practice clinics. In addition, there are PAs in the Air Force Reserves and the Air National Guard. The PAs in the Air Force, part of the Biological Sciences Corps, enjoy strong support from the highest levels of the Air Force medical command. A small number of Air Force PAs also have opportunities in orthopedics, head and neck surgery, emergency medicine, bone marrow transplant/oncology, and as cardiac perfusion specialists.

At one time, the Air Force had its own PA program located at Sheppard Air Force Base in Wichita Falls, Texas (now integrated in the IPAP at Ft. Sam Houston, San Antonio, Texas). Most Air Force PAs are trained in IPAP, but a number are recruited directly from civilian programs and PAs in civilian roles.

Army

The Army, with approximately 610 active duty PAs, 350 National Guard PAs, and 180 PAs in the Army Reserve, has the largest contingent of PAs in the services. From 2004 to 2006, the number of PAs in the Army doubled, largely because of the war in Iraq. This number continues to grow as more batallions are created to meet the expanding role of the Army. The number of PAs filling an Army/National Guard/Reserve role (1,140 as of 2008) is short of the 1,871 total billets (available positions) for PAs.

Army PAs are part of the Medical Specialist Corps and work in the field with operational forces as well as in the primary care setting (O'Hearn, 1991). In addition, Army PAs have opportunities to specialize in occupational medicine, aviation medicine, orthopedic surgery, emergency medicine (Herrera, 1994), cardioperfusion training, and other specialties. In the field, advanced trauma teams that were used in Kosovo were typically overseen by a PA (Henson, 1999). In garrison, the battalion medical officer is usually a PA. Commonly, the forward team of a battalion aid station includes a PA, a staff sergeant medic, and two junior medics.

When sent with units on a mission, PAs are often in the "muddy boots" Army (combat units). These units are often at the point of contact with opposing combat forces at the time of first engagement. Eighty percent of Army PAs are in maneuver units at the division level. There are Army PAs in Korea near the demilitarized zone between North Korea and South Korea. These PAs are somewhat isolated and live in austere conditions. In Iraq, Army PAs are in acute care settings and surgery and hospital units, returning with highly skilled

advanced trauma experience. Because the Army does not have enough PAs to satisfy demand, Army PAs tend to relocate frequently. When Army medical units are detached to war-torn areas such as Afghanistan, they are there not only to care for their own troops, but to provide medical assistance in villages and set up clinics to assist the citizens (Exhibit 17-5).

An example of an advanced trauma managed care team in the Army is described in a paper by Henson (1999). The forward team of a battalion aid station included a PA, a staff sergeant medic, and two junior medics. As a team, they were dispatched to Serbian villages to set up clinics and to provide care to the people who remained. Humanitarian endeavors such as this one will likely be the mission for the military in this century, and PAs will be used increasingly to provide this assistance (Henson, 1999).

Army PAs have opportunities to specialize in a number of areas. The Army has four PA

EXHIBIT 17-5
Army Physician Assistant at Riva Ridge, TMC, Camp Liberty, Iraq, March 2008

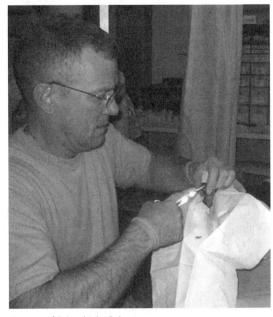

Courtesy of Colonel John Balser.

residency programs: emergency medicine, occupational health, cardiovascular perfusion, and orthopedics. All are located at large Army medical centers. The Army's PA service arose from a desperate need for more doctors during the Vietnam War, and remains the largest such program in the U.S. military service. Beause of their varied missions, Army PAs may have the most diverse skills of any group of PAs.

Navy

Approximately 180 active-duty and 80 reserve Navy PAs are part of the Medical Services Corps. They are used in diverse positions to include shore and overseas hospitals and clinics at home and in foreign lands. They fill needed positions in IPAP and the White House; many work in primary care. A number of operational billets are available for deep-water vessels such as carriers and cruisers, but most are attached to medical centers and shore stations domestically and abroad. Navy PAs are deployed with Marine Corps units around the world; a few serve on independent duty. The Navy PA School was located in San Diego, California, but consolidated with IPAP in San Antonio, Texas, in April 1996. Navy PAs derive from the interservice program and direct civilian procurement, as well as from outside scholarship programs. PAs assigned to the Marines undergo additional training in field medicine.

Coast Guard

Sometimes overlooked as a military branch, the Coast Guard is part of the Department of Homeland Security, rather than the DOD. As such, members of the Coast Guard tend to serve domestically rather than overseas. However, they do serve onboard large ice breakers when deployed to the Arctic and Antarctic and on larger cutters when deployed outside of U.S. waters (Exhibit 17-6). The Coast Guard and the Army utilize specialized PAs such as the Aviation/Aeromedical PA (APA). The APA provides specialized medical care for injured, hypothermic, and evacuees during complicated medical

EXHIBIT 17-6
Physician Assistant During a Medical Evacuation of a Cruise Ship in the Caribbean

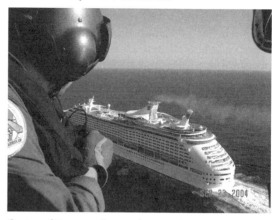

Courtesy of Lieutenant Commander James Cannon.

transports. There are 42 PAs on active duty, 18 in the reserves, and 24 contract civilian PAs. Many of these PAs are at independent-duty stations. Historically, PAs from the enlisted ranks were trained at the Air Force PA training program in Wichita Falls, Texas, as well as in some civilian programs. However, all are now trained at the combined military program in San Antonio, Texas. The USPHS supplies some PAs to the Coast Guard (those PAs wear the USPHS emblem on their uniform), but the majority are recruited and trained by the Coast Guard. Approximately 50% of the medical officers in the Coast Guard are PAs; the others are physicians.

Because there is no specialty corps in the Coast Guard, PAs are line officers and must compete with their operational fellow line officers for promotion. This is in contrast to the promotion process for USPHS-commissioned corps physicians, PAs, and NPs.

PHYSICIAN ASSISTANTS IN COMBAT ROLES

The war in Iraq and Afganistan moved the PA from the garrison, shore station, and base to war-torn areas of the globe. From serving as a medical provider for relatively healthy young men and women to serving as a frontline surgeon, peacekeeper, refugee worker, and combat medical support officer, the PA is deployed in areas never before planned. For the first half of the Iraq and Afghanistan wars, the Army PA was primarily involved. With time and need for skilled medical personnel the Army became so stretched that Navy, Coast Guard, and Air Force PAs were deployed for prolonged tours to Iraq and Afghanistan in Army billets, either supporting the Army directly or working for provisional reconstruction teams. Skilled in life support and combat medicine, the PA in theater is also interacting with military groups from Australia, Canada, Great Britian, Japan, and Europe. With the PA added to the lexicon of military medicine the result has permitted other countries to see the PA functioning in highly trained medical teams (Chitwood, 2008).

NONMILITARY FEDERAL AGENCIES

Within the federal government are numerous nonmilitary agencies that use medical personnel. The following sections describe some of these agencies.

U.S. Department of Health and Human Services

The U.S. Department of HHS includes the USPHS Commissioned Corps, Indian Health Service (IHS), Food and Drug Administration (FDA), Centers for Disease Control and Prevention (CDC), the National Institutes of Health (NIH), the National Health Service Corps (NHSC), and other divisions. Some of the PAs working for this department are commissioned officers; others are civilian or contract workers. All are recruited either as experienced professionals or while they are in PA school. None are trained at the Uniform Services Medical University.

U.S. Public Health Service Commissioned Corps

The mission of the USPHS Commissioned Corps is to protect, promote, and advance the health and safety of the nation. As the U.S.

uniformed service of public health professionals, the USPHS Commissioned Corps achieves its mission through the following:

- Rapid and effective response to public health needs
- Leadership and excellence in public health practices
- Advancement of public health science

The USPHS has 11 operating divisions in the U.S. Department of HHS; over 6,000 personnel are uniformed officers. As of 2009, there were 142 PAs in the USPHS in clinical and administrative positions as well as in posts as a result of being deployed to recent disasters. Roles for PAs are expanding in community health initiatives and the Department of Homeland Security (Zarychta, 2008). In coming years, it is expected that USPHS PAs will fill roles traditionally held by others, such as school-based clinics and managing community-based health programs.

The National Health Service Corps

The NHSC is a division of the Health Resources and Services Administration (HRSA), Bureau of Health Professions. As such, the NHSC has healthcare professionals in more than 500 areas (from urban to rural areas) that suffer from critical shortages of primary healthcare providers.

A number of recruitment funds support programs that offer financial help for PAs and other medical care professionals in exchange for professional services. These NHSC activities for obligated service include scholarships, the Federal Loan Repayment Program, the NHSC State Loan Repayment Program, and the Commissioned Officer Student Extern Program (COSTEP).

Indian Health Service

The IHS is a division within the U.S. Department of HHS responsible for providing federal health services to American Indians and Alaska natives. Established in 1955, the IHS took over health care of American Indian and Alaska natives from the Bureau of Indian Affairs. The provision of health services to members of federally recognized tribes grew out of the special government-to-government relationship between the federal government and Indian tribes. This relationship, established in 1787, is based on Article I, Section 8 of the Constitution, and has been given form and substance by numerous treaties, laws, Supreme Court decisions, and executive orders. The IHS is the principal federal healthcare provider and health advocate for Indian people. Its goal is to raise their health status to the highest possible level. Currently, the IHS provides health services to approximately 1.8 million of the 2.6 million American Indians and Alaska natives who belong to more than 560 federally recognized tribes in 35 states.

The IHS provides health care at more than 600 direct healthcare delivery facilities, including hospitals and health clinics. Thirty-four urban Indian health projects supplement these facilities with various health and referral services.

Within the IHS are approximately 2,700 nurses, 900 physicians, 400 engineers, 500 pharmacists, 300 dentists, 90 PAs, as well as other health professionals, totaling more than 15,000 employees. However, this total is not certain because more health centers are hiring contract or "tribally hired" PAs today as the tribes are "compacted and contracted" under Public Law 638, which allows for Tribal Self-Determination. The senior PA in the IHS is the Chief Clinical Consultant for Physician Assistants.

The IHS has employed PAs to work on Indian reservations since 1975. Most are employed by the federal or tribal government. Some of the PA positions are filled by NHSC scholars and USPHS-commissioned officers. IHS PAs deliver care primarily in family medicine clinics, emergency departments, or urgent care settings. They often work as solo practitioners in rural and remote clinics or Alaskan villages.

From 1971 to 1983, IHS trained community health medics (CHMs) to become PAs through intramural PA training programs at Gallup Indian Medical Center or IHS Clinical Support Center. All CHMs were eligible to take the National Commission on Certification of Physician Assistants (NCCPA) examination upon graduation.

National Institutes of Health

As of September 2008, the NIH is responsible for 28% (about $28 billion) of the total biomedical research funding spent annually in the United States, with the majority of the remaining funding coming from industry. The NIH is divided into two parts: the "extramural" parts of NIH are responsible for the funding of biomedical research outside of NIH, whereas the "intramural" parts of the NIH conduct research. Intramural research is primarily conducted at the main campus in Bethesda, Maryland, and surrounding towns. The National Institute of Aging and the National Institute on Drug Abuse are located in Baltimore, Maryland; the National Institute of Environmental Health Sciences is in Research Triangle, North Carolina.

PAs have been part of the NIH for more than two decades and are recruited to provide healthcare services, commonly in conjunction with research studies. Some of the activities include conducting complete physicals, providing medical treatment, and counseling patients. Most prescribe medication—oftentimes investigational drugs or orphan drugs. Some are subinvestigators of research studies. At least 20 PAs work for the NIH, either in the Maryland office or in other locations.

The Food and Drug Administration

The Food and Drug Administration (FDA) is responsible for regulating food, dietary supplements, drugs, biological medical products, blood products, medical devices, radiation-emitting devices, veterinary products, and cosmetics in the United States. At least two PAs work for the FDA as administrators.

Centers for Disease Control and Prevention

The CDC is an agency based in Atlanta, Georgia, on the campus of Emory University. It works to protect the public health and safety of people by providing information to enhance health decision-making. It also promotes health through partnerships with state health departments and other organizations. The CDC focuses national attention on developing and applying disease prevention and control (especially infectious diseases), environmental health, occupational safety and health, health promotion, injury and disease prevention, and education activities designed to improve the health of the people of the nation. At least one USPHS PA is at the CDC.

Federal Occupational Health

Federal Occupational Health (FOH) is a service that provides for the occupational health of 2.9 million U.S. government employees. FOH was created in 1946 by an amendment to the Public Health Service Act. The agency provides services exclusively to various federal agencies, including the DOD. FOH is currently the largest provider of clinical, wellness/fitness, employee assistance program (EAP), work/life, and environmental health and safety services to the federal government.

There are more than 300 FOH health centers throughout the United States and a network of over 700 private-provider physicians, PAs, and nurses. This system provides clinical services, including emergency response, physical examinations, immunizations, vision and health screenings, and health risk appraisals. It also maintains more than 200 counseling offices in federal buildings as well as a network of affiliate counselors in approximately 11,000 locations across the country and overseas. USPHS PAs, along with doctors and nurses, provide various clinical and administrative roles in the FOH.

National Oceanic and Atmospheric Administration

NOAA is a scientific agency of the U.S. Department of Commerce. This agency is focused on the conditions of the oceans and the atmosphere. NOAA warns of dangerous weather, charts seas and skies, guides the use and protection of ocean and coastal resources, and conducts research to improve understanding and stewardship of the environment. In addition to its civilian employees, 300 uniformed service members, who make up the NOAA Corps, support NOAA research and operations. Sometimes these assignments are in the Arctic or Antarctica for extended periods.

Only a few PAs are assigned to the NOAA. These PAs are part of the USPHS Commissioned Corps and tend to rotate through NOAA for only a few years before moving on to another branch of the USPHS. Rarely do they go afloat.

Federal Aviation Administration

The Federal Aviation Administration (FAA) is an agency of the U.S. Department of Transportation. It has authority to regulate and oversee all aspects of civil aviation in the United States. The Federal Aviation Act of 1958 created the group under the name Federal Aviation Agency, and it adopted its current name in 1967 when it became a part of the U.S. Department of Transportation.

The FAA's major roles include the following:

- Regulating U.S. commercial space transportation
- Encouraging and developing civil aeronautics, including new aviation technology
- Regulating civil aviation to promote safety
- Developing and operating a system of air traffic control and navigation for both civil and military aircraft
- Researching and developing the National Airspace System and civil aeronautics
- Developing and carrying out programs to control aircraft noise and other environmental effects of civil aviation.

Aviation medical officers provide physical examinations for FAA employees and other personnel. A few USPHS PAs are assigned to the FAA and are involved in flight physical examinations and administration.

Federal Bureau of Prisons

The Federal Bureau of Prisons, usually referred to as BOP, is a subdivision of the Justice Department and is responsible for the administration of the federal prison system. The BOP was established in 1930 to provide more progressive and humane care for federal inmates, to professionalize the prison service, and to ensure consistent and centralized administration.

As of 2009, the BOP consisted of more than 106 institutions, 6 regional offices, a central office in Washington, DC, 2 staff training centers, and 28 community corrections offices. It is responsible for the custody and care of approximately 185,000 federal offenders. Approximately 85% of these inmates are confined in BOP-operated correctional facilities or detention centers. The remainder is confined through agreements with state and local governments or through contracts with privately operated community corrections centers, detention centers, prisons, and juvenile facilities.

The BOP has numerous PAs serving in various federal prisons (Chavez, 2008). Because adequate medical services for prisoners is a federal policy, the BOP is an active and growing federal department and is constantly recruiting PAs for correctional medicine (Vause, Beeler, & Miller-Blanks, 1997). At one time, the BOP contracted with the IPAP to train PAs for service in the BOP. There are approximately 40 PAs working in the BOP. All PAs serving in the BOP as members of the USPHS are graduates of an accredited PA program. However, some BOP PAs are international medical graduates and have not graduated from accredited PA programs.

With the establishment of medical referral centers, inmates requiring a high degree of healthcare service are transferred to these institutions. This development gives PAs opportunities to provide specialty services in oncology, orthopedics, surgery, and mental health care and serve as administrators. Today, all PAs hired by the BOP are certified by the NCCPA and have or are eligible for state licensure.

Peace Corps

The Peace Corps is an independent branch of the U.S. Department of State that was established by Executive Order 10924 on March 1, 1961. It was authorized by Congress on September 22, 1961, with passage of the Peace Corps Act (Public Law 87-293). The Peace Corps Act defines its purpose as "to promote world peace and friendship through a Peace Corps, which shall make available to interested countries and areas men and women of the United States qualified for service abroad and willing to serve, under conditions of hardship if necessary, to help the peoples of such countries and areas in meeting their needs for trained manpower." Since 1960, more than 187,000 people have served as Peace Corps volunteers in 139 countries.

The Peace Corps actively recruits PAs, along with physicians and NPs, to be either volunteers or Peace Corps medical officers. Applicants must have and maintain a current license to practice medicine. The Office of Medical Services at the Peace Corps determines the level of provider required at each post before contractor selection. Usually, at least one medical officer who is a staff member in the Peace Corps is deployed to each country where Peace Corps volunteers are located, and PAs are increasingly used in some of these medical officer roles. The first use of a PA as a Peace Corps medical officer was in the Kingdom of Tonga (South Pacific) in 1975, and a PA has been there ever since.

Immigration and Naturalization Service

The U.S. Immigration and Naturalization Service (INS) oversees and enforces the laws that apply to the entry of non-U.S. citizens into the United States. Formerly a part of the Department of Justice (DOJ), it became a part of the Department of Homeland Security in 2003.

The INS oversees the legal entry of non-U.S. citizens who are temporarily or permanently seeking to settle in the United States. It enforces the laws of naturalization, the process by which a foreign-born person becomes a citizen. The INS also tackles illegal entrance into the United States by preventing receipt of benefits, such as social security or unemployment, by those ineligible to receive them and investigating, detaining, and deporting those illegally living in the United States. One of the roles of the INS is to issue certificates for foreign healthcare workers. The list of workers for which certificates are provided includes "physician assistants." Whether this title applies to formally trained PAs or some other use of the word is not clearly stated in INS documents.

The Immigration Health Service actively recruits PAs, along with many other types of healthcare employees, to look after INS workers and detainees. Many of these PAs are under contract to provide local healthcare services. Health care provided to detainees is provided through the Division of Immigration Health Service, a part of the HRSA. USPHS-commissioned officers, including PAs, support this mission of HRSA and the Department of HHS.

DEPARTMENT OF VETERANS AFFAIRS

One of the principal institutional employers of PAs nationwide is the Department of VA. More specifically, the healthcare branch of the VA is the Veterans Health Administration (VHA). The Department of VA was established on March 15, 1989, succeeding the Veterans Administration. It is responsible for providing federal benefits to veterans and their families. Headed by the Secretary of Veterans Affairs, the Department of VA is the second largest of the 15 cabinet departments and operates nationwide programs for health care, financial assistance, and burial benefits.

Of the 24 million veterans alive in 2009, nearly three-quarters served during a war or an official period of conflict. About one-quarter of the nation's population, approximately 70 million people, are potentially eligible for VA benefits and services because they are veterans, family members of veterans, or survivors of veterans.

From the very beginning of the PA profession, the VA saw PAs as potentially useful workers; the VA was the first government agency to employ a PA in 1968 (Fox & Whittaker, 1983). The VA also plays a vital supporting role in education. For example, the VA Medical Center in Durham, North Carolina, has continuously provided clinical education sites, going back to the first PA students at Duke University. The St. Louis University PA program was developed by and initially funded by the VA in St. Louis, Missouri, in 1971.

At first, each VA facility largely determined for itself the role of the PAs it employed. In 1972, however, the VA central office issued Circular 10-7-252, entitled "Utilization Guidelines of Physician Assistants." This document, which represented an effort to standardize the role of the PA within the VA system, defined the areas of the hospital in which the PA could be used, and specified the type and level of tasks assigned to them (Fox & Whittaker, 1983). This standardization seems to have opened the door for PAs. More than 1,800 PAs are working in more than 130 VA locations. However, the VA system is quite large and includes 172 hospitals, 68 satellite outpatient units, and 127 nursing homes. This large system is in a constant state of recruiting PAs.

Several research projects on PAs in the VA have provided a profile of roles and utilization patterns. These evaluations have enhanced the ability of the VA to establish appropriate PA and NP policies. In 1992, a study by Alexander and Lipscomb identified the allocation of time for PAs and NPs.

The VHA is divided into 22 regions designated as Veterans Integrated Service Networks. Not all facilities hire PAs, so the PA presence is larger in some regions than others and the complexity of the VA Medical Center will also determine the rate of PA use. In a VHA survey undertaken in 1998, 1,131 PAs were employed (Lyman, 1999). Approximately two-thirds (68%) were men, the mean age was 47 years, and the mean length of experience was 16 years. Most of the PAs worked in an outpatient setting (58%), but a surprisingly large group also worked inpatient (40%) (Exhibit 17-7). A majority had clinical roles; however, 54% reported working in some administrative capacities (Exhibits 17-8 and 17-9). Almost one-third (31%) indicated they would like their administrative duties increased. At the time of this survey (1998),

EXHIBIT17-7
Ratio of Primary Care Providers by Type of VA Medical Center, 2008

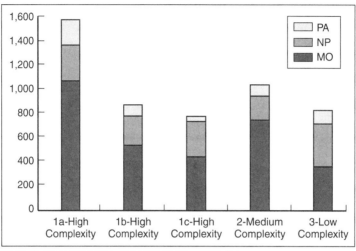

Key: PA, physician assistant; NP, nurse practitioner; MO, medical officer.

EXHIBIT17-8
Growth of Veterans Health Administration Providers, 1999–2008

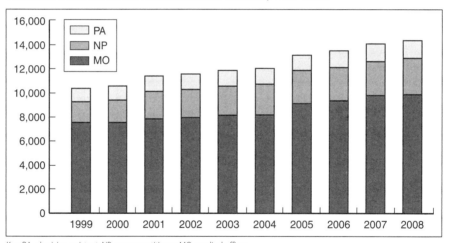

Kay: PA, physician assistant; NP, nurse practitioner; MO, medical officer.

81% had a salary between $50,000 and $70,000. Since then, the salaries of PAs within the VHA has increased, topping out for a GS-13 step 10 is approximately $107,000 (2010).

The VA has a senior PA who reports to the undersecretary of the VA. A VA Association of Physician Assistant (VAAPA) professional society meets annually to discuss policies and practices. The Public Health Service Academy of PAs (PHSAPA), which represents the U.S.

Coast Guard PAs at the AAPA constituent chapter level, are key supporters of the annual VAAPA meeting.

OTHER FEDERAL AGENCIES

Other federal agencies employing PAs include the Federal Bureau of Investigation (FBI), the Central Intelligence Agency (CIA), and the Smithsonian Institution.

EXHIBIT 17-9
Work Assignments for Physician Assistants in the Veterans Health Administration

Work Assignment	No. of Responses	%*
Primary care	287	27
Medicine and subspecialties	234	22
Surgery, anesthesia, and subspecialties	162	15
Mental hygiene/ psychiatry/ substance abuse	118	11
Long-term care/ geriatrics/hospice/ domiciliary	59	6
Employee health	46	4
Administration	36	3
Spinal cord injury	28	3
Rehabilitation	27	3
Community-based clinic/home care/ mobile clinic	25	2
Emergency medicine	13	1
Compensation and pension examinations	9	1
Critical care/urgent care/ transitional care	8	1
Women's health	4	0
Other (research, specialized laboratory, blind rehabilitation, medical informatics, Persian Gulf coordinator)	11	1
TOTAL	1,067	100

*Because of rounding, total percentage does not equal exactly 100%.

Data from Lyman, P., Elli, L., & Gebhart, R. (1999). Physician assistants in the Department of Veterans Affairs. Veterans Health System Journal, 4(3), 25–29.

Federal Bureau of Investigation

The FBI is the primary investigative arm of the U.S. DOJ, serving as a federal criminal investigative body and a domestic intelligence agency. At present, the FBI has investigative jurisdiction over violations of more than 200 categories of federal crimes, making the FBI the de facto lead law enforcement agency of the U.S. government.

Headquartered in Washington, DC, the FBI also has 56 field offices located in major cities throughout the United States, over 400 resident agencies in smaller cities and towns across the nation, and more than 50 international offices called *legal attachés* in U.S. embassies worldwide.

The number of PAs in the FBI is not known, but personal contact with two PAs in the FBI indicates that they travel frequently and are involved in the health care of FBI agents and contract employees.

Central Intelligence Agency

The CIA's primary function is to obtain and analyze information about foreign governments, corporations, and individuals and report information obtained to various branches of the government. Secondary functions include propaganda or public relations, disseminating overt and covert information, and influencing others to decide in favor of the U.S. government. The third function of the CIA is to be the "hidden hand" of the federal government by engaging in covert operations. This is undertaken by direction of the president, with oversight by Congress.

The CIA employs PAs to work with individuals in organizations performing medical care. Responsibilities include establishing and operating independent duty clinics; treating illness and medical emergencies, including managing trauma, performing physical examinations, and interpreting diagnostic tests; teaching in the areas of survival, field medicine, trauma stabilization, first-aid, and cardiopulmonary resuscitation; and performing administrative duties. Although initial assignments and training are usually in the Washington, DC area, travel tends to be extensive and PA employees must be available for worldwide assignment. Entry salary is dependent upon experience. The number of PAs employed in the CIA is not known.

Smithsonian Institution

The Smithsonian Institution is a museum complex as well as an educational and research institute. It is administered and funded by the government of the United States and by funds from its endowment, contributions, and profits from its shops and its magazine. Most of its facilities are located in Washington, DC, but its zoo, 19 museums, and eight research centers include sites in New York City, Virginia, Panama, and elsewhere.

In 2007, the Smithsonian Institution hired two PAs to work at their Washington DC headquarters and museums. They principally work in occupational health and assist the Institute's medical director and nursing staff with expanding roles in travel medicine (care for scientists and researchers who travel throughout the world collecting specimens). A collateral role is assisting the Smithsonian Institute's leadership in emergency planning such as continuity of operations, pandemic influenza preparations, and other activities.

Research and Federal Physician Assistants

The United States is the largest single employer of PAs, yet the various tasks performed by PAs in this setting have not been outlined. Additional research will not only improve health services delivery but will provide information for other countries considering similar roles. Following is a brief review of research areas in need of attention.

- **Case reports:** What does a federal PA do in his or her role? What are the charges of a battalion medical officer PA; a NOAA PA afloat; a BOP PA; or a Peace Corps PA?

- **History:** Who was the first federally employed PA? How did government agencies arrive at the notion to employ a PA?

- **Organization:** How do the VA and the Army organize PAs in terms of structure, influence, staffing ratios, policy development, and leadership?

- **Education:** How does the education of a PA in the IPAP compare with civilian programs in terms of topics, classroom hours, and outcome measures?

- **Supervision:** How does a doctor supervise a remotely deployed PA in the Navy or Coast Guard?

- **Clinic roles:** How does an Air Force PA compare to an NP in terms of characterized patients?

- **Transitions:** What are career trends of PAs when they leave the military?

- **Economics:** Is there a difference in career earnings of PAs in one military service when compared with another?

- **Governance:** How are PAs in the VA staffed and deployed?

- **Attrition:** What is the retention and annulment rate of uniformed PAs?

SUMMARY

Although the federal government remains the largest single employer of PAs, there is no central body that directly recruits PAs for federal service. Each of the military branches of the DOD, as well as federal agencies such as the VHA, Department of HHS, and BOP, have recruitment strategies for ensuring they have enough PAs to care for their members or mission. Collectively, the PAs employed by the federal government are present in more than 15 agencies. The fact that more PAs are employed each year suggests that their use is valued in large part because of their adaptability to changing roles to suit the needs of their employers and to match the demand for various forms of medical care.

Acknowledgments

The authors wish to acknowledge the advice, information, and corrections given to this chapter by the following reviewers: Michael Milner, Denni Woodmansee, William Tozier, Sandra Harding, James Cannon, Robin Hunter Buske, John Chitwood, James Jones, Frances Placides, Angelo Carter, and others.

CHAPTER **18**

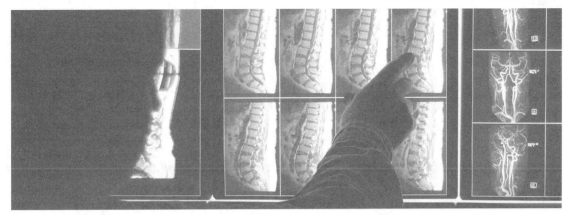

GLOBAL EXPANSION OF THE PHYSICIAN ASSISTANT CONCEPT

RODERICK S. HOOKER ■ JAMES F. CAWLEY ■ DAVID P. ASPREY

All the world's a stage,
And all the men and women merely players.
　—William Shakespeare, As You Like It, *1600*

that the development and evolution of PAs in health systems follow similar steps, suggesting there are lessons learned in the utilization of PAs that may be useful in enactment and expansion.

ABSTRACT

The global expansion of physician assistants (PAs) is a medical workforce trend that began in the 1970s but did not blossom until the turn of the century. As of 2010, at least 10 countries are in various stages of integrating PA-like medical care providers who function under the supervision of a doctor. Countries that have documented their development include Australia, Canada, England, the Netherlands, Scotland, South Africa, and Taiwan. Many of these countries have American-trained PAs working as expatriates and most have developed educational programs aimed at producing healthcare providers functioning as assistants to licensed physicians. Other countries with PAs, but less known in their development, include Eastern Europe, Ghana, Liberia, and India. Each country has made the PA a distinct entity within their health systems, each with their own cultural and educational influences shaping their roles. These PAs have common denominators: They are semi-autonomous clinicians who function under the supervision of a doctor, complementing their capacities to deliver healthcare services. Historical patterns suggest

INTRODUCTION

Shortages of doctors, especially in rural areas; rising healthcare costs; and increases in medical specialization have resulted in a number of countries looking to the physician assistant (PA) concept as one solution to medical workforce problems (Pedersen et al, 2003). For instance, England faces a challenge as a result of meeting the European Union directive to reduce the number of hours house officers are permitted to work. Canada not only has doctor shortages, but also must continue to cope with healthcare access problems for many of its citizens, including those in rural areas. The Netherlands must meet rising numbers of older patients with chronic disease, multiple co-morbidities, and escalating costs of health care. These countries and others have turned their interests to developing a U.S.-modeled PA practitioner to work closely with the doctor and to improve access to care (Exhibit 18-1).

501

EXHIBIT 18-1
Global Advancement of the Physician Assistant Profession

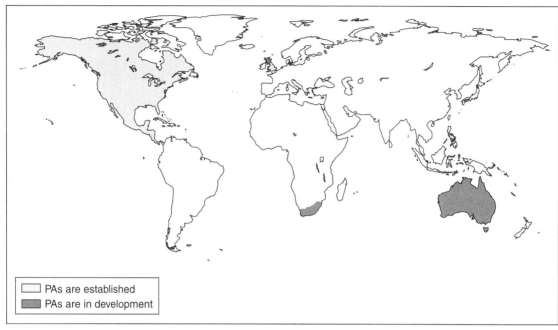

The success of the nurse-midwife, initially developed in the United Kingdom (UK), is an example of how the use of nonmedical clinicians can be optimized. This model found a toehold in other countries and is gradually expanding in the United States and Canada (Cawley & Hooker, 2003). A nonphysician practitioner, such as a nurse-midwife, gives credence to the notion of developing a more rational structure of healthcare personnel— one that makes more efficient use of the training and capabilities of doctors and affords the opportunity to use the skills of different practitioners to maximal benefit (Buchan & Dal Poz, 2002).

In one review of the literature that drew on a wide range of countries that focused on how the role of the doctor can be expanded with additional types of personnel, the authors concluded: "The use of [PA equivalents] does not compromise care quality and could serve to improve access for needy populations" (Buchan, O'May, & Ball, 2007). Although the majority of the studies reviewed by Buchan and colleagues originated in the United States,

the literature contains useful examples of expanded roles of PA-type personnel around the globe. Other authors examining literature under different lenses also conclude that the use of health personnel with different skills remains relatively unexplored but probably has merit (Mullan & Frehywot, 2007). This may be especially the case considering that in the United States the demand for PAs is outpacing supply, suggesting that they must contribute to efficiency or they would not be increasingly employed (Fenn, 2003; Legler, Cawley, & Fenn, 2007).

Australia, Canada, the Netherlands, England, and South Africa, are just some of the countries that have recognized the usefulness of PAs and have developed their own civilian PA programs (Hooker, Hogan, & Leeker, 2007) (Exhibit 18-2). Yet, the concept of assistants to doctors and PA prototypes are not new. Eastern European countries such as Russia and the Ukraine; Asian countries such as China, Malaysia, Australia, and New Guinea; much of Oceania (e.g., Micronesia, Melanesia, and Polynesia); as well as parts of

EXHIBIT 18-2
Global Physician Assistant Programs*

Country	Program (year started)	Length of Program
Canada	Canadian Defense Forces (2002)	24 months
	University of Manitoba in Winnipeg (2008)	24 months
	University of Ontario (2009)	24 months
	McMaster University (2008)	26 months
England (UK)	Kingston University (pilot program) (2002)	24 months
	St. George's University of London (pilot program) (2004)	24 months
	University of Wolverhampton, Birmingham, and Warwick (collaborative) (2004)	24 months
	St. George's University (2004)	24 months
	University of Hertfordshire (2005)	24 months
The Netherlands	Academie Gezondheidszorg in Utrecht (2001)	30 months
	University of Arnhem/Nijmegen (2003)	30 months
	University of Gronengen (2005)	30 months
	University of Leiden (2005)	30 months
Australia	University of Queensland (2009)	24 months
	James Cook University (2009)	24 months
Taiwan	Fooyin University (2004)	36 months
South Africa	University of Witswasterrand (pending)	24 months

*Entry criteria for PA education varies by country, ranging from a prerequisite of a high school education to a bachelor's degree and at least 2 years of direct patient care experience at the other end. Each institution has chosen its prerequisites based on the attainability of qualified applicants in its country.

Africa and South America have had medical aides for decades (Pereira et al, 1996; Garrido, 1997; Vaz et al, 1999). In Puerto Rico, the *practicante* was a PA prototype that lasted for the first third of the 20th century (Strand, 2006). Even in the United States, the Alaskan Community Health Aides project, developed during World War II and continuing through today, constitutes what can be referred to as prototype PAs (Landon et al, 2004). The Medex model of PAs was introduced to 14 countries as long ago as the late 1970s. In a few instances, they continue to flourish in countries such as Lesotho (R. Smith, personal communication, May 25, 2006). The PAs in Liberia and Ghana have been well entrenched for decades, even though little has been written about them. As the PA concept expands its international presence, other countries such as Japan (Haddock, 1971; Gazekpo, 2006), Germany, South Africa, and China have expressed interest in this new medical role for their citizens.

As these countries develop their PA professional, the American Academy of Physician Assistants (AAPA), along with the Physician Assistant Education Association (PAEA), serve as sources of information about PA issues, especially for those desiring to establish new educational programs, abroad or domestically. The PAEA International Affairs Committee has several documents related to international rotations for PA students. The materials provide guidelines that can be used to assist with the development of international rotations for students. This information is located at: http://www.paeaonline.org/iacpage.html.

Information about PA development internationally is fragmented. Although some information exists in reports, much of the information for this chapter was gained in the course of personal communication with knowledgeable informants and visiting the countries of interest. In some instances, representatives of the different countries visited the

EXHIBIT 18-3
Rural Health Is a Challenge for Australia's Development

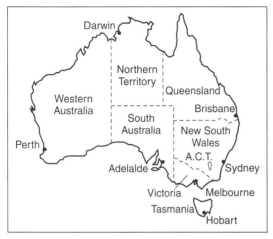

United States for in-depth information on PAs (Hooker, Hogan, & Leeker, 2007).

When the term "physician assistant" is used internationally, it has some ambiguity because in many countries the term "physician" is reserved for internal medicine specialists. Additionally, precise definitions for PAs are in flux because the role of PAs in these countries may lack some of the defining characteristics of their American counterparts (enabling legislation and ability to prescribe, order laboratory or imaging studies, work semi-autonomously, etc.). For the purposes of this chapter the PA is defined as a health professional who is authorized to work under doctor supervision to provide medical care in a delegated role. We purposely avoid framing definitions in American terms but choose instead to examine the similarities of international PA professions by observing the main areas of history, practice, and education. For the most part, the countries that are developing or have developed PA programs similar to those of the U.S. model are mentioned.

AUSTRALIA

The vastness of Australia in geographical terms is daunting. To cope with its great space, Australia has been a major importer of people,

ideas, and technology. However, throughout the last century the effort toward self-sufficiency began paying dividends and a robust population has flourished (Exhibit 18-3). Australia is the about the size of the continental United States in land mass but has a population of only 21 million (compare this to Texas, which has a population of 21 million).

Rural health remains one of the areas that continues to plague Australia's self-sufficiency and development. As of 2009, Australia had 630 rural health clinics, an aging medical workforce, an insufficient number of doctors, and a heavy reliance on the importation of medical graduates (Mullan, 2005; Australian Government of Health & Ageing, 2008). Interest in addressing doctor shortages has been growing. Most of the schemes have centered on expanding the existing supply and have been the outside-of-the-box approach that has been characteristic of other Australian enterprises (Bowman, 2007). About 400 Aboriginal health workers (AHWs) provide some of the care, but the number of doctors serving the rural populations is considered insignificant (Murray & Wronski, 2006; O'Connor & Hooker 2007).

A series of medical workforce conferences held since 2005 have focused on expanding the delegation of doctors using PAs. The idea of recruiting PAs, training AHWs and paramedics as PAs, and expanding some of the medical schools to begin PA programs, has garnered the interests of workforce planners. Visits to the AAPA annual conferences beginning in 2003 have firmed up the conviction that the PA concept is a worthwhile undertaking (Brooks, Robinson, & Ellis, 2008).

Theoretical roles for PAs in Australia have been explored in the literature. In one paper the authors suggest that PAs can be dispersed in many rural settings of Australia to help offset the busy doctor by facilitating access to care and seeing more patients. Employing PAs may also ease the sense of doctor isolation and permit indigenous people an opportunity to enter a higher level of medical care involvement (O'Connor & Hooker, 2007). The Australian College of Rural and Remote Practitioners has endorsed the concept of a PA (Sweet, 2008).

Queensland

In 2006, an Australian medical workforce conference in Mt. Isa, Queensland, concluded that the development of a medical assistant, similar to that of the U.S. PA, could play an important role in addressing the medical workforce shortage in Australia. In the consensus statement, the authors outlined the following:

- Develop sustainable team-based care with medical delegation of clinical tasks
- Allow qualified healthcare workers to obtain, possess, and administer restricted medications when acting under the delegated authority of a doctor
- Expand delegated practice to include the ambulance services, Defence [*sic*] Health Services, Aboriginal health workers, and other assistants to specialists in the private and public sector

In 2009, Queensland Health, the state government health agency, initiated a pilot project to introduce 10 PAs into its medical services as part of a demonstration project to study their feasibility. Two PA programs, one at the University of Queensland and another at James Cook University, began in 2009 and 2011, respectively.

South Australia

The South Australia government in Adelaide recruited a handful of American PAs experienced in surgery and other specialties to work. This pilot study assessed whether PAs are a viable option for the state of South Australia.

Victoria

Melbourne-based Monash University has a rural medical school campus in Bendigo, Victoria, where doctors in training are introduced to rural health medicine. Interest in expanding the rural health component to include PAs has been one of several ideas developed by this university.

CANADA

Canada is the second largest country in the world (Exhibit 18-4). Its 33 million people are spread across a vast land bounded by three

EXHIBIT 18-4

Each Canadian Province and Territory Has Its Own Regulations and Registration Procedure for Physician Assistants

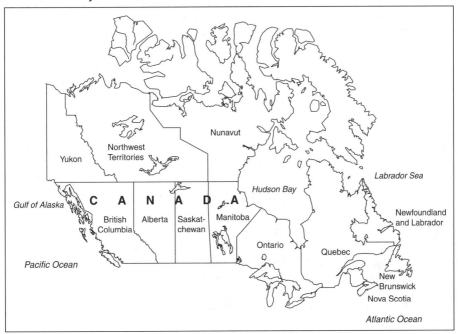

oceans and live as far north as the Arctic Circle. Delivering health care to such distant regions is challenging to say the least. Canada introduced the PA profession as a healthcare occupation in 1984 with the establishment of a military PA program. The Canada Medical Association (CMA) accredited Base Borden, an Ontario military PA program, in 2004. Functioning as the Canadian Forces Medical Services PA Program, this intramilitary institute served as the main producer of Canadian PAs and has graduated more than 200 PAs since the year 2000 (Hooker, MacDonald, & Patterson, 2003). Many military PA retirees have taken up careers in the Canadian health industry, working without the title "PA." A registry of PA graduates is under development.

Of the combined 13 provinces and territories in Canada, each has separate regulations and registration procedures. Only Manitoba has enabling legislation for PAs. Other provinces are exploring whether PAs are viable and whether regulations should be developed for them.

Alberta

Although two medical schools are located in Alberta, a province of only 3 million people, the demands for medical care are outstripping the supply of doctors. Alberta is the fastest growing province and the wealthiest because of its energy resources. One-third of its population lives in rural and underserved areas. The Northern Alberta Institute of Technology (NAIT) in Edmonton is exploring a PA program. The intent of NAIT is to serve the needs of the province and create a primary care PA.

British Columbia

British Columbia has expressed interest in developing PAs since the mid-1990s. The idea started with general practitioners (GPs) in remote locations seeking the employment of retired military PAs. The Justice Institute in Vancouver, which trains emergency medical personnel, also expressed interest in the PA concept by expressing a desire to convert paramedical workers into PAs. Because funding mechanisms were not in place for reimbursement of services, this idea did not gain traction.

In 2005, the British Columbia Medical Association published a study on the use of multidisciplinary primary care and the attitudes of 638 GPs in British Columbia (Exhibit 18-5). The survey showed that 96% of GPs see themselves continuing practice in a multidisciplinary setting within the next 5 years (British Columbia Medical Association, 2005).

A PA program has been discussed at the University of British Columbia, but as of 2008 no development has been put into motion. Students from the Canadian Forces PA program are trained at the Vancouver General Hospital in emergency medicine.

Manitoba

The province of Manitoba passed legislation in 2000 to enable experiments in delegated medical care and restated this in 2007. This was a rare occasion where legislation preceded the use of PAs. The role title was originally termed registered clinical assistants (RCAs). Later, the Minister of Health for Manitoba stated specifically that PAs were welcome to practice in the province (Fleisher, Chan, & McConnell, 2006). This initiative has allowed American PAs to officially practice in Canada. The University of Manitoba opened its doors to the first PA education class in 2008.

Manitoba is one of the latest government agencies to grant legal permission for PAs. The Manitoba Medical Association, in a comfortable arrangement with the provincial government, has provided a guiding policy for PAs, along with a rationale for their endorsement and a commitment to society to remain involved (Exhibit 18-6).

New Brunswick

New Brunswick, one of the Maritime Provinces on the eastern seaboard, is a small region with a widely dispersed population. Initiating a demonstration project that would involve a dozen or more PAs recruited from the United States and Canada has been discussed at the ministerial level. Such a project

EXHIBIT 18-5
Survey of British Columbia General Practitioners, 2005

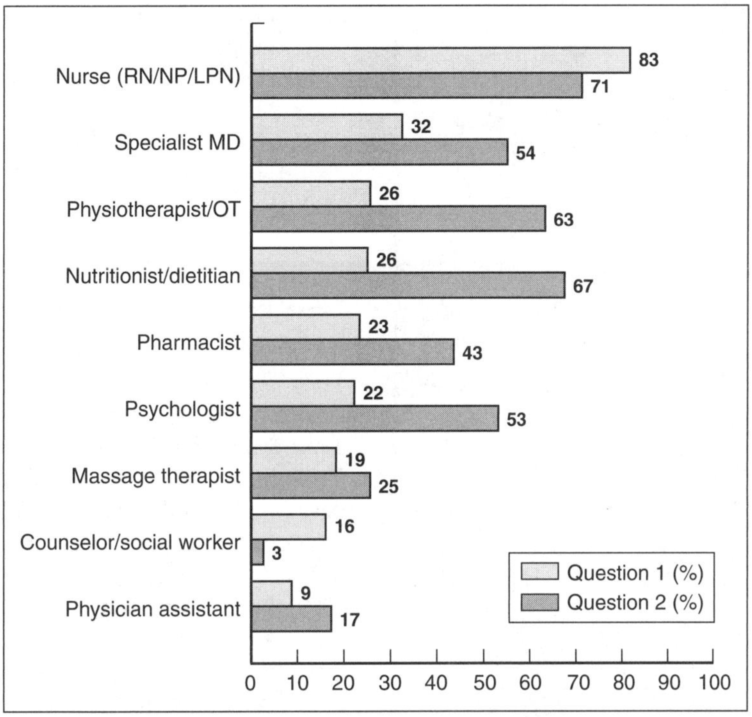

British Columbia Medical Association. (2005). Working Together—Enhancing Multidisciplinary
Primary Care in British Columbia: A Policy Paper by BC's Physicians. *British Columbia, Canada:
Author.*
*1: Types of health professionals you practise with? 2: If in multidisciplinary setting, types of health
professionals you would choose to practice with?*

would deploy PAs in emergency medicine
and assess how the public and healthcare
community views them.

Ontario

In Ontario, the minister of health began
employing civilian PAs within their healthcare
system in 2007 (Kuttler & AAPA, 2006). The
HealthForceOntario pilot project introduced
PAs into Ontario emergency programs, hospitals, and community health clinics (primary
care sites). By establishing demonstration sites
to observe the PA model, this pilot program
allows Ontario to examine the best way to
design an educational system.

The emergency medical project was the
first to be launched. It staffs emergency
medical departments with PAs and nurse
practitioners (NPs) and compares outcomes
of care. One of the assessments was to examine outcomes of ankle injuries managed by
doctors, PAs, and NPs. This diagnosis is a
useful indicator because the management is
straightforward and outcomes can be tested.
Preliminary findings suggest that PAs and
NPs provide near identical care as doctors
and the outcomes are favorable without
incurring a high burden of supervision.

The second of three prongs of this initiative
was to recruit PAs from the United States and
those retired from the Canadian military.
Approximately 40 PAs have been recruited
and dispersed in Ontario. They are deployed
in emergency departments (EDs), community
health clinics, and hospitals.

International medical graduates (IMGs)
are one focus on the *HealthForceOntario's*

EXHIBIT 18-6
Manitoba Medical Association Policy Statement on Physician Assistants

1. There is a chronic shortage of physicians, both in Manitoba and across Canada.

2. This shortage of physicians has resulted in a lack of timely access to medical services and a corresponding decline in the health status/quality of life of countless Manitobans. The shortage has also placed additional stress on the current complement of physicians in the province, as they struggle to provide medical services.

3. For the good of both Manitobans and Manitoba physicians, it is essential that the province's physician supply be increased, both through an increase in the enrollment in our medical school and through concerted efforts to recruit and retain physicians in the province.

4. It is also essential that efforts be made to extend the capacity of Manitoba's physician workforce, in a manner that contributes to the sustainability of the physician workforce and enhances the work life of physicians.

5. The Manitoba Medical Association (MMA) is supportive of the philosophy of physician assistants, in that these professionals can expand the capacity of the physician workforce in a manner that is collaborative, rather than competitive. As such, the MMA is supportive of the University of Manitoba Faculty of Medicine's *Physician Assistant Education Program.*

6. It is crucial that physician assistants be integrated into physician practices, including fee-for-service practices, in a manner whereby issues of medical/legal liability will be appropriately addressed, and whereby all physicians will be appropriately compensated, taking into account such considerations as cost of practice and responsibility issues associated with physician assistants.

7. To ensure that the issues of medical/legal liability and physician compensation be given due consideration, it is imperative that the MMA have representation on the *Physician Assistant Steering Committee Working Group on Remuneration and Liability.*

Adopted by the MMA Board on May 9, 2007.

initiative. Because in Ontario alone there are over 2,000 IMGs without licenses to practice and not always eligible for postgraduate residencies, Ontario decided to see if some of the IMGs could be converted to PAs. A project was undertaken (amidst some controversy) and 24 IMGs underwent 3 months of training to function as PAs. Strict rules govern how these PAs can address and view themselves.

After 2 years working as PAs, these IMGs may compete for residencies with the general pool of postgraduate doctors.

The third initiative of *HealthForceOntario* is to fund two PA programs in medical institutions: McMaster's University (2008) and North Ontario University (2010). Both will produce traditional type 24-month trained PAs, but McMaster's will draw on its renowned experience using problem-based learning.

Canadian Association of Physician Assistants

The Canadian Association of Physician Assistants (CAPA) was established in 1999, with a grant by the Canada Department of National Defence, to serve as a unifying body encompassing both military and civilian PA sectors. In November 2001, CAPA developed a civilian PA profile that the Canadian Forces adopted. As of 2009, the association has more than 70 members and a set of regional chapters. CAPA also developed a certification process and provides consultation to developing programs.

Candidates for certification must be graduates of a PA training program, must be accredited by the Canadian Medical Association, must have previously been practicing as a Canadian PA, or must be certified by the National Commission on Certification of Physician Assistants (NCCPA). New graduates from a CMA-accredited institution must hold CAPA membership and pass the certification examination before they may practice. PAs who have previously practiced in Canada must be graduates of a pre-accreditation Canadian Forces program, hold CAPA membership, have 100 hours of continuing medical education (CME) in the past 3 years, have held direct patient care responsibility in the past 5 years, and have successfully completed the certification examination. The certification period is 3 years.

American-trained PAs must acquire certification in Canada by graduating from an Accreditation Review Commission for Physician Assistant Education (ARC-PA) accredited program, holding CAPA membership, holding a currently valid NCCPA certificate, or successfully completing the Canadian certification examination.

ENGLAND

In England, a directive to reduce the number of hours house officers are permitted to work led to a need for additional medical providers. At the same time, as in other countries, there has been an inexorable trend toward physician specialization, leading to shortages in the number of primary care providers (Fenn, 2003; Hutchinson, 2006). Additionally, as the United Kingdom (UK) adjusts to a reorganization of their health system, titled "Medical Modernization," England (Exhibit 18-7), Scotland, Wales, and Ireland are

EXHIBIT 18-7
Provider Shortages Led England to Initiate Physician Assistant Pilot Programs

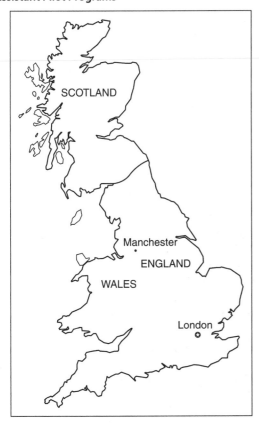

exploring new provider roles in health care (Cameron, 2005). British National Health Service officials see the potential for the PA concept to alleviate some of the time constraints experienced by doctors and to increase staffing in emergency settings, especially those in which patient volume is high relative to the number of providers available.

Although England had an adequate physician workforce at the beginning of the century, it became apparent that they would not be able to sustain access and desired care levels without growing their clinician sector, especially in the hospitals. In response, England initiated a pilot program to test the applicability of American PAs in their healthcare system. The Tipton Care Organization and Great Bridge Partnership for Health recruited two PAs from the United States in 2002 for the pilot program; later, the Rowley Regis and Tipton Primary Care Trust expanded this number to 14. The intent of the demonstration project was to reduce waiting time in the ED to less than 4 hours and to reduce length of stay in hospitals (Buchan, Ball, & O'May, 2006), as well as help meet national targets for waiting times and treatment goals in the general practice setting. There are approximately 40 U.S.-trained PAs in England.

The success of the pilot program influenced the PA-modeled curricula at the University of Birmingham in Southwest England, which started in 2008. This PA program is a collaborative effort with the Universities of Wolverhampton and Warwick. The University of Wolverhampton is the very first program in the UK. It was launched September 2004 and the first graduates finished in June 2006 (Parle, Ross, & Doe, 2006).

Professional Title

Initially, the new providers were given the title of medical care practitioner (MCP). This title was in contrast to the American term of "physician assistant." This initial terminology was in part due to the term "physician" and refers specifically to an internist rather than a general practitioner or a subspecialty practitioner (Westwood & Richardson, 2005). In 2006, the Department of Health replaced the working title of MCP with *physician assistant* after a positive response from public surveys agreed that the PA title was appropriate or not problematic. This title is a working title until the profession is fully established and the regulatory body approves the appropriate protected title.

Education Programs

At first the various practitioner programs in the British medical system developed separately, each falling under the Department of Health. However, all of these programs were being developed to produce workers within various areas of medicine (e.g., emergency medicine, hospitalist roles, surgical role). Later it became apparent there were overlapping educational components. To resolve this issue, the UK brought the various groups together to ensure consistency and transferability nationally of practitioner roles at assistant, senior, and advanced levels. The UK National Health Service (NHS) created the National Practitioner Program (NPP), which was ultimately superseded by two integral groups: the National Reference Panel and the UK Universities Board for the Development of Physician Assistants.

The National Reference Panel, which reports to the Department of Health, is made up of representatives from the Departments of Health, patients, the Royal Colleges of Physicians and General Practitioners, universities (those with and without medical schools), the National Examinations Board (a subgroup of the UK Universities Board), and a PA. Together they form the UK Universities Board for the Development of the Physicians Assistant, which is the educator's board and represents all of the universities in the UK that offer or are interested in offering programs of PA education. The group sets quality standards and has a subgroup that hosts the national written and practical examinations.

Hertfordshire, Kingston/St. George's University of London, London South Bank University, University of Surrey, Wolverhampton University, and the University of Birmingham have established PA programs (Exhibit 18-8). However, as of this writing, some are on hold due to financial

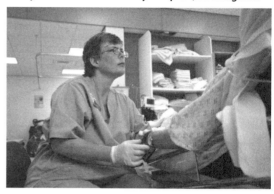

EXHIBIT 18-8
A Physician Assistant at City Hospital, Birmingham

Courtesy of Kirsten Gipson, PA-C.

issues. PA programs in England are 2 years in length, with a third "probationary" year working in a clinical environment. The exception is the Kingston University/St. George's University of London Pilot Program. This program's structure consists of 70% work-based learning in a range of clinical settings, supervised by senior doctors or attending physicians. The remaining 30% of the curriculum is didactic, and includes courses on physical assessment and clinical decision-making. Each program is competency-based. Since publication of the Department of Health curriculum framework, additional knowledge-building and other learning activities have been incorporated into the program.

The remainder of the PA programs, in accordance with the NHS Competence and Curriculum Framework for the Physician Assistant requirements, consist of a total of 3,150 hours (Ross & Parle, 2008). Of these hours, 1,600 (51%) are devoted to clinical learning, 1,400 of which are in a clinical area attached to a unit or doctor (rather than simulation). The remaining 1,550 hours (49%) are didactic (Exhibit 18-9).

Registration Considerations

The NHS Competence and Curriculum Framework for the Physician Assistant has established a National Examination Board to administer a single national assessment of clinical competence, similar to that of the Physician Assistant National Certification

EXHIBIT 18-9
Physician Assistant Program Minimum Requirements in the United Kingdom

1,000 hours of specified clinical experience	600 hours of additional clinical experience	200 hours may be spent in clinical skills centres
Community medicine (Minimum 280 hours)		
General hospital medicine (Minimum 350 hours)		
Accident and emergency (Minimum 160 hours)		
Mental health (Minimum 70 hours)		
Paediatrics (acute) (Minimum 70 hours)		
Obstetrics and gynecology (Minimum 70 hours)		

Data from Ross, N. & Parle, J. (2008). Physician assistants: A UK perspective on clinical need, education and regulation. Clinical Teacher, 5(1), 28–32.

Examination (PANCE). Part one of the examination evaluates general medical knowledge; part two evaluates patient care; and part three evaluates physical examination skills. Upon passing the examination, an individual is subject to a 12-month "probationary" period. After fulfilling the probationary period, the PA is granted registration. Failing any portion of this process warrants an additional period of provisional registration and training.

The United Kingdom Association of Physician Assistants (UKAPA) permits a probationary practice period between the time of the examination and the release of the results. During this probationary period, the practitioner is entitled to practice under strict monitoring and review by the supervising physician, but has limited or no prescriptive or referral authority while waiting for exam results. Only when the PA has received the exam results and has passed all portions of the exam can he or she practice in partnership with the physician and enjoy full prescriptive and referral authority as a qualified PA. Their website is: http://www.ukapa.co.uk/.

It is worth noting that all American PAs and British graduates currently work under Article 54, the Delegation and Referral clause of the General Medical Council's Handbook for Good Medical Practice, despite the fact that registration of the profession has not taken place. The article states that:

> Delegation involves asking a colleague to provide treatment or care on your behalf. Although you will not be accountable for the decisions and actions of those to whom you delegate, you will still be responsible for the overall management of the patient, and accountable for your decision to delegate. When you delegate care or treatment you must be satisfied that the person to whom you delegate has the qualifications, experience, knowledge and skills to provide the care or treatment involved. You must always pass on enough information about the patient and the treatment they need. (General Medical Council, 2006)

The framework gives educational institutions the option to use the national exam for either graduation or registration; any further assessment is left to the discretion of each institution. National recertification will also be required every 6 years, just as it is in the United States. Continuing professional development

(CPD) is also proposed, in a manner similar to the U.S. model of CME, in order to fulfill the professional education requirement of the PA.

THE NETHERLANDS

The Netherlands is a small country adjacent to the North Sea. With 16 million inhabitants in its 400,000 square kilometers, it is one of the more densely populated countries in Europe (Exhibit 18-10). Yet it is an affluent country with a healthy population and a sound healthcare system. Despite debates over the quality and financing of health care and training of healthcare personnel, the Dutch have crafted a high-quality health infrastructure and medical education system (Ten Cate, 2007). The decision to establish PAs was fueled by a need to alleviate the workload of physicians and to prepare for an aging population that would demand more medical services. The consensus was that task redistribution and responsibilities between different categories of healthcare professionals was desirable (RVZ, 2002).

The PA was introduced to the Netherlands in the department of cardiovascular surgery at the University Hospital in Utrecht in 1999. In 2001, a pilot program was launched with four students. After a successful evaluation of the PA program, a set of education initiatives were proposed. The Hogeschool Arnhem/Nijmegen and the Academie Gezondheidszorg in Utrecht developed a national framework for PAs in collaboration with the university hospitals, which was later underwritten by the Department of Education and Science (Verboon, 2005).

Educational Programs

There are four PA training programs in the Netherlands, all fairly uniform in curriculum (van Everdinck et al, 2006). The curricula are modeled in part after the American PA educational design, with the inclusion of a master's research project as a mandatory requirement for program completion (Harbert et al, 2004; Spenkelink-Schut, Koch, & Kort, 2006; van Everdinck et al, 2006). In 2001, the first class of students at the University of Applied Science/Academy of Health Care in Utrecht began their educational process (Exhibit 18-11). Following

EXHIBIT 18-10
The Netherlands Is One of the Most Densely Populated Countries in Europe

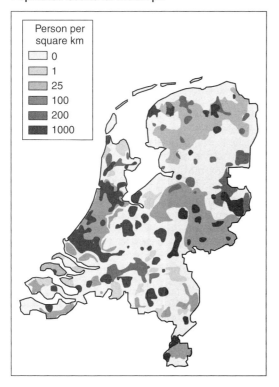

Person per square km

- [ ] 0
- [ ] 1
- [ ] 25
- [ ] 100
- [ ] 200
- [ ] 1000

EXHIBIT18-11
An Inpatient Physician Assistant in the Netherlands

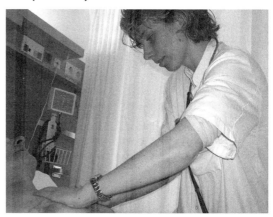

the success of that program, in 2003 the University of Applied Science Arnhem/Nijmegen opened a second 30-month PA program, and graduated its first class in 2006.

In addition to establishing a national curriculum, in 2003 an accreditation process was established by the Dutch Flemish Organization. As a result, the Department of Education and Science in the Netherlands now recognizes PA programs.

Two more programs were established in 2005: at the University of Groningen and the University of Amsterdam. As of 2009, more than 200 PAs have graduated in the Netherlands. The Dutch PAs established their own national organization and governing body for PAs, the Netherlands Association of PAs (NAPA).

In the Netherlands, PA graduates are fully qualified to enter their profession without further study, licensing, or registration. The curriculum design is a competency-based didactic concept, intensely oriented toward the clinical environment. The combined didactic and clinical hours of the program total 4,200 hours or 150 European Credit Points in 2.5 years. Of these hours, 1,400 didactic hours are spent in basic science, patient assessment, clinical medicine courses, tutorial groups, skill labs, lectures, problem-based group activities, and seminars. The remaining 2,800 hours are spent in a clinical setting, under supervision of a designated doctor. This mentorship occurs from the start of the curriculum, beginning in the didactic phase of the program, and continues with clinical rotations with different physician specialists in the later phase of the program (Spenkelink-Schut, Koch, & Kort, 2006).

Within training seminars, students discuss particular self-study topics assigned to them by educators and focused around the current lecture content. Students are also expected to work on specific scientific problems (comparable to case studies) that have been assigned prior to seminars, which directly correlate with classroom material. The coursework is covered in a systems or block format, much like that of American PA programs. However, didactic and clinical portions occur simultaneously.

During the course of the program, students prepare a master's project. The purpose of the master's project is to understand the process of medical research, to interpret the medical literature, and to identify strengths and weaknesses of medical research. Toward the end of the training, students present an oral defense of their research and are given the opportunity to publish their work.

Cost of education in Holland differs from other PA programs in that students receive a government stipend during their clinical training. To qualify for selection all students must have a minimum of 2 years of direct patient care experience before enrollment. In addition, all students remain qualified to perform services in their previous area of expertise.

Accreditation, Certification, and Registration

As of 2009 there is no formal certification system or licensure in the Netherlands for PAs. Instead, the focus has been on the program accreditation process to ensure a competent PA. The Ministry of Health, Welfare, and Sport oversees the Law on Professions in Individual Health Care (known by the Dutch acronym BIG), which sets rules for all healthcare professionals concerning patient protection and quality of care (van Everdinck et al, 2006). The BIG law involves a registry of all healthcare professionals who have graduated from an accredited program. The BIG register includes pharmacists, physicians, physiotherapists, psychologists, psychotherapists, dentists, midwives, nurses, and PAs. The professions listed in this register are the only providers that may use the legally protected titles belonging to these professions. Under Dutch law, anyone is entitled to practice medicine to some extent, but a set of excluded procedures (such as surgical procedures) limits the practice to only those professions designated to carry out select procedures (van Everdinck et al, 2006).

Graduates working as PAs remain registered in their pre-PA profession (e.g., registered nurse or physical therapist), depending on their previous area of expertise (van Everdinck et al, 2006). No annual CME requirements exist for PAs or doctors. In 2007, the Dutch Health Care Inspectorate (IGZ), following an exploratory study, concluded that the transfer of tasks and responsibilities from doctors to PAs has made a positive contribution to safe, effective, patient-focused, and accessible care in the Netherlands.

As PAs develop globally there is anticipation that PAs may be able to move across borders. For example, a Dutch-born, American-trained PA works in family practice in an outpatient setting. This PA has been subject to the same restrictions as Dutch PAs because the Netherlands' programs are considered equivalent to U.S. PA programs (van Everdinck et al, 2006). As long as the Dutch government recognizes the program of study in the United States, then U.S.-trained PAs may qualify for registration in the Netherlands (Simkens et al, 2009).

Prescribing

PAs have not yet been authorized to prescribe medication. A proposal has been made to include the PA and the NP titles in the Law on Prescription of Medicine to grant PAs the authority to prescribe. Securing this legal position requires (1) a demonstrable and adequate teaching process for relevant skills in an area of expertise or specialization, and (2) reliable supervision by a physician. As the PA profession continues to develop, the goal is to be regulated like doctors on a national level. However, some scholars have challenged that stiffer regulation may produce limitations instead of the desired flexibility of the PA concept (Verboon, 2005).

SCOTLAND

Scotland has a population of 5 million and has four medical universities. For more than a century it has been a major exporter of doctors. It also has an inversion of the population pyramid, with an increased number of aging citizens, shrinking numbers of young people to educate, decreasing fertility rates, and an escalating demand for healthcare services. In the medical fields, there is a lack of generalists and an excess of specialists, presenting

challenges to the flexibility of delivery. The National Health Service (NHS) of Scotland believes care should be provided as locally as possible, but also as centrally as needed, moving health care out of hospitals and into communities—adding workforce capacity and capability. In late 2006, a dozen American PAs began working in Scotland as part of a 2-year demonstration project to investigate the potential success of the utilization of PAs in its healthcare system (Exhibit 18-12).

Although there is no PA education system in Scotland, the Scotland NHS has analyzed the demonstration project in terms of the PA roles provided, the impact they made, and the reception of the health system to their inclusion. The creation of a PA training program in Scotland could provide deployment to new posts and have a significant effect on the delivery of patient care, cutting costs, efficiency, teamwork, use of referrals, and patient waiting times (Farmer et al, 2009).

EXHIBIT 18-12
Scotland: Location of the PA Demonstration Projects in 2007–2009

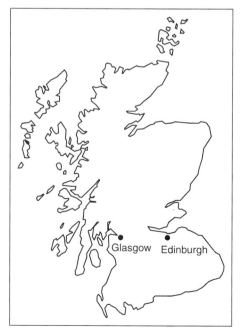

The Accreditation of Prior and Experiential Learning (APEL) facilitates the accreditation of nurses and other healthcare workers in Scotland. Currently, those practitioners who are accredited through this system could potentially transfer their accreditation or registration should they choose to make a career change to become a PA. This approach, however, is subject to change as the PA role becomes more defined.

Regulation for PAs has been somewhat of an obstacle for the NHS, especially due to the fact that the PA role has not been tested and proven to work. Scotland realizes that it is difficult to guarantee that regulation and legislation supports the boundaries and goals of a new role without the education, competencies, accountability, and the role itself being well developed. Thus, there is a paradoxical situation in that there is a great deal of work to do before getting regulation, but it is difficult to create new roles without the reassurance of having regulatory standards already in place.

TAIWAN, REPUBLIC OF CHINA

In the mid-1990s, Taiwan became the first Asian country to enact universal health care for its citizens. Almost overnight a flood of pent-up demand for care was unleashed. Demand for services surged and a shortage of doctors was revealed. Shortly afterward, a group of nurses were allowed to increase their scope of practice in order to help with this swell in medical demand. Doctors who had trained in the United States and knew something about PAs created most of this education. At first the education process was on-the-job training, and each large medical center acted as its own education institution. This advanced training earned the nurses the title of physician assistant or nurse specialist, depending on the center where they worked. In 2004, a survey of 111 hospitals identified approximately 1,400 nurses working in advanced practice roles that could be described as PAs (or NPs) but always under the supervision of a doctor (Exhibit 18-13).

Taiwan has one formal PA program at Fooyin University. It began in 2003 and graduated 40 students in 2006. This program provides a postgraduate-type education for nurses to work as PA equivalents. They are not used in the same context as in the United States or other countries that have introduced the PA concept. The program is 3 years in length and has campuses in three parts of the country. Unlike the U.S. PA model, didactic and clinical learning are integrated. Students spend 2 days per week in the hospital setting and 3 days per week in the classroom. Half of the clinical experience is spent in the student's "current specialty," which is obtained prior to entrance into Fooyin's PA program. When these PAs work in hospitals, they function similar to U.S. NPs and PAs; however, they typically work within nursing departments/services.

PAs can be found in various settings in Taiwan. A 2004 survey by Liu and colleagues

EXHIBIT 18-13

At One Time, Taiwan Had a Physician Assistant Program in Kao-hsiung

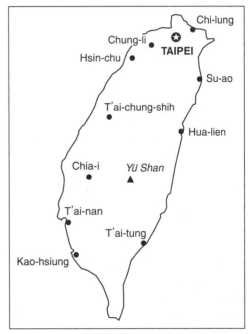

(2005) identified 1,419 PAs who were employed at the 111 responding hospitals. The majority of these PAs worked in surgery (39%) or internal medicine (37%), with the remainder in obstetrics, pediatrics, and emergency medicine. Twenty-four percent of these practicing PAs have a bachelor's or master's degree. The remainder have an associate's degree.

At one time students graduating from Fooyin University received a bachelor's of science in nursing and a PA document. The PA document recognizes graduation from the established PA program at Fooyin, but is not recognized by the government. Promoters of the PA profession, such as Dr. Kao-Lo, worked with the Ministry of Health in Taiwan in order to obtain legal recognition of PAs in the health system and with the Ministry of Education to legitimize the PA degree. Due to political resistance from physicians and government agencies, such recognition has not yet occurred, despite the fact that the PA may prove to be a major health service to the country. As of 2008, Fooyin University has redirected its efforts toward the NP concept.

AFRICA

Over one-half of the 47 countries in sub-Saharan Africa have some form of nonphysician provider (Exhibit 18-14). These providers are trained beyond secondary school and function in some form in the absence of a doctor or as an extension of a doctor. Many are recruited from rural and poor areas, and work in the same region. For some countries, these nonphysician providers are the main conduit for delivering HIV/AIDs treatment and prevention. In about a fifth of the countries, the number of such providers exceeds the number of doctors (Mullan & Frehywot, 2007).

Known by various names, including "sub-assistant surgeons," "senior native medical assistant," "medical auxiliary," "clinical officer," and "medical assistant (MA)," many of these providers have been part of health care in the area for more than a half-century (Exhibit 18-15). For example, in Ethiopia

health officers have been trained at the University of Gonder since 1954. In Ghana, the Rural Health Service trains MAs to deliver care semiautonomously and to function in small villages and rural locations. There are approximately 300 MAs in Ghana, but a new program has been developed that is modeled after the U.S. PA model.

In Liberia, the PA title has already been developed and adopted. The Liberian PA is given 3 years of preservice education and a 1-year clinical internship (Mullan & Frehywot, 2007). They are trained for rural deployment and are capable of handling non-Cesarean deliveries as well as general medical conditions. More recently, South Africa has announced that they are starting a PA program at the University of Witwatersrand in Cape Town.

CENTRAL AND SOUTH AMERICA

Numbers of prototype PAs in Central and South America are difficult to come by. Sometimes national data are distorted by internal inequalities in terms of poverty and health. With regard to income inequalities, the United Nations publication, *The Millennium Development Goals: A Latin American and Caribbean Perspective*, states, "The Latin American countries' poor income distribution has earned the region the dubious distinction of being the least equitable region in the world." Within this region, Panama stands behind only Bolivia, Brazil, and the Dominican Republic as the countries with the most inequitable income distributions (Exhibit 18-16). Only now are some of these inequities being addressed. One of the ideas is that of developing a PA or other nonphysician provider for Latin America. These discussions take place in meetings of the World Health Organization, UNICEF, and the Global Health Initiative.

COMMON DENOMINATORS

At the heart of the expansion of PAs is the need to improve access and healthcare delivery due to new technology, aging citizens, and remote

EXHIBIT 18-14
Over One-Half of the 47 Countries in Sub-Saharan Africa Have Some Form of Nonphysician Provider

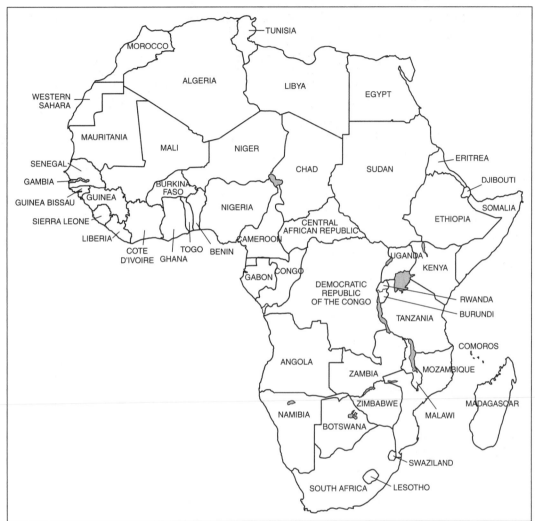

populations. Excluding the Netherlands, every developed country falls short of the 3/1,000 doctor-to-population ratio average (Organization for Economic Cooperation and Development [OECD], 2008). Additionally, many of the countries have reduced the work hours of doctors in training and now need to address doctor shortages more precisely. Exhibit 18-17 shows the population and doctor ratio of these countries. Taiwan has the largest number of "PAs" per capita compared with other countries, and Australia has the smallest number.

In the United States, Australia, South Africa, and Canada, the number of individuals living in rural populations and the remoteness of these populations are substantial (Exhibit 18-18). Although each country defines rural and remote differently (as well as the degree of "rurality"), all have comparatively low doctor-to-rural-population concentrations. The World Health Organization (WHO) estimated that in 2005 75% to 80% of the world's doctors practice in urban localities (Dal Poz et al, 2006). Many countries, like the United States, have difficulty enticing physicians to rural and remote areas, providing additional impetus to develop PA-enabling policies for this citizenry (Jones & Hooker, 2001; Breusch, 2008).

EXHIBIT 18-15
Types of Nonphysician Clinicians in Sub-Saharan African Countries

Country	Clinician Name	Basic Entrance Requirement	Preservice Education (years)	Internship Duration	Scope of Practice	Practice Locale
Angola	Clinical Officer	Secondary School	3	N/A	Medicine, minor surgery, obstetrics (but no caesarean section)	Urban and rural
Burkina Faso	Clinical Officer	Secondary School	3	N/A	Medicine, minor surgery	Urban and rural
Botswana	Nurse Clinicians	RN with experience	1	None	Medicine, obstetrics (but no caesarean section)	Urban and rural
Cape Verde	Health Officer	Secondary School	3	1	Medicine	Urban and rural
Ethiopia	Health Officer	BS or RN	3	1	Medicine, minor surgery, obstetrics including caesarean section	Urban and rural
Gabon	Clinical Officer	Secondary School	3	1	Medicine	Urban and rural
Ghana	Medical Assistant	RN	1	0.5	Medicine, obstetrics (but no caesarean section)	Mostly rural
Guinea-Bissau	Clinical Officer	Secondary School	3	N/A	Medicine	Urban and rural
Kenya	Clinical Officer	Secondary School	3	1	Medicine, minor surgery	Urban and rural
Lesotho	Nurse Officers	RN with 5 years experience	1	1	Medicine, obstetrics (but no caesarean section), public health	Urban and rural
Liberia	Physician Assistant	Secondary School	3	1	Medicine, obstetrics (but no caesarean section)	Rural
Malawi	Clinical Officer	Secondary School	3	1	Medicine, minor surgery, obstetrics including caesarean section	Urban and rural
Mauritius	Community Healthcare Officer	Secondary School	3	1	Medicine, obstetrics (but no caesarean section)	Mostly rural
Mozambique	Clinical Officer	Secondary School	2.5	1	Medicine, minor surgery, obstetrics including caesarean section	Urban and rural
Rwanda	Nurse Clinician	RN with experience	1	None	Medicine, obstetrics (but no caesarean section)	Mostly rural
Senegal	Health Officer	N/A	N/A	N/A	Medicine, minor surgery, obstetrics	Urban and rural
Seychelles	Nurse Clinician	RN	1	None	Medicine	Urban and rural
Sierra Leone	Community Health Officer	Secondary School	2	0.5	Medicine, obstetrics (but no caesarean section)	Mostly rural
South Africa	Physician Assistant	Secondary School	3	N/A	Medicine	Rural
Sudan	Clinical Officer	Secondary School	3	None	Medicine, minor surgery, obstetrics	Rural
Tanzania	Assistant Medical Officer	3 years experience	2	None	Medicine, minor surgery, obstetrics including caesarean section	Urban and rural

EXHIBIT 18-15
Types of Nonphysician Clinicians in Sub-Saharan African Countries—cont'd

Country	Clinician Name	Basic Entrance Requirement	Preservice Education (years)	Internship Duration	Scope of Practice	Practice Locale
Togo	Medical Assistant	RN	2	N/A	Medicine, minor surgery, obstetrics (but no caesarean section)	Urban and rural
Uganda	Clinical Officer	Secondary School	3	2	Medicine, hospice care	Urban and rural
Zambia	Clinical Officer	Secondary School	3	1	Medicine, obstetrics (but no caesarean section), anesthesia, orthopedics	Mostly rural
Zimbabwe	Health Officer	Secondary School	2-3	2	Medicine, obstetrics (but no caesarean section)	Urban and rural

Data from Mullan, F., & Frehywot, S. (2007). Non-physician clinicians in 47 sub-Saharan African countries. Lancet, 370(9605), 2158–2163.

EXHIBIT 18-16
Nonphysician Providers Are Being Considered for Central and South America to Address Inequities in Healthcare

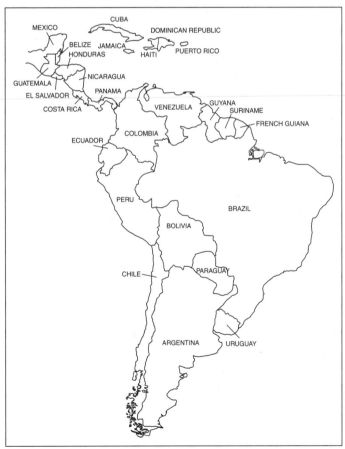

EXHIBIT 18-17
Population Statistics—Doctors and Physician Assistants, 2008

Country	Population	No. of PAs	No. of Doctors	Doctor/Population Ratio
Australia	20,264,082	4	47,875	2.6/1,000
Canada	33,098,932	170	66,583	2.1/1,000
England (UK)	60,609,153	48	133,641	2.3/1,000
Netherlands	16,491,461	75	50,854	3.2/1,000
Scotland	5,062,011	12	12,738	2.5/1,000
South Africa	47,391,900	0	30,740	0.7/1,000
Taiwan	23,036,087	1,400	24,418	1.1/1,000
United States	311,000,000	68,000	650,000	2.1/1,000

Data from Hooker, R. S., Hogan, K., & Leeker, E. (2007). The globalization of the physician assistant profession. Journal of Physician Assistant Education, 18(3), 76–85.

FUTURE OF GLOBAL PHYSICIAN ASSISTANTS

The expansion of the American-type PA model has been underway in various forms and countries for over two decades. A timeline demonstrates this chronological development (Exhibit 18-19). Early data suggest other countries are experiencing similar satisfaction with and acceptance of PAs as has occurred in the United States (Woodin et al, 2005).

EXHIBIT 18-18
Rural Versus Urban Demographics

Country	Percent Rural Population	Percent Urban Population
Australia	7	93
Canada	19	81
England (UK)	11	89
Netherlands	33	67
Scotland	20	80
South Africa	22	78
Taiwan	32	68
United States	14	86

Data from Hooker, R. S., Hogan, K., & Leeker, E. (2007). The globalization of the physician assistant profession. Journal of Physician Assistant Education, 18(3), 76–85.

The U.S. model has been examined by several countries and appears to lend itself to meet workforce needs for some (McCabe, 2007). The use of pilot programs has yet to be proven as a tested strategy in gaining approval officially, but anecdotes abound about the ready acceptance expatriate PAs have received in the communities where they work. Benefits of programs being associated with medical schools have not been reported (although these benefits have not been documented in the United States either).

The implementation of knowledgeable, American-trained PAs may provide some role modeling and assistance to global healthcare settings (Frossard et al, 2008). In addition to their clinical role, PAs can serve as ambassadors of good will and pioneers in novel healthcare delivery, a valuable social role. Lessons can also be learned from the patterns observed with the introduction of PAs into the health systems of various countries. For example, in America, where states confer the right to practice medicine, the movement to introduce PAs into clinical practice took the better part of 40 years to fully accomplish (with the goal of enabling legislation, prescription rights, and reimbursement for services). In other countries, where the impetus to introduce PAs comes from the central government,

EXHIBIT 18-19
Timeline of Physician Assistant Development Globally

Year	Country	Milestone
1967	United States	The first formally trained PAs graduate from Duke University.
1984	Canada	Canadian military graduates first PAs.
1997	Taiwan (Republic of China)	Taiwan enacts universal health care and converts nurses in large medical centers to PAs using advanced training and on-the-job training.
1999	Canada	Manitoba enacts legislation enabling PAs to work in the civilian sector.
2000	The Netherlands	PAs begin training at hospitals for inpatient service.
2002	Taiwan	Fooyin University starts its first PA program.
2002	England	England recruits its first PAs.
2004	England	First PAs graduate from Woolverhampton University.
2004	Canada	Canadian Forces PA Program becomes accredited by the Canadian Medical Association.
2006	Scotland	U.S. PAs begin working in Scotland.
2008	Canada	Ontario employs PAs for emergency medicine, hospital services, and primary care.
2007	Australia	PAs recruited to develop PA education in Queensland.
2007	United States	Profession celebrates the 40th anniversary of the development of formally trained PAs.
2008	Canada	First civilian PA programs begin at the University of Manitoba and McMaster University.
2008	Australia	Adelaide, South Australia, recruits PAs for demonstration project.
2009	South Africa	First PA program begin at the University of Witwatersrand.
2009	Australia	First PA programs begin at University of Queensland.
2010	Canada	University of Toronto begins a PA program.

the legislative process can be much shorter (e.g., Manitoba enacting legislation before there were any PAs). There is more of a potential in such instances to better standardize the practice scope and payment systems of PAs rather than the decentralized pattern observed in the United States.

As each country defines the role and level of autonomy that the PA has or will have, there is no question that there will be modifications and departures from the American version. Every country incorporating the PA profession into the existing healthcare system must endeavor to gain public awareness and acceptance of the new profession and will adapt them to the particulars of their own system. Despite obvious similarities and differences in PAs from country to country, it is apparent that the concept is making a worldwide impact on how healthcare delivery will be constructed in the next decade.

What is not mentioned in this chapter are the many countries that do not have an adequately trained cadre of doctors and instead have a group of nonphysician clinicians who provide clinical functions of medical doctors. In some countries the number of these providers equals or succeeds the number of doctors.

Because of the ever-changing healthcare landscape and the increasing shortages of doctors worldwide, it is likely that the role of the PA globally will grow significantly and become a major force in healthcare delivery by

2020. At a conference in 2002 it was predicted that there would be 15 PA programs outside the United States by 2010; that prediction is now a reality. The nature of organizational change and the doctor's role beyond containing it in one profession are the variables used. Standards of care and standards of education will emerge that will have an international cohesiveness. Education will always need to be refined for the host country and even within regions of the country, but the approach to the patient and basic respect for the individual are already becoming international norms. Another conjecture is that an international forum for PAs will emerge and more information about the profession will become available.

PAs have been shown to be fully capable to assist a variety of developed countries in addressing medical workforce shortages. The clinical versatility of PAs makes them particularly valuable in supplementing doctors in a wide range of roles, as well as replacing doctors in areas of doctor shortage. In some systems, there may be reluctance to create a new category of practitioner—a concern sometimes raised by nurses and by young doctors believing their income will be threatened (Sweet, 2008). However, PAs do not substitute for nurses. Instead, the PA concept may encourage highly qualified people into the health system who may not otherwise have been attracted, and imbues them with a doctor–nurse–PA team approach to healthcare needs (Cawley & Hooker, 2003). The global development of PAs will create dialogues among policymakers, doctors, and citizens that cannot be imagined, and opportunities for healthcare delivery that was only a dream at one time.

Research and the Expansion of Physician Assistants Globally

As PAs expand globally the reasons underlying this professional phenomenon raises many questions. Additional research on these topics may help shed light on the phenomenon.

- **History:** How did each country develop an interest in PAs and implement them? Are there common denominators?

- **Data:** What are the duties of PAs in various countries?

- **Policy:** Globally, how do the policies and laws governing PAs compare in efficiency and implementation?

- **Education:** Compare and contrast the PA education requirements for graduation from each country. Do such education requirements impact outcomes related to patient satisfaction and PA proficiency?

- **Economics:** Does the observed cost effectiveness of PAs in one country translate to other countries?

- **Employment:** Who employs PAs primarily in each country (individual doctors, group practices, community clinics, emergency settings, or hospitals)? Does the employment of PAs by a central government improve access to care?

- **Social:** What is the ratio of underrepresented minorities in each country and are PAs part of this representation?

- **Relationships:** What are the attitudes of different coworkers in each country in regards to PAs, including attitudes of nurses, doctors, and allied health staff?

- **International PA development:** What are the political issues for PAs by country and would an international PA congress be of any utility?

- **Universal:** What are the universal issues for PAs in the 21st century in regard to organization?

SUMMARY

The PA concept of the 21st century has expanded beyond the borders of North America. Since the new century began, the PA profession is flourishing beyond any published expectations. Many American PAs are involved in this expansion, as are academics,

AAPA staff, researchers, and government officials. Work of this type is not undertaken in a vacuum. From these experiments in international healthcare delivery, improved understanding in organizational efficiencies will grow, value will be added in labor costs previously unrealized, and greater knowledge of universal social behaviors regardless of culture will emerge. PAs are poised to bring their professional wares onto the global stage and take jobs in countries different from their educational origins. Additional comparative research is needed to evaluate how these new providers work and what efficiencies they bring to different societies.

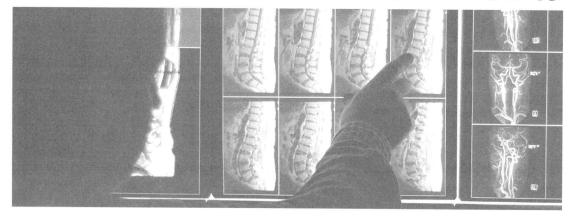

CHAPTER 19

FUTURE DIRECTIONS OF THE PHYSICIAN ASSISTANT PROFESSION

RODERICK S. HOOKER ■ JAMES F. CAWLEY ■ DAVID P. ASPREY

The empires of the future are the empires of the mind.
—Sir Winston Churchill

ABSTRACT

Remarkable changes are underway with the increased use of physician assistants (PAs) domestically and globally. Examining these changes and how they took place provides some perspective that can shed light on the future of PAs. The origin of PAs in the United States was a grassroots activity, with doctors employing PAs at first. Social and political change followed. Eventually, the laws regarding scope of practice were changed on the state level. In other countries, however, this process can be different; legislation may precede innovation in some instances. Enter the PA of the new century. She or he belongs to a robust profession with legislative battles largely behind. Yet extraordinary changes loom for all societies, and the PA is just one more player in a world where there are severe medical workforce shortages and generational shifts that signal a variable healthcare environment.

INTRODUCTION

The role of the physician assistant (PA) in the new millennium is a product of medicine that enjoys an unparalleled success among the health professions. Born in the 1960s, nurtured in the 1970s, and grown in the 1980s, the PA role emerged in the 1990s as a major player in health policy in the United States. By the new century, the PA had become a global phenomenon; by 2015 there will be almost 100,000 PAs worldwide. How did this development come about? Was it the right person at the right time with the right vision? A fluke development? A well-planned evolution in the division of medical labor in the U.S. health system?

Various explanations have been advanced as to why the PA concept is so successful. Clearly, PAs fit well in the entrepreneurial U.S. healthcare system, where their economic advantages, clinical flexibility, and dependent practice stance are considered the most likely responsible factors for their success. Yet it is other countries that are building on the success of the American model, making the future of the global PA look bright. With a worldwide shortage of 4.5 million doctors and an inadequate number of medical schools, the sheer weight of the population growth demands more medical personnel and resources (Dal Poz et al, 2006). Couple these factors with the aging of the population, improvements in childhood survival measures, and the control of archaic diseases that have remained unchanged over thousands of years (e.g., malaria, tuberculosis, dengue fever, smallpox, polio) and the result is that people will live longer and more comfortably than their parents. Technological advancements are limited only by logistics of delivery to remote populations (Scheffler, 2008). The percentage of elderly living longer and more productively means a large cadre of health workers are needed. Without more doctors and nurses, the next group of providers to look to are PAs.

A broad sociological explanation for the success of PAs in America is that they (and similar nonphysicians) represent an evolution in the division of medical labor. Medicine and medical practice have become infinitely more complex over the past several decades. The required knowledge base to practice medicine is enormous and has led to greater levels of specialization and subspecialization. The once-vaunted supremacy of physicians over health and medicine has given way to a sharing of diagnostic and therapeutic tasks, in part because modern physicians cannot know everything and do everything in a field so vast. In the previous century new diagnostic technologies and therapeutic approaches led to the evolution of new professions, such as radiologic technology, physical therapy, and genetics. The expansion of medical activities and capabilites necessitates the inclusion of additional trained personnel who share the domains that once were in the exclusive possession of physicians.

Other reasons for success of the PA profession in American medicine include the major social forces thought to have influenced the PA movement:

- **Changing lifestyles.** The new practice preferences of physicians grew out of the 1960s. Doctors, along with others, realized they did not want to work as hard as their predecessors and needed help.
- **Gender shift.** Women in all professions entered the workforce in a major way, with many seeking a a career in health care. Many were trying out careers that had been traditionally occupied by men, and found them to their liking. For a young woman, a career as a PA is a shorter route than some other professions and a sterling profession to adopt. It also provides an opportunity to raise a family and remain employed.
- **Physician dependency.** The commitment to being a dependent profession that is closely associated with doctors allowed for widespread acceptance of the PA by organized medicine.
- **National competency.** The early establishment of program accreditation and a national board to oversee the specific skills and competency expected of PAs allowed for enabling state legislation.
- **Primary care.** There was a national emphasis on training primary care generalists, with PAs assuming diverse roles after obtaining core competency.

Reflecting on why PAs have succeeded, Fowkes provides the following summary:

In the early part of [the twentieth century] the Flexner report changed the emphasis in our medical schools from a practical approach to a biomedical emphasis as the priority in education. This made medical schools slow to respond to the changing social environment, and less responsive to health care needs. In the 1960s primary care was a new concept. There was a recognized need for these services, a maldistribution of physicians and types of services, and questions about who should do it. A discipline of family medicine was emerging but was not large enough to have much influence. It takes medical schools (and nursing schools for that matter) an enormous amount of time to make critical changes. One of the critical features of the physician assistant movement has been its flexibility and resourcefulness. One only has to look to the way the training programs responded to the early awareness of AIDS, homelessness, drug abuse, and domestic violence by incorporating these conditions in their curriculum. The physician assistant is the only flexible category of health professionals. Both PA programs and PA practitioners have demonstrated their abilities to quickly modify elements of education and practice in response to social need. (Fowkes et al, 1983)

The profession also succeeds in part because of the personal and career attributes of PAs. The first two generations in particular saw themselves as change agents in the health system who were on a mission to prove that individuals trained in the PA model could practice medicine safely and effectively. The profession has been and continues to be one of the most exciting careers in the 21st century.

In looking forward, key questions that arise are: What does the future hold for the PA profession? Will the demand for PA services continue to increase or will it plateau or decrease? Does the past predict the future? How will the changing face of various healthcare systems have an impact on the PA profession? Will the PA trained and certified in Utrecht, Netherlands, be able to work in Mt. Isa, Australia (and be as effective)?

Two phenomena are shaping PAs and their futures: (1) the change of human societies, and (2) the change of healthcare delivery. In this discussion, we examine these directions and then seek a convergence point to make some predictions as they apply to PAs in all settings and in all countries.

THE FUTURE OF SOCIETIES

Forecasts are not so much meant to be predictions but instead glimpses of what is likely to (or should) happen. For many futurists, projections are intended to provoke thought and inspire action. From the world literature we offer some emerging thoughts on what the years ahead may portend for health care in general and PAs in particular.

- **World populations.** World populations are growing larger than predicted due, in part, to people being healthier and living longer

than before. In spite of declines in fertility, the increase in longevity contributes to population growth. The United Nations increased its forecast for global population from 9.1 billion people by 2050 to 9.2 billion (Exhibit 19-1) (United Nations Department of Economic and Social Affairs, Population Division, 2004).
- **Demographics.** Demographics are shifting in ways unexpected only a few years ago. The aging of America will alter society, with one in five individuals being retired by 2030. This factor will change the labor force, the economy, and strain employment-intensive services such as health care, transportation, and food services. Medicare, the U.S. healthcare entitlement for the elderly, will not be adequate to meet demand, and few good ideas have been promoted to address this shortfall. More years in retirement may diminish resources for children and working adults. Special pressures on the elderly will emerge in areas where they are concentrated, such as in Arizona, Nevada, and Florida.
- **Unrealistic expectations of generations X and Y.** Roughly 50% of American high school seniors in 2000 were planning to

EXHIBIT 19-1
World Population Milestones

World Population Reached:		
1 billion in	1804	
2 billion in	1927	(123 years later)
3 billion in	1960	(33 years later)
4 billion in	1974	(14 years later)
5 billion in	1987	(13 years later)
6 billion in	1999	(12 years later)
World Population May Reach:		
7 billion in	2013	(14 years later)
8 billion in	2028	(15 years later)
9 billion in	2054	(26 years later)
10 billion in	2183	(129 years later)

Data from the Department of Economic and Social Affairs, Population Division. (Eds.). (2004). World Population to 2300. *New York: United Nations.*

continue their education after college and obtain an advanced degree. This trend is in contrast to 20% of seniors in 1976. However, the expectations and reality are different; only one-quarter of high school seniors actually obtain a graduate degree, suggesting young people may have unrealistic expectations about the future.

■ **Government.** Burdened by programs that assist society, such as Social Security, medical research, support for the needy, and the courts, government will be strained by a limited tax base and demand for services. People may outlive their savings, having planned for a shorter lifespan.

■ **Education.** Blended learning, virtual classrooms, and online courses will replace much of the classroom. Medicine will be taught using visually stunning graphics and creative courses. New software will portray virtual blackboards and model diseases. In fact, few students may work with real cadavers.

■ **Human knowledge capability.** This factor is the quantity of available knowledge that continues to multiply each decade. The doctor, PA, nurse, and health worker of tomorrow will have access to knowledge in ways that are only rudimentary now. Best practices, evidence-based medicine, and the patient profile will drive standard-of-care templates for a particular patient. Experiences in medicine will enhance knowledge capability by making it more interesting and engaging than just memorizing facts.

■ **Decisions by nonhumans.** Electronically enabled networks will make financial, health, educational, and even political decisions. The power of statistics to make complex decisions based on probability will dictate many new behaviors.

■ **Outsourcing.** Development of many products available electronically, including education and medical care, will be from outsourced systems. Statisticians in India will analyze large databases for firms and healthcare systems in Europe to drive best-fit services. Chinese workers will input data into large systems to fuel these engines. Other systems around the world will be connected seamlessly to enhance all products.

■ **Technology.** New drugs and devices will save and extend lives. They will be delivered by improved communications and technology, and no place on the planet will be logistically isolated. The elderly will provide a growing market for medication and equipment to overcome their disabilities. Understanding senescence may extend lives, creating more demand for healthcare services and technology.

THE FUTURE OF HEALTH CARE

Many experts believe that innovation in every aspect of patient care will be nothing less than astonishing as the new century unfolds. The accelerating pace of technology will bring together healthcare providers who have the ability to adapt to change quickly and adroitly. Futurists have identified some of the technological advances that will likely shape and inform the next generation. They range from fundamental advances in computing and administration, research, nursing, and patient care delivery to minimally invasive surgery, biomolecular therapies, bionics, and beyond. Other advances in technology will emerge in the next decade that existed only in the realm of science fiction.

Some of the changes that will shape how health care is delivered—and with it the fate of the PA—will take place in the next decade. Some of these anticipated changes are already underway:

■ **Epidemics.** Obesity, osteoporosis, diabetes, heart disease, dyslipidemia, arthritis, and dementia are some of the diseases associated with an aging population. These conditions will be sustained and even put into remission due in part to early recognition and early treatment and will contribute to the longevity of populations.

■ **Imaging.** The ability to image the body's metabolism in real time will drive new pharmaceuticals and early aggressive treatments to augment disorders associated with an aging population.

- **Neuroanatomy repair.** The neural processes, long an enigma to researchers, are now being repaired, enhanced, and modified. Cell division and stimulation allows for replacement of neurons and growth of more complicated structures.

- **Robots.** Surgeons are now using robotic instruments and wireless technology as tools to improve the surgical outcome. New technology has allowed robots to feel and visualize areas of surgery more fully while performing delicate procedures. In 2008 alone more than 9,000 robotic operations were performed with excellent outcomes.

- **Neutraceuticals.** The range of food and supplements to enhance wellness or prevent disease is increasing. Vitamin D, more of a hormone than a vitamin, is reemerging as an important food supplement because of the long periods in which people remain indoors and attempts to avoid excessive solar radiation. Enriched foods are being engineered to improve the ability to obtain the mineral and vitamins needed for aging organs, such as bones, that are needed for long lives.

- **Interventional radiology.** The imaging of tiny vessels in healthy, injured, and diseased organs allows new surgical techniques to interrupt the growth of tumors and repair damaged tissue. Using ultrafine lines of plastic and other materials, the interventionist can coil these in remote organs to choke off blood supplies to the neoplasm.

- **No external wound surgery.** Natural orifice translumenal endoscopic surgery (NOTES) involves inserting a fiberoptic endoscope through a natural body opening (such as the mouth or vagina) rather than via an external incision. The most frequently used technique involves inserting the endoscope through the mouth and then through the stomach wall to access the abdomen and remove and repair organs. Surgeons can remove a diseased gallbladder, appendix, or kidney without an external scar.

- **Artificial organs and prosthetics.** The development of eyes, ears, limbs that can sense touch, kidneys, livers, hearts, pancreases, and other organs is nearing perfection. Microelectrodes the size of a human hair are implanted into human brains and robotic/prosthetic arms and legs move with only casual thinking. The cost will be high initially, but will plummet as the manufacture of parts is outsourced and economy of scale produces efficiency.

- **Xenographs.** New animals created through the process of cross-species gene transfer are called xenographs, and the transplanting of organs across species is called xenotransplantation. Genetically engineered animals are being developed as living factories for the production of pharmaceuticals and as sources of organs for transplantation into humans.

- **Genetics.** The understanding of genetics, epigenetics, and proteomics has produced unparalleled growth in new biologically engineered drugs for management of rare conditions. Diseases such as rheumatoid arthritis and lymphoma can now be controlled with genetically engineered proteins not previously known to nature.

- **Genomics.** Humans differ from each other by less than 0.1% genetically. The phenotype and genotype of individuals will merge and single nucleotide pairs that make up the differences between individuals will be known. The HapMap Research Initiative will allow treatment to be tailored to the individual, not to the response of populations.

- **Vaccines.** More than 80 vaccines are approved for human use with more along the way. One vaccine prevents cervical neoplasm, a stunning advancement in the war on cancer. Other vaccines being developed include those for malaria, tuberculosis, HIV, rheumatoid arthritis, Chagas disease, and lymphoma.

- **Rural hospitals.** High-technology monitoring tools will continue to expand expertise to patients in rural intensive care units (ICUs), allowing patients to be under the electronic gaze of specialists at bigger, distant facilities. This process involves a bundle of sensors and software, thus creating an electronic ICU. Preliminary testing in more than 100 hospitals demonstrates that some facilities have been able to cut length of stay and probably save lives.

Healthcare Finance

Forecasting the changing picture of healthcare financing necessitates understanding policy changes at federal and state/provincial levels and movements in the employer and consumer markets. It also requires tracking long-term shifts in demographics and technology. Changes have been underway for some time, and government priorities tend to expand medical coverage for more Americans. It is likely that some form of healthcare reform will occur after 2009 and experts acknowledge that any such measure will necessarily include a workforce component. These policy changes will increase demand on a healthcare system that is struggling with labor costs. PAs offer an opportunity to provide this care at less expensive salaries. The substitutability of PAs for traditional physician services means they are likely to be used in more ways to help fill the gaps in the demand for healthcare access.

Fee-for-service and cost-based reimbursement have been largely replaced with per diems, case rates, and percentage-of-billed charges. New, life-saving technologies and treatments have entered the market, adding to the cost of staffing and equipment. Many stand-alone hospitals have become horizontally integrated systems. Small, autonomous physician practices have, in some markets, given way to large group practices with prescribed treatment protocols. Decades-old challenges continue, including high costs, medical errors, and the complex issue of insurance coverage.

The New Healthcare Consumer

Telecommunications via the Internet is only one example of how the new consumer has fundamentally changed many industries, and health care is next. Newly empowered patients (and their children) are demanding more accountability of their healthcare dollar. However, in the United States, this demand is not well balanced because of its tiered health insurance system. Those with good paying jobs have excellent healthcare coverage compared with those without the benefit of a generous employer. The heavy users of healthcare services are, on average, older, poorer, and less sophisticated than the mainstream baby boomers. As a result, the disenfranchised have less access because those with coverage receive preferential treatment. So, it is unclear exactly who the new healthcare consumer will be and how quickly the healthcare marketplace will change. Increasingly, those who staff healthcare systems are turning to PAs as a solution to meeting the demands of shifting healthcare consumers.

Healthcare Delivery Systems

For many consumers and physicians managed care was not the panacea that was predicted. New organizations and relationships in healthcare delivery systems will be built. At the core of each new experiment will be healthcare providers. Increasingly, health systems realize that diversity of the workforce means not only gender and ethnic diversity, but also various types of providers such as PAs, nurse practitioners (NPs), midwives, and others. Generally, people want and demand choices, and this transcends to nonphysician providers.

Technology

The area of information and medical technologies is where the greatest changes will take place. Emerging technologies and new media impacts patients, delivery networks, insurers, and physicians. How technology will affect the future is difficult to predict, although it will drive up the cost of health care. The role of innovations will be dramatic and the use of these technologies will require a mix of physicians and nonphysician providers such as PAs, nurses, and allied health personnel. Because the growth of physicians is only rising slightly, PAs will increasingly be called to be part of the delivery of new technologies.

Sociodemographic Trends and Health Status

There is a growing realization that medical care alone does not equal a positive health status, and new demands for health care are emerging. For example, consumers are demanding new types of health services such as "complementary and alternative" medicine. On top of this demand will emerge different philosophies about health spending and what contributes to health outcomes. The areas that are likely to dominate U.S. health policy and healthcare delivery are the following:

- Human genomics and the proteins that genes produce
- The empowered consumer
- Internet and telemedicine access
- Complementary and alternative medicine
- Technology developments in electronic information and communication
- Impact on patient access and quality
- Technology (each one of the areas that will open up will require appropriately trained individuals to apply the information)

THE FUTURE FOR PHYSICIAN ASSISTANTS

What does the future hold for PAs? How blue are the skies for the next generation of PAs? Is this a profession that attracts young, bright, and capable people? Although these questions are usually answered in the affirmative, the evidence to support a prediction of a rosy scenario is a mixture of probabilities based on current trends and conjecture. The most solid evidence is that the PA profession is growing in its acceptance and incorporation

into the health system and its demographics are changing. Economic modeling—drawing from an understanding of scarcity of resources relative to human behavior—suggests that if supply exceeds demand, then price goes down. Conversely, if demand exceeds supply, the price increases. The following is an examination of these two fundamental principles as they apply to the future of PAs.

Supply Side

As of 2009, there were 145 accredited PA programs in the United States and more in development. Outside of the United States, there are 14 PA programs in operation and another 12 are in some stage of planning (Exhibit 19-2). At the same time, more than 5,500 new PAs entered the U.S. workforce and 400 PAs entered the workforce in other parts of the world; approximately two-thirds of these new graduates are women. Since the start of the new century, the PA workforce in the aggregate has been largely composed of women. The prevalent theory is that men opt out of joining the labor force or do not remain in one labor market for extended periods. Consequently, there are fewer men applying to PA school and the men in the workforce are older by at least 5 years than their female counterparts. The trend of female PA expansion is calculated to extend to at least 2012.

A swelling of the ranks is expected until at least 2015, when the current number of U.S. PA programs may reach their maximum output. By 2015 there will be an estimated 95,500 clinically active PAs in the U.S. workforce, with an estimated 6,500 U.S. PA graduates per year and 2,000 graduates per year outside of the United States. By 2020 there will be at least 115,000 PAs clinically employed. These numbers take into account retirements of male and female PAs, who are being replaced by more young women than men. The historical 7.5% annual annulment of the U.S. PA cadre will gradually increase to 12.5% by 2015 as more women leave the workforce to pursue families and other careers.

Shifts in gender from historical ratios to new ones may create different work habits. The

EXHIBIT19-2
Accumulative Number of Physician Assistant Programs by Year of Entering Class

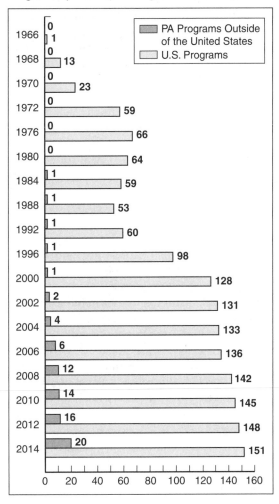

Managers increasingly recognize the value of PAs as a skilled but mobile labor force, able to shift from one area of demand to another. Demand will continue for a while, a slow but steady rise in programs will continue, and from 2000 to 2015 the supply of PAs will double (Orcutt, 2007). Many will welcome this expansion, but the greatest threat to the PA profession is the fickle marketplace. As salaries increase, the cost-effectiveness of PAs will diminish under this invisible hand—pricing oneself out of the market: "If PA income continues to increase at the levels we have seen recently, then cost, value, and productivity differentials will influence hiring decisions" (Jones & Cawley, 1994). Eventually, there may be more PAs than opportunities, and relationships with physicians may suffer.

Until then the dependence of PAs on physicians will probably continue to serve the profession as it continues to reach out to organized medicine for professional guardianship. By demonstrating competence to the physician, the PA's clinical role in practice is ultimately established through a process of ongoing negotiation. Professional autonomy is determined through performance of delegated and negotiated tasks and exists within the practice limits of the supervising physician. Another significant advantage of the PA occupation is the ability to work in different specialties over the course of one's career.

Significant increases in the role of PA and NP use in managed medicine such as health maintenance organizations (HMOs) will be augmented by the degree to which physicians can be persuaded to hire them. Another phenomenon will be the demand for PAs to work globally. The ability to work in another country and experience the culture and diversity of another health system, as well as an adequate salary, will make employment in different countries more attractive—and not just in English-speaking countries. Some of this change will involve PAs coming into the United States, but the majority of global PAs will be U.S. emigrates. Because the shape of the global healthcare workforce is so uncertain, the fundamental question of how many

length of the work week has shrunk. In the United States the doctor's work week is down from 55 hours in 1990 to 50 hours in 2008. In other countries the work week is shorter than 40 hours and not likely to increase. The 45-hour work week for U.S. PAs has remained fairly steady since 1995. A 46-week year is becoming a norm for many doctors.

The obverse side of the PA supply coin is that enterprise and doctor-centerd care continue to be a labor-intensive business. Doctor-centered care is expensive. This factor bodes well for the PA profession in the short run.

PAs will be enough remains unanswered. The demand for healthcare services will exceed supply through 2015, even with a supply of 100,000 clinically active PAs.

Demand Side

The demand side of the equation is more difficult to predict and relies on data from other sectors of the healthcare field. However, the expansion of PA use will likely continue in several sectors of the healthcare system. In fact, the Bureau of Labor Statistics' career outlook projections for healthcare professionals indicate increased demand for PA services through 2018. State survey data of practicing PAs suggest market demand for PAs will increase beyond 2015. The wild card is the role U.S. healthcare reform will play.

In the short run, hospitals will increasingly employ PAs and NPs as more intensive services demand that a permanent, salaried house staff be present 24 hours per day. The number of beds in the United States is growing, but the number of doctors and nurses to tend to those bed patients is not. Teams of hospitalists (physicians and PAs/NPs) will manage inpatient populations that require highly skilled personnel because only the very ill will be hospitalized for any period (Lindenauer et al, 2007). In many teaching institutions, residency program directors have already incorporated PAs (as well as NPs) in resident-substitute roles, in part because of mandated cutbacks in hours worked by residents (Cawley & Hooker, 2006; Dhuper & Choksi, 2009). There is every reason to believe that this trend will continue.

Ambulatory care, where most PAs work, will continue to employ more PAs as physicians become more familiar with their skills and services and demand increases. In the nonprimary care area, advances in technology will create more and more need for skilled providers such as PAs to aid in the application of the technology. This trend will occur in areas such as emergency medicine, dermatology, opthalmology, neurology, nephrology, cardiothoracic surgery, and many other medical and surgical subspecialities.

Other emerging new roles for PAs are wellness and disease prevention; clinical,

biological, and health services research; legal professions; genetics; toxicology; and medical administration. Expanded roles for PAs are in geriatrics, oncology, molecular biology, radiology, and protracted disease management. PAs may also be used to provide effective, humane, and economical care to the millions of individuals with chronic disease. PAs and NPs are probably in a better position than physicians to provide this care because patients will increasingly be absorbed by managed care organizations, and their medical care will require intensive efforts to contain costs through innovative forms of labor. There is also unrealized potential for PAs in the delivery of clinical preventive services. It has long been hypothesized that PAs could become providers that deliver not only medical care services (physician-substitutive) but also clinical preventive services (physician complementary).

A proposed gloomier side of the demand curve is that the number of PAs in the workforce could result in too many clinicians. For example, PAs are in direct competition with NPs and to a lesser extent with nurse-midwives. The majority of NPs are in primary care, and the number of clinically active NPs is almost 50% more than the number of PAs. Such NP activity may prevent a firm foothold in the primary care arena for PAs. There is little evidence, however, to support this scenario. In fact, most observers believe that in the next 5 to 10 years there will be an insufficient number of physicians as well as nonphysicians, particularly in primary care. Physician workforce experts believe that the shortage of physicians will be real and that the nation will require the contributions of both PAs and NPs to meet the demand for medical care services (Cooper, 2007).

One of the nagging issues facing the profession is the appropriate number of PAs to train. How many PAs should there be in America? When considering this issue, it is also necessary to ask: How many primary care physicians should be available to the population and in what ratio? Should PAs, NPs, and midwives be considered part of the equation? Unlike some countries that have developed prescribed physicians/population ratios (e.g., Canada, England, Australia, and the Netherlands), the United States has largely allowed the markets to dictate how many physicians there should be. The only governor of physician supply is the number of medical and osteopathic schools and their ability to turn out graduates. As of 2009, the number of U.S. medical school graduates was approximately 17,000 annually (and the number of U.S. PAs is 5,500). Both are predicted to grow.

There are various responses to the question of how many providers is enough. Some believe there is a surplus of physicians and that PAs and NPs are redundant (Goodman & Grumbach, 2008). This argument is based on counting physician heads and comparing ratios of physicians to populations and comparing these numbers with those of other countries. Others believe there are not enough primary care physicians and that many communities go underserved in terms of access to primary care services. Still, others believe we should mandate primary care quotas in residencies and reduce specialized residencies. Finally, some believe that it is unrealistic to expect that physicians in any appreciable numbers will by themselves reverse the trend of professional specialization (Cawley & Jones, 1997). If this notion holds true, doctors will continue to avoid primary care practices, and it remains doubtful that established specialist physicians will convert to generalist roles in any appreciable numbers. But as we have observed, PAs appear to be emulating this trend of greater specialization creating doubt with regard to the future role for PAs in primary care (Jones & Cawley, 2009).

The continuing decline in interest in primary care and generalist practice careers among young physicians has not yet been reversed, and it will take decades to do so in a way that would impact service delivery— even if the number of medical graduates choosing primary care significantly increases before adjustments in graduate medical education (GME) outcomes. This prospect raises the question of which type of healthcare personnel will provide primary care now and in the future. As physicians become increasingly specialized, moving further away from primary care, PAs are likely to assume a greater profile in delivering primary care services. This is particularly true in settings such as HMOs, other types of managed care systems, and organized healthcare systems such as Veterans Affairs (VA) hospitals, state and federal correctional systems, and the military.

One veteran workforce observer believes that physicians are no longer in the primary care business and that PAs and NPs, working with physician "managers," may be the best providers to meet future primary care needs. In 1992, Meikle was a lone voice in recommending increasing PA educational output and using PAs in primary care roles (Meikle, 1992). A keen health workforce observer, many believe he was right. Some free market economists advocate that as many PAs should be trained as the market will bear because, in the end, competition produces a public good in distributing products and driving down costs (Hooker, 1997).

As of 2009, approximately one-fourth of all U.S. solo practitioners employ a PA or an NP. Of solo and group practices incorporating a PA and/or NP, approximately 14% of patients are seen by an NP or PA (either as the sole provider of record or with the physician). Again, looking just at the population of patients seen by PAs and NPs, approximately one-third of all patients are younger than 18 years, suggesting the physician is delegating a great deal of health care to these providers.

Medical marketplace demand for primary care PAs is anticipated to grow. One estimate of primary care needs suggests that a physician can cover the needs of 1,600 to 1,800 persons annually in a managed care practice setting (Hummel & Pirzada, 1994). Given these figures, the United States will need 150,000 primary care physicians for a population of approximately 330 million in 2015. However, only 88,000 primary care physicians younger than 55 years are in active practice. With the addition of a PA to the practice, the patient panel for a PA-physician primary care team could increase to at least 2,400 (a conservative one-third increase in practice productivity): "This increase in total practice productivity suggests that workforce requirements for primary care physicians could be reduced if more physicians were able to utilize PAs" (Cawley, 1995).

In the future, the demand for PAs and other nonphysician health professions is likely to be determined by political, economic, and legal factors that affect the evolution of their roles in relation to those of physicians. As the U.S. healthcare system changes from one encompassing a disease-oriented and economically open-ended structure to one stressing a more preventive, patient-centered, and cost-conscious direction, PAs or NPs will assume a higher profile than in the past.

The further evolution of the professional roles of PAs and NPs in U.S. health care will be determined by changes in the division of medical labor, higher public expectations in regard to physician response to societal healthcare problem, population-based needs, patient satisfaction, and outcome evidence. In the future, the interdisciplinary team approach to health care may become the standard, while Americans' demand for accountability from its health professionals will increase. This new accountability will require adjustments in the educational preparation of medical and healthcare providers. Approaches will need to extend the biomedical model to encompass the population-based and behavioral sciences.

In response to the charge from the Council on Graduate Medical Education (COGME), the Advisory Group of Physician Assistants and the Workforce (AGPAW) developed a list of recommendations addressing PA education, PA practice characteristics, practice obstacles, and current and anticipated demand. The advisory group called for the following:

- Increasing federal support for PA educational programs to expand the supply of PA graduates
- Increasing National Health Service Corps scholarships and loan repayment programs supporting PA students
- Developing federal policy to support and encourage increased representation from racial and ethnic minorities in the PA profession (Exhibit 19-3)
- Including PAs in national and state health workforce planning activities
- Encouraging states to provide a more uniform regulatory climate for PAs

EXHIBIT 19-3
An Occupational Health Physician Assistant

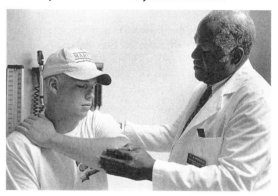

Courtesy of American Academy of Physician Assistants.

The Pew Health Professions Commission predicted that a number of forces will interact to produce a U.S. healthcare system that will be different from the one to which we are accustomed. The obvious changes in health care will be the following:

- More managed care with better integration of services and financing
- More accountability to those who purchase and use healthcare services
- More awareness of and responsiveness to the needs of enrolled populations
- An ability to use fewer resources more effectively
- More innovation and diversity in providing health care
- Less focus on treatment and more concern about education, prevention, and care management
- Orientation to improving the health of the entire population
- Reliance on outcomes data and evidence

Decline in Physician Influence

In 1975, Rick Carlson wrote a book titled *The End of Medicine*. At the time, the author (a lawyer) and his thesis were regarded as being on the radical fringe of healthcare policy. In this futuristic polemic, he asserted that eventually the medical profession, partly because of its arrogant stance of self-regulation, the rise of consumerism and preventive care, and the corporatization of healthcare delivery, would become obsolete. Although actual physician obsolescence is unlikely, it is clear that in today's health system the medical profession is not what it used to be in terms of power and prestige. Over the past decade in particular, physician influence over the health system has eroded to the degree that the number of applicants to medical schools is off once-peak levels, state medical boards are now led by nonphysicians and consumers, and NPs are asserting their roles as independent providers of primary care services. Medicine's power and prestige reached its zenith in the 1960s, the so-called "Golden Age of Medicine," and has since declined, substantially, in the minds of some.

There are a multitude of reasons explaining the decline in physician influence over the health system, but without question an important consequence has been the steady growth over the past quarter century in the numbers and clinical activities of PAs and NPs. Medical sociologists who assert a decline in the power and prestige of the medical profession in the United States refer to this trend as "deprofessionalization" (Hafferty & McKinley, 1993). McKinley in particular is among the more outspoken of the deprofessionalization theorists, and observes that the growing corporatization and bureaucratization of medicine has resulted in effectively eliminating physician self-employment and reduced physician autonomy. As the medical workplace becomes more and more bureaucratized, physicians are increasingly subject to the rules and systems of hierarchical structures that are not of their own making. Physicians are no longer professionally dominant because traditional elements of classic professionalism have been lost. Prerogatives such as control over training content, work autonomy, and the means and remuneration of labor have eroded. Today, the federal government, insurance companies, and consumer groups now hold considerable sway over medical training and practice and the methods by which physicians are paid for their work.

Another important factor in the decline of medicine as a profession is that physicians no longer have a monopoly over medical knowledge. Health consumers and a wide variety of other providers now approach or even exceed physician knowledge in specific areas. The days of the all-knowing, paternalistic physician dispensing medical directives to a subservient patient are gone. As they have become more sophisticated, patients cum consumers now view medical care much as they view other services and are demanding more control, choice, and convenience (Exhibit 19-4).

Delivering medical services in a manner convenient to the patient is a relatively new concept to many physicians. Understandably, accustomed as they are to dealing with life and death situations, physicians in the past have not placed a high priority on customer service and convenience considerations. Yet such adjustments may be required in the future healthcare delivery market. The nature of physician roles in medical work is also changing. It is now clear that health providers such as NPs and PAs can deliver a wide range of medical services as effectively and safely as physicians and at a lower cost (Hooker, 2002). PAs and NPs may be equally knowledgeable in certain clinical disciplines (e.g., primary

EXHIBIT 19-4
Physician Assistant and Patient

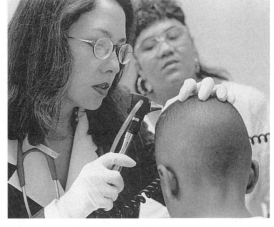

Courtesy of American Academy of Physician Assistants.

care) and have been shown to be as capable as physicians in performing technical procedures in a number of specialty areas, such as cardiac catheterization and sigmoidoscopy.

Consumers and others have come to the realization that physicians may be overtrained for the tasks they perform most of the time. Advances in technology now permit great accuracy and precision in diagnosis, placing less emphasis on physician differential diagnostic and cognitive capabilities. Washington health pundit Daniel Greenberg once said that the system of medical education in the United States was akin to putting all bus drivers through astronaut training. The point is that it may not require 12 years of expensive and federally subsidized education to prepare the medical practitioner of the future, and perhaps this is particularly true in primary care. Physicians have reverted to a movement toward increasing specialization and appear to be abandoning primary care to other providers.

In 2009, fewer U.S. medical school seniors chose primary care residency positions. Among internists, the hospitalist movement has become increasingly popular, driven in part by a desire by physicians to better control the circumstances of their work (Lindenauer et al, 2007). It would be a mistake to believe that physicians as we know them are going to fade from the health delivery scene, yet it is clear that their roles are changing in the division of medical labor (Colwell, Cultice, & Kruse, 2008).

As economics and technology continue to drive medical care, portions of the work that once were exclusively in the domain of physicians will be passed on to others. Familiar examples of this trend are already evident with psychologists and psychiatric social workers working in place of psychiatrists and nurse-midwives working in place of obstetricians. It may very well be that in the future, should such trends continue, NPs and PAs will take on an increasing share of the work of primary care. This occurrence could come about due to a combination of factors:

- practice economics in the delivery system,
- aggressive tactics mounted by some nonphysicians to wrest from physicians dominance in primary care, and

- physicians abrogating primary care and instead seeking inpatient and specialty roles.

It is possible that such a scenario could result in physicians assuming a more medical managerial and care oversight role, with actual clinical care being provided by PAs and NPs. If such a redistribution of medical work were to transpire, a key question will be to what degree will nonphysicians be granted autonomy in their practices. An even more intriguing question would be whether physicians would voluntarily grant such practice prerogatives (Goodman & Grumbach, 2008).

What will happen to the role of the PA in primary care? Can America continue to count on PAs to be generalists? With more than 65% of the profession now practicing in specialties and subspecialties, it is a legitimate question to ask whether PAs can still lay claim to the role of engaging in "big doctoring" (Mullan, 2002).

A discouraging look at modern doctoring sees a deeper more disturbing transformation of the role of the physician as healer (Lantos, 1997). In the book, *Do We Still Need Doctors?*, Lantos, a pediatrician, observes a diminution of the role of the physician from one that is the traditional general doctor who has been supreme in the matters of health and medicine to one that is more narrow, technical, litigious, and shared with many others. The provocative title of the book is meant to reexamine the role of the physician in modern society given the emergence of other healthcare providers, many of whom assume a substantial amount of the work that once was done exclusively by physicians. Lantos notes that the world has assaulted the traditional role of the doctor and as a consequence made it more difficult for physicians to do "big doctoring." This book wonders out loud whether society should entrust physicians with the powers given to them by states and whether doctors are still the best professionals to make judgments on patient problems that extend beyond medical boundaries and far into the socioeconomic, the psychosocial, and the political. This book was described by one reviewer as "a literate and troubled search for the lost soul of doctoring." It raises a number of profound questions in terms of the roles of healthcare professionals of all types, including primary care physicians.

The roles of physicians and PAs have and continue to evolve in our complex healthcare system. Unfortunately, the primary care role seems to be fading. Medical groups remain concerned and have labeled the current circumstances in primary care as a crisis (Kirk, 2006). In this situation, it appears that PAs are more a part of the problem than of the solution. Can or will PAs remain as providers who aspire to do "big doctoring"? It will be a stern professional challenge for PAs to remain primary care providers in a specialized world.

SELF-ACTUALIZATION

Responsibility for administering the profession belongs to the profession. When PAs emerged in the late 1960s, the laws governing the practice of medicine were amended to recognize the physician's ability to delegate tasks to supervised individuals. Most of these laws have been modified and expanded, but the power to regulate PAs has remained, with only a few exceptions, in the hands of the licensing boards, which are predominantly controlled by physicians. If PAs are to seek their own destiny, they must overcome these shortcomings in self-actualization and begin seeking avenues to educate their regulators.

However, if formal participation of PAs in the regulatory process is a worthy goal, it is not a panacea for problems that may exist between physician licensing boards and PAs. Once a PA becomes a board member or sits on a committee that is set up to ensure the benefit of citizens, he or she assumes the role of protector of public health and safety. The responsibilities of that person are to the citizens of the state, not to the PA profession. Advocacy of professional concerns at the state level still rests with state PA associations, often aided by the national organization.

The ability of PAs to effectively identify, attract, and efficiently serve the vagaries of consumers will largely determine their professional future. Organization and financing services will be key variables in these efforts to increase the demand for PAs. Macroeconomic strategies include creative, aggressive, and effective marketing of the quality that PAs bring to society, as well as the recruitment of social scientists into education programs to undertake sorely needed research on the profession. Research must be done on the economic use of PAs and the expansion of PAs into specific client areas such as home health and genomics. These and other macroenocomic and microeconomic strategies are outlined in Exhibit 19-5.

Another approach to self-actualization is to constantly update the knowledge base of what roles PAs play and how well they do them. Collecting demographic data is not enough; research on the healthcare workforce is constantly in demand and needs to be continuously updated. Policymakers want to see data, not opinions.

Taking Stock

After a long period during which medical leaders showed little interest in PA education, attention is now being paid to PA educational policy and the roles that PAs can play in the health workforce (Cawley, 2007). A key issue is whether the PA profession should expand its output of graduates, as has been suggested by

EXHIBIT 19-5
Strategies for Increasing Demand for Physician Assistants

Macro (on the professional organizational level)	Micro (on the individual level)
Aggressive, creative marketing of the profession	Aggressive, creative individual marketing
Research on economic use	Creative self-employment or group employment
Creative organization and financing	Expansion of client areas and contact
Expansion of client areas and contact (scope of practice)	Use of advanced technologies
Use of advanced technologies	Inclusion in policymaking

advocates of the expansion of health professions education. Medicine is counting on PAs to pick up a proportion of the slack in the workforce and the PA profession to raise the output of educational programs, similar to the circumstance underway in medical schools (Whitcomb, 2007). In an attempt to determine the dimensions of current program expansion, the Physician Assistant Education Association (PAEA) has conducted surveys (PAEA, 2009). But thus far, little has been done with the information obtained in response to calls for a greater supply of PA graduates and policy direction (Glicken & Lane, 2006). Even more basic questions can be raised: Who determines PA educational policy? Is it the PA professional organizations or is it left to individual institutions? What is the role of the PAEA in shaping PA educational policy?

U.S. history suggests that it is market forces in higher education, rather than a concerted effort by the professional organizations, that sets the course of PA education. This trend was certainly the case in the second phase of PA program expansion that occurred in the late 1990s, when the number of programs more than doubled. The PA professional organizations have tended to take a passive role by looking forward to tomorrow and refraining from taking any public positions on current program expansion. Over the years, the PAEA has traditionally shied away from taking official positions on workforce policy issues. In view of the recent challenges presented to PA education by prominent leaders in medicine, it seems that the time has come for a more assertive organizational approach. There are many reasons why the United States chooses to be a decentralized system of states rights. However, in other countries central planning is used to to address medical workforce policy issues that ultimately shape the direction for the profession. Perhaps a blend of decentralization and central planning might be in order.

Lessons of PA Models

As changes take place, there are lessons to be learned from other health systems that have installed assistants to physicians, and other systems can learn from the U.S. model of PAs.

Lessons From Other Systems

In projecting the future of PAs in the U.S. healthcare system, it is useful to consider the experiences of PAs in the medical systems of other countries. Practitioners similar to PAs have been used in a number of other nations. Examples include the feldsher in Russia, the barefoot doctor in China, the assistant medical officer in parts of Africa, and a wide range of the variously named healthcare providers working primarily in developing countries throughout the world. As the concept of the PA expands globally, educational approaches have emerged that are different from the U.S. system. How these compare to each other should be a prime focus of research.

The natural history and pertinent experiences of these practitioners have been examined, and when compared with the American experience with nonphysician providers, it is clear that only a few parallels exist. Experience with PAs and their successful (or unsuccessful) integration into a country's healthcare delivery system are based primarily on how these providers fit into the medical, economic, and cultural systems of the nations that employ them. Rarely are experiences with these types of providers exportable to other countries. Each nation that has created and used PAs has fashioned them and their roles to meet specific needs and requirements in that country's systems. However, some overriding patterns do exist that are relevant in the assessment of the American PA.

Nonphysician practitioners are created by the existing cadre of medical providers in a country and emerge from specific perceived needs in healthcare delivery. In nearly all cases, these needs involve a shortage of fully trained physicians to provide adequate medical services to the population. This was in fact the fundamental rationale for the creation of PAs in the United States.

Once nonphysicians enter the delivery system, evolving circumstances and changes in the system affect the roles and perceptions of these providers. As the supply of a country's physician population rises, and as experience with these nonphysician providers accumulates, new perceptions of the roles that these nonphysician providers can assume develop.

In some instances, there is no further need for these providers in the healthcare system. In others, the role of the nonphysician provider changes and becomes more technically oriented. In still other systems, nonphysician clinicians evolve into well-established members of a healthcare delivery team, participating with physicians in a wide variety of clinical functions. The broadest generalization that can be made is that nonphysicians must adjust and adapt to changing forces within the health delivery system in which they work once they outlive the rationale of their initial creation.

As we have seen, this is what has occurred with PAs in the United States. Roles for PAs continue to expand and new employment niches appear regularly. The capability of PAs to adapt to various clinical roles have kept them on the forefront of medical workforce innovations and should continue to expand their utilization in the U.S. system.

Lessons for Other Systems

As we look to other systems to avoid the pitfalls of history lessons ignored, PAs must be cognizant that movements are underway to expand the notion of PAs to other countries. PAs in many ways represent a unique healthcare workforce innovation that has met a number of important needs in the U.S. health system. However, other countries are looking to PAs in American medicine as exportable models to address their own shortages.

Since the 1990s there had been a scattering of reports about the use of PAs in England. The editor-in-chief of the *British Journal of Nursing* reviewed the use of PAs in North America and wrote:

> With the emphasis on reducing doctors' hours and recent concerns about future shortages of doctors and nurses, it could be argued that we should be looking at the feasibility of such a development in the UK. As we do not have a large body of redundant military personnel from which to recruit, perhaps we could gradually convert operating department assistants, technicians and paramedics to the role. It may also be possible to encourage more medically oriented nurse practitioners to enlist! [However, problems exist within a small country with an expanding

> NP presence, where conflict already exists with physicians resenting NPs, much less] introduction of a new species within an established health-care system generating uncertainty and confusion. (Castledine, 1996)

Already, nurses are being tasked with new roles and "the introduction of PAs could cause chaos." Castledine (1996) concluded his editorial by stating, "We must not increase the number of personnel the patient currently comes into contact with. Patients are already confused about the variety of roles that nurses undertake; to add more roles into the healthcare team without proper evaluation of the benefits to the patient would be disastrous."

What Castledine fails to appreciate in his editorial is the apparent desire of patients to have their needs met and the patient satisfaction that occurs when healthcare needs are met regardless of the type of provider. Medicare researchers were able to demonstrate that on a national level the elderly in the United States were satisfied with the care that they received from PAs or NPs and that there were no differences in how they perceived this care in relation to care provided by a doctor. Furthermore, the same study showed that PAs and NPs were more likely to care for the elderly poor and individuals without insurance (Hooker, Cipher, & Sekscenski, 2005).

As of 2009, Canadian PAs are serving the nation's forces and working successfully in the civilian realm. The Canadian Association of Physician Assistants is developing under capable leadership. Two civilian PA programs are underway and more are being considered. Americans are recruited to work in Canada as PAs. Although PAs in the Canadian Forces are warrant officers, their roles are considered valuable and a possible solution to physician shortages throughout the providences (Hooker, MacDonald, & Patterson, 2003).

Interest is expanding in other countries as well. England, frustrated with physician and nurse shortages, has inaugurated four PA programs and Scotland is considering the same. Australia is experiencing workforce shortages, both in physicians and nurses, and has been examining NP and PA models as well (O'Connor & Hooker, 2007). One PA program started in 2009 and others are being considered.

Demonstration programs recruiting American PAs allows citizens to see them in action.

The AAPA reports that at least 83 countries have expressed some interest in the PA model. Many European countries realize that with the development of PAs in the European Union opportunities exist for PA development in their countries as well.

FUTURE ISSUES

No futurist is ever confident of his or her predictions. Making predictions is based on lessons learned; the sciences of history, economics, demographics, and politics; and observations of changes based on technology and sociology. However, every prediction is subject to "wild cards," which are events and movements that are not expected that can produce unanticipated changes. The potential wild cards are PA independence, healthcare reform, doctoral degrees, and international medical graduates (IMGs). Each could change society's attitude toward PAs.

Independence and Professional Recognition

Issues of whether PAs should seek practice independence arise from time to time—typically when there are issues about professional recognition. To some PAs, professional recognition will come only if they gain the legal right to full independence of practice, meaning they would be free to contract and negotiate for services similar to what a small number of NPs do in certain states. To some extent this is already underway as PAs find that there are opportunities to be entrepreneurs and independent owners of healthcare systems (Barnes & Hooker, 2001). Although the push for recognition comes from the PA profession, increased financial pressure on the healthcare industry is also an important substrate for change. A partial list of advantages and disadvantages of independent practice for PAs is listed in Exhibit 19-6.

PAs, however, remain generally satisfied with their dependent practice stance. The matter has not emerged as a concern in any formal sessions of the AAPA or its House of Delegates. PAs have come to realize that it is an ideal circumstance to be able to assume great responsibility for patient care and medical decision-making within a dependent relationship with physicians. Physicians delegate many duties and functions to PAs, who appear to be satisfied with the balance of autonomy and responsibility that the PA role brings. The much-debated independent-dependent issue may represent an outdated paradigm, particularly for PAs who do not see being a dependent provider as an issue.

EXHIBIT 19-6

Advantages and Disadvantages of Physician Assistant Independent Practice

Advantages	Disadvantages
▪ The ability to seek employment and negotiate terms improves.	▪ If physicians are not employers, jobs may not be as plentiful.
▪ Supervising physician can help share the responsibility and fallout in malpractice cases.	▪ PAs may be seen as more vulnerable to plaintiff lawyers.
▪ PAs will have a greater say in standards of care and educational levels.	▪ PAs will constantly have to improve standards of care, seek legislative changes, and improve educational levels on their own.
▪ PAs can negotiate salary with more independence.	▪ Physicians are increasingly opting for salaried work.
▪ A PA can form a business, work for the business, and reap the rewards of one's own labor.	▪ Businesses are increasingly regulated with compliance consuming large amounts of time and resources.
▪ Independent reimbursement from insurance companies will improve return for work.	▪ Many third-seeking reimbursement party payers may resist another group.

International Medical Graduates as Physician Assistants

Nearly all PAs have had extensive contact with IMGs. They make up a considerable part of the medical workforce in several large industrialized nations. IMGs constitute between 23% and 28% of physicians in the United States, the United Kingdom, Canada, and Australia, and lower-income countries supply between 40% and 75% of these IMGs.

The PA profession has sometimes been quick to condemn the capabilities of IMGs, who commonly do not have organizations to speak on their behalf or to reply to criticisms. Even as we face external threats such as international terrorism, we should be careful not to veer carelessly into xenophobia. We also should be careful about generalizing about the IMG-PA comparison, particularly when the existing literature on the topic is far from conclusive.

IMGs have become an important component of the health workforce, particularly serving in rural communities. Bear in mind that not so long ago, serving rural areas was felt to be one of the key social mandates for the PA profession.

There are two types of IMGs: those who are U.S. citizens and have been to medical school outside of the United States and those who are non-U.S. citizens and have not been educated in the United States. When the latter immigrate to the United States and would like to practice as physicians, sometimes those skills are difficult to market. For some, this predicament means undertaking or even repeating a postgraduate training period (residency). Not all can qualify to work as a physician, and some IMGs for whom the door has been closed have sought to attain recognition as PAs as an alternative. This trend has caused some consternation because the National Commission on Certification of Physician Assistants (NCCPA) will not allow some IMGs to take the national certifying examination unless they are graduates of an accredited PA program. Studies performed in two states with high proportions of IMGs have demonstrated that cohorts of IMGs cannot pass the same examinations given to second-year PA students (Fowkes et al, 1996).

IMGs are a unique situation for the United States because there is some evidence that IMGs will accept employment in the health sector that may not be desirable to physicians, such as in the areas of corrections medicine and remote rural health. However, Hagopian and colleagues (2004) showed that after obligated service, IMGs tended to leave underserved areas. The other situation compounding the shortage of providers in underserved areas is that fewer U.S. medical school seniors are choosing primary care residency positions in family practice, pediatrics, internal medicine, and obstetrics and gynecology. Additionally, non-U.S. citizen IMGs are in fewer numbers, while IMGs who are U.S. citizens are in record numbers. These trends are somewhat linked because IMGs who are not U.S. citizens are more likely to choose primary care positions than specialty programs such as surgery, dermatology, or urology. As fewer non-U.S. citizen IMGs enter residency programs over the next several years and more U.S. medical school seniors and U.S-citizen IMGs seek specialty slots, the number of primary care positions filled is expected to further decline.

Specialties such as surgery, anesthesiology, and radiology are attracting more U.S. medical school seniors because the perception of the rewards of primary care has changed. During the past two decades, U.S. medical school seniors began to opt out of primary care for the more lucrative specialties, and primary care residencies began filling open slots with IMGs. Now, however, due to various factors, fewer IMGs are entering the system, so there are fewer opportunities for residency programs in pediatrics, internal medicine, and family practice to fill the open slots that U.S. medical school seniors continue to avoid.

It has become more difficult for IMGs to enter U.S. medicine and medical education. The number of physicians in training with J-1 visa waivers (which IMGs must possess) has fallen by almost one-half over the past decade, from 11,600 in academic year 1996–1997 to fewer than 6,200 in 2004–2005, according to the Government Accountability Office. Federal and state requests for J-1s for physicians dropped from 1,374 in 1995 to 1,012 in 2005. Over each of the past 3 years, about 1,000 practicing physicians have come to the United States on J-1 visa waivers. Many of them are from unstable or undeveloped countries and come here in search of better training, working conditions, and pay.

However, since September 11, 2001, the federal government has made it more difficult for IMGs to qualify for the special visas and to obtain permanent residency. The tests are more difficult, the legal fees are higher, and the Department of Health and Human Services has changed the rules in such a way that fewer counties and clinics are designated as underserved and thus eligible to obtain J-1 doctors. These changes have led to shortages of physicians in rural areas and have hampered access to medical care in many rural communities. PAs may be the only viable alternative for this widening void.

In the past, PAs and the profession have taken a dim view of IMGs attempting to become PAs, particularly if they would attempt to obtain advanced placement in a PA program or try to short-circuit codified steps to PA licensure. To address the issue of unlicensed IMGs, in the past some states enacted legislation that funded so-called "fast-track" educational programs to recruit and matriculate IMGs into PA programs (Fowkes et al, 1996). In such instances, the clinical skills of IMGs were assessed and compared with those of second-year PA students and found to be nonequivalent. Although these experimental tracks in PA programs never became well established, it is upon the basis of this study that many in the PA profession hold that IMGs are inferior in their skills and medical knowledge compared with PA students. It is a risky proposition to generalize about IMGs and to speak definitively about the educational equivalence of PAs versus IMGs.

The Harlem Hospital/CUNY "experiment" was a very shaky tidbit of evidence to put forth in support of the notion that IMGs are incompetent relative to second-year PA students (the comparison used). This study was a small, one-time observation of a selected sample of IMGs,

it had weak internal and external validity, and it was never published in the peer-reviewed literature (Stanhope, Fasser, & Cawley, 1992). Thus, we should hesitate to use it as evidence of the "incompetence" of IMGs. A physician who is an IMG, for example, recently headed the National Institutes of Health.

Ontario, Canada is trying to change the IMG experience with a bold experiment. IMGs who cannot compete for a residency in Canada for whatever reason, are eligible to take a series of orientation courses to become Canadian PAs. By doing so they agree to work as PAs for 2 years before opting to reapply for a residency. This approach is distinctly different from that of many U.S. PA programs, who are not enthusiatic to train or re-train IMGs to become PAs. IMGs represent a very heterogeneous group of physicians, some very well prepared and some not. It is not fair to paint them with a single brush. Canada, in its effort to build its PA profession, decided that IMGs would make very appropriate PA trainees. Most of these candidates will likely make fine PAs and will be appropriately socialized to their dependent role. Also, quite a number of PAs were once IMGs who underwent PA education in the United States, passed the PANCE, and have had successful PA careers.

Healthcare Reform

The wish of so many for so long, of a nation that has access for all citizens, is underway in 2009. It is too early to tell what this will mean for U.S. PAs other than demand will be high for their services. No reform will be as predicted and this movement will be subject to the unintended consequences of policy enactment in ways unanticipated. Predictors of success and failure are abundant. No matter what occurs, the subject will have a prominent place in our fourth edition.

RESEARCH

The research community continues to evaluate the effects of PA employment on quality, cost, access, and other aspects of healthcare delivery. Only by carefully documenting the capabilities of PAs using acceptable research methodologies will policy analysts be able to measure the profession's ability to meet the needs of the medical marketplace. Staffing currently remains a function of physician attitudes instead of administrative rationale (Hooker, 1994). Not until the measured benefits and utility of PAs are reported will change take place. Radical changes in healthcare staffing are not happening (or if so, they are happening slowly) because the data are not available to move managers to act favorably to PA employment. Data proving that PAs can function safely and effectively in healthcare roles are slow in coming and rarely adequate for large structural changes.

Without doubt, there will be encroachments on the homeostasis of the PA in the financial, choice, and professional domain. The girders of physician support of PAs are linked to being less autonomous and more dependent, regardless of skill and outcome. Relative to PAs, economic factors will to a great extent determine their future utilization patterns. Important questions remain for researchers as to how to best use PAs in various societies.

Formulating Research Questions

The essential nature of research is to create new knowledge and information about a subject that was relatively unknown. One of the ways the PA profession can effect change is to help formulate questions that will guide research in ways not only theoretically fruitful, but also historically appropriate. As part of this process the following research questions are offered:

■ **Economics:** Will the market forces remain sufficient to create a long-term demand for PAs? How can the profession document the efficacy, efficiency, and economy of PAs as primary care providers for patients?

■ **Global view:** How will the expansion of PAs globally stimulate interest in PAs?

■ **The next generation:** Should the profession try to recruit more trainees into the PA profession who are trained in economics, psychology, anthropology, and sociology who could stimulate areas of research?

■ **Organizational influences:** Should the AAPA contribute to funding research by supporting proactive, innovative studies that would enhance healthcare delivery?

■ **Leadership:** Should the AAPA help educate and nurture institutional leadership within organizations that have sufficient vision to recognize the pivotal role that PAs can play to more cost-effective healthcare delivery?

■ **History:** What should a time capsule on the profession contain?

■ **Adaptability:** How can PAs continue to demonstrate innovation, high quality, and technical sophistication in primary care medicine?

Some changes are underway that show promise. The AAPA is planning a summit meeting in 2010 aimed at setting research priorities for the PA profession. The PAEA has created a mechanism to stimulate and fund research. The Research Institute arm of the PAEA is organized to use the proceedings of investments to fund small grants for research ideas that examine PA behavior and education.

Research activity on the clinical and professional activities of PAs and other nonphysician providers is now experiencing some resurgence since the extensive health professions investigations conducted in the 1970s. Although much knowledge about PA use and clinical potentials has been learned from this past body of research and widespread empirical observations, many aspects of PA clinical roles and capabilities remain to be explored. For instance, what is the optimal mix of healthcare providers for delivering primary care? How can the economic advantages of these providers be best used in healthcare systems of the future? No data exist to determine how many PAs and NPs, along with physicians and other health professionals, would be required to staff newly emerging types of managed healthcare systems or to meet anticipated health workforce needs in either primary care or GME-related areas. Planning activities regarding the health professions should assess the present capacities of the United States in its healthcare workforce, consider the short-term and long-term population-based need for medical services, and articulate these estimates of need with national goals for providing services required to improve citizen health status. The present lack of reliable information on activities in the healthcare workforce places policymakers at a disadvantage in promoting effective use of PAs or coordinating PA supply and use with those of physicians.

Research on PA practice should focus on the following:

- Determining physician/PA substitutability ratios and task delegation levels in primary care, managed care, and graduate medical education (GME) settings
- Quality of care in chronic disease management such as diabetes, heart disease, renal insufficiency, geriatrics, rheumatic disorders, and disabilities
- Maximal PA/physician substitution potentials and optimal staffing mix in using PAs in GME positions
- Describing current practice characteristics and content of care delivered by PAs in primary care, including clinical preventive services
- Measuring PA levels of clinical productivity and patient care outcomes in various settings and comparing PA practice performance and contributions in primary care delivery with those of physicians and other health practitioners
- Describing the economic aspects of PA practice, including revenue generation, practice costs, and potential for savings
- Educational aspects contributing to minority attrition in PA educational programs
- How the full spectrum of worldwide systems train and deploy PAs

SUMMARY

Growth and *opportunity* are catchwords for the PA profession as it moves along in the new century. Numerous changes are expected, along with stimulating challenges. The 21st century is an exciting time to be a PA, and it is difficult for a profession to be too concerned about the future when it is riding the wave crest of demand. Current focus is on the expansion of the profession to meet the demand of the changing healthcare environment that wants more PAs. For the first time PAs are part of the health policy equation as planners estimate what the health workforce should be like in the years ahead.

An expanding population and an aging population mean greater demand for services. Furthermore, an uninsured population that needs care tends to create demand for services that are unexpected. Excessive health costs, poor access for some citizens, and uneven quality of care bodes well for the PA profession because PAs can help meet this demand quickly.

However, increased penetration and the fickle nature of managed care, coupled with efforts to improve efficiency in delivery, may dampen physician salaries. If rising PA salaries come close to physician salaries, then the surge of new graduates may produce the supply side of the equation that catches up with the demand side sooner than expected. Like all waves, the crest will break and supply will exceed demand. When this event will occur is difficult to predict.

The quality of PAs and medical care in developed countries has never been higher. If PAs want to remain in the great debate about what the medical workforce should look like, they must meet the challenge with the science that shows they are viable players.

RSH JFC DPA

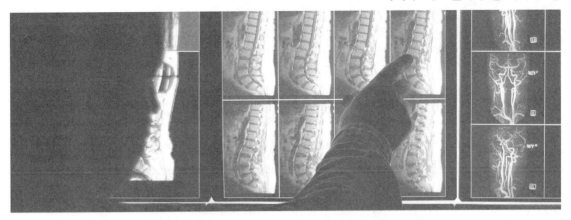

PHYSICIAN ASSISTANT
ORGANIZATIONS

The following information has been obtained from and is provided herein through the American Academy of Physician Assistants.

African Heritage Caucus
858 Saint Johns Place
Brooklyn, NY 11216-4306
(703) 836-2272 ext. 3409
blaqflava23@hotmail.com
http://www.aapa.org/caucus/ahc.html

Alabama Society of Physician Assistants
PO Box 1900
Montgomery, AL 36102-1900
(334) 315-6112
aspa@knology.net
http://www.myaspa.org

Alaska Academy of Physician Assistants
4450 Cordova Street, Suite 110
Anchorage, AK 99503-7273
(907) 646-0588
info@akapa.org
http://www.akapa.org

Alternative and Complementary Health Practices
229 Elizabeth Street, Apt 8
New York, NY 10012-5520
(954) 458-4918
hhpa2001@hotmail.com

American Academy of Nephrology Physician Assistants
2512 Culpeper Road
Alexandria, VA 22308-2133
(703) 360-3100
zuberkim@yahoo.com
http://www.aanpa.org

American Academy of Physician Assistants in Allergy, Asthma and Immunology
950 N Washington Street
Alexandria, VA 22314-1534
(866) 980-2272
aai@aapa.org
http://www.aapa-aai.com

American Academy of Physician Assistants in Legal Medicine
7033 Wellauer Drive
Milwaukee, WI 53213-3734
(474) 727-5467
jeff.g.nicholson@gmail.com
http://www.aapalm.org

American Academy of Physician Assistants in Occupational Medicine
950 N Washington Street
Alexandria, VA 22314-1534
(800) 596-4398
aapaom@aapa.org
http://www.aapaoccmed.org

American Association of Surgical Physician Assistants
4267 NW Federal Highway
PMB 201
Jensen Beach, FL 34957-3600
(888) 882-2772
aaspa@aaspa.com
http://www.aaspa.com

American Society of Endocrine Physician Assistants
8116 Lee Jackson Circle
Spotsylvania, VA 22553-3818
(540) 273-8472
endocrinepa@aol.com
http://www.endocrine-pa.com

Arizona State Association of Physician Assistants
PO Box 37697
Phoenix, AZ 85069-7697
(602) 995-3532
aspa@knology.org
http://www.asapa.org

Arkansas Academy of Physician Assistants
950 N Washington Street
Alexandria, VA 22314-1534
(877) 466-2272
arapa@aapa.org
http://www.arkansaspa.org

Association of Family Practice Physician Assistants
1905 Woodstock Road, Suite 2150
Roswell, GA 30075-5623
(770) 640-7605
afppa@afppa.org
http://www.afppa.org

Association of Neurosurgical Physician Assistants
PMB 202 4267 NW Federal Highway
Jensen Beach, FL 34957
(888) 942-6772
TheANSPA@aol.com
http://www.anspa.org

Association of Physician Assistants in Anesthesia
1322 Walkers Way
San Antonio, TX 78216-7709
(210) 292-5542
surgpa@yahoo.com
http://www.paanesthesiaworld.us

Association of Physician Assistants in Cardiology
950 N Washington Street
Alexandria, VA 22314-1534
(866) 970-2272
apac@aapa.org
http://cardiologypa.org

Association of Physician Assistants in Cardiovascular Surgery
PO Box 4834
Englewood, CO 80155-4834
(303) 221-5651
carol@goddardassociates.com
http://www.apacvs.org/

Association of Physician Assistants in Hospital Medicine
8150 Kraay Avenue
Munster, IN 46321-1423
(219) 201-1299
jsaltzma@medicine.bsd.uchicago.edu
http://www.hospitalistpa.org

**Association of Physician Assistants
in Obstetrics and Gynecology**
PO Box 1109
Madison, WI 53701-1109
(800) 545-0636
apaog@paobgyn.org
http://www.paobgyn.org

**Association of Physician Assistants
in Oncology**
950 N Washington Street
Alexandria, VA 22314-1534
(703) 836-2272
apao@aapa.org
http://www.apao.cc

**Association of Physician Assistants
in Phlebology**
6 Maggie Lane
Gray, ME 04039-7744
(207) 415-1958
cardiacman22@maine.rr.com

**Association of Plastic Surgery Physician
Assistants**
Texas Childrens Hospital
6621 Fannin MC-CC 610.00
Houston, TX 77030
(713) 443-5960
plasticsurgerypas@yahoo.com
http://www.apspa.net

Caduceus Caucus
162 Harrison Avenue
Glenside, PA 19038-4009
(215) 884-6220
bjspaethic@aol.com

California Academy of Physician Assistants
3100 W Warner Avenue, Suite 3
Santa Ana, CA 92704-5331
(714) 427-0321
capa@capanet.org
http://www.capanet.org

**Catholic Organization for Physician
Assistants**
1200 Town Center Drive
#306
Jupiter, FL 33458
(201) 906-1565
padrca@yahoo.com

**Caucus of Community College/Certificate
Physician Assistants**
8400 W Mineral King Avenue
SJVC Primary Care PA Program
Visalia, CA 93291-9283
(559) 651-3478 ext. 350
LesH@sjvc.edu

Colorado Academy of Physician Assistants
PO Box 4834
Englewood, CO 80155-4834
(303) 770-6048
carol@goddardassociates.com
http://www.coloradopas.org

**Connecticut Academy of Physician
Assistants**
1 Regency Drive
PO Box 30
Bloomfield, CT 06002-2310
(860) 243-3977
connapa@ssmgt.com
http://www.connapa.org

Delaware Academy of Physician Assistants
704 Dorcaster Drive
Wilmington, DE 19808-2214
(443) 350-1893
richpac@delawarepas.org
http://www.delawarepas.org

**District of Columbia Academy
of Physician Assistants**
950 N Washington Street
Alexandria, VA 22314-1534
(703) 836-4175
dcapa@aapa.org
http://www.dcapa.org

Downeast Association of Physician Assistants
30 Asssociation Drive
PO Box 190
Manchester, ME 04351-0190
(207) 620-7577
kmiller@deapa.ocom
http://www.deapa.com

Fellowship of Christian Physician Assistants
PO Box 2006
Bristol, TN 37621-2006
(423) 844-1015
fcpa@fcpa.net
http://www.fcpa.net

First Nations Council of Physician Assistants
16 Cloud March E
Santa Fe, NM 87506-2171
(505) 989-1893
wabanang@msn.com
http://home.pacbell.net/kuczek/index.htm

Florida Academy of Physician Assistants
222 S Westmonte Drive, Suite 101
Altamonte Springs, FL 32714-4268
(407) 774-7880
tkautter@kmgnet.com
http://www.fapaonline.org

Gastroenterology Physician Assistants
950 N Washington Street
Alexandria, VA 22314-1534
(703) 836-2272 ext. 3409
gipa@aapa.org
http://www.gipas.org

Georgia Association of Physician Assistants
1905 Woodstock Road, Suite 2150
Roswell, GA 30075-5623
(770) 640-1920
gapa@gapa.net
http://www.gapa.net

Guahan Association of Physician Assistants
PO Box 6578
Tamuning, GU 96931-6578
(671) 646-5824
karynkaufman@mail.com

Hawaii Academy of Physician Assistants
PO Box 30355
Honolulu, HI 96820-0355
(888) 727-4440
opa79@aol.com
http://www.hapahawaii.org

Idaho Academy of Physician Assistants
6057 N Castleton Lane
PO Box 140357
Boise, ID 83714-0357
(208) 343-4818
ssass@idmed.org
http://www.Idahopa.org

Illinois Academy of Physician Assistants
225 E Cook Street
Springfield, IL 62704-2509
(800) 975-9344
info@illinoispa.org
http://www.illinoisPA.org

Indiana Academy of Physician Assistants
950 N Washington Street
Alexandria, VA 22314-1534
(888) 441-0423
iapa@aapa.org
http://www.indianapas.org

Iowa Physician Assistant Society
525 SW 5th Street, Suite A
Des Moines, IA 50309-4501
(515) 282-8192
leann@iapasociety.org
http://www.iapasociety.org

Jewish Association of Physician Assistants
5 N Crest Place
Lakewood, NJ 08701-2967
(732) 886-2997
a_homnick@yahoo.com

Kansas Academy of Physician Assistants
PO Box 597
Topeka, KS 66601-0597
(785) 235-5065
kansaspa@sbcglobal.net
http://www.kansaspa.com

Kentucky Academy of Physician Assistants
950 N Washington Street
Alexandria, VA 22314-1534
(866) 967-4725
kapa@aapa.org
http://www.kentuckypa.org

Lesbian, Bisexual, Gay & Transgender Physician Assistant Caucus
950 N Washington Street
Alexandria, VA 22134
m-cochair@lbgpa.org
http://www.lbgpa.org

Louisiana Academy of Physician Assistants
PMB 177 9655 Perkins Road, Suite C
Baton Rouge, LA 70810-1534
(318) 658-3759
info@ourlapa.org
http://www.ourlapa.org

Maryland Academy of Physician Assistants
PO Box 1726
Annapolis, MD 21404-1726
(888) 357-3360
info@mdapa.org
http://www.mdapa.org

Massachusetts Association of Physician Assistants
PO Box 473
Ludlow, MA 01056-0473
(866) 548-4415
mapa56@msn.com
http://www.mass-pa.com

Michigan Academy of Physician Assistants
120 W Saginaw Street
East Lansing, MI 48823-2605
(517) 336-7505
mapa@michiganpa.org
http://www.michiganpa.org

Minnesota Academy of Physician Assistants
600 S Highway 169 Suite 1680
St. Louis Park, MN 55426-1275
(952) 542-0130
office@mnacadpa.org
http://www.mnacadpa.org

Mississippi Academy of Physician Assistants
950 N Washington Street
Alexandria, VA 22314-1534
(800) 844-4902
missipas@aapa.org
http://www.missipas.org

Missouri Academy of Physician Assistants
950 N Washington Street
Alexandria, VA 22314-1534
(800) 844-4902
mapa@aapa.org
http://www.moapa.org

Montana Academy of Physician Assistants
2475 Village Lane, Suite 300
Billings, MT 59102-2497
(406) 652-0227
holly@cynroc.com
http://www.mtapa.com

Naval Association of Physician Assistants
950 N Washington Street
Alexandria, VA 22314-1534
(703) 836-2272 ext. 3308
napa@aapa.org
http://www.aapacoms.org/napa/index.htm

Nebraska Academy of Physician Assistants
1335 H Street, Suite 100
Lincoln, NE 68508-3790
(402) 476-1528
info@nebraska.org
http://www.nebraskapa.org

Neuroscience Alliance for Physician Assistants
PO Box 18089
Cleveland, OH 44118-0089
(425) 899-3107
sfarris@neurosciencealliance.net
http://www.neurosciencealliance.net

Nevada Academy of Physician Assistants
PO Box 28877
Las Vegas, NV 89126-2877
(702) 777-1765
president@nevada.com
http://www.nevadapa.com

New Hampshire Society of Physician Assistants
PO Box 325
Manchester, NH 03105-0325
(603) 305-0262
nhspa.org@gmail.com
http://www.nh-spa.org

New Jersey State Society of Physician Assistants
760 Alexander Road
Princeton, NJ 08540-6305
(609) 275-4123
njsspa@njha.com
http://www.njsspa.org

New Mexico Academy of Physician Assistants
PO Box 40331
Albuquerque, NM 87196-0331
(505) 342-8023
edamour@salud.unm.edu
http://www.nmapa.com

The New PA
3458 River North Drive
San Antonio, TX 78230-2576
(210) 412-6313
the_new_pa@yahoo.com

New York State Society of Physician Assistants
251 New Karner Road, Suite 10A
Albany, NY 12205-4617
(877) 769-7722
info@nysspa.org
http://www.nysspa.org

North Carolina Academy of Physician Assistants
1121 Slater Road
Durham, NC 27703-8474
(919) 479-1995
mike.borden@ncapa.org
http://www.ncapa.org

North Dakota Academy of Physician Assistants
1412 Cottonwood Avenue
Minot, ND 58707-0001
(701) 838-6394
terri_lang@und.nodak.edu
http://www.ndapahome.org

Ohio Association of Physician Assistants
579 High Street
Worthington, OH 43085-4132
(800) 292-4997
oapa@ohiopa.com
http://www.ohiopa.com

Oklahoma Academy of Physician Assistants
PO Box 1132
Oklahoma City, OK 73101-1132
(405) 236-3161
susan-semtner@ouhsc.edu
http://www.okpa.org

Oregon Society of Physician Assistants
PO Box 2794
Hillsboro, OR 97123-1931
(503) 650-5864
ospa@oregonpa.org
http://www.oregonpa.org

Pennsylvania Society of Physician Assistants
PO Box 128
Greensburg, PA 15601-0128
(724) 836-6411
pspa@pspa.net
http://www.pspa.net

Physician Assistant Academy of Vermont
45 Lyme Road, Suite 304
Hanover, NH 03755-1223
(603) 643-2325
paav@conmx.net
http://www.paav.org

Physician Assistant Administrators, Managers and Supervisors
AAPA 950 North Washington Street
Alexandria, VA 22314
(703) 836-2272 ext. 3414
pspurlock@aapa.org

Physician Assistant Cancer Survivors
210 9th Street SE
Olmsted Medical Center
Rochester, MN 55904-6425
(507) 288-3443
cloversnotes@hotmail.com

Physician Assistants AIDS Network (PAAN)
4N382 Mark Twain Street
Saint Charles, IL 60175-6521
(847) 695-1093
alisont@opendoorclinic.org

Physician Assistants of Asians and Pacific Islanders
105 Old Stewart Avenue
New Hyde Park, NY 11040
(917) 2094175
qycherylann@hotmail.com
http://www.asianpacificpa.org

Physician Assistants in Correctional Health Care
PO Box 546
Las Cruces, NM 88004-0546
(505) 523-3222
emanrique@salud.unm.edu

Physician Assistants in Forensic Medicine
1910 Massachusetts Avenue SE, Building 27
Washington, DC 20003-2542
(202) 698-9016
marybeth.petrasek@dc.gov

Physician Assistants for Global Health
3334 Goat Fell
Ann Arbor, MI 48108-2087
(678) 595-8201
folu@yahoo.com
http://www.pasforglobalhealth.org

Physician Assistants for Health Freedom
306 McCoy Place Road
Sewickley, PA 15143-8854
shayjones@verizon.net
http://www.healthfreedompas.com

Physician Assistants in Infectious Diseases
1210 South Cedar Crest Boulevard
Suite 2700
Allentown, PA 18103-6229
(610) 402-8430 ext 8004
ryann.rood@lvh.com

Physician Assistants for Latino Health
950 N Washington Street
Alexandria, VA 22314-1534
(800) 596-7494
palh@aapa.org
http://pasforlatinohealth.org

Physician Assistants in Orthopedic Surgery
PO Box 10781
Glendale, AZ 85318-0781
(800) 804-7267
info@paos.org
http://www.paos.org

Physician Assistants in Pain Management
8405 E Hampden Avenue, Apt 23C
Denver, CO 80231-4820
(970) 215-0903
ckotten@bigfoot.com

Physician Assistants Pilots Caucus
4916 E Wagoner Road
Scottsdale, AZ 85254-7511
(602) 795-5949
lippincott.randy@mayo.edu

Physician Assistants for Prevention and Public Health
950 N Washington Street
Alexandria, VA 22314-1534
(703) 836-2272 ext. 3416
bmcnellis@aapa.org
http://phsapa.com

Physician Assistants in Psychiatry
4968 400th Street SE
Iowa City, IA 52240-9068
(319) 341-9115
don-stjohn@uiowa.edu
http://www.psychpa.com

Physician Assistants for Puerto Rico/Medico
PO Box 1513
Cidra, PR 00739-1513
(787) 641-7582 ext. 22114/5
manuel.guzman2@med.va.org

Physician Assistants in Research
1616 Millard Street
Bethlehem, PA 18017-5141
(570) 424-1102
christenkutz@yahoo.com
http://www.pa-research.com

Physician Assistants for Social Justice
3917 Linden Avenue
Long Beach, CA 90807-2714
(562) 424-8009
blesofsk@usc.edu

**Public Health Service Academy
of Physician Assistants**
1913 Jenny Wren Road
Lawrence, KS 66047-2226
(785) 749-3287
gcsnowhawk2000@yahoo.com
http://phsapa.com

Radiology Physician Assistants Association
Berkshire Medical Center Radiology
725 North Street
Pittsfield, MA 01201-4109
(413) 447-3222
jeffreykellogg@yahoo.com

**Rhode Island Academy of Physician
Assistants**
1 Regency Drive
Bloomfield, CT 06002-2310
(860) 243-3977
riapa@ssmgt.com
http://www.myriapa.org

**Rural Health Caucus of the American
Academy of Physician Assistants**
111 Mayfair Way
Ada, OK 74820-7238
(580) 759-2336
kubier@cableone.net

Society of Air Force Physician Assistants
PO Box 340838
San Antonio, TX 78234-0838
(972) 333-2315
info@safpa.org
http://www.safpa.org

Society of Army Physician Assistants
PO Box 07490
Fort Myers, FL 33919
(239) 482-2162
hal.slusher@juno.com
http://www.sapa.org

**Society of Dermatology Physician
Assistants**
PO Box 701461
San Antonio, TX 78270-1461
(800) 380-3992
SDPA@dermpa.org
http://www.dermpa.org

**Society of Emergency Medicine Physician
Assistants**
222 S Westmonte Drive, Suite 101
Altamonte Springs, FL 32714-4268
(866) 220-6660
sempa@sempa.org
http://www.sempa.org

**Society of Physician Assistants in Addiction
Medicine**
162 Harrison Avenue
Glenside, PA 19038-4009
(215) 884-6220
bjspaethic@aol.com

Society of Physician Assistants Caring for the Elderly
785 Paul Birch Drive
Crownsville, MD 21032-1501
(410) 766-3115
pwarnock@awcubed.com
http://www.geri-pa.org

Society of Physician Assistants in Otorhinolaryngology/Head and Neck Surgery
950 N Washington Street
Alexandria, VA 22314-1534
(703) 836-2272 ext. 3418
spao@aapa.org
http://www.entpa.org

Society for Physician Assistants in Pediatrics
950 N Washington Street
Alexandria, VA 22314-1534
(800) 596-4398
spap@aapa.org
http://www.spaponline.org/index.php

Society of Physician Assistants in Rheumatology
950 N Washington Street
Alexandria, VA 22314-1534
(866) 980-2272
spar@aapa.org
http://www.aapacoms.org/spar

Society of Physician Assistants in Trauma and (Surgical) Critical Care
9885 SW Ardenwood Street
Portland, OR 97225-4912
(503) 384-0062
sherrys@ohsu.edu

South Carolina Academy of Physician Assistants
PO Box 2054
Lexington, SC 29071-2054
(803) 356-6809
scapa@sc.rr.com
http://www.scapapartners.org

South Dakota Academy of Physician Assistants
120 S Madison Avenue
Pierre, SD 57501-3536
(605) 224-1203
nafmb@dakota2k.net
http://www.sdapa.net

Tennessee Academy of Physician Assistants
PO Box 150785
Nashville, TN 37215-0785
(615) 463-0026
kmoffat@tnpa.com
http://www.tnpa.com

Texas Academy of Physician Assistants
401 W 15th Street
Austin, TX 78701-1670
(800) 280-7655
lisa.jackson@texmed.org
http://www.tapa.org

Urological Association of Physician Assistants
PO Box 955
Farmville, NC 27828-0955
(252) 228-0064
whancock7@nc.rr.com
http://www.uapanet.org

Utah Academy of Physician Assistants
995 Vista View Drive
Salt Lake City, UT 84108-2520
(801) 913-3466
bunnellbob@hotmail.com
http://www.utahapa.org

Veterans Affairs Physician Assistant Association
PO Box 128
Iron Mountain, MI 49801-0128
(866) 828-2722
vapaa1@vapaa.org
http://www.vapaa.org

Veterans Caucus of the American Academy of Physician Assistants
PO Box 362
Danville, PA 17821-0362
(570) 271-0292
skhanley@ptd.net
http://www.veteranscaucus.org

Virginia Academy of Physician Assistants
950 N Washington Street
Alexandria, VA 22314-1534
(703) 836-4207
vapa@vapa.org
http://www.vapa.org

Virgin Islands Academy of Physician Assistants
PMB 163 40193 Diamond Ruby, Suite 7
Christensted, St Croix, VI 00820
(860) 983-5524
petelopez@aya.yale.edu

Washington State Academy of Physician Assistants
2033 6th Avenue, Suite 1100
Seattle, WA 98121-2590
(206) 956-3624
LMK@wsma.org
http://www.wapa.com

West Virginia Association of Physician Assistants
950 N Washington Street
Alexandria, VA 22314-1534
(888) 903-2272
wvapa@aapa.org
http://www.mywvapa.org

Wisconsin Academy of Physician Assistants
PO Box 1109
Madison, WI 53701-1109
(800) 762-8965
wapa@wismed.org
http://www.wapa.org

Women's Association of Physician Assistants
240 E 53rd Street
Savannah, GA 31405-3409
(912) 441-4937
gabesmom@comcast.net

Wyoming Association of Physician Assistants
PO Box 4009
Cheyenne, WY 82003-4009
(307) 635-2424
wyoming_pas@yahoo.com
http://www.wapa.net

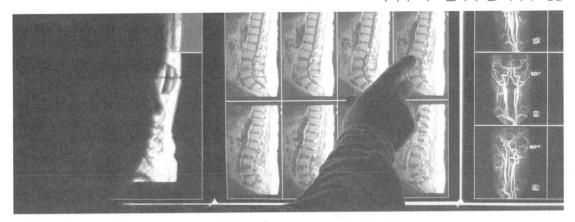

PHYSICIAN ASSISTANT
PROGRAMS

Contact information for various physician assistant programs are listed below. For more information about the status of a program's accreditation, please contact the program directly.

PA programs in the United Sates are accredited by the Accreditation Review Commission for Physician Assistants (ARC-PA). As of October 1, 2009, there were 148 programs accredited through ARC-PA. For a current listing of ARC-PA accredited programs, go to the website: http://www.arc-pa.org/Acc_Programs/acc_programs.html.

AUSTRALIA

James Cook University
Physician Assistant Program
The Registrar
Townsville QLD 4811
Australia
http://www.jcu.edu.au

University of Queensland
Physician Assistant Program
The Registrar
Brisbane QLD 4072
Australia
E-mail: karen.mulitalo@uq.edu.au
http://www.uq.edu.au

CANADA

Manitoba

University of Manitoba
Physician Assistant Education Program
Office of Physician Assistant Studies
University of Manitoba
P127, 770 Bannatyne Avenue
Winnipeg, MB R3E 0W3
Phone: 204-272-3094
http://www.umanitoba.ca/faculties/graduate_studies/admissions/567.htm

Ontario

Canadian Forces
Health Services Education Center
Borden, ON
http://www.forces.gc.ca/health-sante/cfhsco-cssfco/cp/clinicpulse-2009-01-eng.asp

McMaster University
Michael G. DeGroote School of Medicine, Room 2201
1200 Main Street West
Hamilton, ON L8N 3Z5
Fax: 905-528-4727
E-mail: paprogram@mcmaster.ca
http://www.mcmaster.ca

University of Toronto
Physician Assistant Program
Faculty of Medicine
500 University Avenue, Suite 602
Toronto, ON M5G 1V7
Phone: 416-946-7173
E-mail: physician.assistant@utoronto.ca
http://www.PAconsortium.ca

GREAT BRITIAN

St. George's University of London
Post Graduate Diploma Physician Assistant
Studies
St. George's University of London
Cranmer Terrace London, UK SW17 0RE
E-mail: physicianassistant@sgul.ac.uk
http://sgul.ac.uk/postgraduate/taught-
courses/postgraduate-diploma-physician-
assistant-studies-1

University of Birmingham
Post Graduate Diploma Physician Assistant
Studies
Medical School
University of Birmingham
Edgbaston, Birmingham, UK B15 2TT
E-mail: physicianassistant@contacts.bham.ac.uk
http://www.postgraduate.bham.ac.uk/
programmes/taught/medicine/physician-
assistant.shtml

University of Hertfordshire
Master of Science Physician Assistant Studies
Medical Practice
Hatfield, UK AL10 9AB
E-mail: m.p.brennan@herts.ac.uk
http://www.herts.ac.uk/courses/Physician-
Assistant-Studies—Medical-Practice.cfm

University of Wolverhampton
Physician Assistant Studies—Postgraduate
Diploma
School of Health
University of Wolverhampton
Wulfruna Street, Wolverhampton,
UK WV1 1LY
E-mail: M.Humphreys@wlv.ac.uk.
http://www.wlv.ac.uk/default.aspx?
page=17177

THE NETHERLANDS

Rotterdam University (Applied Sciences)
School of Health Care Studies
Master Physician Assistant
Museumpark 40
3015 CX Rotterdam
0031 10 794 53 12
www.hogeschoolrotterdam.nl

**HAN University of Applied Sciences
(Hogeschool van Arnhem en Nijmegen)**
HAN Master Program GGM
Dependance HAN
Sint Annastraat 312
6525 HG NIJMEGEN
Phone: +31(0)24-3530577
E-mail: secretariaat.masterGGM@han.nl
http://www.han.nl/opleidingen/master/
physician-assistant/programma

**Hanze University of Applied Sciences
Groningen (Hanzehogeschool Groningen)**
School of Health Care Studies
Master Physician Assistant
Eyssoniusplein 18
9714 CE GRONINGEN
PO Box 3109
9701 DC GRONINGEN
Phone: +31(0)50-5957750/ +31(0)50-5953818
E-mail: a.van.geer@pl.hanze.nl or
b.draaisma-groenwold@pl.hanze.nl
http://www.hanze.nl/home/Schools/
Academie+voor+Gezondheidsstudies/
Opleidingen/Master/Physician+Assistant/

**InHolland University of Applied Sciences
(Hogeschool InHolland)**
School of Health, Graduate School
Master Physician Assistant
De Boelelaan 1109
1081 HV AMSTERDAM
Phone: +31(0)20-4951465
E-mail: health.masters@inholland.nl
http://www.inholland.nl/Graduate+School/
Opleidingen/Master+Physician+Assistant/

**University of Applied Sciences Utrecht
(Hogeschool Utrecht)**
Master Physician Assistant
Bolognalaan 101
3508 AD Utrecht
Postbus 85182
Phone: +31(0)30-2585307
E-mail: loes.vanbiljouw@hu.nl
http://www.pa.hu.nl

SOUTH AFRICA

University of Pretoria
Clinical Associate Program
http://www.up.ac.za

**University of Witswaterrand in Gauteng
Province**
Clinical Associate Program
http://www.witz.ac.za

**Walter Sisulu University for Technology &
Science, Eastern Cape**
Clinical Associates Program
http://www.wsu.ac.za/admissions/
prospectus/genindex.htm

TAIWAN, REPUBLIC OF CHINA

Fooyin University
151, Chinhsueh Rd.
Ta-liao, Kaohsiung, Taiwan, R.O.C
Phone: +886-7-7811151, ext. 186
E-mail: sn@mail.fy.edu.tw
http://english.fy.edu.tw

UNITED STATES

Alabama
University of Alabama at Birmingham
Surgical Physician Assistant Program
School of Health Related Professions
SHPB 481; 1530 3rd Avenue South
Birmingham, AL 35294-1212
Phone: 205-934-4605
E-mail: kpeoples@uab.edu

University of South Alabama
Department of Physician Assistant Studies
1504 Springhill Avenue, Suite 4410
Mobile, AL 36604-3273
Phone: 251-434-3641
E-mail: pastudies@usouthal.edu

Arizona
Arizona School of Health Sciences
Physician Assistant Program
5850 East Still Circle
Mesa, AZ 85206
Phone: 480-219-6000
E-mail: paprogram@atsu.edu

Midwestern University
PA Program
Office of Admissions
Physician Assistant Program
19555 North 59th Avenue
Glendale, AZ 85308-6813
Phone: 623-572-3215
Email: klohen@midwestern.edu

Arkansas
Harding University
Physician Assistant Program
915 East Market Avemue
HU 12231
Searcy, AR 72149-2231
Phone: 501-279-5642
E-mail: paprogram@harding.edu

California
**Charles R. Drew University of Medicine
and Science**
Physician Assistant Program
The College of Allied Health Keck Building
1731 East 120th Street
Los Angeles, CA 90059
Phone: 323-563-5950
E-mail: caspauld@cdrewu.edu

Keck School of Medicine of the University of Southern California
Physician Assistant Program
Department of Family Medicine
1000 South Fremont Avenue, Unit 7, Bldg.
A-6, Rm. 6429
Alhambra, CA 91803-8897
Phone: 626-457-4240
E-mail: uscpa@usc.edu

Loma Linda University
Department of Physician Assistant Sciences
School of Allied Health Professions
Nichol Hall, Room 2033
Loma Linda, CA 92350
Phone: 909-558-7295
E-mail: RJWilliams@llu.edu

Riverside County Regional Medical Center/Riverside Community College
Physician Assistant Program
16130 Lasselle Street
Moreno Valley, CA 92551
Phone: 951-571-6166
Email: pa@rcc.edu

Samuel Merritt College
Physician Assistant Program
450 30th Street, Suite 4708
Oakland, CA 94609
Phone: 510-869-6623
E-mail: admission@samuelmerritt.edu

San Joaquin Valley College
Primary Care PA Program
Visalia Campus
8400 West Mineral King Avenue
Visalia, CA 93291
Phone: 559-651-2500, ext. 351
E-mail: monicau@sjvc.edu

Stanford University School of Medicine
Primary Care Associate Program
Family Nurse Practitioner/Physician
Assistant Program
1215 Welch Road, Modular G
Palo Alto, CA 94305-5408
Phone: 650-725-6959
E-mail: pcap-information@lists.stanford.edu

Touro University—California College of Health Sciences
Joint MSPAS/MPH Program
College of Health Sciences
1310 Johnson Lane
Vallejo, CA 94592
Phone: 888-652-7580
E-mail: sdavis@touro.edu

University of California—Davis
Physician Assistant Program/Family Nurse Practitioner Program
Department of Family and Community Medicine
2516 Stockton Boulevard, Suite 254
Sacramento, CA 95817-2208
Phone: 916-734-3551
E-mail: fnppa@ucdavis.edu

Western University of Health Sciences
Primary Care Physician Assistant Program
309 East Second Street
Pomona, CA 91766-1854
Phone: 909-469-5378
E-mail: admissions@westernu.edu

Colorado

Red Rocks Community College
Red Rocks Community College PA Program
Campus Box 38
13300 West 6th Avenue
Lakewood, CO 80228-1255
Phone: 303-914-6386
E-mail: ruth.fry@rrcc.edu

University of Colorado at Denver and Health Sciences Center
Child Health Associate/Physician Assistant Program
Mail Stop F543, P.O. Box 6508
Aurora, CO 80045
Phone: 303-724-1344
E-mail: chapa-info@ucdenver.edu

Connecticut

Quinnipiac University
Physician Assistant Program
Office of Graduate Admissions (AB-GRD)
275 Mount Carmel Avenue
Hamden, CT 06518-1908
Phone: 203-582-8672
E-mail: graduate@quinnipiac.edu

Yale University School of Medicine
Physician Associate Program
Harkness Office Building, Second Floor
367 Cedar Street
New Haven, CT 06510-3222
Phone: 203-785-2860
E-mail: pa.program@yale.edu

District of Columbia

George Washington University
Physician Assistant Program
Department of Health Care Sciences,
School of Medicine and Health Sciences
900 23rd Street NW, Suite 6148
Washington, DC 20037
Phone: 202-994-6661
E-mail: paadm@gwumc.edu

Howard University
Physician Assistant Program
College of Pharmacy, Nursing and Allied
Health Sciences
6th & Bryant Street, NW, Annex Il, #119
Washington, DC 20059
Phone: 202-806-7536
E-mail: Spowers@howard.edu

Florida

Barry University
Physician Assistant Program
11300 NE Second Avenue, Box SGMS
Miami Shores, FL 33161
Phone: 305-899-3296
E-mail: mweiner@mail.barry.edu

Keiser University
Physician Assistant Program
1500 NW 49th Street
Ft. Lauderdale, FL 33309
http://www.keiseruniversity.edu/
graduateschool/PA/packet.php

Miami Dade College
Physician Assistant Program
Medical Center Campus
950 NW 20th Street
Miami, FL 33127-4693
Phone: 305-237-4124
E-mail: Jhernan7@mdc.edu

Nova Southeastern University—
Ft. Lauderdale
Physician Assistant Program
3200 South University Drive
Ft. Lauderdale, FL 33328
Phone: 954-262-1250
800-356-0026
E-mail: melissa.colffman@nova.edu

Nova Southeastern University—
Jacksonville
Physician Assistant Program
6675 Corporate Center Parkway, Suite 112
Jacksonville, FL 32216
Phone: 904-245-8990
E-mail: dgerbert@nova.edu

Nova Southeastern University—Naples
Physician Assistant Program
2655 Northbrooke Drive
Naples, FL 34119
Phone: 239-591-4528, ext. 20
E-mail: jkeena@nsu.nova.edu

Nova Southeastern University—Orlando
Physician Assistant Program
4850 Millenia Boulevard
Orlando, FL 32839
Phone: 407-264-5150
E-mail: asantiag@nova.edu

University of Florida
Physician Assistant Program
P.O. Box 100176
Gainesville, FL 32610-0176
Phone: 352-265-7955
E-mail: taryn.stoffs@medicine.ufl.edu

Georgia

Emory University School of Medicine
Physician Assistant Program
Department of Family and Preventive
Medicine
1462 Clifton Road, Suite 280
Atlanta, GA 30322
Phone: 404-727-7825
E-mail: emory-pa-admit@learnlink.emory.edu

Medical College of Georgia
Physician Assistant Program
Physician Assistant Department EC-3304
Augusta, GA 30912
Phone: 706-721-3246
E-mail: underadm@mail.mcg.edu

Mercer University College of Pharmacy and Health Sciences
Physician Assistant Program
3001 Mercer University Drive
Davis Building, Suite 213
Atlanta, GA 30341
Phone: 678-547-6214
E-mail: paprogram@mercer.edu

South University
Physician Assistant Program
709 Mall Boulevard
Savannah, GA 31406
Phone: 912-201-8171
E-mail: paprogram@southuniversity.edu

Idaho

Idaho State University
Department of Physician Assistant Studies
921 South 8th Avenue, Stop-8253
Pocatello, ID 83209-8253
Phone: 208-282-4726
E-mail: pa@isu.edu

Illinois

John H. Stroger, Jr. Hospital of Cook County/Malcolm X College
Physician Assistant Program
1900 West Van Buren, #3241
Chicago, IL 60612
Phone: 312-850-7255

Midwestern University Downers Grove
Physician Assistant Program
555 31st Street
Downers Grove, IL 60515
Phone: 800-458-6253
E-mail: admissil@midwestern.edu

Rosalind Franklin University of Medicine and Science
Physician Assistant Program
3333 Green Bay Road
North Chicago, IL
60064-3095
Phone: 847-578-8686
E-mail: pa.admissions@rosalindfranklin.edu

Southern Illinois University Carbondale
Physician Assistant Program
Lindegren Hall, Room 129, Mail Code 6516
Carbondale, IL 62901-6516
Phone: 618-453-5527
E-mail: pa_advisement@siumed.edu

Indiana

Bethel College
1001 West McKinley Avenue
Mishawaka, IN 46545
Phone: 574-259-8511

Butler University/Clarian Health
Physician Assistant Program
College of Pharmacy and Health Sciences
4600 Sunset Avenue
Indianapolis, IN 46208
Phone: 317-940-9969
E-mail: dpearson@butler.edu

University of Saint Francis
Department of Physician Assistant Studies
2701 Spring Street
Fort Wayne, IN 46808
Phone: 260-434-7737
E-mail: jcashdollar@sf.edu

Iowa

Des Moines University
Physician Assistant Program
3200 Grand Avenue
Des Moines, IA 50312
Phone: 515-271-1685
E-mail: paadmit@dmu.edu

University of Iowa
Physician Assistant Program
Carver College of Medicine
5167 Westlawn
Iowa City, IA 52242-1100
Phone: 319-335-8922
E-mail: paprogram@uiowa.edu

Kansas

Wichita State University
Physician Assistant Program
College of Health Professions
1845 North Fairmount, Box 43
Wichita, KS 67260-0043
Phone: 316-978-3011
E-mail: dee.mcdaniel@wichita.edu

Kentucky

University of the Cumberlands
Physician Assistant Program
6191 College Station Drive
Williamsburg, KY 40769
E-mail: pa@ucumberlands.edu

University of Kentucky
Physician Assistant Program
College of Health Sciences
900 South Limestone Street, Suite 205
Lexington, KY
40536-0200
Phone: 859-323-1100
E-mail: laalle1@uky.edu

Louisiana

Louisiana State University Health Sciences Center
Physician Assistant Program
School of Allied Health Professions
1501 Kings Highway
Shreveport, LA 71130-3932
Phone: 318-813-2920 675-7317
E-mail: kmeyer1@lsuhsc.edu

Our Lady of the Lake College
Physician Associate Program
7443 Picardy Avenue
Baton Rouge, LA 70808
Phone: 225-214-6988
E-mail: egrant@ololcollege.edu

Maine

The University of New England
Physician Assistant Program
716 Stevens Avenue
312 Hersey Hall
Portland, ME 04103-7688
Phone: 207-221-4529
E-mail: GradAdmissions@une.edu

Maryland

Anne Arundel Community College
Physician Assistant Program
School of Health Professions, Wellness and
Physical Education
101 College Parkway
Arnold, MD 21012
Phone: 410-777-7310
E-mail: mjbondy@aacc.edu

Towson University—CCBC Essex
Physician Assistant Program
7201 Rossville Boulevard
Baltimore, MD 21237-1899
Phone: 410-780-6159
E-mail: sshaw@ccbcmd.edu

University of Maryland—Eastern Shore
Physician Assistant Department
Hazel Hall, Room 1034
Princess Anne, MD 21853
Phone: 410-651-7584
E-mail: pa@mail.umes.edu

Massachusetts

Massachusetts College of Pharmacy and Health Sciences
Physician Assistant Studies Program
179 Longwood Avenue, W110
Boston, MA 02115
Phone: 617-732-2918
E-mail: admissions@mcphs.edu

Northeastern University
Physician Assistant Program
360 Huntington Avenue
202 Robinson Hall
Boston, MA 02115
Phone: 617-373-3195
E-mail: paprogram@neu.edu

Springfield College
Physician Assistant Program
263 Alden Street
Springfield, MA 01109
Phone: 413-748-3554
http://www.springfieldcollege.edu

Michigan

Central Michigan University
Physician Assistant Program
1222 Health Professions Building
Mount Pleasant, MI 48859
Phone: 989-774-2478
E-mail: chpadmit@cmich.edu

Grand Valley State University
Physician Assistant Studies Program
301 Michigan Street, NE, Suite 200 CHS
Grand Rapids, MI 49503
Phone: 616-331-3356
E-mail: pas@gvsu.edu

University of Detroit—Mercy
Physician Assistant Program
4001 West McNichols Road
Detroit, MI 48221
Phone: 313-993-2474
E-mail: warnimsk@udmercy.edu

Wayne State University
Physician Assistant Studies Program
259 Mack Avenue, Suite 2590
Detroit, MI 48201
Phone: 313-577-1368
E-mail: ac2605@wayne.edu

Western Michigan University
Physician Assistant Program
1903 West Michigan Avenue
Kalamazoo, MI 49008-5138
Phone: 269-387-5314

Minnesota

Augsburg College
Physician Assistant Program
Campus Box 149
2211 Riverside Avenue
Minneapolis, MN 55454
Phone: 612-330-1399
E-mail: paprog@augsburg.edu

Missouri

Missouri State University
Department of Physician Assistant Studies
901 South National Avenue
PTPA 112
Springfield, MO 65897
Phone: 417-836-6151
E-mail:
physicianasststudies@missouristate.edu

Saint Louis University
Physician Assistant Program
Doisy College of Health Sciences
3437 Caroline Street
St. Louis, MO 63104-1111
Phone: 314-977-8521
E-mail: paprog@slu.edu

Montana

Rocky Mountain College
Master of Physician Assistant Studies
Program
1511 Poly Drive
Billings, MT 59102-1739
Phone: 406-657-1190
E-mail: pa@rocky.edu

Nebraska

Union College
Physician Assistant Program
3800 South 48th Street
Lincoln, NE 68506
Phone: 402-486-2527
E-mail: paprog@ucollege.edu

University of Nebraska Medical Center
Physician Assistant Program
984300 Nebraska Medical Center
Omaha, NE 68198-4300
Phone: 402-559-9495
E-mail: dklandon@unmc.edu

Nevada

Touro University—Nevada
Master of Physician Assistant Studies
Program
874 American Pacific Drive
Henderson, NV 89014-8800
Phone: 702-777-1770
E-mail: dPastudiesnv@touro.edu

New Hampshire

**Massachusetts College of Pharmacy
and Health Sciences—Manchester**
Physician Assistant Studies Program
School of Health Sciences
1260 Elm Street
Manchester, NH 03101
Phone: 603-314-1763
E-mail: admissions.manchester@mcphs.edu

New Jersey

Seton Hall University
Physician Assistant Program
400 South Orange Avenue
South Orange, NJ 07079-2689
Phone: 973-275-2596
E-mail: codelljo@shu.edu

**University of Medicine and Dentistry
of New Jersey**
Physician Assistant Program
Robert Wood Johnson Medical School
675 Hoes Lane
Piscataway, NJ 08854-5635
Phone: 732-235-4445
E-mail: pa-info@umdnj.edu

New Mexico

University of New Mexico
Physician Assistant Program
Department of Family & Community
Medicine
MSC 09 5040, 1 University of New Mexico
Albuquerque, NM 87131-0001
Phone: 505-272-9678
E-mail: paprogram@salud.unm.edu

**University of St. Francis,
Albuquerque Campus**
Physician Assistant Program
4401 Silver Avenue, SE, Suite B
Albuquerque, NM 87108
Phone: 505-266-5565 888-446-4657
E-mail: weiesterer@stfrancis.edu

New York

**Albany Medical College Physician
Assistant Program**
Center for Physician Assistant Studies
47 New Scotland Avenue, Mail Code 4
Albany, NY 12208-3412
Phone: 518-262-5251
E-mail: greenr@mail.amc.edu

CUNY York College
Physician Assistant Program
94-20 Guy Brewer Blvd, Room 112 SC
Jamaica, NY 11451
Phone: 718-262-2823
E-mail: paprogram@york.cuny.edu

Daemen College
Physician Assistant Department
4380 Main Street
Amherst, NY 14226-3592
Phone: 716-839-8563
E-mail: physician_assistant@daemen.edu;
and mmoore@daemen.edu

D'Youville College
Physician Assistant Program
320 Porter Avenue
Buffalo, NY 14201
Phone: 716-829-7713
E-mail: harrison@dyc.edu

Hofstra University
Physician Assistant Studies Program
113 Monroe Lecture Center
127 Hofstra University
Hempstead, NY 11549
Phone: 516-463-4074
E-mail: paprogram@hofstra.edu

Le Moyne College
Department of Physician Assistant Studies
1419 Salt Springs Road
Syracuse, NY 13214-1399
Phone: 315-445-4265
E-mail: Physassist@lemoyne.edu

Long Island University
Physician Assistant Program
1 University Plaza
Brooklyn, NY 11201
Phone: 718-488-1505
E-mail: pastudies@brooklyn.liu.edu

Mercy College
Graduate Program in Physician Assistant
Studies
1200 Waters Place
Bronx, NY 10461
Phone: 914-674-7635
E-mail: paprogram@mercy.edu

New York Institute of Technology
Physician Assistant Program
Riland Building, Suite 352, Northern
Boulevard
P.O. Box 8000
Old Westbury, NY 11568-8000
Phone: 516-686-3881
E-mail: pa@nyit.edu

Pace University—Lenox Hill Hospital
Physician Assistant Program
One Pace Plaza, Room Y-31
New York, NY 10038
Phone: 212-346-1357
E-mail: paprogram@pace.edu; and
paprogram_admissions@pace.edu

Rochester Institute of Technology
Physician Assistant Program
Building 75-CBET, 153 Lomb Memorial Drive
Rochester, NY 14623-5603
Phone: 585-475-5151 716-475-2978
E-mail: hbmscl@rit.edu

**Sophie Davis School of Biomedical
Education at the City College of New York/
Harlem Hospital Center**
Physician Assistant Program
160 Convent Avenue
New York, NY 10031
Phone: 212-650-7745
E-mail: paprog@ccny.cuny.edu

**State University of New York Downstate
Medical Center**
Physician Assistant Program
450 Clarkson Avenue Box 1222
Brooklyn, NY 11203
Phone: 718-270-2324
E-mail: admissions@downstate.edu

St. John's University
Physician Assistant Program
Andrew Bartilucci Center
175-05 Horace Harding Expressway
Fresh Meadows, NY 11365
Phone: 718-990-8400
E-mail: simoneg@stjohns.edu

Stony Brook University
Physician Assistant Program
School of Health Technology & Management
SHTM-HSC, L2-424
Stony Brook, NY 11794-8202
Phone: 631-444-3190, ext. 6
E-mail: paprogram@stonybrook.edu

Touro College of Health Sciences
Physician Assistant Program—Winthrop
Extension Center, Mineola, NY
1700 Union Boulevard
Bay Shore, NY 11706
Phone: 631-665-1600
E-mail: enrollhealth@touro.edu

Touro College—Manhattan Campus
Physician Assistant Program
School of Health Sciences
27-33 West 23rd Street
New York, NY 10010
Phone: 212-463-0400, ext. 7
E-mail: ngraff@touro.edu

Upstate Medical Uniersity
Physician Assistant Program
College of Health Professions
788 Irving Avenue, Room 1103
Syracuse, NY 13210
E-mail:admiss@upstate.edu

Wagner College PA Program
Physician Assistant Program
1 Campus Road
Staten Island, NY 10301
Phone: 718-420-4142
E-mail: admissions@wagner.edu

Weill Cornell Medical College
Physician Assistant Program (A Surgical Focus)
575 Lexington Avenue, Suite 600
New York, NY 10022
Phone: 646-962-7277
E-mail: dav2009@med.cornell.edu

North Carolina
Duke University Medical Center
Physician Assistant Program
Department of Community and Family Medicine
DUMC 3848
Durham, NC 27710
Phone: 919-681-3161
E-mail: paadmission@mc.duke.edu

East Carolina University
Physician Assistant Program
Department of Physician Assistant Studies; SAHS
College of Allied Health Sciences
4310 Health Science Building
Greenville, NC 27858-4353
Phone: 252-744-1100
E-mail: pastudies@ecu.edu

Methodist University
Physician Assistant Program
5107 College Centre Drive
Fayetteville, NC 28311
Phone: 910-630-7495
E-mail: paprog@methodist.edu

Wake Forest University
Department of Physician Assistant Program
Medical Center Boulevard
Winston-Salem, NC 27157-1006
Phone: 336-716-4356
E-mail: paadmit@wfubmc.edu

Wingate University
Department of PA Studies
Campus Box 5010
Wingate, NC 28174
Phone: 704-233-8051
E-mail: pa@wingate.edu
Website: http://www.wingate.edu

North Dakota
University of North Dakota
Physician Assistant Program
School of Medicine and Health Sciences, Department of Family Medicine
501 North Columbia Road-Stop 9037
Grand Forks, ND 58202-9037
Phone: 701-777-2344
E-mail: painfo@medicine.nodak.edu

Ohio
Cuyahoga Community College
Physician Assistant Program
11000 Pleasant Valley Road
Parma, OH 44130
Phone: 216-987-5123
E-mail: Daniel.mcdermott@tri-c.edu

Kettering College of Medical Arts
Physician Assistant Program
3737 Southern Boulevard
Kettering, OH 45429
Phone: 937-296-7238
E-mail: sue.wulff@kcma.edu

Marietta College
Physician Assistant Program
215 Fifth Street
Marietta, OH 45750
Phone: 740-376-4458
E-mail: paprog@marietta.edu

Mount Union College
Physician Assistant Program
1972 Clark Avenue
Alliance, OH 44601
Phone: 330-823-4685 and 800-334-6682
Email: scarpill@muc.edu

University of Findlay
Physician Assistant Program
1000 North Main Street
Findlay, OH 45840-3695
Phone: 419-434-4529
E-mail: mcbride@findlay.edu

University of Toledo Health Science Campus
Physician Assistant Program
HSC Mail Stop 1027
3000 Arlington Avenue
Toledo, OH 43614-2598
Phone: 419-383-5408
E-mail: Kristi.hayes@utoledo

Oklahoma

University of Oklahoma
Physician Assistant Program
Health Sciences Center
P.O. Box 26901
Oklahoma City, OK 73190
Phone: 405-271-2058

University of Oklahoma—Tulsa
Physician Assistant Program
4502 East 41st Street
Suite 1C22
Tulsa, OK 74135-2512
Phone: 918-619-4760
E-mail: outulsapa@ouhsc.edu

Oregon

Oregon Health Sciences University
Physician Assistant Program
3181 SW Sam Jackson Park Road
GH219
Portland, OR 97239-3098
Phone: 503-494-1484
E-mail: paprgm@ohsu.edu

Pacific University
Physician Assistant Program
School of Physician Assistant Studies
222 SE 8th Avenue, Suite 551
Hillsboro, OR 97123
Phone: 503-352-7272
E-mail: pa@pacificu.edu

Pennsylvania

Arcadia University
Physician Assistant Program
Brubaker Hall, Health Science Center
450 South Easton Road
Glenside, PA 19038
Phone: 215-572-2082
E-mail: daysc@arcadia.edu

Chatham College
Physician Assistant Program
Woodland Road
Dilworth Hall
Pittsburgh, PA 15232
Phone: 412-365-1412
E-mail: admissions@chatham.edu

DeSales University
Physician Assistant Program
2755 Station Avenue
Center Valley, PA 18034-9568
Phone: 610-282-1100, ext. 1
E-mail: paprog@desales.edu

Drexel University
Hahnemann PA Program
College of Nursing and Health Professions
1505 Race Street, 8th Floor, MS 504
Philadelphia, PA 19102-1192
Phone: 215-762-7135
E-mail: dml26@drexel.edu

Duquesne University
Physician Assistant Program
John G. Rangos, Sr., School of Health Sciences
418 Health Sciences Building
Pittsburgh, PA 15282
Phone: 800-456-0590
E-mail: calhoun@duq.edu

Gannon University
Physician Assistant Program
109 University Square
Erie, PA 16541-0001
Phone: 814-871-7474
E-mail: gillespi002@gannon.edu

Kings College
Department of Physician Assistant Studies
133 North River Street
Wilkes-Barre, PA 18711
Phone: 570-208-5853
E-mail: sharonkaminski@kings.edu

Lock Haven University of Pennsylvania
Physician Assistant Program
432 Railroad Street
Lock Haven, PA 17745
Phone: 570-484-2929
E-mail: weisenha@lhup.edu

Marywood University
Physician Assistant Program
2300 Adams Avenue
Scranton, PA 18509
Phone: 570-348-6298
E-mail: paprogram@marywood.edu

Pennsylvania College of Technology
Department of Physician Assistant Studies
DIF #123
One College Avenue
Williamsport, PA 17701-5799
Phone: 800-367-9222
E-mail: pa@pct.edu

Philadelphia College of Osteopathic Medicine
Department of Physician Assistant Studies
4190 City Avenue, Rowland Hall
Philadelphia, PA 19131
Phone: 215-871-6772
E-mail: admissions@pcom.edu

Philadelphia University
Physician Assistant Program
School House Lane & Henry Avenue
Philadelphia, PA 19144
Phone: 215-951-2908
E-mail: fieldsg@philau.edu

Saint Francis University
Department of Physician Assistant Sciences
117 Evergreen Drive
Loretto, PA 15940-0600
Phone: 814-472-3020
E-mail: pa@francis.edu

Salus University
Physician Assistant Program
8360 Old York Road
Elkins Park, PA 19027
Phone: 215-780-1515
E-mail: admissions@pco.edu

Seton Hill University
Physician Assistant Program
Seton Hill Drive
Greensburg, PA 15601
Phone: 724-838-4283
E-mail: gadmit@setonhill.edu

University of Pittsburgh
Physician Assistant Program
School of Health and Rehabilitation Sciences
4020 Forbes Tower
Pittsburgh, PA 15261
http://www.shrs.pitt.edu/pa.aspx

South Carolina

Medical University of South Carolina
Physician Assistant Program
Medical University of South Carolina
151 B Rutledge Avenue, Suite B-102
(MSC 962)
Charleston, SC 29425
Phone: 843-792-3789
E-mail: simmshe@musc.edu

South Dakota

University of South Dakota
Physician Assistant Studies Program
School of Health Sciences
414 East Clark Street, Julian #120
Vermillion, SD 57069-2390
Phone: 605-677-5128 and 877-269-6837
E-mail: usdpa@usd.edu

Tennessee

Bethel College
Physician Assistant Program
P.O. Box 329
325 Cherry Avenue
McKenzie, TN 38201
Phone: 731-352-5708
E-mail: atwills@bethel-college.edu

Lincoln Memorial University—DeBusk College of Osteopathic Medicine
Physician Assistant Program
6965 Cumberland Gap Parkway
Herrogate, TN 37752
Phone: 423-869-6691
E-mail: paadmissions@lmunet.edu

South College
Physician Assistant Program
3904 Lonas Drive
Knoxville, TN 37909-3323
Phone: 865/251-1880
E-mail: pa_program@southcollegetn.edu

Trevecca Nazarene University
Physician Assistant Program
333 Murfreesboro Road
Nashville, TN 37210-2877
Phone: 615-248-1225
E-mail: admissions_pa@trevecca.edu

Texas

Baylor College of Medicine
Physician Assistant Program
Room 107 BTXX, One Baylor Plaza
Houston, TX 77030-3498
Phone: 713-798-4842
E-mail: wthomas@bcm.edu

Interservice Physician Assistant Program
Physician Assistant Program
Attn: MCCS-HE-PA
3151 Scott Road, Suite 1202
Fort Sam Houston, TX 78234-6138
Phone: 210-221-8004

Texas Tech University Health Sciences Center
School of Allied Health Sciences, Department of Laboratory Sciences
Physician Assistant Program
3600 North Garfield
Midland, TX 79705
Phone: 432-620-9905
E-mail: allied.health@ttuhsc.edu

University of North Texas Health Science Center at Fort Worth
Physician Assistant Studies
Health Science Center at Fort Worth
3500 Camp Bowie Boulevard
Fort Worth, TX 76107-2699
Phone: 817-735-2301
E-mail: PAStudies@hsc.unt.edu

University of Texas Health Science Center at San Antonio
Department of Physician Assistant Studies
7703 Floyd Curl Drive, MC 6249
San Antonio, TX 78229-3900
Phone: 210-567-8810
E-mail: pastudies@uthscsa.edu

University of Texas Medical Branch
Physician Assistant Program
School of Allied Health Services
301 University Boulevard
Galveston, TX 77555-1145
Phone: 409-772-3046
E-mail: rrahr@utmb.edu

University of Texas, Southwestern Medical Center
Department of Physician Assistant Studies
5323 Harry Hines Boulevard, Suite V4.114
Dallas, TX 75390-9090
Phone: 214-648-1701
E-mail: isela.perez@utsouthwestern.edu

University of Texas—Pan American
Physician Assistant Studies Program
1201 West University Drive
Edinburg, TX 78539
Phone: 956-316-7049
E-mail: pastudies@utpa.edu

Utah

University of Utah
Physician Assistant Program
375 Chipeta Way, Suite A
Salt Lake City, UT 84108
Phone: 801-581-7766
E-mail: admissions@upap.utah.edu

Virginia

Eastern Virginia Medical School
Master of Physician Assistant Program
700 West Olney Road, Suite 1110
Norfolk, VA 23501-1980
Phone: 757-446-7158
E-mail: paprog@evms.edu

James Madison University
Graduate Studies in Physician Assistant
Program
Department of Health Sciences, MSC 4301
Harrisonburg, VA 22807
Phone: 540-568-2395
E-mail: paprogram@jmu.edu

Jefferson College of Health Sciences
Physician Assistant Program
920 South Jefferson Street
P.O. Box 13186
Roanoke, VA 24031-3186
Phone: 540-985-4016
E-mail: admissions@mail.jchs.edu

Shenandoah University
Division of Physician Assistant Studies
1460 University Drive
Winchester, VA 22601
Phone: 540-542-6208
E-mail: pa@su.edu

Washington

University of Washington
MEDEX Northwest Physician Assistant
Program
Physician Assistant Program
4311 11th Avenue NE, Suite 200
Seattle, WA 98105-4608
Phone: 206-616-4001
E-mail: medex@u.washington.edu

West Virginia

Alderson-Broaddus College
Physician Assistant Program
101 College Hill Drive. P.O. Box 2036
Philippi, WV 26416
Phone: 304-457-6290
E-mail: holtmw@ab.edu

Mountain State University
The Physician Assistant Program
609 South Kanawha Street
P.O. Box 9003
Beckley, WV 25802-9003
Phone: 304-929-1598
E-mail: mprince@mountainstate.edu

Wisconsin

Marquette University
Department of Physician Assistant Studies
College of Health Sciences
1700 Building
Milwaukee, WI 53201-1881
Phone: 414-288-5688

University of Wisconsin—LaCrosse
Gundersen Lutheran Medical Foundation,
Mayo School of Health
Physician Assistant Program
1725 State Street, 4031 Health Science Center
LaCrosse, WI 54601-3788
Phone: 608-785-8470
E-mail: paprogram@uwlax.edu

University of Wisconsin—Madison
Physician Assistant Program
Room 1278 Health Sciences Learning Center
750 Highland Avenue
Madison, WI 53705
Phone: 800-442-6698
E-mail: paprogram@mailplus.wisc.edu

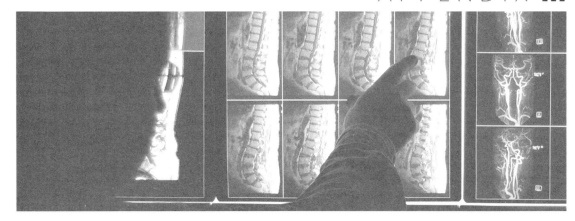

MODEL STATE LEGISLATION REGARDING PHYSICIAN ASSISTANTS

The government affairs department of the American Academy of Physician Assistants (AAPA) developed this model legislation to provide a foundation for achieving national consensus regarding state legislation. It was most recently updated in July 2009. For more information visit http://www.aapa.org/advocacy-and-practice-resources/state-advocacy/490-model-state-legislation.

INTRODUCTION

The model legislation reflects two principal concepts: that physician assistants (PAs) should be licensed to practice medicine with physician supervision and that PA scope of practice should be determined by supervising physicians.

Licensure is the most appropriate level of PA regulation in order to protect the public health and safety. Some states have been using a de facto licensing system; that is, permission to practice is dependent on presentation of appropriate qualifications and approval by the state regulatory agency. However, rather than calling this licensure, it has been called "certification" or "registration."

Experts have defined state **certification** as regulation of the use of a specific occupational title; that is, it is illegal to use a professional title without state approval, but anyone may deliver the service if they refrain from using the protected title.

Registration creates an official list of persons. Registration presumes the existence of the right to engage in activity and makes it illegal to practice in a regulated occupation without being registered. It generally is not intended to assure the public of qualified practitioners.

The Pew Health Commission's Taskforce on Health Care Workforce Regulation issued a report in December 1995 recommending, among other things, that the term "licensure" be used for state regulation of health professions. The taskforce stated that the term "certification" should be reserved for voluntary private sector programs that attest to the competency of individual health professionals. For PAs, such a system is administered by the National Commission on Certification of Physician Assistants (NCCPA).

Thus, to eliminate confusion between private and state certification, as well as to identify the true level of regulation, the AAPA recommends that state laws use the term "license." The majority of state laws conform to this recommendation. Forty-five states use licensure as the regulatory term for physician assistants; just three states use the term "certification," and two others "register," with a handful "registering" physician assistants.

The model state legislation proposes an administrative process in which a PA presents his or her credentials to a state regulatory agency and receives a license in return. The license is renewable, based on meeting state requirements. Obtaining a license should occur independently of a PA's employment status. One analogy is a driver's license—you get one before you buy a car so that you can start driving as soon as you are ready. This system should be attractive to state licensing boards because it eliminates a lot of paperwork. Many of the early statutes either granted permission to physicians to utilize specific PAs or required PAs to submit all transcripts, test scores, references, and so on every time they changed employers or supervisors. Under such systems, PAs legally ceased to exist between jobs.

The model legislation does not propose that the regulatory authority approve or register supervising physicians. Any licensed physician (M.D. or D.O.) may supervise a PA unless the physician's ability to supervise has been limited by specific disciplinary action.

The scope of PA practice under the model legislation is dependent on what the supervising physician wishes to delegate. This is consistent with the original concept of PA utilization and reflects a movement away from a regulatory micromanagement of physician/PA practices.

The model legislation allows physicians to delegate prescriptive authority, including controlled substances in Schedules II through V, as well as limited dispensing authority. Also included is language clarifying a PA's authority to request, receive, and distribute professional samples. PAs who are delegated prescribers of controlled medications are required to register with the federal Drug Enforcement Administration (DEA).

It is stated quite clearly that a physician need not be physically on the premises as long as the PA and physician can contact one another easily. The details of supervision are left to the physician-PA team.

The "Optional Replacement Parts" are offered as substitutes for some of the provisions described above. If the delegatory system contained in the model legislation is not feasible, language is provided to give a licensing board more control over the supervising physician and PA. Two options (the more preferable presented first) are included. They would be inserted in place of the "Supervising Physician" section.

If a description of PA scope of practice must be included, an alternative section is proposed that is intended to discourage the development of lists of tasks. This optional replacement section would take the place of "Scope of Practice—Delegatory Authority," although it is recommended that the paragraph that describes PAs as agents of physicians be retained.

Locum tenens language is not necessary in the model legislation as the proposed licensure system allows for easy substitution of one licensed PA for another. However, if the "Practice Agreement" concept is included, then the recommended section on locum tenens may be needed. The definition of locum tenens should be inserted in the "Definitions" section and the rest of the locum tenens provision placed elsewhere in the bill.

The final set of optional replacement parts deals with the regulatory structure—control by a medical licensing board without PA input; a voting PA on the medical board; a separate PA board; and the most popular model, regulation by a medical board with a PA committee.

This model law was first drafted in 1991 and revised in 1994, 1998, 2001, 2002, 2004, and 2005 to reflect changes in the PA program accrediting agencies and to incorporate other new provisions. The APA's government affairs staff is available to assist with revisions and additions as needed and to explain what and why the model bill contains what it does. We hope the ideas are clear and can be transformed into the appropriate style and format to be compatible with your existing state code.

MODEL STATE LEGISLATION—PHYSICIAN ASSISTANTS

Definitions

"Physician assistant" means a health professional who meets the qualifications defined in this chapter and is licensed under this chapter to practice medicine with physician supervision.

"Board" means the Medical Licensing Board.

"Supervising physician" means an M.D. or D.O. licensed by the board who supervises physician assistants [hereinafter PAs].

"Supervision" means overseeing the activities of, and accepting responsibility for, the medical services rendered by a PA. The constant physical presence of the supervising physician is not required as long as the supervising physician and PA are in contact or can be easily in contact with each other by telecommunication.

Qualifications for Licensure

Except as otherwise provided in this chapter, an individual shall be licensed by the board before the individual may practice as a PA. The board may grant a license as a PA to an applicant who:

1. submits an application on forms approved by the board;
2. pays the appropriate fee as determined by the board;
3. has successfully completed an educational program for physician assistants accredited by the Accreditation Review Commission on Education for the Physician Assistant or, prior to 2001, by either the Committee on Allied Health Education and Accreditation, or the Commission on Accreditation of Allied Health Education Programs;
4. has passed the Physician Assistant National Certifying Examination administered by the National Commission on Certification of Physician Assistants;
5. is mentally and physically able to engage safely in practice as a physician assistant;
6. has no licensure, certification, or registration as a PA under current discipline, revocation, suspension, or probation for cause resulting from the applicant's practice as a physician assistant, unless the board considers such condition and agrees to licensure;
7. is of good moral character;
8. submits to the board any other information the board deems necessary to evaluate the applicant's qualifications; and
9. has been approved by the board.

The board may also grant a license to an applicant who does not meet the educational requirement specified in subsection 3, but who passed the Physician Assistant National Certifying Examination administered by the National Commission on Certification of Physician Assistants prior to 1986.

Temporary License

A temporary license may be granted to an applicant who meets all the qualifications for licensure but is awaiting the next scheduled meeting of the board.

Inactive License

Any PA who notifies the board in writing on forms prescribed by the board may elect to place his or her license on an inactive status. A PA with an inactive license shall be excused from payment of renewal fees and shall not practice as a physician assistant. Any licensee who engages in practice while his or her license is lapsed or on inactive status shall be considered to be practicing without a license, which shall be grounds for discipline under section _____ of this Act. A PA requesting restoration from inactive status shall be required to pay the current renewal fee and shall be required to meet the criteria for renewal as specified in section _____ of this Act.

Renewal

Each person who holds a license as a PA in this state will, upon notification from the board, renew said license by:

1. submitting the appropriate fee as determined by the board;
2. completing the appropriate forms; and
3. meeting any other requirements set forth by the board.

Exemption From Licensure

Nothing herein shall be construed to require licensure under this Act of:

1. a PA student enrolled in a PA educational program accredited by the Accreditation Review Commission on Education for the Physician Assistant;
2. a PA employed in the service of the federal government while performing duties incident to that employment; or
3. technicians or other assistants or employees of physicians who perform physician-delegated tasks but who are not rendering services as PAs or identifying themselves as a PA.

Scope of Practice—Delegatory Authority—Agent of Supervising Physician

PAs practice medicine with physician supervision. PAs may perform those duties and responsibilities, including the ordering, prescribing and dispensing, and administration of drugs and medical devices that are delegated by their supervising physician(s).

PAs may provide any medical service that is delegated by the supervising physician when the service is within the PA's skills, forms a component of the physician's scope of practice, and is provided with supervision. A PA may perform a task not within the scope of practice of the supervising physician as long as the supervising physician has adequate training, oversight skills, and supervisory and referral arrangements to ensure competent provision of the service by the PA.

PAs may pronounce death and may authenticate with their signature any form that may be authenticated by a physician's signature.

PAs shall be considered the agents of their supervising physicians in the performance of all practice-related activities including, but not limited to, the ordering of diagnostic, therapeutic, and other medical services.

Prescriptive Authority

A PA may prescribe, dispense, and administer drugs and medical devices to the extent delegated by the supervising physician.

Prescribing and dispensing of drugs may include Schedules II through V substances as described in [the state controlled drug act] and all legend drugs.

All dispensing activities of PAs shall:

1. comply with appropriate federal and state regulations; and
2. occur when pharmacy services are not reasonably available, or when it is in the best interest of the patient, or when it is an emergency.

PAs may request, receive, and sign for professional samples and may distribute professional samples to patients.

PAs authorized to prescribe and/or dispense controlled substances must register with the federal Drug Enforcement Administration [and any applicable state-controlled substance regulatory authority].

Supervision

Supervision shall be continuous but shall not be construed as necessarily requiring the physical presence of the supervising physician at the time and place that the services are rendered.

It is the obligation of each team of physician(s) and PAs to ensure that the PA's scope of practice is identified; that delegation of medical tasks is appropriate to the PA's level of competence; that the relationship of, and access to, the supervising physician is defined; and that a process for evaluation of the PA's performance is established.

Supervising Physician

A physician wishing to supervise a PA must:

1. be licensed in this state;
2. be free from any restriction on his or her ability to supervise a PA that has been imposed by board disciplinary action; and
3. maintain a written agreement with the PA. The agreement must state that the physician will exercise supervision over the PA in accordance with any rules adopted by the board and will retain professional and legal responsibility for the care rendered by the PA. The agreement must be signed by the physician and the PA and updated annually. The agreement must be kept on file at the practice site and made available to the board upon request.

Satellite Settings

Nothing contained herein shall be construed to prohibit the rendering of services by a PA in a setting geographically remote from the supervising physician.

Exclusions of Limitations on Employment

Nothing herein shall be construed to limit the employment arrangement of a PA licensed under this Act.

Violations

The board may, following the exercise of due process, discipline any PA who:

1. fraudulently or deceptively obtains or attempts to obtain a license;
2. fraudulently or deceptively uses a license;
3. violates any provision of this chapter or any regulations adopted by the board pertaining to this chapter or any other laws or regulations governing licensed health professionals or any stipulation or agreement of the board;
4. is convicted of a felony;
5. is a habitual user of intoxicants or drugs to such an extent that he or she is unable to safely perform as a PA;
6. has been adjudicated as mentally incompetent;
7. is physically or mentally unable to engage safely in practice as a PA;
8. is negligent in practice as a PA or demonstrates professional incompetence;
9. violates patient confidentiality except as required by law;
10. engages in conduct likely to deceive, defraud, or harm the public;
11. engages in unprofessional or immoral conduct;
12. prescribes, sells, administers, distributes, orders, or gives away any drug classified as a controlled substance for other than medically accepted therapeutic purposes;
13. has committed an act of moral turpitude;
14. is disciplined or has been disciplined by another state or jurisdiction based upon acts or conduct similar to acts or conduct that would constitute grounds for disciplinary action as defined in this section;
15. fails to cooperate with an investigation conducted by the board; or
16. represents himself or herself as a physician.

Disciplinary Authority

The board, upon finding that a PA has committed any offense described in section _____, may:

1. refuse to grant a license;
2. administer a public or private reprimand;
3. revoke, suspend, limit, or otherwise restrict a license;

4. require a PA to submit to the care or counseling or treatment of a physician or physicians designated by the board;
5. impose corrective measures;
6. impose a civil penalty or fine;
7. suspend enforcement of its finding thereof and place the PA on probation with the right to vacate the probationary order for noncompliance; or
8. restore or reissue, at its discretion, a license and remove any disciplinary or corrective measure which it may have imposed.

Impaired Physician Assistant Program

The board shall establish and administer a program for the rehabilitation of PAs whose competency is impaired due to the abuse of drugs or alcohol. The board may contract with any other state agency or private corporation to perform duties under this section. The program shall be similar to that available to other health professionals licensed in this state.

Title and Practice Protection

Any person not licensed under this Act is guilty of a [felony or misdemeanor] and is subject to penalties applicable to the unlicensed practice of medicine if he or she:

1. holds himself or herself out as a PA;
2. uses any combination or abbreviation of the term "physician assistant" to indicate or imply that he or she is a PA; or
3. acts as a PA without being licensed by the board.

An unlicensed physician shall not be permitted to use the title of "physician assistant" or to practice as a PA unless he or she fulfills the requirements of this [Act].

Identification Requirements

PAs licensed under this Act shall keep their license available for inspection at their primary place of business and shall, when engaged in their professional activities, identify themselves as a "physician assistant."

Participation in Disaster and Emergency Care

A PA licensed in this state or licensed or authorized to practice in any other U.S. jurisdiction or who is credentialed as a PA by a federal employer who is responding to a need for medical care created by an emergency or a state or local disaster (not to be defined as an emergency situation which occurs in the place of one's employment) may render such care that they are able to provide without supervision as it is defined in this section of law, or with such supervision as is available.

Any physician who supervises a PA providing medical care in response to such an emergency or state or local disaster shall not be required to meet the requirements set forth in this section of law for a supervising physician.

No PA licensed in this state or licensed or authorized to practice in other states of the United States who voluntarily and gratuitously, and other than in the ordinary course of employment or practice, renders emergency medical assistance shall be liable for civil damages for any personal injuries which result from acts or omissions by those persons in rendering emergency care which may constitute ordinary negligence. The immunity granted by this section shall not apply to acts or omissions constituting gross, willful, or wanton negligence or when the medical assistance is rendered at any hospital, physician's office, or other healthcare delivery entity where those services are normally rendered. No physician who supervises a PA voluntarily and gratuitously providing emergency care as described in this subsection shall be liable for civil damages for any personal injuries which result from acts or omissions by the physician assistant rendering emergency care.

Rule-Making Authority

The board shall promulgate, in accordance with the provisions of the [state] Administrative Procedures Act, all rules that are reasonable and necessary for the performance of the various duties imposed upon the board by the provisions of this Act, including but not limited to:

1. setting licensure fees; and
2. establishing renewal dates.

OPTIONAL REPLACEMENT PARTS FOR MODEL LEGISLATION SUPERVISING PHYSICIAN—PRACTICE AGREEMENT

Option 1

A physician wishing to supervise a PA must:

1. be licensed in this state;
2. notify the board of his intent to supervise a PA;
3. submit a statement to the board that he will exercise supervision over the PA in accordance with any rules adopted by the board and that he will retain professional and legal responsibility for the care rendered by the PA.

NOTIFICATION OF INTENT TO PRACTICE

A PA licensed in this state, prior to initiating practice, will submit, on forms approved by the board, notification of such intent. Such notification shall include:

1. the name, business address, and telephone number of the supervising physician(s); and
2. the name, business address, and telephone number of the PA.

A PA will notify the board of any changes or additions in supervising physicians within _____ days.

SUPERVISING PHYSICIAN—PRACTICE AGREEMENT

Option 2

Any physician licensed in this state may apply to the board for permission to supervise a PA. The application shall be jointly submitted by the physician and the PA(s) and may be accompanied by a fee as determined by the board.

The joint application shall describe the manner and extent to which the PA will practice and be supervised, including identification of additional licensed physicians who will supervise the PA; the education, training, and experience of the primary supervisor and the PA; and other such information as the board may require.

The board may approve, modify, or reject such applications.

Whenever it is determined that a physician or PA is practicing in a manner inconsistent with the approval granted, the board may demand modification of the practice, withdraw approval of the practice agreement, or take other disciplinary action as defined in section _____ of this Act.

PHYSICIAN ASSISTANT SCOPE OF PRACTICE

The practice of a PA shall include medical services within the education, training, and experience of the PA that are delegated by the supervising physician.

Medical services rendered by PAs may include, but are not limited to:

1. obtaining patient histories and performing physical examinations;
2. ordering and/or performing diagnostic and therapeutic procedures;
3. formulating a diagnosis;
4. developing and implementing a treatment plan;
5. monitoring the effectiveness of therapeutic interventions;
6. assisting at surgery;
7. offering counseling and education to meet patient needs; and
8. making appropriate referrals.

The activities listed above may be performed in any setting authorized by the supervising physician, including but not limited to: clinics, hospitals, ambulatory surgical centers, patient homes, nursing homes, and other institutional settings.

LOCUM TENENS PERMIT

The board may grant a locum tenens permit to any applicant who is licensed in the state. The permit may be granted by an authorized representative of the board. Such applications for locum tenens permits will be reviewed at the next scheduled board meeting. The maximum duration of a locum tenens permit is one year. The permit may be renewed annually on a date set by the board.

Definition: "Locum tenens means the temporary provision of services by a substitute provider."

REGULATORY OPTIONS

I. Regulation by the Medical Board

The state board of medical examiners shall administer the provisions of this Act under such procedures as it considers advisable and may adopt rules that are reasonable and necessary to implement the provisions of this Act.

II. Regulation by a PA Board

To administer this Act, there is hereby established a Board of Physician Assistant Examiners. The board shall consist of five members appointed by the governor, each of whom shall be residents of this state, four of whom shall be PAs who meet the criteria for licensure as established by this Act, and one of whom shall be a licensed physician experienced in supervising PAs.

Initial appointments shall be made as follows:

1. two members shall be appointed for terms of four years;
2. one member shall be appointed for a term of three years;
3. one member shall be appointed for a term of two 2 years; and
4. one member shall be appointed for a term of one year.

Each regular appointment thereafter shall be for a term of four years. Any vacant term shall be filled by the governor for the balance of the unexpired term. No member shall serve more than two consecutive four-year terms, and each member shall serve on the board until his or her successor is appointed.

While engaged in the business of the board, each member shall receive a per diem of $_____ and shall also receive compensation for actual expenses paid in accordance with [other state regulations].

The board shall elect a chair and a secretary from among its members at the first meeting of each fiscal year. The board shall meet on a regular basis. A board meeting may be called, upon reasonable notice, at the discretion of the chair and shall be called at any time, upon reasonable notice, by a petition of three board members to the chair.

Powers and duties of the board shall include the following:

1. promulgation of all rules reasonable and necessary to implement the provisions of this Act;
2. review and approval or rejection of applications for licensure;
3. review and approval or rejection of applications for renewal;
4. issuance of all licenses;
5. denial, suspension, revocation, or other discipline of a licensee; and
6. determination of the amount and collection of all fees.

III. Regulation by a Medical Board With a Physician Assistant Advisory Committee

There is hereby created a PA committee which shall review and make recommendations to the board regarding all matters relating to PAs that come before the board. Such matters shall include, but not be limited to:

1. applications for licensure;
2. practice agreements (if applicable);
3. disciplinary proceedings;
4. renewal requirements; and
5. any other issues pertaining to the regulation and practice of PAs in this state.

Committee Membership

The committee shall consist of three PAs, one physician experienced in supervising PAs, and one member of the board. All committee members must be residents of this state and hold a license in good standing in their respective disciplines.

The chair of the committee shall be elected by a majority vote of the committee members.

Committee members shall receive reimbursement for time and travel expenditures [consistent with usual state practices].

Appointments

The PA and supervising physician members of the committee shall be appointed by the governor. The board of medical examiners shall designate one member to serve on the board. All appointments shall be made within 60 days of the effective date of this Act. All appointments shall be for four-year terms, at staggered intervals. Members shall serve no more than two consecutive terms. Reappointments of the PA and supervising physician members of the committee shall be made by the governor.

Meetings

The committee shall meet on a regular basis. A committee meeting may be called, upon reasonable notice, at the discretion of the chair and shall be called at any time, upon reasonable notice, by petition of three committee members to the chair.

IV. Adding a Physician Assistant to the Medical Board

To assist in the administration of this Act, the governor shall appoint a licensed PA to the board of medical examiners for a term of ____ years, [etc., in accordance with existing law]. The PA member will have full voting privileges.

Reprinted with permission from the American Academy of Physician Assistants.

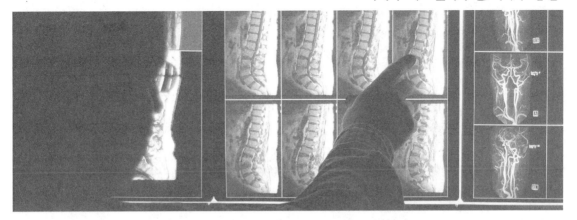

AAPA GUIDELINES FOR ETHICAL CONDUCT FOR THE PHYSICIAN ASSISTANT

(Adopted 2000, amended 2004, 2006, 2007, and 2008)

INTRODUCTION

The physician assistant (PA) profession has revised its code of ethics several times since the profession began. Although the fundamental principles underlying the ethical care of patients have not changed, the societal framework in which those principles are applied has. Economic pressures of the healthcare system, social pressures of church and state, technological advances, and changing patient demographics continually transform the landscape in which PAs practice.

Previous codes of the profession were brief lists of tenets for PAs to live by in their professional lives. This document departs from that format by attempting to describe ways in which those tenets apply. Each situation is unique. Individual PAs must use their best judgment in a given situation while considering the preferences of the patient and the

supervising physician, clinical information, ethical concepts, and legal obligations.

Four main bioethical principles broadly guided the development of these guidelines: autonomy, beneficence, nonmaleficence, and justice. *Autonomy*, strictly speaking, means self-rule. Patients have the right to make autonomous decisions and choices, and physician assistants should respect these decisions and choices. *Beneficence* means that PAs should act in the patients' best interest. In certain cases, respecting the patients' autonomy and acting in their best interests may be difficult to balance. *Nonmaleficence* means to do no harm, to impose no unnecessary or unacceptable burden upon the patient. *Justice* means that patients in similar circumstances should receive similar care. Justice also applies to norms for the fair distribution of resources, risks, and costs.

PAs are expected to behave legally and morally. They should know and understand the laws governing their practice. Likewise, they should understand the ethical responsibilities of being healthcare professionals.

Legal requirements and ethical expectations will not always be in agreement. Generally speaking, the law describes minimum standards of acceptable behavior, and ethical principles delineate the highest moral standards of behavior.

When faced with an ethical dilemma, PAs may find the guidance they need in this document. If not, they may wish to seek guidance elsewhere—possibly from a supervising physician, a hospital ethics committee, an ethicist, trusted colleagues, or other American Academy of Physician Assistant (AAPA) policies. PAs should seek legal counsel when they are concerned about the potential legal consequences of their decisions.

The following sections discuss ethical conduct of PAs in their professional interactions with patients, physicians, colleagues, other health professionals, and the public. The "Statement of Values" within this document defines the fundamental values that the PA profession strives to uphold. These values provide the foundation upon which the guidelines rest. The guidelines were written with the understanding that no document can encompass all actual and potential ethical responsibilities, and PAs should not regard them as comprehensive.

Statement of Values of the Physician Assistant Profession

- PAs hold as their primary responsibility the health, safety, welfare, and dignity of all human beings.
- PAs uphold the tenets of patient autonomy, beneficence, nonmaleficence, and justice.
- PAs recognize and promote the value of diversity.
- PAs treat equally all persons who seek their care.
- PAs hold in confidence the information shared in the course of practicing medicine.
- PAs assess their personal capabilities and limitations, striving always to improve their medical practice.

- PAs actively seek to expand their knowledge and skills, keeping abreast of advances in medicine.
- PAs work with other members of the healthcare team to provide compassionate and effective care of patients.
- PAs use their knowledge and experience to contribute to an improved community.
- PAs respect their professional relationship with physicians.
- PAs share and expand knowledge within the profession.

The Physician Assistant and the Patient

Physician Assistant Role and Responsibilities

PA practice flows out of a unique relationship that involves the PA, the physician, and the patient. The individual patient-PA relationship is based on mutual respect and an agreement to work together regarding medical care. In addition, PAs practice medicine with physician supervision; therefore, the care that a PA provides is an extension of the care of the supervising physician. The patient-PA relationship is also a patient-PA-physician relationship.

The principal value of the PA profession is to respect the health, safety, welfare, and dignity of all human beings. This concept is the foundation of the patient-PA relationship. PAs have an ethical obligation to see that each of their patients receives appropriate care. PAs should recognize that each patient is unique and has an ethical right to self-determination. PAs should be sensitive to the beliefs and expectations of the patient but are not expected to ignore their own personal values, scientific or ethical standards, or the law.

A PA has an ethical duty to offer patients the full range of information on relevant options for their health care. If personal moral, religious, or ethical beliefs prevent a PA from offering the full range of treatments available or care the patient desires, the PA has an ethical duty to refer an established patient to another qualified provider. PAs are obligated to care for patients in emergency situations and to responsibly transfer established patients if they cannot care for them.

The Physician Assistant and Diversity

The PA should respect the culture, values, beliefs, and expectations of the patient.

Discrimination

PAs should not discriminate against classes or categories of patients in the delivery of needed health care. Such classes and categories include gender, color, creed, race, religion, age, ethnic or national origin, political beliefs, nature of illness, disability, socioeconomic status, or sexual orientation.

Initiation and Discontinuation of Care

In the absence of a pre-existing patient-PA relationship, the PA is under no ethical obligation to care for a person unless no other provider is available. A PA is morally bound to provide care in emergency situations and to arrange proper follow-up. PAs should keep in mind that contracts with health insurance plans might define a legal obligation to provide care to certain patients.

A PA and supervising physician may discontinue their professional relationship with an established patient as long as proper procedures are followed. The PA and physician should provide the patient with adequate notice, offer to transfer records, and arrange for continuity of care if the patient has an ongoing medical condition. Discontinuation of the professional relationship should be undertaken only after a serious attempt has been made to clarify and understand the expectations and concerns of all involved parties.

If the patient decides to terminate the relationship, he or she is entitled to access appropriate information contained within his or her medical record.

Informed Consent

PAs have a duty to protect and foster an individual patient's free and informed choices. The doctrine of informed consent means that a PA provides adequate information that is able to be comprehended by a competent patient or patient surrogate. At a minimum, this should include the nature of the medical condition, the objectives of the proposed treatment, treatment options, possible outcomes, and the risks involved. PAs should be committed to the concept of shared decision-making, which involves assisting patients in making decisions that account for medical, situational, and personal factors.

In caring for adolescents, the PA should understand all of the laws and regulations in his or her jurisdiction that are related to the ability of minors to consent to or refuse health care. Adolescents should be encouraged to involve their families in healthcare decision-making. The PA should also understand consent laws pertaining to emancipated or mature minors. (See the next section on confidentiality.)

When the person giving consent is a patient's surrogate, a family member, or other legally authorized representative, the PA should take reasonable care to assure that the decisions made are consistent with the patient's best interests and personal preferences, if known. If the PA believes the surrogate's choices do not reflect the patient's wishes or best interests, the PA should work to resolve the conflict. This may require the use of additional resources, such as an ethics committee.

Confidentiality

PAs should maintain confidentiality. By maintaining confidentiality, PAs respect patient privacy and help to prevent discrimination based on medical conditions. If patients are confident that their privacy is protected, they are more likely to seek medical care and more likely to discuss their problems candidly.

In cases of adolescent patients, family support is important but should be balanced with the patient's need for confidentiality and the PA's obligation to respect the patient's emerging autonomy. Adolescents may not be of age to make independent decisions about their health, but providers should respect that they soon will be. To the extent they can, PAs should allow these emerging adults to participate as fully as possible in decisions about their care. It is important that PAs be familiar with and understand the laws and regulations in their jurisdictions that relate to the confidentiality rights of adolescent patients. (See the section on informed consent.)

Any communication about a patient conducted in a manner that violates confidentiality is unethical. Because written, electronic, and verbal information may be intercepted or overheard, the PA should always be aware of anyone who might be monitoring communication about a patient.

PAs should choose methods of storage and transmission of patient information that minimize the likelihood of data becoming available to unauthorized persons or organizations. Modern technologies such as computerized record-keeping and electronic data transmission present unique challenges that can make the maintenance of patient confidentiality difficult. PAs should advocate for policies and procedures that secure the confidentiality of patient information.

Patient and the Medical Record

PAs have an obligation to keep information in the patient's medical record confidential. Information should be released only with the written permission of the patient or the patient's legally authorized representative. Specific exceptions to this general rule may exist (e.g., workers compensation, communicable disease, HIV, knife/gunshot wounds, abuse, substance abuse). It is important that a PA be familiar with and understand the laws and regulations in his or her jurisdiction that relate to the release of information. For example, stringent legal restrictions on release of genetic test results and mental health records often exist.

Both ethically and legally, a patient has certain rights to know the information contained in his or her medical record. While the chart is legally the property of the practice or the institution, the information in the chart is the property of the patient. Most states have laws that provide patients access to their medical records. The PA should know the laws and facilitate patient access to the information.

Disclosure

A PA should disclose to his or her supervising physician information about errors made in the course of caring for a patient. The supervising physician and PA should disclose the error to the patient if such information is significant to the patient's interests and well-being. Errors do not always constitute improper, negligent, or unethical behavior, but failure to disclose them may.

Care of Family Members and Coworkers

Treating oneself, coworkers, close friends, family members, or students whom the PA supervises or teaches may be unethical or create conflicts of interest. PAs should be aware that their judgment might be less than objective in cases involving friends, family members, students, and colleagues and that providing "curbside" care might sway the individual from establishing an ongoing relationship with a provider. If it becomes necessary to treat a family member or close associate, a formal patient-provider relationship should be established, and the PA should consider transferring the patient's care to another provider as soon as it is practical. If a close associate requests care, the PA may wish to assist by helping him or her find an appropriate provider.

There may be exceptions to this guideline; for example, when a PA runs an employee health center or works in occupational medicine. Even in those situations, PAs should be sure they do not provide informal treatment, but provide appropriate medical care in a formally established patient-provider relationship.

Genetic Testing

Evaluating the risk of disease and performing diagnostic genetic tests raise significant ethical concerns. PAs should be knowledgeable about the benefits and risks of genetic tests. Testing should be undertaken only after the patient's informed consent is obtained. If PAs order or conduct the tests, they should assure that appropriate pre- and post-test counseling is provided.

PAs should be sure that patients understand the potential consequences of undergoing genetic tests—from impact on patients themselves, possible implications for other family members, and potential use of the information by insurance companies or others who might have access to the information. Because of the potential for discrimination by insurers, employers, or others, PAs should be particularly aware of the need for confidentiality concerning genetic test results.

Reproductive Decision-Making
Patients have a right to access the full range of reproductive healthcare services, including fertility treatments, contraception, sterilization, and abortion. PAs have an ethical obligation to provide balanced and unbiased clinical information about reproductive health care.

When the PA's personal values conflict with providing full disclosure or providing certain services, such as sterilization or abortion, the PA need not become involved in that aspect of the patient's care. By referring the patient to a qualified provider, the PA fulfills his or her ethical obligation to ensure the patient access to all legal options.

End of Life
PAs have an obligation to optimize care and maximize quality of life for patients at the end of life. PAs are encouraged to facilitate open discussion with patients and their family members concerning end of life treatment choices. PAs should involve the physician in all near-death planning. The PA should only withdraw life support with the supervising physician's agreement and in accordance with the policies of the healthcare institution.

PAs should be aware of the medical, legal, social, and ethical issues in end-of-life decision-making. Advance directives, living wills, and organ donation should be discussed during routine patient visits.

The Physician Assistant and Individual Professionalism

Conflict of Interest
PAs should place service to patients before personal material gain and should avoid undue influence on their clinical judgment. Trust can be undermined by even the appearance of improper influence. Examples of excessive or undue influence on clinical judgment can take several forms. These may include financial incentives, pharmaceutical or other industry gifts, and business arrangements involving referrals. PAs should disclose any actual or potential conflict of interest to their patients.

Acceptance of gifts, trips, hospitality, or other items is discouraged. Before accepting a gift or financial arrangement, PAs might consider the guidelines of the Royal College of Physicians, "Would I be willing to have this arrangement generally known?" or of the American College of Physicians–American Society of Internal Medicine, "What would the public or my patients think of this arrangement?"

Professional Identity
PAs should not misrepresent directly or indirectly their skills, training, professional credentials, or identity. PAs should uphold the dignity of the PA profession and accept its ethical values.

Competency
PAs should commit themselves to providing competent medical care and extend to each patient the full measure of their professional ability as dedicated, empathetic healthcare providers. PAs should also strive to maintain and increase the quality of their healthcare knowledge, cultural sensitivity, and cultural competence through individual study and continuing education.

Sexual Relationships
It is unethical for PAs to become sexually involved with patients. It also may be unethical for PAs to become sexually involved with former patients or key third parties. Key third parties are individuals who have influence over the patient, including spouses or partners, parents, guardians, or surrogates. Such relationships generally are unethical because of the PA's position of authority and the inherent imbalance of knowledge, expertise, and

status. Issues such as dependence, trust, transference, and inequalities of power may lead to increased vulnerability on the part of the current or former patients or key third parties.

Gender Discrimination and Sexual Harassment

It is unethical for PAs to engage in or condone any form of gender discrimination. Gender discrimination is defined as any behavior, action, or policy that adversely affects an individual or group of individuals due to disparate treatment, disparate impact, or the creation of a hostile or intimidating work or learning environment.

It is unethical for PAs to engage in or condone any form of sexual harassment. Sexual harassment is defined as unwelcome sexual advances, requests for sexual favors, or other verbal or physical conduct of a sexual nature when:

- such conduct has the purpose or effect of interfering with an individual's work or academic performance or creating an intimidating, hostile, or offensive work or academic environment, or
- accepting or rejecting such conduct affects or may be perceived to affect professional decisions concerning an individual, or
- submission to such conduct is made either explicitly or implicitly a term or condition of an individual's training or professional position.

The Physician Assistant and Other Professionals

Team Practice

PAs should be committed to working collegially with other members of the healthcare team to ensure integrated, well-managed, and effective care of patients. PAs should strive to maintain a spirit of cooperation with other healthcare professionals, their organizations, and the general public.

Illegal and Unethical Conduct

PAs should not participate in or conceal any activity that will bring discredit or dishonor to the PA profession. They should report illegal or unethical conduct by healthcare professionals to the appropriate authorities.

Impairment

PAs have an ethical responsibility to protect patients and the public by identifying and assisting impaired colleagues. "Impaired" means being unable to practice medicine with reasonable skill and safety because of physical or mental illness, loss of motor skills, or excessive use or abuse of drugs and alcohol. PAs should be able to recognize impairment in physician supervisors, PAs, and other healthcare providers and should seek assistance from appropriate resources to encourage these individuals to obtain treatment.

Physician Assistant-Physician Relationship

Supervision should include ongoing communication between the physician and the PA regarding patient care. The PA should consult the supervising physician whenever it will safeguard or advance the welfare of the patient. This includes seeking assistance in situations of conflict with a patient or another healthcare professional.

Complementary and Alternative Medicine

A patient's request for alternative therapy may create conflict between the PA and the patient. Though PAs are under no obligation to provide an alternative therapy, they do have a responsibility to be sensitive to the patient's needs and beliefs and to help the patient understand their medical condition. The PA should gain an understanding of the alternative therapy being considered or being used, the expected outcome, and whether the treatment would clearly be harmful to the patient. If the treatment would harm the patient, the PA should work diligently to dissuade the patient from using it and advise other treatment.

The Physician Assistant and the Healthcare System

Workplace Actions

PAs may face difficult personal decisions to withhold medical services when workplace actions (e.g., strikes, sick-outs, slowdowns) occur. The potential harm to patients should be carefully weighed against the potential improvements to working conditions and, ultimately, patient care that could result. In general, PAs should individually and collectively work to find alternatives to such actions in addressing workplace concerns.

Managed Care

The focus of managed care organizations on cost containment and resource allocation can present particular ethical challenges to clinicians. When practicing in managed care systems, PAs should always act in the best interests of their patients and as advocates when necessary. PAs should actively resist managed care policies that restrict free exchange of medical information. For example, a PA should not withhold information about treatment options simply because the option is not covered by a particular managed care organization.

PAs should inform patients of financial incentives to limit care, use resources in a fair and efficient way, and avoid arrangements or financial incentives that conflict with the patient's best interests.

Physician Assistants as Educators

All PAs have a responsibility to share knowledge and information with patients, other health professionals, students, and the public. The ethical duty to teach includes effective communication with patients so that they will have the information necessary to participate in their health care and wellness.

Physician Assistants and Research

The most important ethical principle in research is honesty. This includes assuring subjects' informed consent, following treatment protocols, and accurately reporting findings. Fraud and dishonesty in research should be reported so that the appropriate authorities can take action.

PAs involved in research must be aware of potential conflicts of interest. The patient's welfare takes precedence over the desired research outcome. Any conflict of interest should be disclosed.

In scientific writing, PAs should report information honestly and accurately. Sources of funding for the research must be included in the published reports. Plagiarism is unethical. Incorporating the words of others, either verbatim or by paraphrasing, without appropriate attribution is unethical and may have legal consequences. When submitting a document for publication, any previous publication of any portion of the document must be fully disclosed.

Physician Assistants as Expert Witnesses

The PA expert witness should testify to what he or she believes to be the truth. The PA's review of medical facts should be thorough, fair, and impartial. The PA expert witness should be fairly compensated for time spent preparing, appearing, and testifying. The PA should not accept a contingency fee based on the outcome of a case in which testimony is given or derive personal, financial, or professional favor in addition to compensation.

The Physician Assistant and Society

Lawfulness

PAs have the dual duty to respect the law and to work for positive change to laws that will enhance the health and well-being of the community.

Executions

PAs, as healthcare professionals, should not participate in executions because to do so would violate the ethical principle of beneficence.

Access to Care/Resource Allocation

PAs have a responsibility to use healthcare resources in an appropriate and efficient manner so that all patients have access to needed health care. Resource allocation should be based on societal needs and policies, not the circumstances of an individual patient-PA encounter. PAs participating in policy decisions about resource allocation should consider medical need, cost-effectiveness, efficacy, and equitable distribution of benefits and burdens in society.

Community Well-Being

PAs should work for the health, well-being, and the best interest of both the patient and the community. Sometimes there is a dynamic moral tension between the well-being of the community in general and the individual patient. Conflict between an individual patient's best interest and the common good is not always easily resolved. In general, PAs should be committed to upholding and enhancing community values, be aware of the needs of the community, and use the knowledge and experience acquired as professionals to contribute to an improved community.

CONCLUSION

The AAPA recognizes its responsibility to aid the PA profession as it strives to provide high quality, accessible health care. PAs wrote these guidelines for themselves and other PAs. The ultimate goal is to honor patients and earn their trust while providing the best and most appropriate care possible. At the same time, PAs must understand their personal values and beliefs and recognize the ways in which those values and beliefs can impact the care they provide.

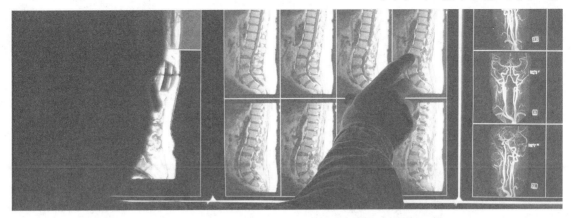

ACCREDITATION STANDARDS FOR PHYSICIAN ASSISTANT EDUCATION

The Accreditation Review Commission on Education for the Physician Assistant (ARC-PA) only accredits qualified physician assistant (PA) programs offered by, or located within institutions chartered by, and physically located within, the United States, and where students are geographically located within the United States for their education. (The United States are defined as "the fifty States, the District of Columbia, the Commonwealth of Puerto Rico, the Commonwealth of the Northern Mariana Islands, Guam, the Virgin Islands, American Samoa, Wake Island, the Midway Islands, Kingman Reef, and Johnston Island.")

The ARC-PA does not accredit educational programs leading to the PA credential in institutions that are chartered outside the United States or programs provided in foreign countries by ARC-PA accredited U.S. PA programs.

Approved by the ARC-PA March 2005.
Effective date September 28, 2007.
Next revision of the Standards anticipated in late fall 2009.
(*Note:* Sections A2.06, A2.07, and A2.13 edition become effective March 1, 2006.)
Reprinted with permission from the Accreditation Review Commission on Education for the Physician Assistant.

These Standards were initially adopted in 1971; revised in 1978, 1985, 1990, 1997, 2000, and 2005, and endorsed by the following organizations:

- American Academy of Family Physicians (AAFP)
- American Academy of Pediatrics (AAP)
- American Academy of Physician Assistants (AAPA)
- American College of Physicians (ACP)
- American College of Surgeons (ACS)
- American Medical Association (AMA)
- Physician Assistant Education Association (PAEA; formerly Association of Physician Assistant Programs)

These Standards constitute the minimum requirements to which an accredited program is held accountable and provide the basis on which the ARC-PA will confer or deny program accreditation.

INTRODUCTION

The AAFP, the AAP, the AAPA, the ACP, the ACS, the AMA, and the PAEA cooperate with the ARC-PA to establish, maintain, and promote appropriate standards of quality for entry-level education of PAs and to provide recognition for educational programs that meet the minimum requirements outlined in these Standards. These Standards are to be used for the development, evaluation, and self-analysis of PA programs.

PAs are academically and clinically prepared to practice medicine with the direction and responsible supervision of a doctor of medicine or osteopathy. The physician-PA team relationship is fundamental to the PA profession and enhances the delivery of high quality health care. Within the physician-PA relationship, PAs make clinical decisions and provide a broad range of diagnostic, therapeutic, preventive, and health maintenance services. The clinical role of PAs includes primary and specialty care in medical and surgical practice settings. PA practice is centered on patient care and may include educational, research, and administrative activities.

The role of the PA demands intelligence, sound judgment, intellectual honesty, appropriate interpersonal skills, and the capacity to respond to emergencies in a calm and reasoned manner. An attitude of respect for self and others, adherence to the concepts of privilege and confidentiality in communicating with patients, and a commitment to the patient's welfare are essential attributes of the graduate PA. The professional curriculum for PA education includes basic medical, behavioral, and social sciences; patient assessment and clinical medicine; supervised clinical practice; and health policy and professional practice issues.

The Standards acknowledge the ongoing evolution of the PA profession and continue to endorse competency-based education as a fundamental tenet of PA education. They reflect the realization that a commonality in the core professional curriculum of programs remains desirable and necessary in order to offer curricula of sufficient depth and breadth to prepare all PA graduates for practice in a dynamic and competitive healthcare arena. The Standards allow programs to remain creative and innovative in program design and the methods used to enable students to achieve program goals and acquire the competencies needed for entry into clinical practice. They support the underlying rights of the sponsoring institution as it works with the program to meet the Standards. Program mission statements should be consistent with the Standards and the mission of the sponsoring institution.

The ARC-PA supports the sponsoring institution's prerogative in awarding credentials and degrees, and encourages sponsoring institutions to recognize the evolution of the profession as one that requires a graduate level of curricular intensity. Institutions that sponsor PA programs are also encouraged to incorporate this higher level of academic rigor into their programs and acknowledge it with an appropriate degree.

The ARC-PA acknowledges ongoing change in the delivery of health care and in the education of health professionals. The needs of patients and society at large should be considered by the ARC-PA, the sponsoring institutions, and the programs. Establishing an environment that will foster and promote diversity is considered essential to educating PAs to provide service to others that is not exclusionary of any group, race, or culture. The various insights and resources offered by a diverse faculty, staff, and student body will increase the overall impact the PA profession can have on the future of the global community. PA programs are encouraged to have policies and practices addressing diversity of their student bodies and faculty.

PROGRAM REVIEW

Accreditation of PA programs is a voluntary process that includes a comprehensive review of the program relative to the Standards. Accreditation decisions are based on the ARC-PA's review of information contained in the accreditation application and self-study report, the report of site visit evaluation teams, any additional requested reports or documents submitted to the ARC-PA by the PA program, and the program's past accreditation history. Additional data to clarify information submitted with the application may be requested at the time of the site visit associated with the comprehensive review. New information submitted after a site visit will not be accepted or considered by the ARC-PA.

DEFINITIONS

Note: Where terms are not defined, their definitions are at the discretion of the ARC-PA.

ABMS: American Board of Medical Specialties

Accurately: Free from error

All sites: Sites used for supervised clinical practice in the curriculum, to include those for program-required rotations or preceptorships, as well as elective rotations or preceptorships throughout the program

Analysis: Study of compiled or tabulated data interpreting cause-and-effect relationships and trends, with the subsequent understanding and conclusions used to validate current practices or make changes as needed for program improvement

AOA: American Osteopathic Association

Comparable: Similar but not necessarily identical

Competencies: The knowledge; interpersonal, clinical, and technical skills; professional behaviors; and clinical reasoning and problem-solving abilities required for PA practice

Core faculty: The program director, medical director, and at least two additional full-time equivalent (FTE) positions occupied by no more than four individuals who must be currently NCCPA-certified PAs

Course director: Faculty member primarily responsible for the organization, delivery, and evaluation of a course

Distant campus: A campus geographically separate from the main PA program at which didactic or preclinical instruction occurs for all or some of the students enrolled

Diversity: Differences within and between groups of people that contribute to variations in habits, practices, beliefs, and values

Equivalent: Resulting in the same outcomes or end results

Formative evaluation: Intermediate or continuous evaluation that may include feedback to help in achieving goals

Geographic scope: The ARC-PA only accredits qualified PA programs offered by, or located within institutions chartered by, and physically located within, the United States, and where students are geographically located within the United States for their education. (The United States are defined as "the fifty States, the District of Columbia, the Commonwealth of Puerto Rico, the Commonwealth of the Northern Mariana Islands, Guam, the Virgin Islands, American Samoa, Wake Island, the Midway Islands, Kingman Reef, and Johnston Island.") The ARC-PA does not accredit educational programs leading to the PA credential in institutions that are chartered outside the United States or programs provided in foreign countries by ARC-PA accredited U.S. PA programs.

Health record(s): The primary legal record documenting the healthcare services provided to a person in any aspect of the healthcare system. (This term includes routine clinical or office records, records of care in any health-related setting, preventive care, lifestyle evaluation, research protocols, and various clinical databases.)

Instructional faculty: Individuals providing instruction or supervision during the didactic and clinical phases of the program, regardless of length of time of instruction or faculty rank

Instructional objectives: A statement that describes what the learner will be able to do after completing a unit of instruction. Instructional objectives are related to intended outcomes, not to the process for achieving those outcomes.

Long-term care settings: Facilities for patients who require assistance with activities of daily living or are unable to live independently

Maximum aggregate student enrollment: The maximum potential number of students enrolled simultaneously at any point in time

Maximum class size: Maximum potential number of students enrolled for each admission cycle

Must: A term used to designate requirements that are compelled or mandatory. "Must" indicates an absolute requirement.

NCCPA: National Commission on Certification of Physician Assistants

PANCE: Physician Assistant National Certification Exam (administered by the National Commission on Certification of Physician Assistants)

Prospective students: Individuals who have requested information about the program or submitted information to the program

Published: Presented in written or electronic format

Readily available: Made accessible to others in a timely fashion via defined program or institution procedures

Recognized Regional or Specialized and Professional Accrediting Agencies:
- Liaison Committee on Medical Education
- American Osteopathic Association
- Middle States Association of Colleges and Schools—Commission on Higher Education (MSA-CHE)
- New England Association of Schools and Colleges—Commission on Institutions of Higher Education (NEASC-CIHE)
- North Central Association of Colleges and Schools—The Higher Learning Commission (NCA-HLC)
- Northwest Commission on Colleges and Universities (NWCCU)
- Southern Association of Colleges and Schools—Commission on Colleges (SACS)
- Western Association of Schools and Colleges—Accrediting Commission for Senior Colleges and Universities (WASC-ACSCU)

Remediation: The program's defined process for addressing deficiencies in a student's knowledge and skills, such that the correction of these deficiencies is measurable and can be documented

Should: The term used to designate requirements that are so important that their absence must be justified

Succinctly: Marked by compact, precise expression without wasted words

Sufficient: Enough to meet the needs of a situation or proposed end

Student(s): Individuals enrolled in the professional phase of a PA program

Summative evaluation: An assessment of the learner conducted by the program to assure that the learner has the knowledge, interpersonal skills, patient care skills, and professionalism required for entry into the profession

Supervised clinical practice experiences: Supervised student encounters with patients that include comprehensive patient assessment and involvement in patient care decision-making, and which result in a detailed plan for patient management

Timely: Without undue delay; as soon as feasible after giving considered deliberation

REQUIREMENTS FOR ACCREDITATION

Section A: Administration

A1 Sponsorship Institution Accreditation

A1.01 The sponsoring institution must
a) be accredited by a recognized regional or specialized and professional accrediting agency to award graduates of the PA program a baccalaureate or higher degree.[1]
b) be authorized under applicable law to provide a program of post secondary education.

---

[1] Programs sponsored by the military branches of the federal government or accredited prior to January 1, 2006, will not be held to this Standard.

Institution Sponsorship

A1.02 One sponsor must be clearly identified as being ultimately responsible for the program.

A1.03 When more than one institution is involved in the provision of academic and clinical education, responsibilities of the respective institutions for instruction and supervision must be clearly described and documented in a manner signifying agreement by the involved institutions.

A1.04 The sponsoring institution, together with its affiliates, must be capable of providing clinically oriented basic science education as well as clinical instruction and experience requisite to PA education.

Program Location[2]

A1.05 Accredited PA programs must be established in:

a) schools of allopathic or osteopathic medicine, or

b) colleges and universities affiliated with appropriate clinical teaching facilities, or

c) medical education facilities of the federal government.

Institution Responsibilities

A1.06 The sponsoring institution has primary responsibility for:

a) supporting curriculum planning and course selection by program faculty and staff.

b) appointment of faculty and staff.

c) maintaining student transcripts permanently.

d) granting the degree and/or credential documenting satisfactory completion of the educational program.

e) assuring that appropriate security and personal safety measures are addressed for students and faculty in all locations where instruction occurs.

Institution Resources

A1.07 The sponsoring institution must assure that the program has the following fiscal, human, and academic resources:

a) sufficient financial resources to operate the educational program and to fulfill obligations to matriculating and enrolled students.

b) the human resources needed to operate the program.

c) the human resources needed to process admission applications.

d) sufficient computer hardware, software, and audio/visual equipment for the faculty and staff to perform their duties.

e) sufficient office equipment and supplies for the faculty and staff to perform their duties.

f) sufficient instructional materials for the faculty and staff to perform their duties.

g) access to and training in the use of the Internet, including medical and other health-related electronic databases, for core faculty and students.

h) readily available access to the full text of current books, journals, periodicals, and other reference materials related to the curriculum for students and faculty.

A1.08 The sponsoring institution must assure that the program has:

a) classroom and laboratory environments conducive to student learning.

b) appropriate space for confidential academic counseling of students by core faculty.

c) offices sufficient for core faculty to perform their duties.

d) space for program conferences and meetings.

e) secure storage for student files and records.

---

[2] Programs accredited prior to January 1, 2001, "should" be established in the settings indicated. Programs accredited on or after January 1, 2001, "must" be established in the settings indicated.

A2 Program Personnel
Core Program Faculty

A2.01 Core program faculty must possess the qualifications by education and experience to perform their assigned duties.

A2.02 Core program faculty must include, at a minimum, the program director, medical director, and two additional faculty positions for individuals currently NCCPA-certified as PAs.

The latter two FTE positions cannot be occupied by more than four individuals.

A2.03 Core faculty must be sufficient in number to meet the academic needs of enrolled students.

A2.04 Core program faculty should have appointments and privileges comparable to other faculty who have similar responsibilities within the institution.

A2.05 Core program faculty must have responsibility for:
  a) developing the mission statement for the program.
  b) selecting applicants for admission to the PA program.
  c) providing student instruction.
  d) evaluating PA student performance.
  e) academic counseling of PA students.
  f) assuring the availability of remedial instruction.
  g) designing, implementing, coordinating, and evaluating curriculum.
  h) administering and evaluating the program.

Program Director

A2.06 The program director should be a PA or a physician
  a) If the program director is a PA, he or she must hold current NCCPA certification or current PA licensure by the state in which the program exists.[3]
  b) If the program director is a physician, he or she must hold current licensure as an allopathic or osteopathic physician in the state in which the program exists, and must be certified by an ABMS- or AOA-approved specialty board.[4]

A2.07 The program director must not be the medical director.[3]

A2.08 The program director should be assigned to the program on a full time basis.

A2.09 The program director must provide effective leadership and management.

A2.10 The program director must be knowledgeable about and responsible for the accreditation process.

A2.11 The program director must be knowledgeable about and have primary responsibility for the program's:
  a) organization.
  b) administration.
  c) fiscal management.
  d) continuous review and analysis.
  e) planning.
  f) development.

A2.12 The program director must supervise the medical director, faculty, and staff in all activities that directly relate to the PA program.

Medical Director

A2.13 The medical director must be:
  a) a currently licensed allopathic or osteopathic physician.[5]

---

[3] Programs accredited prior to March 1, 2006, will be held to this Standard only when a new program director is appointed.

[4] Physician program directors appointed before March 1, 2006, "should" be board certified; those appointed on or after March 1, 2006, "must" be board certified.

[5] Medical directors appointed on or after March 1, 2006, "should" have their current licensure in the state in which the program exists.

b) certified by an ABMS- or AOA-approved specialty board.[6]

c) knowledgeable in current practice standards and the PA role.

d) an advocate for the program within the medical and academic community.

e) responsible for supporting the program director to ensure that both didactic and supervised instruction meets current practice standards.

A2.14 If the position of medical director is shared, each individual must have defined roles and responsibilities.

Professional Development

A2.15 The program must provide the opportunity for continuing professional development of the core faculty by supporting development of their clinical, teaching, scholarly, and administrative skills/abilities.

A2.16 The program must support core PA faculty in maintaining their NCCPA certification status.

Instructional Faculty

A2.17 In addition to the core program faculty, there must be sufficient faculty and instructors to provide students with the necessary attention, instruction, and supervised practice experiences to acquire the knowledge and competence needed for entry into the profession.

A2.18 Instructional faculty must be:

a) qualified through academic preparation and experience to teach assigned subjects.

b) knowledgeable in course content and effective in teaching assigned subjects.

A2.19 Instructional faculty should participate in the evaluation of student performance and the identification of students who are not achieving course and program objectives.

A2.20 Instructional faculty for the supervised clinical practice portion of the educational program must consist primarily of practicing physicians and PAs.

A2.21 The program should not rely principally on resident physicians for didactic or clinical instruction.

A2.22 In each location to which a student is assigned for didactic or supervised practice instruction, there must be an individual designated by core faculty to supervise and assess the student's progress in achieving program requirements.

Administrative Support Staff

A2.23 There must be sufficient administrative and technical support staff so that faculty can accomplish the tasks required of them.

A2.24 Student workers may be used by, but must not be substituted for administrative and technical support staff.

A3 Operations
Administration

A3.01 Program policies must apply to all students and faculty regardless of location.

A3.02 The program must provide students and faculty at geographically distant locations access to services and resources equivalent to those on the main campus.

Fair Practices and Admissions

A3.03 Announcements and advertising must accurately reflect the program offered.

A3.04 All personnel and student policies must be consistent with federal and state statutes, rules, and regulations.

---

[6] Medical directors appointed before March 1, 2006, "should" be board certified, those appointed on or after March 1, 2006, "must" be board certified.

A3.05 Admission of students must be made in accordance with clearly defined and published practices of the institution and program.

A3.06 The program should not require that students supply their own clinical sites or preceptors for program-required clinical rotations.

A3.07 The following must be defined, published, and readily available to prospective and enrolled students:
  a) any institutional policies and practices that favor specific groups of applicants.
  b) requirements for prior education or work experience.
  c) policies regarding advanced placement.
  d) required academic and technical standards.
  e) all required curricular components.
  f) academic credit offered by the program.
  g) estimates of all costs related to the program.
  h) ARC-PA accreditation status.
  i) first time PANCE pass rates for the five most recent graduating classes.
  j) policies and procedures for student withdrawal.
  k) policies and procedures for refunds of tuition and fees.
  l) policies that limit or prevent students from working during the program.
  m) policies and procedures for processing student grievances.

A3.08 Programs granting advanced placement must document that students receiving advanced placement have:
  a) met program-defined criteria for such placement.
  b) met institution-defined criteria for such placement.
  c) demonstrated appropriate competencies for the curricular components in which advanced placement is given.

A3.09 The following must be defined, published, and readily available to faculty:
  a) policies and procedures for processing student grievances.
  b) policies and procedures for processing faculty grievances.

A3.10 PA students must not have access to the records or other confidential information of other PA students.

A3.11 PA students must not be required to work for the program.

A3.12 During clinical experiences, PA students must not be used to substitute for clinical or administrative staff.

Student Records

A3.13 Student files kept by the program must include documentation:
  a) that the student has met published admission criteria.
  b) of the evaluation of student performance while enrolled.
  c) of remediation.
  d) of disciplinary action.
  e) that the student has met institution and program health screening and immunization requirements.

Faculty Records

A3.14 Core faculty records must include:
  a) current job descriptions that include duties and responsibilities specific to each core faculty member.
  b) current curriculum vitae.

A3.15 The program must have current curriculum vitae for each course director.

Section B: Curriculum

B1 Instruction

B1.01 The curriculum must include core knowledge about the established and evolving biomedical and clinical sciences and the application of this knowledge to patient care.

B1.02 The curriculum must be of sufficient breadth and depth to prepare the student for the clinical practice of medicine.

B1.03 The curriculum design must reflect sequencing that enables students to develop the competencies necessary for current and evolving clinical practice.

B1.04 The program must assist students in becoming critical thinkers who can apply the concepts of medical decision-making and problem-solving.

B1.05 The program must provide students with published expectations of student outcomes and behaviors required for successful completion of the program.

B1.06 For each didactic and clinical course, the program must provide a published syllabus that defines expectations and guides student acquisition of expected competencies.

B1.07 The program must orient instructional faculty and preceptors to the specific educational competencies expected of PA students.

B1.08 Programs must educate students regarding issues related to intellectual honesty and academic and professional misconduct.

B1.09 The program must prepare students to provide medical care to patients from diverse populations.

B1.10 The program must assure educational equivalency of course content, student experience, and access to didactic and laboratory materials when instruction is:
a) conducted at geographically separate locations.
b) provided by different means for some students.

B2 Basic Medical Sciences

B2.01 While programs may require basic sciences as prerequisites to enrollment, those prerequisites must not substitute for the basic medical sciences in the professional component of the program.

B2.02 Instruction in the professional phase of the program must include instruction in the following basic medical sciences:
a) anatomy.
b) physiology.
c) pathophysiology.
d) pharmacology and pharmacotherapeutics.
e) the genetic and molecular mechanisms of health and disease.

B3 Clinical Preparatory Sciences

B3.01 The program must provide instruction in interpersonal and communication skills that result in the effective exchange of information and collaboration with patients, their families, and other health professionals.

B3.02 The program must provide students with instruction in patient assessment and management, including:
a) techniques of interviewing and eliciting a medical history.
b) performance of physical examinations across the life span.
c) generation of differential diagnoses.
d) ordering and interpretation of diagnostic studies.
e) development and implementation of treatment plans.
f) presentation of patient data in oral form.
g) documentation of patient data.
h) appropriate referral of patients.

B3.03 The program must provide instruction in clinical medicine covering all organ systems.

B3.04 The program must provide instruction in the important aspects of patient care including:
a) preventive.
b) acute.
c) chronic.
d) rehabilitative.
e) end-of-life.

B3.05 The program must provide instruction in technical skills and procedures based on current professional practice.

B4 Behavioral and Social Sciences

B4.01 The program must provide instruction in basic counseling and patient education skills necessary to help patients and families:
  a) cope with illness and injury.
  b) adhere to prescribed treatment plans.
  c) modify their behaviors to more healthful patterns.

B4.02 The program must provide instruction in:
  a) normal psychological development of pediatric, adult, and geriatric patients.
  b) detection and treatment of substance abuse.
  c) human sexuality.
  d) end-of-life issues.
  e) response to illness, injury, and stress.
  f) principles of violence identification and prevention.

B5 Information Literacy

B5.01 The program must provide instruction to equip students with the necessary skills to search, interpret, and evaluate the medical literature in order to maintain a critical, current, and operational knowledge of new medical findings including its application to individualized patient care.

B6 Health Policy and Professional Practice

B6.01 The program must provide instruction in:
  a) the impact of socioeconomic issues affecting health care.
  b) healthcare delivery systems and health policy.
  c) reimbursement, including documentation, coding, and billing.
  d) quality assurance and risk management in medical practice.
  e) legal issues of health care.
  f) cultural issues and their impact on healthcare policy.

B6.02 The program must provide instruction in medical ethics to include:
  a) the attributes of respect for self and others.
  b) professional responsibility.
  c) the concepts of privilege, confidentiality, and informed patient consent.
  d) a commitment to the patient's welfare.

B6.03 The program must provide instruction on:
  a) the history of the PA profession.
  b) current trends of the PA profession.
  c) the physician-PA team relationship.
  d) political and legal issues that affect PA practice.
  e) PA professional organizations.
  f) PA program accreditation.
  g) PA certification and recertification.
  h) licensure.
  i) credentialing.
  j) professional liability.
  k) laws and regulations regarding prescriptive practice.

B7 Supervised Clinical Practice

B7.01 The program must provide medical and surgical clinical practice experiences that enable students to meet program expectations and acquire the competencies needed for clinical PA practice.

B7.02 The program must assure that all sites used for students during supervised clinical practice meet the program's prescribed expectations for student learning and performance evaluation measures, regardless of location.

B7.03 The program must document that every student has supervised clinical practice experiences with patients seeking:
  a) medical care across the life span to include infants, children,

adolescents, adults, and the elderly.

b) prenatal care and women's health care.

c) care for conditions requiring inpatient surgical management, including preoperative, intra-operative, and postoperative care.

d) care for conditions requiring emergency management.

e) care for psychiatric/behavioral conditions.

B7.04 Supervised clinical practice experiences should be provided in the following settings:

a) outpatient.

b) emergency room/department.

c) inpatient.

d) operating room.

e) long-term care.

B7.05 Supervised clinical practice experiences should occur with residency-trained physicians or other licensed healthcare professionals experienced in the following disciplines:

a) emergency medicine.

b) family medicine.

c) general internal medicine.

d) general surgery.

e) general pediatrics.

f) psychiatry.

g) obstetrics and gynecology.

Section C: Evaluation

C1 Ongoing Program Self-Assessment

C1.01 The program must regularly collect and analyze the following qualitative and quantitative information to support an ongoing process of monitoring and documenting program effectiveness:

a) student attrition, deceleration, and remediation.

b) faculty attrition.

c) student failure rates in individual courses and rotations.

d) student evaluations of individual didactic courses, clinical experiences, and faculty.

e) graduate evaluations of curriculum and program effectiveness.

f) preceptor evaluations of student performance and suggestions for curriculum improvement.

g) graduate performance on the PANCE

C1.02 The program must apply the results of ongoing program assessment to the curriculum and other dimensions of the program.

C2 Periodic Self-Study Report[7]

C2.01 The program must prepare a self-study report as part of the application for continuing accreditation that accurately and succinctly documents the process and results of ongoing self-assessment. The report must follow the guidelines provided by the ARC-PA and, at a minimum, must document:

a) the program's process of ongoing self assessment.

b) outcome data and critical analysis of:

1) student attrition, deceleration, and remediation.

2) faculty attrition.

3) student failure rates in individual courses and rotations.

4) student evaluations of individual didactic courses, clinical experiences, and faculty.

5) graduate evaluations of curriculum and program effectiveness.

6) preceptor evaluations of student performance and suggestions for curriculum improvement.

7) the most recent 5-year first time and aggregate graduate performance on the PANCE.

---

[7] Programs applying for provisional accreditation must complete a descriptive report, as opposed to a self-study report, as described in section E and the application for provisional accreditation.

c) self-identified program strengths and areas in need of improvement.

d) modifications that occurred as a result of self-assessment.

e) plans for addressing areas needing improvement.

C3 Student Evaluation

C3.01 The program must use objective evaluation methods that are administered equitably to all students in the program.

C3.02 Objective evaluation methods must be related to expected student competencies for both didactic and supervised clinical education components.

C3.03 The program must conduct frequent, objective, and documented formative evaluations of students to assess their acquisition of knowledge, problem-solving skills, and psychomotor and clinical competencies.

C3.04 The program must assess and document student demonstration of professional behaviors.

C3.05 The program must monitor the progress of each student in such a way that deficiencies in knowledge or skills are promptly identified and means for remediation established.

C3.06 The program must document a summative evaluation of each student toward the end of the program to assure that students are prepared to enter clinical practice.

C4 Clinical Site Evaluation

C4.01 The program must define and maintain consistent and effective processes for the initial and ongoing evaluation of all sites and preceptors used for students' clinical practice experiences.

C4.02 The program must apply comparable evaluation processes to clinical sites regardless of geographic location.

C4.03 The program must ensure and document that each clinical site provides the student access to the physical facilities, patient populations, and supervision necessary to fulfill the program's expectations of the clinical experience.

Section D: Student Services

D1 Student Health

D1.01 Student health records are confidential and must not be accessible to or reviewed by program faculty and staff except for immunization and tuberculosis screening results, which may be maintained and released with written permission from the student.

D1.02 Health screening and immunization of students must:
a) be based on current Centers for Disease Control recommendations for health professionals.
b) not be conducted by program personnel.

D1.03 The program must inform students of and provide access to equivalent student healthcare services that the sponsoring institution makes available to students enrolled in other courses of instruction.

D1.04 Core program faculty must not participate as healthcare providers for students in the program.

D2 Student Guidance

D2.01 The program must assure that guidance is available to assist students in understanding and abiding by program policies and practices.

D2.02 The program must assure that students have timely access to faculty for assistance and counseling regarding their academic concerns and problems.

D2.03 The program must provide referral for students with personal problems that may interfere with their progress in the program.

D3 Student Identification

D3.01 The program must assure that PA students are clearly identified as such in the clinical setting to distinguish them from physicians, medical students, and other health profession students and graduates.

Section E: Provisional Accreditation

Provisional accreditation is recognition granted for a limited period of time to a new program that, at the time of the initial provisional site visit, has demonstrated to the ARC-PA's satisfaction its preparedness to initiate a program in accordance with the Standards. The provisional accreditation process involves a thorough review of the planning, organization, and proposed content of a program that is in the advanced planning stages, but not yet operational.

Provisional accreditation status indicates the ARC-PA's determination that the plans and resources allocated for the program, if fully implemented as proposed, demonstrate an ability to meet the Standards. In all cases, provisional accreditation of the program must precede the matriculation of students.

Initial provisional accreditation visits are conducted during the year prior to enrollment of the charter class of students. Follow-up provisional visits are conducted at programs that have successfully achieved provisional accreditation. Follow-up visits must occur no sooner than 4 months after students have entered the clinical phase of the program and no later than 6 months after graduation of the first class.

Failure of a program to achieve accreditation after its follow-up provisional visit requires that the program enter the accreditation process again via the provisional pathway.

E1 Provisional Accreditation Requirements

E1.01 The sponsoring institution must authorize the development of the PA program.

E1.02 The program must submit a needs assessment with its provisional application materials.

E1.03 The program must have a defined mission statement, which is consistent with its needs assessment and the mission of the sponsoring institution.

E1.04 There must be a qualified program director and a qualified medical director responsible for the development of the program.

E1.05 If provisional accreditation status is granted, the program must not admit more students than the number for which it has been approved by the ARC-PA, based on its application.

E1.06 The program must agree to inform, in writing, everyone who requests information, applies, or plans to enroll that the program is not yet accredited and must convey the implications of non-accreditation to applicants.

E1.07 The program must submit, with its application for provisional accreditation, a descriptive narrative report as described in the application materials.

E1.08 The chief academic officer of the sponsoring institution, or his or her designee, must sign the provisional accreditation application and descriptive narrative report, thus approving its content and verifying the institution's intent to implement and support the program as planned.

E1.09 The program must provide a detailed line item budget for the first 3 years of the program as part of its application.

E1.10 The program must provide a copy of current or proposed promotional literature including the course of study and course descriptions, proposed tuition, and fees. Documentation must include the date that the information will be included in the institution's literature and must describe the current method for disseminating the information.

E1.11 The program must have a completed curriculum design, course sequence, and evaluation methods for all didactic and clinical components of the program.

E1.12 For each course offered in the first 12 months of the program, the program must:

a) provide course descriptions.
b) provide a written syllabus that defines expectations and guides student acquisition of expected competencies.
c) describe methods of student evaluation.
d) provide examples of student evaluation instruments.
e) describe methods of instructor and course evaluation.
f) have identified qualified faculty in sufficient number to provide instruction.

E1.13 While all aspects of the program beyond the first 12 months are not required to be in place at the time of the site visit for provisional accreditation, the program must have clearly articulated plans and mechanisms for bringing the program into compliance with the Standards as required within the application.

E1.14 The program must have identified prospective clinical sites sufficient in number to meet the needs of students.

E1.15 The program must have a written plan describing its ongoing self-assessment process.

E1.16 Although no outcome data will be available at the time of the initial review of materials, the program must submit a full plan for comprehensive program evaluation, including an assessment of outcomes.

E1.17 Programs preparing for their follow-up provisional site visit must submit their applications and self-study reports to the ARC-PA at least 8 weeks before the follow-up site visit for accreditation occurs.

Section F: Accreditation Maintenance

F1 Program and Sponsoring Institution Responsibilities

F1.01 In accordance with ARC-PA policy, failure of a program to meet administrative requirements for maintaining accreditation will result in the program being placed on Administrative Probation and, if not corrected as directed by the ARC-PA, ultimately to an accreditation action of Accreditation Withdrawn.

F1.02 The program must inform the ARC-PA within 30 days of the date of notification of any adverse accreditation action (probation, withdrawal of accreditation) received from the sponsoring institution's regional or specialized and professional accrediting agency.

F1.03 The program must agree to periodic comprehensive review that may include a site visit as determined by the ARC-PA.

F1.04 The program must submit self-study reports or progress reports as required by the ARC-PA.

F1.05 The program must inform the ARC-PA in writing of changes in the program director, medical director, or other core program faculty within 30 days of the date of the effective change.

F1.06 The program must demonstrate active recruitment to fill vacated core faculty positions.

F1.07 If an interim program director (IPD) is appointed, this person should meet the qualifications of the PD.

F1.08 The appointment of an IPD should not exceed 12 months.

F1.09 The program must obtain ARC-PA approval 6 months prior to implementing any intended program expansion to a distant campus.

F1.10 The program must inform the ARC-PA in writing, no less than 6 months prior to implementation, of proposed changes in the following:
a) degrees or certificate granted at program completion.
b) requirements for graduation.
c) program length.
d) maximum class size.
e) maximum aggregate student enrollment that will result in an increase of 15% or greater in

maximum aggregate student enrollment, as compared to the program's most recent application for accreditation or as approved by the ARC-PA.

F1.11 The sponsoring institution must inform the ARC-PA in writing of the intent to transfer program sponsorship as soon as it begins considering transfer.

F1.12 The program and the sponsoring institution must pay ARC-PA accreditation fees as determined by the ARC-PA.

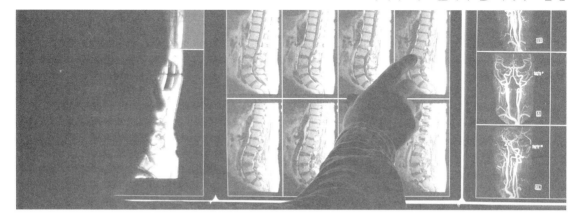

SUMMARY OF U.S. LAWS FOR PHYSICIAN ASSISTANTS, ABRIDGED VERSION

A detailed summary of all state laws is available by purchasing the latest edition of *Physician Assistants: State Laws and Regulations*, published by the American Academy of Physician Assistants (AAPA). To account for ongoing changes to laws and regulations, updated summaries are available on the AAPA's website.

ALABAMA

Qualifications: Graduation from accredited PA program and NCCPA examination.

Application: By PA for license. PA must be registered to licensed physician prior to practice. Job description must be approved by the board.

Scope of practice: Obtaining histories, performing physical exams, ordering and/or performing diagnostic and therapeutic procedures, formulating a working diagnosis, developing and implementing a treatment plan, monitoring the effectiveness of therapeutic interventions, assisting at surgery, offering counseling and education, making referrals. PA may not perform any medical service, procedure, function or activity which is not approved by the board.

Prescribing/dispensing: PAs may prescribe, administer, authorize for administration, or dispense controlled substances listed in Schedules III–V (regulations necessary to implement the law have not yet been adopted), and noncontrolled drugs from board-approved formulary.

Supervision: Oversight and direction but not direct, on-site physician supervision.

Participation in regulation: Four PAs serve on an eight-member Physician Assistant Advisory Committee.

Alabama State Board of Medical Examiners, P.O. Box 946, Montgomery, AL 36101-0946; (334) 242-4116.

ALASKA

Qualifications: Graduation from accredited PA program and current NCCPA certificate.

Application: PA applies for license. Licensed PA applies on board forms for authorization to practice; must have file documentation of established collaborative relationship(s) with the board within 14 days of commencing practice.

Scope of practice: Medical diagnosis and treatment within the scope of practice of the collaborating physician.

Prescribing/dispensing: PA may prescribe and dispense noncontrolled drugs and Schedules II–V controlled drugs. Prescriptions for controlled medications must include collaborating physician's name and Drug Enforcement Administration (DEA) number and PA's name and DEA number.

Supervision: Periodic assessment by physician and at least monthly telephone or radio review of patient care and records. PAs in remote locations with less than two years of experience must first work 160 hours in direct patient care under immediate, direct supervision of collaborating or alternate collaborating physician within 90 days of starting practice in remote location. First 40 hours must be completed before PA works in remote location. Periodic assessment for PAs with less than two years of experience must include at least one direct personal contact visit from supervising physician at least every four months for at least four hours.

Participation in regulation: One PA serves on medical board.

Alaska Division of Occupational Licensing, 550 West 7th Avenue, Suite 1500, Anchorage, AK 99501; (907) 269-8163.

ARIZONA

Qualifications: Graduation from accredited PA program and passage of NCCPA examination.

Application: PA applies for license. Interview, physical examination, mental evaluation, and oral competency examination may be required. PA and supervising physician must submit notification of supervision.

Scope of practice: Histories and physicals; diagnostic and therapeutic procedures; treatment plans; assisting in surgery; patient education and counseling; referrals; minor surgery (not including surgical abortion) and other nonsurgical tasks as approved by the board.

Prescribing/dispensing: PA may prescribe noncontrolled and controlled drugs. Schedules II and III drugs limited to 72-hour supply or an NCCPA certified PA or a PA with 45 hours of pharmacology in the preceding 3 years may prescribe a Schedule II or III drug for up to 14 days; Schedules IV and V drugs may not be prescribed more than five times in a six-month period for an individual patient. No refills of Schedules II and III drugs. Except for samples, dispensed drugs must be prepackaged by physician or pharmacist.

Supervision: Physician need not be present on-site; weekly meeting required. Board may approve PA utilization in a location geographically separate from supervising physician; specific supervision provisions required.

Participation in regulation: Four PAs serve on ten-member PA regulatory board.

Arizona Regulatory Board of Physician Assistants, 9545 E. Doubletree Ranch Road, Scottsdale, AZ 85258, (480) 551-2700.

ARKANSAS

Qualifications: Graduation from accredited PA program, passage of NCCPA examination and bachelor's degree (some exceptions apply).

Application: PA applies for license. Physician notifies board of intent to supervise. Personal interview of PA and physician required. Board must approve protocol describing PA scope of practice and supervision. Must pass jurisprudence exam on PA laws and regulations.

Scope of Practice: Duties and responsibilities assigned by supervising physician.

Prescribing/dispensing: PA may prescribe noncontrolled and Schedules III–V controlled medications as delegated by supervising physician. PAs authorized to prescribe controlled medications must register with the DEA. All PA prescriptions and orders must identify the supervising physician.

Supervision: Constant physical presence of supervising physician not required as long as PA and supervising physician can be in contact via telecommunication.

Participation in Regulation: Two PAs serve on six-member advisory committee.

Arkansas State Medical Board, 2100 Riverfront Drive, Suite 200, Little Rock, AR 72202-1793; (501) 296-1802.

CALIFORNIA

Qualifications: Graduation from accredited PA program and NCCPA examination.

Application: By PA for license.

Scope of practice: Medical services delegated in writing, within supervising physician's customary practice and within PA's competence. PA may take histories; perform physical examinations; perform or assist with laboratory, screening, and therapeutic procedures; counsel patients; and assist physician in institutional settings.

Prescribing/dispensing: PA may transmit orally or in writing on patient record or in a drug order, an order to a person who may lawfully furnish the medication. Authority limited by delegation from supervising physician. Physician must adopt a practice-specific formulary. "Drug order" means an order for medication which is dispensed to or for a patient issued and signed by a PA and is treated in the same manner as a prescription or order of the supervising physician. PA signing the drug order is deemed a prescriber. Schedules II–V medications administered, provided or for which a drug order is issued require a patient-specific order from a supervising physician (unless PA has taken an approved course). Drug orders for controlled medications require PA's DEA registration number. Medical record of patient receiving prescription for Schedule II

medication must be countersigned by supervising physician within 7 days. PA may hand to a patient a properly labeled drug prepackaged by pharmacist, physician, or manufacturer.

Supervision: Physician must be available in person or by electronic communication at all times PA is caring for patients. Written guidelines for supervision must include one or more of the following: same-day examination of patient by physician; countersignature of all medical records within 30 days; protocols for some or all tasks. Supervising physician must review, countersign and date at least 5% of medical records within 30 days for patients treated by PA when PAs working under protocols.

Participation in regulation: Four PAs serve on nine-member PA regulatory body.

California Physician Assistant Committee, Medical Board of California, 2005 Evergreen Street, Suite 1100, Sacramento, CA 95815-3831, (916) 561-8780.

COLORADO

Qualifications: Graduation from accredited PA program (or equivalent) and NCCPA examination.

Application: By PA for licensure; supervising physician must register with the board.

Scope of practice: PA may perform acts that constitute the practice of medicine, as delegated by the supervising physician. (After July 1, 1990, state-licensed Child Health Associates are eligible for licensure as PAs, but practice is restricted to patients under the age of 21 years.)

Prescribing/dispensing: PA may prescribe controlled (Schedules II–V) and noncontrolled substances. Each prescription must include the name of the supervising physician as well as the PA's name. All drugs dispensed by PAs must be unit doses prepackaged by pharmacist or physician. PA prescribing controlled substances must be registered with DEA.

Supervision: PA must practice with personal and responsible supervision of physician. In acute care hospital PA may practice without physical presence of physician if physician regularly practices in hospital or if hospital is located in a health professional shortage area; physician must review medical records every 2 working days. In other settings, physician must be available via telecommunication. New graduate PAs require on-site presence of physician for first 1,000 working hours; for first 6 months of employment and a minimum of 500 patient encounters charts must be co-signed within 7 days. Experienced PAs new to practice require chart review within 14 days for first three months of employment and minimum of 500 patient encounters. All other PAs are required to meet with supervising physician at least twice during each 12 month period for performance assessment.

Participation in regulation: None

Colorado Board of Medical Examiners, 1560 Broadway, Suite 1350, Denver, CO 80202; (303) 894-7690.

CONNECTICUT

Qualifications: Graduation from accredited PA program, current NCCPA certification, a bachelor's degree and documentation of 60 hours of pharmacology education.

Application: By PA for license.

Scope of practice: Medical functions delegated by supervising physician that are within the normal scope of the physician's practice and in accordance with written protocols.

Prescribing/dispensing: PA may be delegated the authority to prescribe and administer drugs, including controlled substances, in all settings. Supervising physician must document physician's approval of order for Schedule II or III drugs within 1 calendar day. Each prescription must include the name, license number, and address of the supervising physician and physician assistant.

Supervision: Includes, but is not limited to, the continuous availability of direct communication between PA and physician either in person or by radio, telephone, or telecommunication; at least weekly personal review of PA's practice, and face-to-face meetings between supervising physician and PA in non-hospital settings; regular chart review with documentation of review to be kept at practice site; existence of predetermined plan for emergency situations; and designation of an alternate physician in absence of supervisor.

Participation in regulation: One PA serves on medical examining board. One physician on medical board must supervise PAs.

Connecticut Division of Medical Quality Assurance, Dept. of Public Health, PA Licensing, 410 Capitol Avenue, MS#12APP, P.O. Box 340308, Hartford, CT 06134-0308; (860) 509-7603.

DELAWARE

Qualifications: Graduation from accredited PA program and passage of national certifying exam.

Application: By PA for license.

Scope of practice: Medical acts delegated by supervising physician. PA may take histories; perform physicals; record progress notes in outpatient setting; relay, transcribe, or execute diagnostic and therapeutic orders (orders must be countersigned within 72 hours); and perform delegated medical acts of diagnosis and prescription of therapeutic drugs and treatments.

Prescribing/dispensing: PA may prescribe up to a 6-month supply of noncontrolled drugs and up to a 3-month supply of controlled Schedules II–V drugs. PA must have both a state controlled substance number and a DEA number to prescribe controlled drugs.

Supervision: Physician need not be present as long as is readily accessible by electronic communication and can be present within 30 minutes if necessary. Patients seen by PA receiving controlled drugs should be seen by physician every

3 months; patients receiving other prescriptions should be seen by physician every 6 months.

Participation in regulation: Four PAs serve on PA Advisory Council.

Delaware Board of Medical Practice: Cannon Building, Suite 203, 861 Silver Lake Boulevard, Dover, DE 19904-2467; (302) 744-4500.

DISTRICT OF COLUMBIA

Qualifications: Graduation from accredited PA program and NCCPA examination.

Application: PA applies for license; PA and supervising physician file delegation agreement with board prior to practice.

Scope of practice: Acts of medical diagnosis and treatment, prescription, preventive health care, and other functions authorized by the board.

Prescribing/dispensing: PA may prescribe Schedules II–V and noncontrolled medications.

Supervision: Physician must be available in person or by communication device; need not be physically present on premises. Physician must countersign all outpatient medical orders and progress notes within 10 days. In hospitals, physician must countersign medical orders within 30 days.

Participation in regulation: One PA serves on three-member PA advisory committee.

District of Columbia Board of Medicine, 717 14th Street NW, Suite 600, Washington, DC 20005; (877) 672-2174.

FLORIDA

Qualifications: Graduation from accredited PA program and NCCPA examination; two letters of recommendation from physicians.

Application: By PA for license; includes information about supervising physician.

Scope of practice: PA may perform delegated tasks and procedures for which he or she is skilled that are within supervising physician's scope of practice. Some duties may only be performed if the physician is on the premises, such as insertion of chest tubes and monitoring cardiac stress tests. Final diagnoses may not be delegated.

Prescribing/dispensing: Negative formulary; PAs may prescribe or dispense drugs not listed on the formulary established by Council on PAs and adopted by medical and osteopathic boards. PAs may not prescribe controlled substances. Medical record of prescription or dispensing must be countersigned by supervising physician. Prior to prescribing, PA must complete a 3-hour course in prescriptive practice, 3 months of clinical experience in the specialty area of the supervising physician, and 10 hours of CME in the specialty area of practice. The Board issues a prescriber number to the PA.

Supervision: Physical presence or easy availability (by telecommunications) of physician is required.

Participation in regulation: One PA serves on five-member PA Council.

Florida Board of Medicine, 4052 Bald Cypress Way, Bin #C03, Tallahassee, FL 32399; (850) 488-0595.

Florida Board of Osteopathic Medical Examiners, 4052 Bald Cypress Way, Bin #C06, Tallahassee, FL 32399; (850) 245-4161.

GEORGIA

Qualifications: Graduation from accredited PA program and NCCPA examination. Personal interview may be required.

Application: By PA for license; by physician for approval to utilize PA (includes job description and description of locations where PA will practice).

Scope of practice: Delegated medical tasks contained in job description and approved by board.

Prescribing/dispensing: PAs may issue a prescription drug order for Schedules III–V and noncontrolled drugs as delegated by physician. Dispensing authorized in public or nonprofit health facilities. PAs who are authorized to prescribe controlled medications must register with the DEA.

Supervision: Supervising physician must be readily available. Board approval required for utilization of PA in satellite clinic where there is a shortage of healthcare professionals.

Participation in regulation: Four PAs serve on eight-member PA advisory committee. Committee appoints PA to serve as nonvoting medical board member.

Georgia Composite Medical Board, 2 Peachtree Street NW, 36th floor, Atlanta, GA 30303-3465; (404) 656-3913.

HAWAII

Qualifications: Graduation from accredited PA program and NCCPA examination; current NCCPA certificate required for biennial renewal.

Application: By PA for license. Must include signed statement from supervising physician(s) that will direct and supervise PA.

Scope of practice: Medical services including histories and physicals, ordering, interpreting or performing diagnostic and therapeutic procedures, formulating a diagnosis, implementing a treatment plan, patient counseling, making referrals and assisting at surgery.

Prescribing/dispensing: PAs may prescribe Schedules III–V controlled drugs and all legend drugs as delegated by supervising physician. Dispensing activities must comply with federal and state regulations. PA prescribers of controlled medications must register with DEA. Prescription must include both the PA's DEA number and the physician's DEA number. Medical record of controlled substance prescription must be initialed by the physician within 7 working days. PAs employed or extended privileges by hospital or extended care facility may write orders for Schedules II–V medications as allowed by facility policy.

Supervision: Physical presence of physician or physician availability via telecommunication. Physician must review PA records within 7 working days and must designate a supervising physician in his or her absence.

Participation in regulation: Five PAs serve on advisory committee.

Hawaii Board of Medical Examiners, Dept. of Commerce and Consumer Affairs, Division of Professional Licensing, P.O. Box 3469, Honolulu, HI 96801; (808) 586-3000.

IDAHO

Qualifications: Graduation from accredited PA program, baccalaureate degree, and NCCPA examination.

Application: By PA for license. Delegation of Services Agreement with supervising physician required for practice. Personal interview of PA, supervising physician, or both may be required.

Scope of practice: PA may take histories, perform physical examinations, initiate and interpret laboratory and diagnostic tests, and perform other duties that are included in the supervising physician's scope of practice and are delineated in the Delegation of Services Agreement.

Prescribing/dispensing: PA may apply for approval to prescribe Schedules II–V and noncontrolled medications. Application to prescribe must include documentation of all pharmacology course content completed (at least 30 hours). PAs who are authorized to prescribe controlled medications must register with the DEA and Idaho Board of Pharmacy. Dispensing limited to times when pharmacist is not available. PAs in family planning, communicable disease, or chronic disease clinics under government contract or grant may also dispense medications.

Supervision: Supervising physician must conduct on-site visit at least monthly. Must be available by phone or in person, hold regularly scheduled conferences, and review sampling of charts. Supervising physician must designate an alternate supervising physician in his or her temporary absence.

Participation in regulation: Three PAs serve on PA advisory committee.

Idaho Board of Medicine, P.O. Box 83720, Boise, ID 83720; (208) 327-7000.

ILLINOIS

Qualifications: Completion of approved program or verification from NCCPA that applicant has substantially equivalent training and experience. NCCPA examination; current NCCPA certificate required for renewal. No one holding medical degree eligible.

Application: By PA for license. Physician must file notice of supervision.

Scope of practice: Delegated medical duties within the supervising physician's scope of practice, consistent with the PA's education and experience.

Prescribing/dispensing: Physician may delegate prescriptive authority for noncontrolled and Schedules III–V medications to PA. Physician may delegate limited Schedule II prescribing authority to PA (effective August 17, 2009; rules to implement law not yet adopted). Medication orders issued by PA must be periodically reviewed by supervising physician. Physician must file notice of delegation of prescriptive authority to PA with Department of Professional Regulation. Physician and PA must include prescribing authority within a written supervision agreement. PAs who prescribe controlled medications must register with state controlled substance authority and the DEA.

Supervision: PAs shall practice in accordance with a written supervision agreement that is kept on file at the practice site (effective August 17, 2009; rules to implement law not yet adopted). Physician need not be physically present

at all times provided consultation available by radio, telephone, or telecommunications. Supervising physician may designate alternate supervising physician in accordance with statute. Physicians within a practice group of the supervising physician may supervise the PA with respect to their patients without being deemed an alternate supervising physician.

Participation in regulation: Three PAs serve on seven-member PA advisory committee.

Illinois Division of Professional Regulation, 320 West Washington Street, Springfield, IL 62786; (217) 785-0800.

INDIANA

Qualifications: Graduation from accredited PA program and current NCCPA certificate.

Application: By PA for license by the committee. Supervising physician must file supervisory agreement to the board for approval.

Scope of practice: Medical tasks delegated by supervising physician.

Prescribing/Dispensing: PA may apply for approval to prescribe Schedules III–V and noncontrolled medications. Application to prescribe must include documentation of all pharmacology course content completed (at least 30 contact hours), and proof that PA has practiced for at least 1 year. Supervisory agreement to include medications PA is authorized to prescribe, and protocol PA must follow when prescribing. PAs who prescribe controlled medications must register with the state and the DEA.

Supervision: Must be continuous but does not require the physical presence of the physician. Physician shall review all patient encounters within 24 hours. Supervision must meet one of the following requirements: (1) supervising physician is physically present at the location which PA practices; (2) supervising physician is immediately available for consultation and is in the same county or a county adjacent to the location in which PA practices; or (3) PA (or physician) is practicing at a hospital or other health-care facility or is traveling to or from the facility.

Participation in regulation: Three PAs serve on a five-member PA committee.

Indiana Health Professions Bureau, Attn: PA Committee, Professional Licensing Board, 402 West Washington Street, Suite W072, Indianapolis, IN 46204; (317) 234-2060.

IOWA

Qualifications: Graduation from accredited PA program (or equivalent education and training) and NCCPA examination.

Application: By PA for license. PA must supply information on supervising physician to PA board prior to beginning practice.

Scope of practice: Medical services that are within the supervising physician's scope of practice and for which the PA is qualified by training to perform that are delegated by the supervising physician.

Prescribing/dispensing: PA may prescribe noncontrolled and controlled substances (except Schedule II depressants). May dispense under certain conditions. PAs who prescribe controlled medications must register with the DEA.

Supervision: Physician need not be physically present, but must be readily available by telecommunication.

Participation in regulation: Five PAs serve on nine-member PA regulatory board.

Iowa Board of Physician Assistants, Bureau of Professional Licensure, Lucas State Office Building, 321 East 12th Street, Capitol Complex, Des Moines, IA 50319-0075; (515) 281-4401.

KANSAS

Qualifications: Graduation from an accredited PA program (or military experience that meets medical board requirements) and NCCPA examination.

Application: By PA for license, including designation of the responsible physician.

Scope of practice: Delegated acts constituting the practice of medicine and surgery that can be competently performed by the PA, based on his or her education, skill, and experience. Physician is required to submit utilization plan.

Prescribing/dispensing: PAs may prescribe Schedules II–V and noncontrolled medications as authorized in a written protocol with a supervising physician. PA prescribers of controlled medications must register with the DEA.

Supervision: Physician need not be physically present, but must be immediately available for consultation by telecommunication. Biweekly review of patient records and annual evaluation of PA performance and protocols required. PA may work in different practice location after completing at least 80 hours of on-site supervision with supervising physician, physician periodically sees patients at the same location, and a notice is posted.

Participation in regulation: Three PAs serve on a five-member advisory council.

Kansas State Board of Healing Arts, 235 SW Topeka Boulevard, Topeka, KS 66603-3068; (785) 296-7413 or (888) 886-7205.

KENTUCKY

Qualifications: Graduation from board-approved or accredited PA program and NCCPA examination; current NCCPA certificate required for biennial renewal.

Application: By PA for license; by physician for approval to supervise (includes job description).

Scope of practice: PA considered to practice medicine or osteopathy with physician supervision. PA may perform duties and responsibilities described in the initial application or supplemental application received by the board. PA may initiate evaluation and treatment in emergency situations without specific approval. PA may not practice in hospitals or other facilities without permission of facility's governing body.

Prescribing/Dispensing: PAs may prescribe noncontrolled medications as delegated to do so by supervising physician.

Supervision: Physician need not be physically present provided there is reliable means of direct communication. All records of service must be cosigned by physician in a timely manner. Newly graduated PAs must practice with on-site physician supervision for 18 months before they may practice in location separate from supervising physician. Certain exceptions apply.

Participation in regulation: Five PAs serve on nine-member PA advisory committee.

Kentucky State Board of Medical Licensure, 310 Whittington Parkway, Suite 1B, Louisville, KY 40222; (502) 429-7150.

LOUISIANA

Qualifications: Graduation from accredited PA program and current NCCPA certification.

Application: By PA for license; by physician for approval to supervise. Possible interview for initial license, if discrepancies exist.

Scope of practice: Medical services within the PA's education, training, and experience, which are delegated by the supervising physician.

Prescribing/dispensing: PAs may prescribe Schedules III–V and noncontrolled medications if delegated by supervising physician to do so and approved by the board. To be approved for prescribing, PA must have had a minimum of 1 year of clinical rotations during training and have practiced for a minimum of 1 year (PAs with less than a full year of clinical rotations may substitute 2 years of practice). In order to prescribe controlled medications, PA must register with state controlled drug agency and DEA.

Supervision: Continuous but does not require the physical presence of supervisor at time and place services are rendered. All written entries by PAs shall be cosigned by physician within 24 hours for inpatients, acute care settings, and hospital emergency departments; 48 hours for nursing home patients; 72 hours in all other cases.

Participation in regulation: Three PAs serve on a five-member PA advisory committee.

Louisiana State Board of Medical Examiners, P.O. Box 30250, New Orleans, LA 70190-0250; (504) 568-6820.

MAINE

Qualifications: Graduation from accredited PA program and/or passage of NCCPA exam.

Application: By PA for license. Supervising physician must submit affidavit stating written plan of supervision is on file in practice setting.

Scope of practice: Delegated medical services within supervising physician's proficiency and scope of practice.

Prescribing/dispensing: PA may prescribe and dispense drugs and medical devices, including noncontrolled and Schedules III–V controlled substances. PA and physician may request authorization to prescribe Schedule II drugs under specific individual guidelines. Registration with DEA required. PAs supervised by osteopathic physicians can prescribe noncontrolled and Schedules III–V controlled drugs.

Supervision: Physician must be available by radio, telephone, or telecommunication device. PA and physician establish supervision plan.

Participation in regulation: Two PAs serve on four-member PA Advisory Committee to the Board of Licensure in Medicine.

Maine Board of Licensure in Medicine, 137 State House Station, 161 Capitol Avenue, Augusta, ME 04333; (207) 287-3601.

Board of Osteopathic Examiners, 142 State House Station, 161 Capitol Avenue., Augusta, ME 04333, (207) 287-2480.

MARYLAND

Qualifications: Graduation from accredited PA program and NCCPA examination. Applicant who graduates from PA program after October 1, 2003, must have bachelor's degree or equivalent.

Application: By PA for certification; PA and physician apply for approval of delegation agreement.

Scope of Practice: Delegated medical acts within the physician's customary practice; appropriate to the PA's education, training, and experience; and consistent with delegation agreement submitted to board.

Prescribing/dispensing: Physician may delegate prescriptive authority including Schedules II–V and noncontrolled medications to PA. Must be consistent with delegation agreement. PAs prescribing controlled medications must register with the DEA and state controlled substance agency. Prescribing PAs must have passed NCCPA exam within previous 2 years or have completed 8 hours of Category I pharmacology CME within previous 2 years and have bachelor's degree or its equivalent, or 2 years work experience as a PA.

Supervision: Physician oversight of patient services rendered by PA, including continuous availability to PA in person, through written instructions, or by electronic means.

Participation in regulation: PA serves on medical board. Three PAs serve on seven-member PA advisory committee.

Maryland Board of Physicians, 4201 Patterson Avenue, Baltimore, MD 21215-0095; (410) 764-4777 or (800) 492-6836.

MASSACHUSETTS

Qualifications: Graduation from accredited PA program, baccalaureate degree, and NCCPA exam.

Application: By PA to PA board for registration.

Scope of practice: Medical services delegated by the supervising physician.

Prescribing/dispensing: PA may prescribe noncontrolled drugs and controlled substances (Schedules II–V). Prescriptions or orders for Schedule II drugs must be reviewed by the physician within 96 hours.

Supervision: Physician need not be physically present when PA renders medical services; patient records must be reviewed in a timely manner.

Participation in regulation: Four PAs and one PA educator serve on the nine-member PA board.

Massachusetts Board of Registration of Physician Assistants, Division of Registration, 239 Causeway Street, Suite 200, Boston, MA 02114; (617) 973-0806 or (800) 414-0168.

MICHIGAN

Qualifications: Graduation from accredited PA program and NCCPA examination.

Application: By PA for license.

Scope of practice: Medical care services delegated by the supervising physician, within the physician's usual scope of practice, and approved by the board.

Prescribing/dispensing: PA may prescribe noncontrolled and Schedules III–V drugs as delegated by supervising physician. PA may prescribe 7-day supply of Schedule II drugs as discharge medications. Supervising physician's and PA's names must be indicated on prescription. PA prescribers of controlled medications must register with the DEA.

Supervision: Physician must be continuously available for direct communication in person or by radio, telephone, or telecommunication and must regularly review PA performance and patient records, consult, and educate.

Participation in regulation: Five PAs serve on nine-member PA regulatory task force. Task force sends one PA to serve as member of medical board and one PA to serve on osteopathic board.

Michigan Task Force on Physician Assistants, Bureau of Health Professions,

P.O. Box 30670, Lansing, MI 48909-7518; (517) 335-0918.

MINNESOTA

Qualifications: Current NCCPA certification.

Application: By PA for license; by PA and supervising physician for approval of their practice agreement. Effective August 10, 2009, PA and supervising physician will not need approval of practice agreement, but PA to file a notice of intent to practice prior to beginning practice.

Scope of practice: Effective August 10, 2009, physician and PA must maintain a delegation agreement outlining delegated patient services within supervising physician's customary practice consistent with PA's training or experience. Specifically allowed are taking histories, doing physical examinations, data interpretation and evaluation to determine treatment, ordering or performing diagnostic and therapeutic procedures, patient counseling, assisting in surgery, and assisting physician in healthcare institutions and patient homes.

Prescribing/dispensing: NCCPA-certified PAs may prescribe controlled (Schedules II–V) and noncontrolled drugs. Delegation of prescribing authority must be outlined in delegation agreement (effective August 10, 2009). PAs authorized to prescribe controlled medications must register with the DEA.

Supervision: Constant presence of supervising physician is not required so long as the PA and supervising physician can be in touch via telecommunication.

Participation in regulation: Three PAs serve on seven-member PA advisory council.

Minnesota Board of Medical Practice, 2829 University Avenue SE, Suite 500, Minneapolis, MN 55414-3246; (612) 617-2130.

MISSISSIPPI

Qualifications: Graduation from accredited PA program, current NCCPA certificate, and bachelor's degree until December 31, 2004; master's degree in a science or health-related field required as of January 1, 2005. Temporary licensure available for PA applicants seeking masters degree.

Application: By PA for license. Board approval of protocol submitted by PA and supervising physician required prior to PA beginning practice. Interview and passage of jurisprudence exam required.

Scope of practice: Any delegated medical service within the PA's training and skills that forms a component of the physician's scope of practice and is provided with supervision. Board must approve protocol outlining delegated duties.

Prescribing/dispensing: PA may prescribe those noncontrolled medications outlined in board-approved protocol. PA must apply to board for authority to prescribe controlled substances (Schedules II–V); must complete board approved educational program prior to application; must comply with physician regulations on maintenance of records, prescription of diet medication, prescription of controlled substances for chronic pain, and prescription guidelines. PAs authorized to prescribe controlled medications must register with the DEA.

Supervision: On-site presence of physician required for first 120 days. Thereafter, supervision must be continuous but does not require physical presence of supervising physician. Supervising physician must review and initial 10% of PA charts monthly.

Participation in regulation: Any board-appointed task force or committee must include at least one PA.

Mississippi State Board of Medical Licensure, 1867 Crane Ridge Drive, Suite 200B, Jackson, MS 39216; (601) 987-3079.

MISSOURI

Qualifications: Graduation from accredited PA program and current NCCPA certification. Person employed as PA for three years prior to August 28, 1989, who has passed NCCPA exam and has current certification also eligible. Applicants for licensure who have graduated from a PA program after January 1, 2008, must have a master's degree from a PA program.

Application: By PA for license, includes form signed by supervising physician. Personal appearance may be required.

Scope of practice: Histories and physicals, routine office laboratory and screening procedures, routine therapeutic procedures, counselling, assisting at surgery, writing orders, and other delegated tasks.

Prescribing/dispensing: Physician assistants shall not prescribe nor dispense any drug, medicine, device, or therapy independent of consultation with the supervising physician. PAs may prescribe Schedules III–V drugs and non controlled drugs pursuant to supervision agreement with supervising physician (changes to laws pertaining to controlled medication effective August 28, 2009). Prescriptions shall include name, address, and telephone number of PA and supervising physician. Dispensing is limited to 72-hour starter dose supply of medication.

Supervision: PA must practice in same facility as supervising physician. Supervising physician must be present 66% of the time (per calendar quarter) PA is providing patient care. Physician must be immediately available in person or via telecommunication for consultation, assistance, and intervention. PA is limited to practicing in locations where the supervising physician is no further than 30 miles away. PA and physician practicing in certain settings may apply for a waiver for alternative supervision and distance requirements.

Participation in regulation: Two PAs serve on a five-member Advisory Commission for Physician Assistants.

Missouri Board of Registration for the Healing Arts, State Advisory Commission for Physician Assistants, P.O. Box 4, Jefferson City, MO 65102; (573) 751-0098 or (866) 289-5753.

MONTANA

Qualifications: Graduation from accredited PA program and current NCCPA certificate.

Application: By PA for license; PA submits physician supervision agreement prior to beginning practice. Interview may be required.

Scope of practice: Duties delegated by the supervising physician that are within his or her scope of practice and the PA's training and experience.

Prescribing/dispensing: PA may prescribe and dispense drugs, including Schedules II–V controlled substances, as delegated by physician. Schedule II prescriptions may be up to a 34-day supply.

Supervision: On-site supervision of PA not required if supervising physician has provided a means of communication or an alternate means of supervision. PA and supervising physician must meet in person once every 30 days. Physician must review and sign 10% of PA charts; greater percentage in specific circumstances.

Participation in regulation: One PA appointed to medical board; one nonvoting PA acts as liaison to the Board of Medical Examiners.

Montana State Board of Medical Examiners, P.O. Box 200513, Helena, MT 59620-0513; (406) 841-2364.

NEBRASKA

Qualifications: Graduation from accredited PA program and NCCPA examination.

Application: By PA for state licensure; by physician for approval to supervise (physician approval not required after September 30, 2009).

Scope of practice: Medical services that are delegated by and provided under the supervision of a licensed physician, appropriate to the level of competence of the physician assistant, form a component of the supervising physician's scope of practice, and are not otherwise prohibited by law (effective September 30, 2009).

Prescribing/dispensing: PA may prescribe medications as delegated to do so by supervising physician. Delegated authority may include legend drugs and Schedules II–V controlled drugs. PAs authorized to prescribe controlled medications must register with the DEA.

Supervision: Supervision should be continuous but not require the personal presence of the supervising physician. Board may place limitations on amount of on-site supervision required for PAs with less than 2 years experience; may apply for a waiver for this requirement (effective September 30, 2009; rules to implement this law not yet adopted).

Participation in regulation: Two PAs serve on five-member PA committee.

Nebraska Health Department, Board of Examiners in Medicine and Surgery, P.O. Box 94986, Lincoln, NE 68509-4986; (402) 471-2118.

NEVADA

Qualifications: Graduation from accredited PA program and current NCCPA certificate.

Application: By PA for license (PA must send in supervision form signed by physician prior to initiating practice).

Scope of practice: Medical services delegated by the supervising physician; within his or her specialty; within the PA's training, experience, and competence; and approved by the board.

Prescribing/dispensing: With board approval, PA may prescribe and dispense drugs and devices, including Schedules II–V controlled substances, as delegated by the supervising physician. Registration with pharmacy board and pharmacy law exam required. PAs who prescribe controlled medications must register with the DEA.

Supervision: Supervising physician must be available at all times for consultation, which may be indirect (by telecommunication); physician shall regularly review

and initial selected patient records. Supervising physician shall spend part of a day at least once a month at any location where PA provides medical services to act as consultant to PA and to monitor quality of care.

Participation in regulation: Three PAs serve on PA advisory committee.

Nevada State Board of Medical Examiners, P.O. Box 7238, Reno, NV 89510; (775) 688-2559 or (888) 890-8210.

Nevada State Board of Osteopathic Medicine, 2860 East Flamingo Road, Suite D, Las Vegas, NV 89121-5208, (702) 732-2147.

NEW HAMPSHIRE

Qualifications: Graduation from accredited PA program and current NCCPA certificate.

Application: By PA for license, must include statement from supervising physician that he or she accepts supervisory responsibility for PA.

Scope of practice: PA's scope of practice is defined by agreement with the registered supervising physician. Scope of practice is limited to and no broader than the scope of practice and privileges of the supervising physician.

Prescribing/dispensing: PA may prescribe and dispense legend drugs and controlled substances (Schedules II–V).

Supervision: Supervising physician(s) must file a written acceptance of supervisory responsibility with the board. Physician must be available for consultation at all times in person or via electronic communications device and provide regular ongoing evaluation of representative sample of charts. Alternate designated by supervising physician assumes responsibility for PA when supervising physician is unavailable.

Participation in regulation: One PA serves on eight-member medical board.

New Hampshire Board of Medicine, 2 Industrial Park Drrive, Suite 8, Concord, NH 03301-8520; (603) 271-1203.

NEW JERSEY

Qualifications: Graduation from accredited PA program and NCCPA exam.

Application: By PA for license; file notice of employment within 10 days of commencing employment.

Scope of practice: Delegated tasks such as histories and physicals, assisting at surgery, patient education, and determining and implementing therapeutic plans.

Prescribing/dispensing: PAs may prescribe noncontrolled drugs as delegated by supervising physician. PAs may order or prescribe controlled medications in Schedules II–V, if authorized by supervising physician and controlled drug is to continue or reissue order or prescription of controlled drug issued by supervising physician; adjust dose of controlled drug prescribed by physician with prior consultation; initiate order or prescription for controlled drug with prior consultation with supervising physician; or initiate order or prescription for controlled drug as part of treatment plan for patient with terminal illness.

Supervision: Constant availability through electronic communication; intermittent physical presence; and regular review of records. 24-hour countersignature of inpatient medical orders. Outpatient chart countersignature in 7 days; 48 hours if chart has medication order or prescription.

Participation in regulation: Three PAs named to five-member PA advisory committee; one PA on medical board.

New Jersey Board of Medical Examiners, PA Advisory Committee, P.O. Box 45035, Newark, NJ 07101; (973) 504-6580.

NEW MEXICO

Qualifications: Graduation from accredited PA program; current NCCPA certificate.

Application: By PA for license; by supervising physician for approval. Personal interview with board member or designee and attendance at orientation required. PAs supervised by DOs must attend board meeting when application is discussed.

Scope of practice: Medical services delegated by supervising physician within PA's skills and forming a usual component of physician's practice. Written utilization plan must be developed.

Prescribing/dispensing: PA may prescribe, administer, and distribute noncontrolled medications and Schedules II–V drugs under direction of supervising physician and within parameters of board-approved formulary and guidelines. PA prescribers of controlled medications must register with the DEA.

Supervision: Must be immediate communication between physician and PA, which can be through telecommunication. Quality assurance program must be in place and reviewed on an ongoing basis.

Participation in regulation: One PA serves on medical board.

New Mexico Medical Board, 2055 South Pacheco Street, Building 400, Santa Fe, NM 87505; (505) 476-7220 or (800) 945-5845.

Board of Osteopathic Medical Examiners, 2550 Cerrillos Road, Santa Fe, NM 87505; (505) 476-4695.

NEW YORK

Qualifications: Graduation from approved PA program and NCCPA examination.

Application: By PA for state registration.

Scope of practice: Medical acts and duties delegated by the supervising physician, within the physician's scope of practice and appropriate to the PA's education, training, and experience.

Prescribing/dispensing: PA may prescribe Schedules II–V and noncontrolled medications.

Supervision: Physician is not required to be physically present at time and place where PA performs services.

Participation in regulation: At least two PAs appointed to medical examining board.

New York State Board for Medicine, Office of the Professions, 89 Washington Avenue, Albany, NY 12234; (518) 474-3817 ext. 560.

NORTH CAROLINA

Qualifications: Graduation from accredited PA program and NCCPA exam.

Application: By PA for license; physician submits statement of supervision.

Scope of practice: Medical acts and tasks delegated by supervising physician and within the PA's training.

Prescribing/dispensing: PA may prescribe noncontrolled and controlled drugs in Schedules II–V (Schedules II and III limited to 30-day supply). Pharmacy Board approval required for compounding and dispensing drugs. PA prescribers of controlled medications must register with the DEA.

Supervision: Supervision continuous but physical presence of physician not required at all times. PA must meet with supervising physician monthly for first 6 months of employment and every 6 months thereafter to discuss clinical problems and quality improvement measures.

Participation in regulation: Physician extender (PA or NP) serves on medical board. PAs serve in the majority on a 15-member PA Advisory Council.

North Carolina Medical Board, P.O. Box 20007, Raleigh, NC 27619-0007; (919) 326-1100 or (800) 253-9653.

NORTH DAKOTA

Qualifications: Current NCCPA certification.

Application: By PA for license; includes copy of contract.

Scope of practice: Patient services delegated by supervising physician and approved by board.

Prescribing/dispensing: PAs may prescribe noncontrolled drugs and Schedules II–V controlled substances (Schedule II effective August 1, 2009). PA may dispense prepackaged medications (Schedules IV and V and noncontrolled substances) prepared by pharmacist acting on physician's written order and labeled to show names of PA and physician. Dispensing must be authorized by and within preestablished guidelines of supervising physician. PA prescribers of controlled drugs must register with the DEA.

Supervision: Physician must be continuously available for contact personally or by telephone or radio.

North Dakota State Board of Medical Examiners, 418 East Broadway Avenue, Suite 12, Bismarck, ND 58501; (701) 328-6500.

OHIO

Qualifications: Current NCCPA certificate needed for initial registration and for change of employment and renewal. After January 1, 2008, PAs are required to possess a master's degree in a health-related field. Those already licensed as PAs in any jurisdiction are exempt from this requirement.

Application: By PA for certificate of registration (license); by physician for approval.

Scope of practice: Taking histories and performing physical examinations, assisting in surgery, and other tasks approved by the board in a physician supervisory plan. Scope of practice in a licensed health facility is determined by physician delegation and the policies of the health facility.

Prescribing/dispensing: PAs may prescribe noncontrolled and controlled drugs in Schedules III–V. PA prescribers must apply for a certificate, issued by the state medical board, to prescribe. PA prescribers of controlled medications are required to register with the DEA.

Supervision: Physician not required to be physically present but must be available for consultation and within 60 minutes travel time of PA's location. Physician to develop a quality assurance plan to ensure proper PA supervision. During first 500 hours of the provisional pre-scribing period, physician provides on-site supervision of PA prescribing.

Participation in regulation: Three PAs serve on seven-member PA policy committee.

Ohio State Medical Board, 77 South High Street, 17th Floor, Columbus, OH 43215-6127; (614) 466-3934.

OKLAHOMA

Qualifications: Graduation from accredited PA program, which for graduates after July 1, 2007, must include minimum of 1 year of classroom instruction and 1 year of clinical experience (including at least 1-month rotations each in family medicine, emergency medicine, and surgery). Passage of NCCPA examination required.

Application: By PA for license. Board must approve PA and physician (includes job description). Passage of jurisprudence exam required.

Scope of practice: Diagnostic and therapeutic procedures common to the physician's practice.

Prescribing/dispensing: PAs may prescribe noncontrolled and Schedules III–V drugs on board-approved formulary. Schedules III–V drugs are limited to 30-day supply or 40 dosage units with one refill, whichever is smaller. PAs who prescribe controlled medications must register with the DEA and the Oklahoma Bureau of Narcotics and Dangerous Drugs.

Supervision: Physician not required to be physically present when, nor specifically consulted before, PA performs delegated task. Board approval required for PA utilization in remote site. In the remote setting, physician shall be present at least half a day each week.

Participation in regulation: Two PAs serve on seven-member PA committee.

Oklahoma State Board of Medical Licensure and Supervision, P.O. Box 18256, Oklahoma City, OK 73154-0256; (405) 848-6841.

OREGON

Qualifications: Graduation from accredited PA program and NCCPA examination. New graduate PAs, PAs new to the state, and supervising physicians not previously approved must pass an open-book exam on the Medical Practice Act.

Application: By PA and physician (includes job description). Interview may be required.

Scope of practice: Medical services delegated by the physician and included in the board-approved job description.

Prescribing/dispensing: PA may prescribe medications, including Schedules II–V controlled substances, as determined by physician and approved by board. PAs prescribing Schedule II drugs must have current NCCPA certification. DEA registration is required. PA may apply for emergency dispensing authority for medications prepackaged by pharmacist.

Supervision: Physician must always be available for verbal communication. Board approval required for PA utilization at remote site. Supervising physician must provide 4 hours of on-site supervision every 2 weeks.

Participation in regulation: Three PAs serve on five-member PA committee.

Oregon Board of Medical Examiners, 1500 SW First Avenue, Suite 620, Portland, OR 97201; (971) 673-2700 or (877) 254-6263.

PENNSYLVANIA

Qualifications: Graduation from accredited PA program and NCCPA examination (current NCCPA certificate required for renewal), baccalaureate or higher degree from a college or university and not less than 60 clock hours of didactic instruction in pharmacology or other related courses as the board may approve by regulation.

Application: By PA for license; supervising physician must register with board.

Scope of practice: Medical procedures delegated by supervising physician, within

PHYSICIAN ASSISTANTS: POLICY AND PRACTICE

normal scope of physician's practice, and within the training and expertise of the PA.

Prescribing/dispensing: PAs may prescribe and dispense drugs including Schedules II–V controlled substances. Schedule II drugs are limited to a 72-hour supply for initial therapy; 30-day supply if given prior approval by supervising physician. Written agreement specifying PA prescribing and dispensing privileges, and categories of drugs which the PA is not permitted to prescribe, must be kept on file and available for review. PAs supervised by osteopathic physicians may not prescribe.

Supervision: Physician's constant physical presence not required as long as contact is available through radio, telephone, or telecommunication. Board approval required for satellite office. Supervising physician must review and sign medical record of patient cared for by PA within 10 days. If at a satellite location, supervising physician must visit location at least weekly to provide supervision.

Participation in regulation: One medical board seat reserved for, and rotates among, PA, nurse practitioner, respiratory care practitioner, acupuncturist, and nurse midwife. One PA, certified athletic trainer, or respiratory care practitioner on osteopathic board.

Pennsylvania State Board of Medicine, P.O. Box 2649, Harrisburg, PA 17105-2649; (717) 783-1400.

Pennsylvania State Board of Osteopathic Medicine, same address as above; (717) 783-4858.

RHODE ISLAND

Qualifications: Graduation from accredited PA program and NCCPA examination.
Application: By PA for license.
Scope of practice: Health-care services delegated by supervising physician consistent with the physician's and the PA's expertise.

Prescribing/dispensing: PAs may prescribe legend and Schedules II–V drugs. PA prescribers of controlled medications must register with state drug control office and the DEA.

Supervision: Physician not required to be physically present but must be available for easy communication.

Participation in regulation: Two PAs serve on seven-member PA regulatory board.

Rhode Island Board of Physician Assistants, Division of Health Services Regulation, Health Professionals, 3 Capitol Hill, Room #104, Providence, RI 02908; (401) 222-3855.

SOUTH CAROLINA

Qualifications: Graduation from accredited PA program; current NCCPA certificate required for licensure and license renewal. Must pass examination on state laws governing PA practice.

Application: By PA for license; interview of PA and supervising physician by board member or board designee required.

Scope of practice: Medical acts, tasks, or functions delegated by supervising physician in written scope of practice guidelines.

Prescribing/dispensing: PA may prescribe noncontrolled and Schedules III–V drugs as delegated by supervising physician in scope of practice guidelines. PAs who prescribe controlled drugs must register with the DEA. PA and supervising physician must read and sign a document approved by the board describing the management of expanded controlled substances prescriptive authority for PAs, which must be kept on file for review.

Supervision: Supervising physician must be available by telecommunication. Supervising physician must be present at least 75% of the time PA is providing services; PA must have 6 months clinical experience with supervising physician before off-site supervision authorized; PA may not provide services in the absence of supervising physician for more than 7 consecutive days per month. PA may not practice in any location more than 45 miles or 60 minutes from supervising physician without board approval, and supervising physician must be physically present at least 20% of the time PA is providing services. Supervising physician must review, initial, and date the off-site physician assistant's charts not later than 5 working days from the date of service, as proportionate to the acuity of care and practice setting (board may authorize exceptions to these provisions).

Participation in regulation: Three PAs serve on a nine-member PA committee.

South Carolina Board of Medical Examiners, P.O. Box 11289, Columbia, SC 29211-1289; (803) 896-4500.

SOUTH DAKOTA

Qualifications: Graduation from an accredited PA program and NCCPA examination.

Application: By PA for license; includes copy of practice agreement and personal interview. Physician interviewed in person or by telephone.

Scope of practice: PA may perform delegated tasks which are within the PA's skills and the supervising physician's scope of practice.

Prescribing/dispensing: PA may prescribe medication including Schedules II–V, limited to 30 days for Schedule II drugs. PAs who prescribe controlled medications must register with the state and the DEA.

Supervision: May be by personal contact or via telecommunication. If PA utilized in satellite office, physician must provide intermittent on-site personal supervision. PA and supervising physician must maintain jointly written and signed supervisory agreement, which is filed with the board prior to commencing practice.

Participation in regulation: Board has established PA advisory committee with three PA members.

South Dakota Board of Medical and Osteopathic Examiners, 125 South Main Avenue, Sioux Falls, SD 57104; (605) 367-7781.

TENNESSEE

Qualifications: Graduation from accredited PA program and NCCPA examination.

Application: By PA for license; includes name of supervising physician.

Scope of practice: Medical services delegated in writing by supervising physician and form a usual component of the physician's scope of practice.

Prescribing/dispensing: PAs may prescribe noncontrolled and Schedules II–V drugs. PA prescribers of controlled drugs must register with the DEA. Supervising physician must review all controlled substance prescriptions within 30 days.

Supervision: Active and continuous overview, but physician not required to be physically present at all times. Physician shall review 20% of chart notes written by PA every 30 days and must visit remote site once every 30 days.

Participation in regulation: Five PAs serve on five-member PA regulatory committee.

Tennessee Committee on Physician Assistants, Department of Health-Related Boards, 227 French Landing, Suite 300, Nashville, TN 37243, (615) 532-3202 or (800) 778-4123.

TEXAS

Qualifications: Graduation from accredited PA program and current NCCPA certification; must also pass board-approved jurisprudence exam on state PA law and regulations.

Application: By PA for license.

Scope of practice: Medical services delegated by the supervising physician within education, training, and experience of PA.

Prescribing/dispensing: PA may carry out or sign a prescription drug order if delegated this task under standing orders. Limited to medically underserved areas, practices with preponderance of medically indigent patients, a physician's primary practice site, hospital, location when physician is present, or an alternate site when specified conditions are met. Authority includes Schedules III–V and noncontrolled medications. PAs who prescribe controlled medications must register with the DEA.

Supervision: Supervision shall be continuous but constant physical presence of physician not required. Establishment of office practice setting separate from that of supervising physician limited to site serving medically underserved, and physician must be on-site to provide medical direction and consultation at least once every 10 business days and randomly review and cosign at least 10% of the charts.

Participation in regulation: Three PAs serve on nine-member PA board.

Texas Physician Assistant Board, c/o Texas Medical Board, P.O. Box 2018, Austin, TX 78768-2018; (512) 305-7022.

UTAH

Qualifications: Graduation from accredited PA program and NCCPA examination, as well as exam on state laws and rules.

Application: By PA for license; to practice in Utah, PA must have a delegation of services agreement with a Utah-licensed physician.

Scope of practice: Delegated medical services within supervising physician's scope of practice, within PA's skills, and included on the delegation of services agreement.

Prescribing/dispensing: PA may prescribe Schedules II–V and non-scheduled drugs. Any limitations on prescribing may be made in the delegation agreement. Prescriptions for Schedules II and III drugs require chart cosignature. PAs who prescribe controlled medications must register with the DEA and hold a state controlled substance license.

Supervision: Physician must be available for consultation by electronic means if not on-site; shall cosign sufficient number of charts to ensure patient health, safety, and welfare.

Participation in regulation: One PA and one PA educator serve on seven-member PA board.

Utah Physician Assistant Licensing Board, P.O. Box 146741, Salt Lake City, UT 84114-6741; (801) 530-6628 or (866) 275-3675.

VERMONT

Qualifications: Graduation from an accredited PA program and passage of NCCPA examination, or completion of board-approved apprenticeship program.

Application: By PA for state certification and by physician (includes employment contract and job description).

Scope of practice: Delegated medical acts within supervising physician's normal scope of practice, consistent with PA education and experience, and approved by board. Separate approval required for each practice site.

Prescribing/dispensing: PA may prescribe those drugs authorized by physician in job description and approved by board. (May include legend drugs and Schedules II–V medications.) PAs who prescribe controlled medications must register with the DEA.

Supervision: Physician must be available for consultation and review. Separate board approval required for each site where physician supervises PA.

Participation in regulation: One PA serves on medical board.

Vermont Board of Medical Practice, P.O. Box 70, Burlington, VT 05402-0070; (802) 657-4220 or (800) 745-7371.

VIRGINIA

Qualifications: Graduation from accredited PA program and NCCPA examination; current NCCPA certificate required for renewal.

Application: By PA for license; prior to practice, PA and physician submit description of practice.

Scope of practice: Medical care services delegated by supervising physician, included in a delegation agreement, and approved by the board. Physician must see patient on follow-up visit if condition has not improved and must see patient with continuing illness at least every fourth visit.

Prescribing/dispensing: PAs may prescribe noncontrolled drugs and devices and Schedules II–V controlled drugs. PAs who prescribe controlled substances must register with the DEA.

Supervision: Continuous supervision, but supervising physician is not required to be present; physician must review PA record of services proportionate to acuity of care and practice setting.

Participation in regulation: Three PAs serve on five-member Advisory Board.

Virginia State Board of Medicine, Perimeter Center, 9960 Mayland Drive, Suite 300 Richmond, VA 23233-1463; (804) 367-4600.

WASHINGTON

Qualifications: Graduation from accredited PA program and NCCPA examination.

Application: By PA for license. Practice arrangement plan must be filed with the board.

Scope of practice: Medical services delegated by supervising physician and approved by board.

Prescribing/dispensing: PAs may write and sign prescriptions, including controlled substances in Schedules II–V. PAs who prescribe controlled medications must register with the DEA. PAs supervised by osteopathic physicians may prescribe controlled substances in Schedules II–V (NCCPA certification required for Schedule II prescription privileges).

Supervision: Physician is not required to be physically present where PA services are

rendered. Board approval required for PA utilization in remote site. PA supervised by osteopathic physicians require chart review within 1 week.

Participation in regulation: Two PAs serve on medical quality assurance commission. Commission has established PA Advisory Committee.

Washington State Department of Health, Medical Quality Assurance Commission, P.O. Box 47865, Olympia, WA 98504-7865; (360)236-4700.

Board of Osteopathic Medicine and Surgery, Health Professions Quality Assurance, P.O. Box 47865, Olympia, WA 98504; (360) 236-4700.

WEST VIRGINIA

Qualifications: Graduation from accredited PA program and NCCPA examination. Bachelor's or master's degree required.

Application: By PA for license; by supervising physician for approval to supervise (includes job description).

Scope of practice: Medical procedures delegated by supervising physician, within physician's normal scope of practice, included on PA's job description, and approved by the board.

Prescribing/dispensing: PAs with 2 years of experience who have completed board-approved pharmacology course and maintain NCCPA certification may prescribe controlled (Schedules III–V) and noncontrolled drugs from formulary. Schedule III drugs limited to 72-hour supply. Schedules IV–V drugs limited to 90 dosage units or 30 days. Other drugs not to exceed 6-month supply. Registration with the DEA required. Under certain conditions PAs may dispense legend drugs.

Supervision: Physician's constant physical presence not required provided consultation available by radio, telephone, or telecommunication.

Participation in regulation: One PA serves on medical board.

West Virginia Board of Medicine, 101 Dee Drive, Suite 103, Charleston, WV 25311; (304) 558-2921.

West Virginia State Board of Osteopathy, 334 Penco Road, Weirton, WV 26062; (304) 723-4638 or (800) 206-6625.

WISCONSIN

Qualifications: Graduation from accredited PA program and current NCCPA certification.

Application: By PA for license

Scope of practice: Patient services include taking histories; physical examinations, routine diagnostic studies, and therapeutic procedures; counseling; monitoring treatment and therapy plans; referrals; and assisting the physician in a hospital or other facility.

Prescribing/dispensing: PA may prescribe Schedules II–V and noncontrolled drugs in situations specified in written guidelines developed by supervising physician. Guidelines must be reviewed annually. Supervising physician must sign patient record within 72 hours, review patient record within 72 hours, or review by telephone within 48 hours and sign patient record within 1 week. PA prescribers of controlled medications must register with the DEA. (*Note:* Chart cosignature and record review requirement repealed, effective September 1, 2009.)

Supervision: Physician must be available at all times for consultation either in person or within 15 minutes of contact by telephone, two-way radio, or television. Physician must visit and review on-site any facilities attended by PA at least once a month.

Participation in regulation: Three PAs serve on five-member advisory council.

Wisconsin Medical Examining Board, P.O. Box 8935, Madison, WI 53708-8935; (608) 266-2112.

WYOMING

Qualifications: Graduation from accredited PA program and current NCCPA certification.

Application: By PA for license; by physician for approval to supervise.

Scope of practice: Medical services delegated by supervising physician and approved by the board in the specialty area(s) for which physician and PA are trained or experienced.

Prescribing/dispensing: Physicians may delegate prescribing of noncontrolled and Schedules II–V medications to PAs; also dispensing of prepackaged medications in rural areas when pharmacy services unavailable. PAs must register with the DEA if they prescribe controlled medications.

Supervision: Physician must be readily available for consultation, in person or by telecommunication.

Participation in regulation: One PA serves on medical board; two PAs serve on four-member advisory committee.

Wyoming Board of Medical Examiners, 211 West 19th St., 2nd Floor, Colony Building, Cheyenne, WY 82002; (307) 778-7053 or (800) 438-5784.

Reprinted with permission from the American Academy of Physician Assistants.

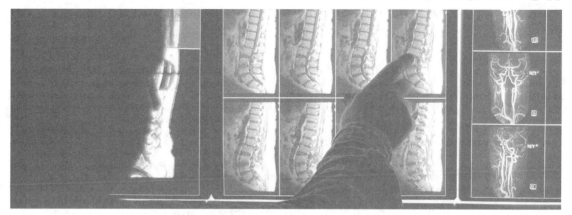

COMPETENCIES FOR THE PHYSICIAN ASSISTANT PROFESSION

Version 3.5 (March 22, 2005)

PREAMBLE

In 2003, the National Commission on Certification of Physicians Assistants (NCCPA) initiated an effort to define physician assistant (PA) competencies in response to similar efforts being conducted within other health-care professions and growing demand for accountability and assessment in clinical practice. The following year, representatives from three other national PA organizations, each bringing a unique perspective and valuable insights, joined the NCCPA in that effort. Those organizations were the Accreditation Review Commission for Education of the Physician Assistant (ARC-PA), the body that accredits PA educational programs; the Association of Physician Assistant Programs (APAP), the membership association for PA educators and program directors; and the American Academy of Physician Assistants (AAPA), the only national membership association representing all PAs.

The resultant document, *Competencies for the Physician Assistant Profession*, is a foundation from which each of those four organizations, other PA organizations, and individual PAs themselves can chart a course for advancing the competencies of the PA profession.

INTRODUCTION

The purpose of this document is to communicate to the PA profession and the public a set of competencies that all PAs regardless of specialty or setting are expected to acquire and maintain throughout their careers. This document serves as a map for the individual PA, the physician-PA team, and organizations that are committed to promoting the development and maintenance of these professional competencies among physician assistants.

Source: http://www.nccpa.net/PAC/Competencies_home.aspx.
See also: Kohlhepp, B., Rohrs, R., & Robinson, P. (2005). Charting a course to competency. *Journal of the American Academy of Physician Assistants, 18,* 14–18.

The clinical role of PAs includes primary and specialty care in medical and surgical practice settings. Professional competencies for PAs include the effective and appropriate application of medical knowledge, interpersonal and communication skills, patient care, professionalism, practice-based learning and improvement, systems-based practice, as well as an unwavering commitment to continual learning, professional growth, and the physician-PA team, for the benefit of patients and the larger community being served. These competencies are demonstrated within the scope of practice, whether medical or surgical, for each individual PA as that scope is defined by the supervising physician and appropriate to the practice setting.

In 1999, the Accreditation Council for Graduation Medical Education (ACGME) endorsed a list of general competencies for medical residents. NCCPA's Eligibility Committee, with substantial input from representatives of the AAPA, the APAP, and the ARC-PA, has modified the ACGME's list for PAt practice, drawing from several other resources, including the work of Drs. Epstein and Hundert; research conducted by the AAPA's EVP/CEO, Dr. Steve Crane; and the NCCPA's own examination content blueprint.

The PA profession defines the specific knowledge, skills, and attitudes required and provides educational experiences as needed in order for PAs to acquire and demonstrate these competencies.

MEDICAL KNOWLEDGE

Medical knowledge includes an understanding of pathophysiology, patient presentation, differential diagnosis, patient management, surgical principles, health promotion, and disease prevention. PAs must demonstrate core knowledge about established and evolving biomedical and clinical sciences and the application of this knowledge to patient care in their area of practice. In addition, PAs are expected to demonstrate an investigatory and analytic thinking approach to clinical situations. PAs are expected to:

- understand etiologies, risk factors, underlying pathological process, and epidemiology for medical conditions;
- identify signs and symptoms of medical conditions;
- select and interpret appropriate diagnostic or laboratory studies;
- manage general medical and surgical conditions to include understanding the indications, contraindications, side effects, interactions, and adverse reactions of pharmacological agents and other relevant treatment modalities;
- identify the appropriate site of care for presenting conditions, including identifying emergent cases and those requiring referral or admission;
- identify appropriate interventions for prevention of conditions;
- identify the appropriate methods to detect conditions in an asymptomatic individual;
- differentiate between the normal and the abnormal in anatomic, physiological, laboratory findings, and other diagnostic data;
- appropriately use history and physical findings and diagnostic studies to formulate a differential diagnosis; and
- provide appropriate care to patients with chronic conditions

INTERPERSONAL AND COMMUNICATION SKILLS

Interpersonal and communication skills encompass verbal, nonverbal, and written exchange of information. PAs must demonstrate interpersonal and communication skills that result in effective information exchange with patients, their patients' families, physicians, professional associates, and the healthcare system. PAs are expected to:

- create and sustain a therapeutic and ethically sound relationship with patients;

- use effective listening; nonverbal, explanatory questioning; and writing skills to elicit and provide information;
- appropriately adapt communication style and messages to the context of the individual patient interaction;
- work effectively with physicians and other healthcare professionals as a member or leader of a healthcare team or other professional group;
- apply an understanding of human behavior;
- demonstrate emotional resilience and stability, adaptability, flexibility, and tolerance of ambiguity and anxiety;
- accurately and adequately document and record information regarding the care process for medical, legal, quality, and financial purposes

PATIENT CARE

Patient care includes age-appropriate assessment, evaluation, and management. PAs must demonstrate care that is effective, patient-centered, timely, efficient, and equitable for the treatment of health problems and the promotion of wellness. PAs are expected to:

- work effectively with physicians and other healthcare professionals to provide patient-centered care;
- demonstrate caring and respectful behaviors when interacting with patients and their families;
- gather essential and accurate information about their patients;
- make informed decisions about diagnostic and therapeutic interventions based on patient information and preferences, up-to-date scientific evidence, and clinical judgment;
- develop and carry out patient management plans;
- counsel and educate patients and their families;
- competently perform medical and surgical procedures considered essential in the area of practice;

- provide healthcare services and education aimed at preventing health problems or maintaining health

PROFESSIONALISM

Professionalism is the expression of positive values and ideals as care is delivered. Foremost, it involves prioritizing the interests of those being served above one's own. PAs must know their professional and personal limitations. Professionalism also requires that PAs practice without impairment from substance abuse, cognitive deficiency, or mental illness. PAs must demonstrate a high level of responsibility, ethical practice, sensitivity to a diverse patient population, and adherence to legal and regulatory requirements. PAs are expected to demonstrate:

- understanding of legal and regulatory requirements, as well as the appropriate role of the PA;
- professional relationships with physician supervisors and other healthcare providers;
- respect, compassion, and integrity;
- responsiveness to the needs of patients and society;
- accountability to patients, society, and the profession;
- commitment to excellence and ongoing professional development;
- commitment to ethical principles pertaining to provision or withholding of clinical care;
- confidentiality of patient information, informed consent, and business practices;
- sensitivity and responsiveness to patients' culture, age, gender, and disabilities;
- self-reflection, critical curiosity, and initiative

PRACTICE-BASED LEARNING AND IMPROVEMENT

Practice-based learning and improvement includes the processes through which clinicians engage in critical analysis of their own practice experience, medical literature, and other information resources for the purpose of self-improvement. PAs must be able to assess, evaluate, and improve their patient care practices. PAs are expected to:

- analyze practice experience and perform practice-based improvement activities using a systematic methodology in concert with other members of the healthcare delivery team;
- locate, appraise, and integrate evidence from scientific studies related to their patients' health problems;
- obtain and apply information about their own population of patients and the larger population from which their patients are drawn;
- apply knowledge of study designs and statistical methods to the appraisal of clinical studies and other information on diagnostic and therapeutic effectiveness;
- apply information technology to manage information, access online medical information, and support their own education;
- facilitate the learning of students and/or other healthcare professionals;
- recognize and appropriately address gender, cultural, cognitive, emotional, and other biases; gaps in medical knowledge; and physical limitations in themselves and others

SYSTEMS-BASED PRACTICE

Systems-based practice encompasses the societal, organizational, and economic environments in which health care is delivered. PAs must demonstrate an awareness of and responsiveness to the larger system of health care to provide patient care that is of optimal value. PAs should work to improve the larger healthcare system of which their practices are a part. PAs are expected to:

- use information technology to support patient care decisions and patient education;
- effectively interact with different types of medical practice and delivery systems;
- understand the funding sources and payment systems that provide coverage for patient care;
- practice cost-effective health care and resource allocation that does not compromise quality of care;
- advocate for quality patient care and assist patients in dealing with system complexities;
- partner with supervising physicians, healthcare managers, and other healthcare providers to assess, coordinate, and improve the delivery of health care and patient outcomes;
- accept responsibility for promoting a safe environment for patient care and recognizing and correcting systems-based factors that negatively impact patient care;
- apply medical information and clinical data systems to provide more effective, efficient patient care;
- use the systems responsible for the appropriate payment of services

BIBLIOGRAPHY

Aaronson, W. E. (1991). The use of physician extenders in nursing homes: A review. *Medical Care Review, 48,* 411–447.

Aaronson, W. E. (1992). Is there a role for physician extenders in nursing homes? *Journal of Long Term Care Administration, 20*(3), 18–22.

Abbott, S., Dadabhoy, S., Dalphinis, J., Hill, M., & Smith, R. (2007). Professionalization in new primary care roles. *Practice Nursing, 18*(8), 413–417.

Accreditation Review Commission on Education for the Physician Assistant. (2006). *Accreditation Standards for Physician Assistant Education* (3rd ed.). Duluth, GA: Author. Retrieved September 14, 2006, from http://www.arcpa.org/General/standards/newStandards3.31.05.pdf

Ackermann, R. J., & Kemle, K. A. (1998). The effect of a physician assistant on the hospitalization of nursing home residents. *Journal of the American Geriatrics Society, 46*(5), 610–614.

Acuna, H. R. (1977a). The medical assistant (editorial). *Boletin de la Oficina Sanitaria Panamericana. Pan American Sanitary Bureau, 82*(6), 473–477.

Acuna, H. R. (1977b). The physician's assistant and extension of health services. *Bulletin of the Pan American Health Organization, 11*(3), 189–194.

Alaska State Medical Board, Department of Community and Economic Development. (2008). *Application for a license to practice as a physician assistant-certified.* Retrieved June 25, 2008, from http://www.dced.state.ak.us/occ/pub/med4226a.pdf

Alexander, D., Waters, V., McQueen, K., & Basinger, S. (2006). Utilizing a substance use attitudes, practices and knowledge survey for multidisciplinary curriculum development. *Substance Abuse, 26*(3–4), 63–66.

Alexander, B. J., & Lipscomb, J. (1992). Nonphysician practitioners panel report. In: J. Lipscomb & B. J. Alexander (Eds.), *Physician Staffing for the VA.* National Academy Press, Washington, DC.

Allen, M., Sargeant, J. Mann, K. Fleming, M., & Premi, J. (2003). Videoconferencing for practice-based small-group continuing medical education: Feasibility, acceptability, effectiveness, and cost. *Journal of Continuing Education in Health Professions, 23*(1), 38–47.

Alliance for Aging Research. (2006). *Ageism: How Healthcare Fails the Elderly.* Washington, DC: Author.

Amann, H. J. (1973). Physician's assistants: An extension of the physician. *U.S. Navy Medicine, 62,* 36–38.

American Academy of Family Physicians. (2007a). *National residency matching program.* Retrieved March 8, 2008, from http://www.aafp.org/online/en/home/residents/match.html.

American Academy of Family Physicians. (2007b). *2007 match summary and analysis.* Retrieved March 8, 2008, from http://www.aafp.org/online/en/home/residents/match/summary.html#Parsys0005

American Academy of Pediatrics. Committee on Hospital Care. (1999). The role of the nurse practitioner and physician assistant in the care of hospitalized children. *Pediatrics, 103*(5 Pt 1), 1050–1052.

American Academy of Physician Assistants. (2000). *2000 AAPA Physician Assistant Census Report.* Alexandria, VA: Author.

American Academy of Physician Assistants. (2001). *2001 Survey of new enrollees in physician assistant programs.* Retrieved July 31, 2008, from http://www.aapa.org/research/enrollees01/index.html

American Academy of Physician Assistants. (2002). *2002 AAPA Physician Assistant Census Report.* Alexandria, VA: Author.

American Academy of Physician Assistants. (2005). Maintaining professional flexibility: The case against accreditation of postgraduate physician assistant programs. *Journal of the American Academy of Physician Assistants, 18*(8), 14–16.

American Academy of Physician Assistants. (2006a). *2006 AAPA Physician Assistant Census Report.* Alexandria, VA: Author.

American Academy of Physician Assistants. (2006b). *Physician Assistants: State Laws and Regulations.* (10th ed.). Alexandria, VA: Author.

American Academy of Physician Assistants. (2006c). *Physician Assistant Prescribing and Dispensing.* Alexandria, VA: Author.

American Academy of Physician Assistants. (2007a). *2007 AAPA Physician Assistant Census Report.* Alexandria, VA: Author.

American Academy of Physician Assistants. (2007b). *Demographics and Characteristics of Physician Assistants, Results of the 2006 Census.* Alexandria, VA: Author.

American Academy of Physician Assistants. (2007c). *AAPA physician assistant census report for cardiovascular/cardiothoracic surgery.* Retrieved June 6, 2008, from http://www.aapa.org/research/SpecialtyReports07/cardiovascularsurgery07C.pdf

American Academy of Physician Assistants. (2007d). *Information update: Number of visits to physician assistants for select disorders in 2007.* Retrieved June 7, 2008, from http://www.aapa.org/research/InformationUpdates07/IUDisorders2007.pdf

American Academy of Physician Assistants. (2007e). *Regional Report of the 2006 Student Census Survey.* Alexandria, VA: Author.

American Academy of Physician Assistants. (2007f). *Insurance—Risky business: The ins and outs of liability insurance.* Retrieved September 4, 2008, from http://www.aapa.org/gandp/risky.html

American Academy of Physician Assistants. (2008a). *2008 AAPA Physician Assistant Census Report.* Alexandria, VA: Author.

American Academy of Physician Assistants. (2008b). *Physician assistants and hospital practice.* Retrieved June 29, 2008, from http://www.aapa.org/gandp/pdf/pahpman.pdf

American College of Physicians. (2006, March). College warns of looming collapse of nation's primary care. Retrieved August 28, 2008, from http://www.acponline.org/journals/news/march06/advocacy.htm

American Geriatrics Society. (1999). *Position statement: Geriatric rehabilitation.* Retrieved June 7, 2008, from http://www.americangeriatrics.org/products/positionpapers/gerrehab.html

American Hospital Association. (2006). *Chartbook 2006: Trends affecting hospitals and health systems, April 2006.* Retrieved May 25, 2008, from http://www.aha.org/aha/research-and-trends/chartbook/2006chartbook.html

American Medical Association. (2001). *Guidelines for Physician/Physician Assistant Practice.* Chicago: Policy Compendium.

Anderson, D. M., & Hampton, M. B. (1999). Physician assistants and nurse practitioners: Rural-urban settings and reimbursement for services. *Journal of Rural Health, 15*(2), 252–263.

Anderson, K. H., & Powers, L. (1970). The pediatric assistant. *North Carolina Medical Journal, 31,* 1–8.

Andrews, B. T. (1999). [Letter to the editor]. *Journal of Trauma, 47*(2), 438.

Angel, M. (2004). *The Truth About the Drug Companies.* New York: Random House.

Anonymous. (2000). Cultural perspectives: Treating patients from other cultures. *Perspective on Physician Assistant Education, 11*(2), 129–130.

Anonymous. (2002). Suit arising from physician assistant's services raises supervision questions. Rockefeller v. Kaiser Foundation Health Plan of Georgia. *Hospital Law Newsletter, 19*(6), 1–3.

Anonymous. (2004). Nonphysician providers play larger role in dermatology practice. *Dermatology Nursing, 16*(2), 191–192.

Anonymous. (2006, October 11). Verispan reports: Nurse practitioner and physician assistant retail prescriptions increasing substantially. *Business Wire.* Retrieved September 4, 2008, from http://findarticles.com/p/articles/mi_m0EIN/is_2006_Oct_11/ai_n27041539

Anthony, M. (2000). It's all in the name: The case for associate physicians. *ADVANCE for Physician Assistants, 8*(6), 16.

Arbett, S., Lathrop, J., & Hooker, R. S. (2009). Using practice analysis to improve the certifying examinations for PAs. *Journal of the American Academy of Physician Assistants, 22*(2), 31–36.

Arnopolin, S. L., & Smithline, H. A. (2000). Patient care by physician assistants and by physicians in an emergency department. *Journal of the American Academy of Physician Assistants, 13*(12), 39–40, 49–50, 53–54, 81.

Ashton, C. W., Aiken, A., & Duffie, D. (2007). Physician Assistants—A solution to wait times in Canada? *Healthcare Management Forum/Forum Gestion Des Soins De Santé, 20*(2), 38–42.

Asprey, D. (2006). Clinical skills utilized by physician assistants in rural primary care settings. *Journal of Physician Assistant Education, 17*(2), 45–47.

Asprey, D. (2008). Postgraduate residency programs. In R. M. Ballweg, E. M. Sullivan, D. Brown, & D. Vetrosky (Eds.), *Physician Assistant: A Guide to Clinical Practice.* Philadelphia: Elsevier.

Asprey, D., Dehn, R., & Kreiter, C. (2004a). The impact of program characteristics on the Physician Assistant National Certifying Examination scores and pass rates. *Perspectives on Physician Assistant Education, 15*(1), 33–37.

Asprey, D., Dehn, R., & Kreiter, C. (2004b). The impact of age and gender on the Physician Assistant National Certifying Examination scores and pass rates. *Perspective on Physician Assistant Education 15*(1), 38–41.

Asprey, D., Hegmann, T., & Bergus, B. (2007). Comparison of medical student and physician assistant student performance on standardized-patient assessments. *Journal of Physician Assistant Education, 18*(4), 16–19.

Asprey, D., & Helms, L. (1999). A description of physician assistant post-graduate residency training: The director's perspective. *Perspectives on Physician Assistant Education, 10*(3), 124–131.

Asprey, D., & Helms, L. (2000). A description of physician assistant post-graduate residency training: The resident's perspective. *Perspectives on Physician Assistant Education, 11*(2), 79–86.

Asprey, D., Zollo, S., & Kienzle, M. (2001). Implementation and evaluation of a telemedicine course for physician assistants. *Academic Medicine, 76*(6), 652–655.

Association of American Medical Colleges. (2008). *Industry funding of medical education: A report from the AAMC task force*. Washington, DC: Author.

Association of Family Practice Physician Assistants. (n.d.) *Mission statement*. Retrieved March 5, 2008, from http://www.afppa.org/mission_statement.html

Atwater, J. B. (1980). Must local health officers be physicians? *American Journal of Public Health, 70*, 11.

Austin, G., Foster, W., & Richards, J. C. (1968). Pediatric screening examinations in private practice. *Pediatrics, 41*, 115–119.

Australian Government of Health and Ageing. (2008). *Report on the audit of health workforce in rural and regional Australia, April 2008*. Commonwealth of Australia, Canberra.

Ayanian, J. Z., Landrum, M. B., Guadagnoli, E., & Gaccione P. (2002). Specialty of ambulatory care physicians and mortality among elderly patients after myocardial infarction. *New England Journal of Medicine, 347*, 1678–1686.

Baer, L. D., Geslera, W. M., & Konrad, T. R. (2000). The wineglass model: Tracking the locational histories of health professionals. *Social Science & Medicine, 50*(3), 317–329.

Baker, K. E. (2000). Will a physician assistant improve your dermatology practice? *Seminars in Cutaneous Medicine and Surgery, 19*(3), 201–203.

Baker, J. A., Oliver, D., Donahue, W., et al. (1989). Predicting role satisfaction among practicing physician assistants. *Journal of the American Academy of Physician Assistants, 2*, 461–470.

Baker, T. (2005). *The Medical Malpractice Myth*. Chicago: The University of Chicago Press.

Baldwin, K. A., Sisk, R. J., Watts, P., McCubbin, J., Brockschmidt, B., & Marion, L. N. (1998). Acceptance of nurse practitioners and physician assistants in meeting the perceived needs of rural communities. *Public Health Nurse, 15*(6), 389–397.

Ball, J. C., Corty, E., Petroski, S. P., Bond, H., Tommasello, A., & Graff, H. (1986). Medical services provided to 2,394 patients at methadone programs in three states. *Journal of Substance Abuse Treatment, 3*(3), 203–209.

Ballenger, M. D. (1971). The physician's assistant: Legal considerations. *Hospitals, 45*(11), 58–61.

Ballenger, M. D., & Estes, E. H., Jr. (1971). Licensure of responsible delegation? *New England Journal of Medicine, 284*(6), 330–332.

Ballweg, R. M. (2003). Federal funding of the physician assistant profession. *Perspective on Physician Assistant Education, 14*(1), 4–5.

Ballweg, R. M. (2008). *Physician Assistant: A Guide to Clinical Practice* (4th ed.). Philadelphia: Saunders/Elsevier Science.

Ballweg, R. M., Cawley, J., Crane, S. C., et al. (1998). *Physician assistant task force on the impact of managed care*. A joint report of the Pew Health Professions Commission and the Center for the Health Professions. San Francisco: University of California, San Francisco, Center for the Health Professions.

Ballweg, R. M., Hooker, R. S., & Cawley, J. F. (2006). *Dick Smith: Interviews of the Founder of the Medex Physician Assistant Movement*. Honolulu, HI: Unpublished.

Ballweg, R. M., Stolberg, S., Sullivan, E.M. (1999). *Physician Assistant: A Guide to Clinical Practice* (2nd ed.). Philadelphia: Saunders/Elsevier Science.

Ballweg, R. M., Stolberg, S., Sullivan, E.M. (2004). *Physician Assistant: A Guide to Clinical Practice* (3rd ed.). Philadelphia: Saunders/Elsevier Science.

Ballweg, R. M., & Wick, K. H. (1999). Decentralized didactic training for physician assistants: Academic performance across training sites. *Journal of Allied Health, 28*, 220–225.

Banja, J. (2005). *Medical Errors and Medical Narcissism*. Boston: Jones & Bartlett.

Barnes, D., & Hooker, R. S. (2001). Physician assistant entrepreneurs. *Physician Assistant, 25*(10), 36–41.

Beattie, D. S. (2000). Expanding the view of scholarship: Introduction. Guest Eds.: The Council of Academic Societies Task Force on Scholarship. *Academic Medicine, 75*, 871–876.

Begely, B. (1993). PA-C: PA-SEE or passe. *Journal of the American Academy of Physician Assistants, 4*(4), 297.

Benjamin, R., Bigby, J. A., Blessing, D., et al, for the Bureau of Health Professions. (1999). Into the future: Physician assistants look to the 21st century: A strategic plan for the physician assistant profession. *Perspective on Physician Assistant Education, 10*(2), 73–81.

Benzie, K., Miller, K., Cawley, J. F., & Heinrich, J. (2003). Interest in physician assistant/public health dual-degree programs. *Perspective on Physician Assistant Education, 14*(1), 40–41.

Berg, R. H. (1966). More than a nurse, less than a doctor. *Look, 30*(18), 58–61.

Bergeron, J., Neuman, K., & Kinsey, J. (1999). Do advanced practice nurses and physician assistants benefit small rural hospitals? *Journal of Rural Health, 15*(2), 219–232.

Bergeson, J., Cash, R., Boulger, J., & Bergeron, D. (1997). The attitudes of rural Minnesota family physicians toward nurse practitioners and physician assistants. *Journal of Rural Health, 13*(3), 196–205.

Bergman, A. B. (1971). Two views on the latest health manpower issue: Physician's assistants belong in the nursing profession. *American Journal of Nursing, 71*(5), 975.

Berlin, L. E., Harper, D., Werner, K. E., & Stennett, J. E. (2002). *Master's level nurse practitioner educational programs. Findings from the 2000–2001 collaborative curriculum survey*. Washington, DC: American Association of Critical Care Nurses and National Organization of Nurse Practitioner Faculties.

Bernzweig, J., Takayama, J. I., Phibbs, C., Lewis, C., & Pantell, R. H. (1997). Gender differences in physician-patient communication: Evidence from pediatric visits. *Archives of Pediatrics & Adolescent Medicine, 151*(6), 586–591.

Blake, R. L., Jr., & Guild, P. A. (1978). Mid-level practitioners in rural health care: A three-year experience in Appalachia. *Journal of Community Health, 4*(1), 15–22.

Blaser, L. (1993). The business of clinical practice. *Journal of the American Academy of Physician Assistants, 6,* 402–406.

Blendon, R. J. (1979). Can China's health care be transplanted without China's economic policies? *New England Journal of Medicine, 300,* 1453–1458.

Blessing, J. D., & Davis, N. L. (1988). Marketing and medicine. A basic guide for PAs. *Physician Assistant, 12*(7), 91–98.

Blessing, J. D., Askin, D. G., Cook, P. A., Diamond, M. A., Huntington, C. G., & Kaplan, M. E. (1998). Physician views on the PA profession. *Physician Assistant, 22*(6), 1100–1116.

Blessing, J. D., Hooker, R. S., Jones, P. E., & Rahr, R. R. (2001). An investigation of potential criteria for ranking physician assistant programs. *Perspective on Physician Assistant Education, 12*(3), 160–166.

Bliss, A. A., & Cohen, E. D. (1978). Issues confronting the new health professionals. *Journal of Allied Health, 7*(1), 64–71.

Blumenthal, D. (2004). New steam from an old cauldron—The physician supply debate. *New England Journal of Medicine, 350*(17), 1780–1787.

Blumenthal, D., & Hsiao, W. (2005). Privatization and its discontents—The evolving Chinese health care system. *New England Journal of Medicine, 353*(11), 1165–1170.

Bodenheimer, T. (2006). Primary care—will it survive? *New England Journal of Medicine, 355*(9), 861–864.

Borland, B. L., Williams, F. E., & Taylor, D. (1972). A survey of attitudes of physicians on proper use of physician's assistants. *Health Services Reports, 87*(5), 467–472.

Bottom, W. D. (1988). Geriatric medicine in the United States: New roles for physician assistants. *Journal of Community Health, 13*(2), 95–103.

Bottom, W. D., & Evans, H. A. (1994). Who should be called "physician assistants?" *Journal of the American Academy of Physician Assistants, 7,* 19A–20A.

Bowman, R. C. (2007). New models or remodeling students or both? *Rural Remote Health, 7*(1), 722.

Boyer, E. L. (1990). *Scholarship Reconsidered: Priorities of the Professoriate.* Lawrenceville, NJ: Princeton University Press.

Brenneman, A., Hemminger, C., & Dehn, R. (2007). Surgical graduates' perspectives on postgraduate physician assistant training programs. *Journal of Physician Assistant Education, 18*(1), 42–44.

Breslau, N., & Novack, A. H. (1979). Public attitudes toward some changes in the division of labor in medicine. *Medical Care, 17*(8), 859–867.

Breusch, J. (2008). Gatekeepers outdated. *Australian Financial Review, 88*(264), 1.

Brock, R. (1998). The malpractice experience: How PAs fare. *Journal of the American Academy of Physician Assistants, 11*(6), 93–94.

Brooks, P. M., Robinson, L., & Ellis, N. (2008). Options for expanding the health workforce. *Australian Health Review, 32*(1), 156–160.

Brotherton, P. (2000). Administrator, consultant credit PA background for success. *AAPA News 21,* 7.

Broughton, B. (1996). A delineative study of physician assistants in orthopaedic surgery: Tasks, professional relationships, and satisfaction [PhD dissertation]. Columbia Pacific University, California.

Brown-Benedict, D. J. (2008). The doctor of nursing practice degree: Lessons from the history of the professional doctorate in other health disciplines. *Journal of Nursing Education, 47*(10), 448–457.

Brugna, R., Cawley, J. F., & Baker, M. D. (2007). Physician assistants in geriatric medicine. *Clinical Geriatrics, 15,* 2–9.

Brutsche, R. L. (1975). Medicine and penology. Problems of health care delivery in penal institutions. *New York State Journal of Medicine, 75*(7), 1082–1084.

Brutsche, R. L. (1986). Utilization of PAs in federal correctional institutions. *Physician Assistant, 10*(9), 60–66.

Buchan, J., Ball, J., & O'May, F. (2006). *Physician assistants in the National Health Service (NHS) Scotland: Reviewing the issues.* Commissioned by the Scottish Executive Health Department to review the implementation of the physician assistant pilot program. (Unpublished). Edinburgh, Scotland: Queen Margaret University College.

Buchan, J., & Dal Poz, M. R. (2002). Skill mix in the health care workforce: Reviewing the evidence. *Bulletin of the World Health Organization, 80*(7), 575–580.

Buchan, J., O'May, F., & Ball, J. (2007). New role, new country: Introducing U.S. physician assistants to Scotland. *Human Resources for Health, 5,* 13.

Buchanan, J. L., Kane, R. L., & Garrard, J. (1989). *Results of the Massachusetts Nursing Home Connection.* Santa Monica, CA: RAND Corporation.

Bunn, W. B., III, Holloway, A. M., & Johnson, C. E. (2004). Occupational medicine: The use of physician assistants and the changing role of the occupational and environmental medicine provider. *Occupational Medicine, 54,* 3145–3146.

Buppert, C. (2004). *Nurse Practitioner's Business Practice and Legal Guide.* (2nd ed.). Sudbury, MA: Jones & Bartlett.

Bureau of Health Manpower Education. (1971). *Selected training programs for physician support personnel.* Washington, DC: National Institutes of Health, Department of Health, Education and Welfare.

Burgess, S. E., Pruitt, R. H., Maybee, P., Metz, A. E., Jr., & Leuner, J. (2003). Rural and urban physicians' perceptions regarding the role and practice of the nurse practitioner, physician assistant, and certified nurse midwife. *Journal of Rural Health, 19*(Suppl), 321–328.

Burnett, W. H. (1980). Building the primary health care team: The state of California approach. *Family & Community Health, 3*(2), 49–61.

Burt, C. W., McCaig, L. F., & Rechtsteiner, E. A. (2007). Ambulatory medical care utilization estimates for 2005. *Advance Data, 29*(388), 1–15.

Bush, T., Cherkin, D., & Barlow, W. (1993). The impact of physician attitudes on patient satisfaction with care for low back pain. *Archives of Family Medicine, 2*(3), 301–305.

Byrnes, J. F., Jr. (1991). The evolution of surgical PAs . . . physician assistants. *Journal of the American Academy of Physician Assistants, 4*(6), 449–451.

Calabrese, W. J., Crane, S. C., & Legler, C. F. (1997). Issues in quality care. The two-sided coin of PA credentialing. *Journal of the American Academy of Physician Assistants,10*(5), 121–122.

Calhoun, B. C., Vrbin, C. M., & Grzybicki, D. M. (2008). The use of standardized patients in the training and evaluation of physician assistant students. *Journal of Physician Assistant Education, 19*(1), 18–23.

Callahan, E. (2007). *Limits on resident duty hours promote collaboration between medical staff and physician extenders*. Medical Staff Briefing. Retrieved May 28, 2008, from http://www.healthleadersmedia.com/content/89842/topic/WS_HLM2_HOM/Limits-on-resident-duty-hours-promote-collaboration-between-medical-staff-and-physician-extenders.html

Camargo, C. A., Jr., Ginde, A. A., Singer, A. H., Espinola, J. A., Sullivan, A. F., Pearson, J. F., et al. (2008). Assessment of emergency physician workforce needs in the United States, 2005. *Academic Emergency Medicine, 5*(12), 1317–1320.

Cameron, I. (2005). Physician assistants can do majority of GPs' work. *Pulse, 65*(19), 8.

Camp, B. (1984). PA prescriptive privileges: An ongoing controversy. *Physician Assistant, 8*, 11, 14.

Campbell, J. C., & Soeken, K. L. (1999). Women's responses to battering: A test of the model. *Research in Nursing and Health, 22*, 49–58.

Canadian Institute for Health Information. (2005). *Rising number of nurse practitioners in Canada*. Retrieved August 22, 2008, from http://www.icis.ca/cihiweb/dispPage.jsp?cw_page=media_07sep2005_e

Caprio, T. V. (2006). Physician practice in the nursing home: Collaboration with nurse practitioners and physician assistants. *Annals of Long Term Care, 14*(3), 17–24.

Cardenas, A. P. (1993). Forensic pathology and the PA [Letter to the editor]. *Journal of the American Academy of Physician Assistants, 6*, 77.

Cargill, V. A., Conti, M., Neuhauser, D., & McClish, D. (1991). Improving the effectiveness of screening for colorectal cancer by involving nurse clinicians. *Medical Care, 29*(1), 1–5.

Carlson, R. (1975). *The End of Medicine*. New York: John Wiley and Sons.

Carter, R., Emelio, J., & Perry, H. (1984). Enrollment and demographic characteristics of physician's assistant students. *Journal of Medical Education, 59*, 316–322.

Carter, R. D. (2000). An office to study, preserve, and present the history of the physician assistant profession. *Perspective on Physician Assistant Education, 11*(3), 185–187.

Carter, R. D., & Fasser. C. E. (2003). The American registry of physicians' associates—Forerunner of the Association of Physician Assistant Programs. *Perspective on Physician Assistant Education, 14*(2), 114–115.

Carter, R., Emelio, J., & Perry, H. (1984). Enrollment and demographic characteristics of physician's assistant students. *Journal of Medical Education, 59*(4), 316–322.

Carter, R. D., & Strand, J. (2000). Physician assistants: A young profession celebrates the 35th anniversary of its birth in North Carolina. *North Carolina Medical Journal, 61*(5), 249–256.

Carter, R., Thompson, A., & Stanhope, B. (2008). *People v. Whitaker:* The trial and its aftermath in California. *Journal of Physician Assistant Education, 19*(2), 44–51.

Carzoli, R. P., Martinez-Cruz, M., Cuevas, L. L., Murphy, S., & Chiu, T. (1994). Comparison of neonatal nurse practitioners, physician assistants, and residents in the neonatal intensive care unit. *Archives of Pediatrics & Adolescent Medicine, 148*(12), 1271–1276.

Cassard, S. D., Weisman, C. S., Plichta, S. B., & Johnson, T. L. (1997). Physician gender and women's preventive services. *Journal Women's Health, 6*(2), 199–207.

Castledine, G. (1996). Do we need physician assistants in the UK? *British Journal of Nursing, 5*, 124.

Cawley, J. F. (1982). Foreign medical graduates and physician assistants [Letter]. *Journal of the American Medical Association, 247*(7), 977.

Cawley, J. F. (1988). Physician assistants as alternatives to foreign medical graduates [Letter]. *Health Affairs (Milwood), 7*(1), 152–156.

Cawley, J. F. (1992). Federal health policy and PAs. *Journal of the American Academy of Physician Assistants, 5*(9), 679–688.

Cawley, J. F. (1995). *Physician assistants in the health workforce, 1994: Final report of the Advisory Group on Physician Assistants and the Workforce submitted to Council on Graduate Medical Education (COGME)*. Rockville, MD: Health Resources and Services Administration, Council on Graduate Medical Education.

Cawley, J. F. (2000). *The Obsolete Physician?* Clifton, NJ: Clinicians Publishing Group.

Cawley, J. F. (2003). Physician assistant education and PANCE performance: A passing controversy? *Perspective on Physician Assistant Education, 13*, 79–80.

Cawley, J. F. (2007a). Physician assistant education: An abbreviated history. *Journal of Physician Assistant Education, 18*(3), 6–15.

Cawley, J. F. (2007b). No longer invisible: Challenges to physician assistant education. *Journal of Physician Assistant Education, 18*(4), 7–8.

Cawley, J. F. (2008a). Physician assistants and title VII support. *Academic Medicine, 83,* 1049–1056.

Cawley, J. F. (2008b). Doctoral degrees for physician assistants. *Journal of the American Academy of Physician Assistants, 21,* 13.

Cawley, J. F., Andrews, M. D., Barnhill, G. C., Webb, L., & Hill, K. (2001). What makes the day: An analysis of the content of physician assistant's practice. *Journal of the American Academy of Physician Assistants, 14*(5), 41–42, 44, 47–50, 55–56.

Cawley, J. F., & Golden, A. S. (1983). Nonphysicians in the United States: Manpower policy in primary care. *Journal of Public Health Policy, 4*(1), 69–82.

Cawley, J. F., & Hooker, R. S. (2003). Physician assistants: Does the U.S. experience have anything to offer other countries? *Journal of Health Services Research & Policy, 8*(2), 65–67.

Cawley, J. F., & Hooker, R. S. (2006). The effect of resident work hour restrictions on physician assistant hospital utilization. *Journal of Physician Assistant Education, 17*(3), 41–43.

Cawley, J. F., & Jones, P. E. (1997). The possibility of an impending health professions glut. *Journal of the American Academy of Physician Assistants, 10,* 80–92.

Cawley, J. F., & Perry, H. B., III. (1988). Who is that house officer? The shifting roles of personnel in graduate medical education. *Journal of the American Academy of Physician Assistants, 1*(4), 255–257.

Cawley, J. F., Rohrs, R., & Hooker, R. S. (1998). Physician assistants and malpractice risk: Findings from the National Practitioner Data Bank. *Federal Bulletin, 85*(4), 242–247.

Cawley, J. F., Simon, A., Blessing, J. D., Pedersen, D. M., & Link, M. S. (2000). Marketplace demand for physician assistants: Results of a national survey of 1998 graduates. *Perspective on Physician Assistant Education, 11*(1), 12–17.

Chaffee, D. (1988). Do PAs have a future in cardiothoracic surgery? *Physician Assistant, 12,* 107–108.

Chaikin, E. J., Thornby, J. I., & Merrill, J. (2000). Caring for terminally ill patients: A comparative analysis of physician assistant and medical students' attitude. *Perspective on Physician Assistant Education, 11*(2), 87–94.

Chavez, R. S. (2008). Correctional medicine. In R. Ballweg, E. M. Sullivan, D. Brown, & D. Vetrosky (Eds.), *Physician Assistant: A Guide to Clinical Practice* (4th ed., pp. 828–850). Philadelphia: Saunders/Elsevier.

Cherry, D. K., Woodwell, D. A., & Rechtsteiner, E. A. (2007). National Ambulatory Medical Care Survey (NHAMCS): 2005 summary. *Advance Data from Vital and Health Statistics, 387.* Hyattsville, MD: Centers for Disease Control and Prevention, National Center for Health Statistics.

Cherry, D. K., Hing, E., Woodwell, D. A., & Rechtsteiner, E. A. (2008). National Ambulatory Medical Care Survey (NHAMCS): 2006 summary. *National Health Statistics Report, 3.* Hyattsville, MD: Centers for Disease Control and Prevention, National Center for Health Statistics.

Chidley, E. (1997). PA profiles: A New York PA directs a clinic in Kenya. *PA Today, 5,* 10–13.

Chitwood, J. L. (2008). Military medicine. In R. Ballweg, E. M. Sullivan, D. Brown, & D. Vetrosky (Eds.), *Physician Assistant: A Guide to Clinical Practice* (4th ed., pp. 851–860). Philadelphia: Saunders/Elsevier.

Christian, C., Dower, C., & O'Neil, E. (2007). *Overview of Nurse Practitioner Scopes of Practice in the United States.* San Francisco: University of California San Francisco Center for the Health Professions.

Christman, L. (1979). The relationship of the physician's assistant to nursing. *Journal of Advanced Nursing, 4*(2), 215–218.

Christman, L. (1998). Advanced practice nursing: Is the physician's assistant an accident of history or a failure to act? *Nursing Outlook, 46*(2), 56–59.

Christmas, A. B., Reynolds, J., Hodges, S., Franklin, G. A., Miller, F. B., Richardson, J. D., & Rodriguez, J. L. Physician extenders impact trauma systems. *Journal of Trauma, 58*(5), 917–920.

Clark, A. R., Monroe, J. R., Feldman, S. R., Fleischer, A. B., Hauser, D. A., & Hinds, M. A. (2000). The emerging role of physician assistants in the delivery of dermatological health care. *Dermatologic Clinics, 18*(2), 297–302.

Council on Graduate Medical Education. (1994). *Physician Assistants in the Health Workforce 1994: Final report of the Advisory Group on Physician Assistants and the Workforce Subcommittee to the Council on Graduate Medical Education.* Rockville, MD: Health Resources and Services Administration, Division of Medicine. Special Projects and Data Analysis Branch.

Cohen, H. (1996). *Physician Assistant Pursuit of Prescriptive Authority: A Five State Analysis.* Master's thesis, the Johns Hopkins School of Public Health, Baltimore, MD.

Cohen, S. (2000). Treating patients from other cultures. *Perspective on Physician Assistant Education, 11*(2), 129–130.

Colver, J. E., Blessing, D., & Hinojosa, J. (2007). Military physician assistants; their background and education. *Journal of Physician Assistant Education, 18*(3), 40–45.

Colwill, J. M., Cultice, J. M., & Kruse, R. L. (2008). Will generalist physician supply meet demands of an increasing and aging population? *Health Affairs, 27*(3), 232–241.

The Competence and Curriculum Framework Steering Group on behalf of the Medical Care Practitioner National Programme Board. (2006). *The Competence and Curriculum Framework for the Medical Care Practitioner Consultation Document.* Surrey, England: Department of Health.

Conant, L., Jr., Robertson, L. S., Kosa, J., & Alpert, J. J. (1971). Anticipated patient acceptance of new nursing roles and physicians' assistants. *American Journal of Diseases and Children, 122*(3), 202–205.

Condit, D. (1977). PAs: Russian style. *Health Practitioner Physician Assistant, 1*(1), 37–40.

Condit, D. (1992). A quarter century of surgical physician assistants. *Physician Assistant, 15*(4), 3–13.

Condit, D. (1993). Our military heritage . . . The physician assistant profession. *Physician Assistant, 17*(11), 58–62.

Condit, D. (2000). Credentialing. *Surgical Physician Assistant, 6*(8), 7–8.

Coniglio, D., Menezes, P., Moorman, P., Morgan, P., & Schmidt, M. (2007). Evaluation of student confidence in utilizing EBM skills following completion of an EBM curriculum. *Journal of Physician Assistant Education, 18*(2), 7–13.

Cooke, M., Irby, D. M., Sullivan, W., & Ludmerer, K. (2006). American medical education 100 years after the Flexner report. *New England Journal of Medicine, 355*(13), 1339–1344.

Cooper, R. A. (2007). New directions for nurse practitioners and physician assistants in an era of physician shortages. *Academic Medicine, 82*(9), 827–828.

Cooper, R. A., Henderson, T., & Dietrich, C. L. (1998). Roles of nonphysician clinicians as autonomous providers of patient care. *Journal of the American Medical Association, 280*(9), 795–802.

Cooper,R. A., Laud, P., & Dietrich, C. L. (1998). Current and projected workforce of nonphysician clinicians. *Journal of the American Medical Association, 280*(9), 788–794.

Cooper, J. K., & Willig, S. H. (1971). Nonphysicians for coronary care delivery: Are they legal? *The American Journal of Cardiology, 28*(2), 363–365.

Cornell, S. (1998). You say assistant, I say associate, we can't call the whole thing off. *ADVANCE for Physician Assistants, 6*(4), 12.

Cornell, S. (2000a). Care and convictions: PA practice in corrections medicine. *ADVANCE for Physician Assistants, 8*, 60–61.

Cornell, S. (2000b). A dinosaur on the ticket: PA Rick Hillegas bids for state senate seat. *ADVANCE for Physician Assistants, 8*(8), 58–59.

Cornell, S. (2007). PA specialties: Society for physician assistants in pediatrics. *ADVANCE for Physician Assistants, 15*(10), 18.

Corso, T. (2001). A literature and medicine course in the physician assistant studies curriculum. *Perspective on Physician Assistant Education, 12*(1), 17–23.

Coryell, W., Cloninger, C. R., & Reich, T. (1978). Clinical assessment: Use of nonphysician interviewers. *Journal of Nervous & Mental Disease, 166*(8), 599–606.

Coulter, I., Jacobson, P., & Parker, L. E. (2000). Sharing the mantle of primary female care: Physicians, nurse practitioners, and physician assistants. *Journal of the American Medical Womens Association, 55*(2), 100–103.

Counselman, F. L., Graffeo, C. A., & Hill, J. T. (2000). Patient satisfaction with physician assistants (PAs)

in an ED fast track. *American Journal of Emergency Medicine, 18*(6), 661–665.

Coye, R. D., & Hansen, M. F. (1969). The "doctor's assistant:" A survey of physicians' expectations. *Journal of the American Medical Association, 209*, 529–533.

Crandall, L. A., Haas, W. H., & Radelet, M. L. (1986). Socioeconomic influences in patient assignment to PA or MD providers. *Physician Assistant, 10*, 164, 167–168, 170.

Crandall, L. A., Santulli, W. P., Radelet, M. L., Kilpatrick, K. E., & Lewis, D. E. (1984). Physician assistants in primary care. Patient assignment and task delegation. *Medical Care, 22*(3), 268–282.

Crane, S. C. (1995). PAs/NPs: Forging effective partnerships in managed-care systems. *Physician Executive, 21*(10), 23–27.

Crane, S. C. (2006). Perspectives on the physician assistant specialty credentialing debate: "Mountains beyond mountains." *Journal of the American Academy of Physician Assistants, 19*(8), 16.

Crane, S. C., & Carpenter, D. (2006). Perspectives on the physician assistant specialty credentialing debate. Mountains beyond mountains. *Journal of the American Academy of Physician Assistants, 19*(8), 16.

Crile, G., Jr. (1987). Cleveland Clinic: The supporting cast 1920–1940. *Cleveland Clinic Journal of Medicine, 54*(4), 344–347.

Curran, J. (2007). Nurse practitioners and physician assistants: Do you know the difference? *Medsurg Nursing, 15*(6), 404–407.

Curran, W. J. (1972). Legal responsibility for actions of physicians' assistants. *New England Journal of Medicine, 286*(5), 254.

Currey, R. (1992). *Medicine for Sale: Commercialism vs. Professionalism.* Knoxville, TN: Grand Rounds Press.

Curry, R. H., Fasser, C. E., & Schafft, G. (1987). Physician assistant training and practice in geriatric medicine. *Gerontology & Geriatrics Education, 7*(3/4), 55–66.

Cyr, K. A. (1985). Physician-PA practice in a military clinic: A statistical comparison of productivity/availability. *Physician Assistant, 9*(4), 112–114.

Dacey, M. J., Mirza, E. R., Wilcox V., Doherty, M., Mello, J., Boyer, A., et al. (2007). The effect of a rapid response team on major clinical outcome measures in a community hospital. *Critical Care Medicine, 35*(9), 2076–2082.

Dal Poz, M. R., Kinfu Y., Drager, S., Kunjumen T., & Diallo K. (2006). *Counting health workers: Definitions, data, methods and global results.* Geneva, Switzerland: World Health Organization.

Davis, A. (2002). State regulations of the physician assistant profession. *Journal of the American Academy of Physician Assistants, 15*(10), 27–32.

Dawley, K. (2003). Origins of nurse-midwifery in the United States and its expansion in the 1940s. *Journal of Midwifery & Women's Health, 48*(2), 86–95.

Dawley, K. (2005). Doubling back over roads once traveled: Creating a national organization for nurse-midwifery. *Journal of Midwifery & Women's Health, 50*(2), 71–82.

Dawley, K., & Burst, H. V. (2005). The American College of Nurse-Midwives and its antecedents: A historic time line. *Journal of Midwifery & Women's Health, 50*(1), 16–22.

Deal, C. L., Hooker, R. S., Harrington, T., Birnbaum, N., Hogan, P., Bouchery, E., et al. (2007). The United States rheumatology workforce: Supply and demand, 2005–2025. *Arthritis and Rheumatism, 56*(3), 722–729.

DeBarth, K. (1996). Outer banks PA: Medicine at the edge. *Clinician Reviews, 6,* 148–158.

D'Ercole, A., Skodol, A. E., Struening, E., Curtis, J., & Millman, J. (1991). Diagnosis of physical illness in psychiatric patients using axis III and a standardized medical history. *Hospital Community Psychiatry, 42,* 395–400.

Dehn, R. W. (2002). Does experience count? *The Clinical Advisor, 5*(1), 98.

Dehn, R. (2007). 2006 national survey of PA program admission prerequisites. *Journal of Physician Assistant Education, 18*(1), 45–47.

Dehn, R., & Hooker, R. S. (1999). Procedures performed by Iowa family practice physician assistants. *Journal of the American Academy of Physician Assistants, 12*(4), 63–77.

DeMaria, W. J., Cherry, W. A., & Treusdell, D. H. (1971). Evaluation of the marine physician assistant program. *HSMHA. Health Reports, 86*(3), 195–201.

Demory-Luce, D. K., & McPherson, R. S. (1999). Current clinical nutrition issues. Nutrition knowledge and attitudes of physician assistants. *Topics in Clinical Nutrition, 14*(2), 71–82.

DeMots, H., Coombs, B., Murphy, E., & Palac, R. (1987). Coronary arteriography performed by a physician assistant. *American Journal of Cardiology, 60*(10), 784–787.

DeNicola, L., Kleid, D., Brink, L., van Stralen, D., Scott, M., Gerbert, D., & Brennan, L. (1994). Use of pediatric physician extenders in pediatric and neonatal intensive care units. *Critical Care Medicine, 22*(11), 1856–1864.

Department of Health, Education, and Welfare. (1977). *An evaluation of physician assistants in diagnostic radiology.* Rockville, MD: U.S. Public Health Service, Health Resources Administration, National Center for Health Services, Research Digest Series.

Detmer, L.M. (1973). The American Medical Association Council on Medical Education Accreditation Program for the Education of Assistants to the Primary Care Physician. *Physician's Associate, 3,* 4–9.

DeVore, L., & Shapiro, S. (1978). The physician assistant: A new breed of dental educator. *Journal of Dental Education, 42,* 568–571.

Dhuper, S., & Choksi, S. (2009). Replacing an academic internal medicine residency program with a physician assistant-hospitalist model: A comparative analysis study. *American Journal of Medical Quality, 23*(2), 132–139.

Dial, T. H., Palsbo, S. E., Bergsten, C., Gabel, J. R., & Weinder, J. (1995). Clinical staffing in staff- and group-model HMOs. *Health Affairs (Millwood), 14*(2), 168–180.

Diekema, D. J., Ferguson, K. J., & Doebbeling, B. N. (1995). Motivation for hepatitis B vaccine acceptance among medical and physician assistant students. *Journal of General Internal Medicine, 10*(1), 1–6.

Dieter, P. M., & Fasser, C. E. (1989). Physician assistants in geriatrics: Meeting the demand. *Journal of the American Academy of Physician Assistants, 2*(1), 49–51.

DiMatteo, M. R. (2004). Evidence-based strategies to foster adherence and improve patient outcomes. *Journal of the American Academy of Physician Assistants, 17*(11), 18–21.

Donaldson, M. S., et al. (1996a). *Primary Care: America's Health in a New Era.* Washington, DC: National Academy Press.

Donaldson, M. S., et al. (1996b). Defining primary care. In *Primary Care: America's Health in a New Era.* Washington, DC: National Academy Press.

Doescher, M. P., Ellsbury, K. E., & Hart, L. G. (2000). The distribution of rural female generalist physicians in the United States. *Journal of Rural Health, 16*(2), 111–118.

Dowling, B., & Glendinning, C. (2003). *The New Primary Care.* Berkshire, United Kingdom: Open University Press.

Dracup, K., DeBusk, R. F., De Mots, H., Gaile, E. H., Sr., Norton, J. B., Jr., & Rudy, E. B. (1994). Task force 3: Partnerships in delivery of cardiovascular care. *Journal of the American College of Cardiology, 24*(2), 296–304.

Drozda, P. F. (1992). Physician extenders increase healthcare access. *Health Progress, 73*(4), 46–48, 74.

Dubaybo, B. A., Samson, M. K., & Carlson, R. W. (1991). The role of physician-assistants in critical care units. *Chest, 99*(1), 89–91.

Duffy, K. (2003). PAs filling the gap in patient care in academic hospitals. *Perspective on Physician Assistant Education, 14,* 158–162.

Dungy, C. I. (1974). The child health associate in a rural setting. *Journal of the National Medical Association, 66*(1), 32–34.

Dungy, C. I. (1975). The child health associate. The new image in the nursery. *American Journal of Public Health, 65*(11), 1179–1183.

Dungy, C. I., & Sander, D. L. (1977). Evaluation of a child health associate program. *Journal of Medical Education, 52*(5), 413–415.

Dungy, C. I., & Silver, H. K. (1977). Pediatricians' perceptions: Competence of child health associates. *Rocky Mountain Medical Journal, 74*(1), 25–27.

Duryea, W. R., & Hooker, R. S. (2000). Elder physician assistants and their practices. *Journal of the American Academy of Physician Assistants, 13*(4), 67–68, 71–72, 74, 80, 82, 85.

Duttera, M. J., & Harlan, W. R. (1978). Evaluation of physician assistants in rural primary care. *Archives of Internal Medicine, 138,* 224–228.

Dychtwald, K., & Zitter, M. (1988). Changes during the next decade will alter the way elder-care is provided, financed. *Modern Healthcare, 18*(16), 38.

Earle-Richardson, G. B., & Earle-Richardson, A. F. (1998). Commentary from the front lines: Improving the National Health Service Corps' use of nonphysician medical providers. *Journal of Rural Health, 14*(2), 91–97.

Edwards, J. B., Wilson, J. L., Behringer, B. A., Smith, P. L., Ferguson, K. P., Blackwelder, R. B., et al. (2006). Practice locations of graduates of family physician residency and nurse practitioner programs: Considerations within the context of institutional culture and curricular innovation through Titles VII and VIII. *Journal of Rural Health, 22*(1), 69–77.

Ehrenberg, R. G., Goldhaber, D. D., & Brewer, D. J. (1995). Do teachers' race, gender, and ethnicity matter? Evidence from the National Educational Longitudinal Study of 1988. *Industrial and Labor Relations Review, 48*(3), 547–561.

Ekwo, E., Daniels, M., Oliver, D., & Fethke, C. (1979). The physician assistant in rural primary care practices: Physician assistant activities and physician supervision at satellite and non-satellite practice sites. *Medical Care, 17*, 787–795.

Elizondo, E., & Blessing, J. D. (1990). The ability of PAs to solve patients' psychosocial problems. A preliminary report on patient expectations. *Physician Assistant, 14*(2), 75–82.

Elliott, C. H. (1984a). The physician assistant—Newest member of the corporate health care team: A guide to hiring a PA and cutting health care costs. *The Personnel Administrator, 29*(12), 87–92.

Elliott, C. H. (1984b). The physician assistant in occupational medicine. *PA Drug Update, 4*(9), 42–48.

Ellis, B. I. (1991). Physician's assistants in radiology: Has the time come? [Letter]. *Radiology, 180*(3), 880–881.

Ellis, G. L., & Brandt, T. E. (1997). Use of physician extenders and fast tracks in United States emergency departments. *American Journal of Emergency Medicine, 15*(3), 229–232.

Emelio, J. (1994). Barriers to physician assistant practice. In *Health Personnel in the United States*. Washington, DC: U.S. Department of Health and Human Services, Health Resources and Services Administration.

Enns, S. M., Muma, R. D., & Lary, M. J. (2000). Examining referral practices of primary care physician assistants. *Journal of the American Academy of Physician Assistants, 13*(5), 81, 84, 86, 118.

Erikson, C., Salsberg, E., Forte, G., Bruinooge, S., & Goldstein, M. (2007). Challenges to assuring access to oncology services. *Journal of Oncology Practice, 3*(2), 87–88.

Erkert, J. D. (1985). Nurses' attitudes toward PAs. *Physician Assistant, 9*(12), 41–44.

Estes, E. H., Jr. (1968a). The critical shortage—Physicians and supporting personnel. *Annals of Internal Medicine, 69*, 957–962.

Estes, E. H., Jr. (1968b). The Duke physician assistant program: A progress report. *Archives of Environmental Health, 17*(5), 690–691.

Estes, E. H., Jr. (1993). Training doctors for the future: Lessons from 25 years of physician assistant education. In D. K. Clawson & M. Osterweis (Eds.), *The Roles of Physician Assistants and Nurse Practitioners in Primary Care*. Washington, DC: Association of Academic Health Centers.

Estes, E. H., Jr., & Howard, D. R. (1969). The physician's assistant in the university center. *Annals of the New York Academy of Sciences, 166*, 903–910.

Estes, E. H., Jr., & Howard, D. R. (1970). Potential for newer classes of personnel: Experiences of the Duke physician's assistant program. *Journal of Medical Education, 45*, 149–155.

Ewing, G. B., Selassie, A. W., Lopez, C. H., & McCutcheon, E. P. (1999). Self-report of delivery of clinical preventive services by U.S. physicians: Comparing specialty, gender, age, setting of practice, and area of practice. *American Journal of Preventive Medicine, 17*, 62–72.

Expert Committee on Professional and Technical Education of Medical and Auxiliary Personnel (WHO). (1968). *Training of medical assistants and similar personnel*. Geneva: World Health Organization, Technician Report Service.

Fang, D., Wilsey-Wisniewski, S., & Bednash, G. D. (2006). *2005–2006 Enrollment and Graduations in Baccalaureate and Graduate Programs in Nursing. Annual Report*. Washington, DC: American Association of Colleges of Nursing.

Farmer, J., Currie, M., West, C., Hyman, J., & Arnott, N. (2009). Evaluation of Physician Assistants to NHS Scotland: Final Report. Centre for Rural Health UHI Millennium Institute The Centre for Health Science Perth Road, Inverness, Scotland IV2 3JH.

Fasser, C. E., Andrus, P., & Smith, Q. (1984). Certification, registration and licensure of physician assistants. In R. D. Carter & H. B. Perry, III (Eds.), *Alternatives in Health Care Delivery*. St. Louis, MO: Warren H. Green.

Fawcett, J. (2004). *Contemporary Nursing Knowledge: Analysis and Evaluation of Nursing Models and Theories* (2nd ed.). Philadelphia: F.A. Davis.

Feldstein, P. J. (2004). *Health Care Economics* (6th ed.). Albany, NY: Thomson Delmar Learning; Delmar Series in Health Services Administration.

Fenn, P. A. (1987). Acceptance of physician assistants in western North Carolina. *Physician Assistant, 11*(5), 161–162.

Fenn, W. H. (2002). Physician assistants. American idea of physician assistants can be Anglicized. *British Medical Journal (Clinical Research Ed.), 324*(7339), 735.

Fenn, W. H. (2003). The English patient. *Journal of the American Academy of Physician Assistants, 16*(2), 43–47.

Fincham, J. E. (1985). Prescriptive authority: The physician assistants' views. *Journal of the Medical Association of Georgia, 74*(2), 81–83.

Fincham, J. E. (1986). How pharmacists are rated as a source of drug information by physician assistants. *Drug Intelligence & Clinical Pharmacy, 20*(5), 379–383.

Fine, L. L. (1977a). The pediatric practice of the child health associate. *American Journal of Diseases of Children (1960)*, 131(6), 634–637.

Fine, L. L. (1977b). Pediatrician receives more than a helping hand from child health associate. *Commitment*, 3(1), 14–18.

Fine, L. L., & Machotka, P. (1973). Role identity development of the child health associate. *Journal of Medical Education*, 48(7), 670–675.

Fine, L. L., & Scriven, S. S. (1977). The child health associate: A nonphysician primary care practitioner for children. *PA Journal*, 7(3), 137–142.

Fine, L. L., & Silver, H. K. (1973). Comparative diagnostic abilities of child health associate interns and practicing pediatricians. *Journal of Pediatrics*, 83(2), 332–335.

Fischer, J. (1995). PAs committed to practice with physician supervision [Letter]. *Texas Medicine*, 91(6), 7.

Fisher, D. W., & Horowitz, S. M. (1977). The physician's assistant: Profile of a new health profession. In A. A. Bliss & E. Cohen (Eds.), *The New Health Professionals: Nurse Practitioners and Physician's Assistants.* Germantown, MD: Aspen System Corporation.

Fishfader, V., Henning, B., & Knott, P. (2002). Physician assistant student and faculty perceptions of physician assistant residency training programs. *Perspective on Physician Assistant Education*, 13(1), 34–38.

Fleisher, W. P., Chan, M. K., & McConnell, K. (2006). Issues regarding the development of a physician assistant program in Manitoba. *Journal of Physician Assistant Education*, 17(1), 53–54.

Ford, L. C. (1979). Nurse practitioner education. In J. Hamburg (Ed.), *Review of Allied Health Education.* Lexington, KY: University Press of Kentucky.

Foreman, S. (1993). *Oral Testimony Before the Physician Payment Review Commission.* Washington, DC: Physician Payment Review Commission.

Fowkes, V., Cawley, J. F., Herlihy, N., & Cuadrado, R. R. (1996). Evaluating the potential of international medical graduates as physician assistants in primary care. *Academic Medicine*, 71(8), 886–892.

Fowkes, V. K., Hafferty, F. W., Goldberg, H. I., & Garcia, R. D. (1983). Educational decentralization and deployment of physician's assistants. *Journal of Medical Education*, 58, 194–200.

Fox, D. P., & Whittaker, R. G. (1983). PAs in the Veterans Administration: A report of a national survey. *Physician Assistant*, 7(2), 106.

Frampton, J., & Wall, S. (1994). Exploring the use of NPs and PAs in primary care. *HMO Practice/HMO Group*, 8(4), 165–170.

Frary, T. N., Fleming, D. K., Kemle, K., Segal-Gidan, F., & Simon, B. (2000). Health care for a legion of aging baby boomers. *Journal of the American Academy of Physician Assistants*, 13(4), 23–24, 27–28, 31.

Franks, P., Clancy, C. M., & Nutting, P. A. (1992). Gatekeeping revisited: Protecting patients from overtreatment. *New England Journal of Medicine*, 327(21), 424–429.

Freeborn, D. K., & Hooker, R. S. (1995). Satisfaction of physician assistants and other nonphysician providers in a managed care setting. *Public Health Reports (Washington, D.C. 1974)*, 110(6), 714–719.

Freeborn, D. K., Hooker, R. S., & Pope, C. R. (2002). Satisfaction and well-being of primary care providers in managed care. *Evaluation & The Health Professions*, 25(2), 239–254.

Freeborn, D. K., & Pope, C. R. (1994). *Promise and Performance in Managed Care: The Prepaid Group Practice Model.* Washington, DC: Johns Hopkins University Press.

Freeman, G. M., & Rose, C. P. (1981). Vicarious liability and the ophthalmologist. *Canadian Journal of Ophthalmology*, 16(4), 203–204.

Freidson, E. (2001). *Professionalism, the Third Logic: On the Practice of Knowledge.* Chicago: University of Chicago Press.

Frick, J. C. (1983). Physician assistants as house officers: Our experience. *Physician Assistant*, 7(11), 13.

Frick, J. C. (1986). The urban health care setting: The Harper-Grace hospital experience. In S. F. Zarbock & K. Harbert (Eds.), *Physician Assistants: Present and Future Models of Utilization.* New York: Praeger.

Friedman, E. (1978). Staff privileges for nonphysicians. Part 2: A sampling of hospital programs and privileges for nurse practitioners and physician's assistants. *The Hospital Medical Staff*, 7, 22–28.

Frossard, L. A., Liebich, G., Hooker, R. S., Brookes, P. M., & Robinson, L. (2008). Introducing physician assistants into new roles: International experiences. *Medical Journal of Australia*, 188(4), 199–201.

Fox, D. M. (1996). The political history of health workforce policy. In M. Osterweis, C. J. McLaughlin, H. R. Manasse, & C. Hopper, C. (Eds.) *The U.S. Health Workforce: Power, Politics, and Policy.* Washington, DC: Association Academic Health Centers.

Fuchs, V. R. (1998). *Who Shall Live?: Health, Economics, and Social Choice (Economic Ideas Leading to the 21st Century)* (3rd ed.). River Edge, NJ: World Scientific.

Fulop, T., & Roemer, M. I. (1982). International development of health manpower policy. *WHO Offset Publication*, 61, 1–168.

Gale, J. A., & Coburn A. F. (2003). *The Characteristics and Roles of Rural Health Clinics in the United States: A Chartbook.* Portland, ME: University of Southern Maine, Edmund S. Muskie School of Public Service.

Gamm, L. D., Hutchison, L. L., Dabney, B. J., & Dorsey A. M. (Eds.) (2003). *Rural Healthy People 2010: A Companion Document to Healthy People 2010.* Volume 1. College Station, TX: The Texas A&M University System Health Science Center, School of Rural Public Health, Southwest Rural Research Center. Retrieved June 22, 2008, from http://www.srph.tamhsc.edu/centers/rhp2010/Volume1.pdf

Ganley, O. H., Pendergrast, W. J., Wilkerson, M. W., & Mattingly, D. E. (2005). Outcome study of substance impaired physicians and physician assistants under contract with North Carolina Physicians Health Program for the period 1995–2000. *Journal of Addictive Diseases, 24*(1), 1–12.

Gara, N. (1989). State laws for physician assistants. *Journal of the American Academy of Physician Assistants, 2,* 303–313.

Gara, N. (1990). Regulation of physician assistant prescribing. *Journal of the American Academy of Physician Assistants, 3,* 71–78.

Gara, N. (1995). AMA adopts guidelines on PA practice. *AAPA News, 3,* 303–313.

Gara, N., & Davis, A. (2008). The political process. In R. Ballweg, E. Sullivan, D. Brown, & D. Vetrosky (Eds.), *Physician Assistant: A Guide to Clinical Practice* (4th ed., pp. 44–91). Philadelphia: Elsevier/Saunders.

Garrido, P. I. (1997). Training of medical assistants in Mozambique for surgery in a rural setting. *South African Journal of Surgery, 35*(3), 144–145.

Gaudry, C. L., Jr., & Nicholas, N. C. (1977). The USAF/USN physician assistant program. *Military Medicine, 142*(1), 29–31.

Gaufberg, S. (2007). *Emergency medicine in Russia.* Retrieved May 12, 2008, from http://www.emedicine.com/emerg/topic725.htm

Gazekpo, V. (2006). The state of the physician assistant profession in Ghana. *Journal of Physician Assistant Education, 17*(1), 55.

General Accounting Office. (1993). *Health care access: Innovative programs using nonphysicians.* GAO/HRD-93-128, General Accounting Office.

General Medical Council. (2006). *Good Medical Practices.* London: Author.

Genova, N. J. (1995). *The influence of market factors on physician assistant practice settings* [Master's thesis]. University of Southern Maine, Edmund S. Muskie Institute of Public Affairs.

Gentile, C. A. (1976). Development of an emergency medical physician's assistant program in North Carolina. *Emergency Medical Services, 5,* 36–37, 64.

Gerchufsky, M. (1996). Inside the gritty world of PAs in the New York City ME's office. *ADVANCE for Physician Assistants, 4*(9–10), 23–28.

Giardino A. P., Giardino E. R., & Burns K. M. (1994). Same place, different experience: Nurses and residents on pediatric emergency transport. *Holistic Nursing Practice, 8*(3), 54–63.

Gifford, J. F., Jr. (1987a). Prototype PA (Amos Johnson and Henry Treadwell). *North Carolina Medical Journal, 48*(11), 601–603.

Gifford, J. F., Jr. (1987b). The fate of America's prototype PA. *Physician Assistant, 11*(7) 95–96.

Gittins, P. (1996). Physician assistants in plastic and reconstructive surgery. *NEWS-Line for Physician Assistants, 5*(9), 4–7.

Glazer-Waldman, H. R. (1984). Perceptions of patient-provider relationships in allied health education textbooks. *Journal of Allied Health, 13*(2), 104–111.

Glenn, J. K., & Hofmeister, R. W. (1976). Will physicians rush out and get physician extenders? *Health Services Research, 11*(1), 69–74.

Glicken, A. D., & Lane, S. (2007). Results of the PAEA 2006 survey of PA program expansion plans. *Journal of Physician Assistant Education, 18*(1), 48–53.

Glicken, A. D., Merenstein, G., & Arthur, M. S. (2007). The child health associate physician assistant program—An enduring educational model addressing the needs of families and children. *Journal of Physician Assistant Education, 18*(3), 24–29.

Gofin, J., & Cawley, J. F. (2004). The physician assistant and community-oriented primary care. *Perspective on Physician Assistant Education, 2*(15), 126–128.

Goldberg, D. J. (2005). Laser physician legal responsibility for physician extender treatments. *Lasers in Surgery and Medicine, 37*(2), 105–107.

Goldberg, H. (1983). Role of the PA in a prepaid medical care group. *Physician Assistant, 7*(10), 127–128, 131, 135.

Golden, A. S., & Cawley, J. F. (1983). A national survey of performance objectives of physician's assistant training programs. *Journal of Medical Education, 58*(5), 418–424.

Golden, A. S., Hagan, J. L., & Carlson, D. (1981). *The Art of Teaching Primary Care.* New York: Springer Publishers.

Golden, R. M. (1986). Physician assistants in forensic pathology. *Physician Assistant, 10,* 101–102.

Goldfrank, L., Corso, T., & Squillacote, D. (1980). The emergency services physician assistant: Results of two years' experience. *Annals of Emergency Medicine, 9*(2), 96–99.

Goldgar, C. (2006). A new rating system applied to "tips for learning and reaching evidence-based medicine." *Journal of Physician Assistant Education, 17*(3), 48–50.

Goldman, M. B., Occhiuto, J. S., Peterson, L. E., Zapka, J. G., & Palmer, R. H. (2004). Physician assistants as providers of surgically induced abortion services. *American Journal of Public Health, 94*(8), 1352–1357.

Goldstein, E. T. (1996). Outcomes of anorectal disease in a health maintenance organization setting. The need for colorectal surgeons. *Diseases of the Colon and Rectum, 39*(11), 1193–1198.

Goldstein, N. (2005). Look what's next in telemedicine: The physician assistant and telemedicine. *Hawaii Medical Journal, 64*(5), 116.

Golladay, F. L., Miller, M., & Smith, K. R. (1973). Allied health manpower strategies: Estimates of the potential gains from efficient task delegation. *Medical Care, 11*(6), 457–469.

Goode, W. (1960). Encroachment, charlatanism and the emerging profession: Psychology, sociology, and medicine. *American Sociological Review, 25,* 902–914.

Goodman, D. C., & Fisher, S. F. (2008). Physician workforce crisis? Wrong diagnosis, wrong prescription. *New England Journal of Medicine, 358*(16), 1658–1661.

Gordon, C. R., Axelrad, A., Alexander, J. B., Dellinger, R. P., & Ross, S. E. (2006). Care of critically ill surgical patients using the 80-hour accreditation Council of Graduate Medical Education

Work-Week Guidelines: A survey of current strategies. *American Surgeon, 72(6)*, 497–499.

Gore, C. L. (2000). A physician's liability for mistakes of a physician assistant. *Journal of Legal Medicine, 21*, 125–142.

Gorman, P. N., Yao, P., & Seshadri, V. (2004). Finding the answers in primary care: Information seeking by rural and nonrural clinicians. *Medinfo, 11(2)*, 1133–1137.

Gould, S. H., & Gould, J. S. (1984). The microsurgical assistant. *Journal of Reconstructive Microsurgery, 1(2)*, 113–117.

Grabenkort, W. R., & Ramsay, J. G. (1991). Role of physician assistants in critical care units. *Chest, 99(1)*, 89–91.

Grant, J. K., & Sullivan, E. M. (2008). Obstetrics and gynecology. In R. M. Ballweg, E. M. Sullivan, & D. Vetrosky (Eds.), *Physician Assistant: A Guide to Clinical Practice* (4th ed., pp. 398–410). Philadelphia: Elsevier/Saunders.

Gray, D. (1997). What is the association of PAs in cardiovascular surgery? *Surgical Physician Assistant, 3(5)*, 38.

Gray, J., & Fryer, G. E. (1991). Physician assistants as members of social service child protection units. *Child Abuse & Neglect, 15(4)*, 415–421.

Gray, J., Lacey, C., Alexander, S., & Andresen, M. (1995). Colorado survey: Do PAs use the procedures and skills they learn? *Journal of the American Academy of Physician Assistants, 8*, 45–51.

Green, B. A., & Johnson, T. (1995). Replacing residents with midlevel practitioners: A New York City-area analysis. *Health Affairs (Milwood), 14(2)*, 192–198.

Green, H. (2000). Student forum. Physician assistant students' guide to paying for school. *Perspective on Physician Assistant Education, 11*, 131–133.

Green, L. A., Fryer, G. E., Jr., Yawn, B. P., Lanier, D., & Dovey, S. M. (2001). The ecology of medical care revisited. *New England Journal of Medicine, 344(26)*, 2021–2025.

Greenfield, S., Komaroff, A. L., Pass, T. M., Anderson, H., & Nessim, S. (1978). Efficiency and cost of primary care by nurses and physician assistants. *New England Journal of Medicine, 298(6)*, 305–309.

Greenlee, R. L., Levy, J. W., & Allen, A. J. (1977). Utilization of a physician assistant in a comprehensive community mental health center. *PA Journal, 7(3)*, 143–147.

Griffiths, S. E. (1986). Medicine behind bars: Medical professionals "practicing" in prisons. *Dissertation Abstracts Iinternational, 47(10A)*, 3875.

Grumbach, K., & Coffman, J. (1998). Physicians and nonphysician clinicians: Complements or competitors? *Journal of the American Medical Association, 280(9)*, 825–826.

Grumbach, K., Hart, L. G., Mertz, E., Coffman, J., & Palazzo, L. (2003). Who is caring for the underserved? A comparison of primary care physicians and nonphysician clinicians in California and Washington. *Annals of Family Medicine, 1(2)*, 97–104.

Grumbach, K., Selby, J. V., Damberg, C., Bindman, A. B., Quesenberry, C., Jr., Truman, A. et al. (1999). Resolving the gatekeeper conundrum: What patients value in primary care and referrals to specialists. *Journal of the American Medical Association, 282(3)*, 261–266.

Grumbach, K., Selby, J. V., Schmittdiel, J. A., & Quesenberry, C. P., Jr. (1999). Quality of primary care practice in a large HMO according to physician specialty. *Health Services Research, 34(2)*, 485–502.

Guerra, P. (2007). Achieving mastery through the competencies. *Journal of the American Academy of Physician Assistants, 20(12)*, 12.

Gunderson, C. H., & Kampen, D. (1988). Utilization of nurse clinicians and physician assistants by active members and fellows of the American Academy of Neurology. *Neurology, 38(1)*, 156–160.

Gunneson, T. J., Menon, K. V., Wiesner, R. H., Daniels, J. A., Hay, J. E., Charlton, M. R., et al. (2002). Ultrasound-assisted percutaneous liver biopsy performed by a physician assistant. *American Journal of Gastroenterology, 97(6)*, 1472–1475.

Grzybicki, D. M., & Vrbin C. M. (2003). Pathology resident attitudes and opinions about pathologists' assistants. *Archives of Pathology & Laboratory Medicine, 127(6)*, 666–672.

Grzybicki, D. M., Vrbin, C. M., Reilly, T. L., Zarbo, R. J., & Raab, S. S. (2004). Use of physician extenders in surgical pathology practice. *Archives of Pathology & Laboratory Medicine, 128(2)*, 165–172.

Gwinn, D. H., & Keller, J. E. (1999). Military medicine. In R. M. Ballweg, S. Stolberg, & E. Sullivan (Eds.), *Physician Assistant: A Guide to Clinical Practice* (2nd ed.). Philadelphia: W. B. Saunders.

Haddock, D. R. (1971). Letter: Medical auxiliaries. *Ghana Medical Journal, 10(1)*, 62–63.

Hafferty, F. W., & McKinley, J. B. (Eds). (1993). *The Changing Medical Profession*. New York: Oxford University Press.

Hagopian, A., Thompson, M. J., Kaltenbach, E., & Hart L. G. (2004). The role of international medical graduates in America's small rural critical access hospitals. *Journal of Rural Health, 20(1)*, 52–58.

Hammond, J. (2003). Education. In R. M. Ballweg, S. Stolberg, & E. M. Sullivan (Eds.), Physician Assistant: A Guide to Clinical Practice (3rd ed.). Philadelphia: Saunders/Elsevier Science.

Hankins, G. D., Shaw, S. B., Cruess, D. F., Lawrence, H. C., III, & Harris, C. D. (1996). Patient satisfaction with collaborative practice. *Obstetrics and Gynecology, 88(6)*, 1011–1015.

Hanna, K. M. (1993). Effect of nurse-client transaction on female adolescents' oral contraceptive adherence. *Image Journal of Nursing Scholarship, 25(4)*, 285–290.

Hansen, C. (1992). *Access to rural health care: Barriers to practice for nonphysician providers*. Rockville, MD: Bureau of Health Professions, Health Resources and Services Administration (HRSA-240-89-0037), Department of Health and Human Services.

Hansen, J. P., Stinson, J. A., & Herpok, F. J. (1980). Cost effectiveness of physician extenders as compared to family physicians in a university health clinic. *Journal of the American College Health Association, 28*(4), 211–214.

Harbert, K. (1978). PAs and the coke oven industry. *Newsletter of Maryland Academy of Physician Assistants, 5*(2), 6–8.

Harbert, K. (1993). *The role of physician assistants as health educators: A national study.* Unpublished doctoral dissertation. Pennsylvania State University.

Harbert, K., Shipman, R. A., & Conrad, W. (1994). The utilization of physician extenders. Mid-level providers in a large group practice within a tertiary health care setting. *Medical Group Management Journal/MGMA, 41*(6), 26, 28, 49–50 passim.

Harbert, K., van den Brink, G., Smith, R., & van Bergen, B. (2004). Best practice approach to the development of an international physician assistant program: The University of Arnhem-Nijmegen model. *Perspective on Physician Assistant Education, 15*(2), 106–115.

Harper, D., & Johnson J. (1998). The new generation of nurse practitioners: Is more enough? *Health Affairs, 17*(5), 158–164.

Harty-Golder, B. (1995). Physician extenders. *Journal of the Florida Medical Association, 82,* 417–420.

Haselkorn, A., Coyle, M., & Doarn, C. R. (2007). The future of remote health services: Summary of an expert panel discussion. *Telemedicine and e-Health, 13,* 341–347.

Hathaway, D., Jacob, S., Stegbauer, C., Thompson, C., & Graff, C. (2006). The practice doctorate: Perspectives of early adopters. *Journal of Nursing Education, 45*(12), 487–496.

Haug Associates, Inc., for the Board of Medical Examiners. (1973). *Attitudes Toward the Physician's Assistant Program Among the Public, Physicians, and Allied Health Professionals.* California: Board of Medical Examiners.

Hayden, R. J., Salley, M. A., Brasseur, J., Kircher, J. R., & Ross, R. R. (1995). Provider-assisted suicide: A survey of PA attitudes. Results of the 1994 Michigan survey conducted by the Michigan Academy of Physician Assistants Public Policy Committee. *Physician Assistant, 19*(6), 73–76, 78.

Hayward, K. S., Kochniuk, L., Powell, L., & Peterson, T. (2005). Changes in students' perceptions of interdisciplinary practice reaching the older adult through mobile service delivery. *Journal of Allied Health, 34*(4), 192–198.

Health Resources and Services Administration, Division of Medicine, Bureau of Health Professions. (1990). *Annual Report: Grants Program for Physician Assistants.* Rockville, MD: U.S. Government Printing Office.

Heinerich, J. (2000). International rotations: An informal survey of PA schools. *ADVANCE for Physician Assistants, 8,* 30.

Heinrich, J. J., Fichandler, B. C., Beinfield, M., Frazier, W., Krizek, T. J., & Baue, A. E. (1980). The physician's assistant as resident on surgical service. An example of creative problem solving in surgical manpower. *Archives of Surgery, 115*(3), 310–314.

Heller, R. (1978). Officiers de santé: The second-class doctors of nineteenth-century France. *Medical History, 22*(1), 25–43.

Heller, L. E., & Fasser, C. (1978). Physicians' assistants: The new prescribers. *American Pharmacy, 18*(13), 12–17.

Henning G. F., Graybill, M., & George, J. (2008). Reason for visit: Is migrant health care that different? *Journal of Rural Health, 24*(2), 219–220.

Henry, R. A. (1974). Evaluation of physician's assistants in Gilchrist County, Florida. *Public Health Reports, 89*(5), 428–432.

Henry, L. R., & Hooker, R. S. (2007). Retention of physician assistants in rural health clinics. *Journal of Rural Health, 23*(3), 207–214.

Henson, K. E. (1999). In Kosovo, making a difference. *Journal of the American Academy of Physician Assistants, 12*(12), 77–79.

Herrera, J., Gendron, B. P., & Rice, M. M. (1994). Military emergency medicine physician assistants. *Military Medicine, 159*(3), 241–242.

Herrick, T. (2000). PA union movement flourishes in NY. *Clinician News, 4,* 19–20.

Hillman, B. J., Fajardo, L. L., Hunter, T. B., Mockbee, B. C., Cook, E. R., Hagaman, M., Bjelland, J. C., Frey, C. S., & Harris, C. J. (1987). Mammogram interpretation by physician assistants. *American Journal of Roentgenology, 149*(5), 907–912.

Hing, E., Cherry, D. K., & Woodwell, D. A. (2006). National ambulatory medical care survey: 2004 summary. *Advance Data From Vital and Health Statistics, 374,* Hyattsville, MD: National Center for Health Statistics.

History of the navy corpsman. (December 2006). Retrieved March 2, 2008, from http://www.jeffreywiener.com/pamphlet.htm

Holmes, S. E., & Fasser, C. E. (1993). Occupational stress among physician assistants. *Journal of the American Academy of Physician Assistants, 6*(3), 172–178.

Holt, N. (1998). "Confusion's masterpiece:" The development of the physician assistant profession. *Bulletin of the History of Medicine, 72*(2), 246–278.

Hooker, R. S. (1986). Medical care utilization: MD-PA/NP comparisons in an HMO. In S. F. Zarbock & K. Harbert (Eds.), *Physician Assistants: Present and Future Models of Utilization.* New York: Praeger.

Hooker, R. S. (1987). Coast Guard physician assistants. *AAPA News, 8*(7), 4.

Hooker, R. S. (1989). A comparison of rank and pay structure for military physician assistants. *Journal of the American Academy of Physician Assistants, 2*(4), 293–300.

Hooker, R. S. (1991a). The military physician assistant. *Military Medicine, 156*(12), 657–660.

Hooker, R. S. (1991b). The Coast Guard medical service. *Navy Medicine, 82*(1), 18–21.

Hooker, R. S. (1992). Employment specialization in the PA profession. *Journal of the American Academy of Physician Assistants, 5*(8), 695–704.

Hooker, R. S. (1993). The roles of physician assistants and nurse practitioners in a managed care organization. In D. K. Clawson & M. Osterweis (Eds.), *The Roles of Physician Assistants and Nurse Practitioners in Primary Care.* Washington, DC: The Association of Academic Health Centers.

Hooker, R. S. (1994). PAs and NPs in HMOs [Editorial]. *HMO Practice, 8,* 148–150.

Hooker, R. S. (1995). Job satisfaction: Physician assistants versus nurse practitioners [Abstract]. *Journal of the American Academy of Physician Assistants, 8*(8), 15.

Hooker, R. S. (1997). Is there an undersupply of PAs? *Journal of the American Academy of Physician Assistants, 10*(9), 81, 94, 97–98, 101–102 passim.

Hooker, R. S. (1998). Educating PAs in an HMO: A 15-year experience. *Journal of the American Academy of Physician Assistants, 11*(11), 45–56.

Hooker, R. S. (1999). *Cost-benefit analysis of physician assistants* [Dissertation]. Portland State University.

Hooker, R. S. (2000). The economics of physician assistant employment. *Physician Assistant, 24*(4), 67–85.

Hooker, R. S. (2001). The economics basis of physician assistant practice. *Physician Assistant, 24*(4), 51–71.

Hooker, R. S. (2002). A cost analysis of physician assistants in primary care. *Journal of the American Academy of Physician Assistants, 15*(11), 39–42, 45, 48 passim.

Hooker, R. S. (2004). Physician assistants in occupational medicine: How do they compare to occupational physicians? *Occupational Medicine (Oxford, England), 54*(3), 153–158.

Hooker, R. S. (2006). Physician assistants and nurse practitioners: The United States experience. *The Medical Journal of Australia, 185*(1), 4–7.

Hooker, R. S. (2007). Understanding the roles of PAs and NPs in rheumatology. *Arthritis Practitioner, 3*(5), 42.

Hooker, R. S. (2008a). *The Use of Physician Assistants and Nurse Practitioners in Rheumatology. Principles of Non-Pharmacological Management of Musculoskeletal Conditions.* Sussex, UK: Rapid Medical Media, 2008.

Hooker, R. S. (2008b). Federally employed physician assistants. *Military Medicine, 173*(9), 895–899.

Hooker, R. S. (2008c). Ambulatory care. In R. M. Ballweg, E. M. Sullivan, D. Brown, & D. Vetrosky (Eds.), *Physician Assistant: A Guide to Clinical Practice* (4th ed.). Philadelphia: Elsevier/Saunders.

Hooker, R. S. (2009). Physician assistant postgraduate education arguments. *Journal of the American Academy of Physician Assistants, 22*(5), 13.

Hooker, R. S., & Berlin, L. (2002). Trends in the supply of physician assistants and nurse practitioners in the American health care system. *Health Affairs, 21*(5), 174–181.

Hooker, R. S., & Brown, J. B. (1985). Rheumatology referrals. *HMO Practice/HMO Group 4, 4*(2), 61–65.

Hooker, R. S., Carter, R., & Cawley, J. F. (2004). The national commission on certification of physician assistants: History and role. *Perspective on Physician Assistant Education, 15*(1), 8–15.

Hooker, R. S., & Cawley, J. F. (1995). Clinical staffing in HMOs [Letter to the editor]. *Health Affairs (Milwood) 14,* 282.

Hooker, R. S., & Cawley, J. F. (1997). *Physician Assistants in American Medicine.* New York: Churchill Livingstone.

Hooker, R. S., & Cawley, J. F. (2003). *Physician Assistants in American Medicine* (2nd ed.). New York: Churchill Livingstone.

Hooker, R. S., & Cipher, D. J. (2005). Physician assistant and nurse practitioner prescribing: 1997–2002. *Journal of Rural Health, 21*(4), 355–360.

Hooker, R. S., Cipher, D. J., Cawley, J. F., Herrmann, D., & Melson, J. (2008). Emergency medicine services: Interprofessional care trends. *Journal of Interprofessional Care, 22*(2), 167–178.

Hooker, R. S., Cipher, D. J., & Sekscenski, E. (2005). Patient satisfaction with physician assistant, nurse practitioner, and physician care: A national survey of Medicare beneficiaries. *Journal of Clinical Outcomes Management, 12*(2), 88–92.

Hooker, R. S., & Freeborn, D. K. (1991). Use of physician assistants in a managed health care system. *Public Health Reports (Washington, DC: 1974), 106*(1), 90–94.

Hooker, R. S., Hess, B., & Cipher, D. (2002). A comparison of physician assistant programs by national certification examination scores. *Perspective on Physician Assistant Education, 13*(2), 81–86.

Hooker, R. S., Hogan, K., & Leeker, E. (2007). The globalization of the physician assistant profession. *Journal of Physician Assistant Education, 18*(3), 76–85.

Hooker, R. S., MacDonald, K., & Patterson, R. (2003). Physician assistants in the Canadian forces. *Military Medicine, 168,* 948–950.

Hooker, R. S., & McCaig, L. F. (1996). Emergency department uses of physician assistants and nurse practitioners: A national survey. *American Journal of Emergency Medicine, 14*(3), 245–249.

Hooker, R. S., & McCaig, L. F. (2001). Use of physician assistants and nurse practitioners in primary care, 1995–1999. *Health Affairs (Milwood), 20*(4), 231–238.

Hooker, R. S., Nicholson, J., & Le, T. (2008). *Physician assistant and nurse practitioner: Malpractice claims and compensation 1991 to 2008.* Unpublished manuscript.

Hooker, R. S., Nicholson, J., & Le, T. (2009). Does the employment of physician assistants and nurse practitioners increase liability? *Journal of Medical Licensure and Discipline, 95*(2), 6–16.

Hooker, R. S., Potts, R., & Ray, W. (1997). Patient satisfaction: Comparing physician assistants, nurse practitioners and physicians. *Permanente Journal, 1*(1), 38–42.

Hooker, R. S., & Rangan, B.V. (2008). Role delineation of rheumatology physician assistants. *Journal of Clinical Rheumatology, 14*(4), 202–205.

Hooker, R. S., & Warren, J. (2001). Comparison of physician assistant programs by tuition costs. *Perspective on Physician Assistant Education, 12*, 87–91.

Hormann, B. M., Bello, S. J., Hartman, A. R., & Jacobs, M. (2004). The effects of a full-time physician assistant staff on postoperative outcomes in the cardiothoracic ICU: 1-year results. *Surgical Physician Assistant, 10*(10), 38–41.

Horton, K., Reffel, A., Rosen, K., & Farraye, F. A. (2001). Training of nurse practitioners and physician assistants to perform screening flexible sigmoidoscopy. *Journal of the American Academy of Nurse Practitioners, 13*(10), 455–459.

Houston, E. A., Bork, C. E., Price, J. J., Jordan, T. R., & Dake, J. A. (2001). How physician assistants use and perceive complementary and alternative medicine. *Journal of the American Academy of Physician Assistants, 14*(1), 29–30, 33–34, 39–40, 44–46 passim, 46.

Howard, D. R. (1969). The physician's assistant. *Journal of the Kansas Medical Society, 70*(10), 411–416.

Howard, P. L. (2000a). PA clinical analyst and researcher find nonclinical jobs rewarding. *AAPA News, 21*, 4–10.

Howard, P. L. (2000b). Beyond the clinic: PAs in forensic medicine. *AAPA News, 12*(21), 1, 10, 11.

Hsiao, W. C. (1984). Transformation of health care in China. *New England Journal of Medicine, 310*(14), 932–936.

Hsu, R. C. (1974). The barefoot doctors of the People's Republic of China—Some problems. *New England Journal of Medicine, 291*(3), 124–127.

Huch, M. H. (1992). Nurse practitioners and physician assistants: Are they the same? *Nursing Science Quarterly, 5*(2), 52–53.

Hudson, C. L. (1961). Expansion of medical professional services with nonprofessional personnel. *Journal of the American Medical Association, 176*, 839–841.

Hughbanks, J., & Freeborn, D. K. (1971). Review of 22 training programs for physician's assistants 1969. *HSMHA Health Reports, 86*(10), 857–862.

Hughes, N. (2000). PA on bargaining team for Kaiser Permanente strike. *AAPA News, 21*, 1–10.

Hugo, J. (2005). *Health workers in South Africa: Not an easy option.* Retrieved August 28, 2008, from www.hst.org.za/uploads/files/sahr05_chapter11.pdf

Hugo, J., & Mfenyana, K. (2007). Midlevel workers: High level bungling? *South African Medical Journal, 97*(03), 147–148.

Hummel, J., & Pirzada, S. (1994). Estimating the cost of using non-physician providers in primary care teams in an HMO: Where would the savings begin? *HMO Practice, 8*, 162–164.

Hutchinson, L. (2006). Challenges of training doctors in the new English NSH. *British Medical Journal, 332*(7556), 1502–1504.

Iglehart, J. (2008). Medicare, graduate medical education, and new policy directions. *New England Journal of Medicine, 359*(6), 643–650.

Institute of Medicine. (1978). *A manpower policy for primary health care: Report of a study/Institute of Medicine.* Washington, DC: National Academy of Sciences, Division of Health Manpower and Resources Development.

Intrator, O., Zinn, J., & Mor, V. (2004). Nursing home characteristics and potentially preventable hospitalizations of long-stay residents. *Journal of the American Geriatrics Society, 52*(10), 1730–1736.

Isberner, F. R., Lloyd, L., Simon, B., Joyce, M. S., & Craven, J. M. (2003). Utilization of physician assistants: Incentives and constraints for rural physicians. *Perspective on Physician Assistant Education, 14*(2), 69–73.

Isiadinso, O. O. (1979). Physician's assistant in geriatric medicine. *New York State Journal of Medicine, 79*(7), 1069–1071.

Jacobson, P. D., Parker, L. E., & Coulter, I. D. (1998). Nurse practitioners and physician assistants as primary care providers in institutional settings. *Inquiry, 35*(4), 432–446.

Jameson, K. P. (2000). Address to the 1995 graduating class of the Utah PA Program. *Perspective on Physician Assistant Education, 11*(2), 125–128.

Janis, I. L. (1980). An analysis of psychological and sociological ambivalence: Nonadherence to courses of action prescribed by health-care professionals. *Transactions of the New York Academy of Sciences, 39*, 91–110.

Jacques, P. (2004). Cultural competency curriculum: Components for inclusion in physician assistant education. *Perspective on Physician Assistant Education, 15*, 102–105.

Jarmul, D. B., & Chavez, R. S. (1991). On "ethics of PAs' work" . . . Role in cavity searches within a correctional facility. *Journal of the American Academy of Physician Assistants, 4*(7), 602–603.

Jarski, R. W. (1988). An investigation of physician assistant and medical student empathic skills. *Journal of Allied Health, 17*, 211–219.

Jarski, R. W. (2001). Introduced into evidence. PAs are recommending, and using, CAM [Editorial]. *Journal of the American Academy of Physician Assistants, 14*(1), 6–12.

Jekel, J. F., Dunaye, T. M., Siker, E., & Rossetti, M. (1980). The impact of non-physician health directors on full-time public health coverage in Connecticut. *American Journal of Public Health, 70*, 73–74.

Johnson, B. X. (1998). The 5 R's of becoming a psychiatric nurse practitioner: Rationale, readying, roles, rules, and reality. *Journal of Psychosocial Nursing and Mental Health Services, 36*(9), 20–24, 38–39.

Johnson, R.E., & Freeborn, D. K. (1986). Comparing HMO physicians' attitudes towards NPs and PAs. *Nurse Practitioner, 11*(1), 39–43.

Johnson, R. E., Hooker, R. S., & Freeborn, D. K. (1988). The future role of physician assistants in prepaid group practice health maintenance organizations. *Journal of the American Academy of Physician Assistants, 1*(2), 88–90.

Joiner, C. L., & Harris, A. M. (1974). Physician's assistants and rural health care: A study of physician's attitudes. *Journal of the Medical Association of the State of Alabama, 44*(5), 251, 255, 258.

Jolly, R. (2008). *Health workforce: A case for physician assistants?* Report no. 24, Parliamentary Library, Commonwealth of Australia, Canberra, 1–36.

Johnstone, D. E. (1977). The idenitity crisis of the allergy nurse associate-physician's assistant. *Annals of Allergy, 38*(5), 311–315.

Jones, J. M. (2002). *A Kernel in the Pod: The Adventures of a "Midlevel" Clinician in a Top-Level World.* Philadelphia: Xlibris Corporation.

Jones, P. E. (1994). A descriptive study of doctorally prepared physician assistants. *Journal of the American Academy of Physician Assistants, 7*(5), 353.

Jones, P. E. (2007). Physician assistant education in the United States. *Academic Medicine, 82,* 882–887.

Jones, P. E. (2008). Doctor and physician assistant distribution in rural and remote Texas counties. *Australian Journal of Rural Health, 16*(2), 12.

Jones, P. E., & Cawley, J. F. (1994). Physician assistants and health system reform. Clinical capabilities, practice activities, and potential roles. *Journal of the American Medical Association, 271*(16), 1266–1272.

Jones, P. E., & Cawley, J. F. (2009). Workweek restrictions and specialty-trained physician assistants: Potential opportunities. *Journal of Surgical Education, 66*(3), 152–157.

Jones, P. E., & Hooker, R. S. (2001). Physician assistants in Texas. *Texas Medicine, 97*(1), 68–73.

Jones, P. E., & Miller, A. A. (2003). Physician assistant education: A call for standardized prerequisites. *Perspective on Physician Assistant Education, 13,* 114.

Jonsson, M., Norden, S. L., & Hanson, U. (2007). Analysis of malpractice claims with a focus on oxytocin use in labour. *Acta Obstetricia et Gynecologica Scandinavica, 86*(3), 315–319.

Joslin, V. H., Cook, P., Ballweg, R., Cawley, J. F., Miller, A. A., Sewell, D., Somers, J. E., et al. (2006). Value added: Graduate-level education in physician assistant programs. *Journal of Physician Assistant Education, 17*(2), 16–30.

Joyner, S. L., & Easley, D. (1984). Organ donation: Who holds the key? *Physician Assistant, 8*(11), 109–116, 119.

Judd, C. R., & Hooker, R. S. (2001). Physician assistant education in substance abuse. *Perspective on Physician Assistant Education, 12*(3), 172–176.

Kahn, L., Wirth, P., & Perkoff, G. T. (1978). The cost of a primary care teaching program in a prepaid group practice. *Medical Care, 16*(1), 61–71.

Kane, R. L., Gardner, J., Wright, D. D., Woolley, F. R., Snell, G. F., Sundwall, D. N., & Castle, C. H. (1978). Differences in the outcomes of acute episodes of care provided by various types of family practitioners. *Journal of Family Practice, 6*(1), 133–138.

Kane, R. L., Garrard, J., Buchanan, J. L., Rosenfeld, A., Skay, C., & McDermott, S. (1991). Improving primary care in nursing homes. *Journal of the American Geriatrics Society, 39*(4), 359–367.

Kane, R. L., Olsen, D. M., & Castle, C. H. (1978). Effects of adding a Medex on practice costs and productivity. *Journal of Community Health, 3*(3), 216–226.

Kappes, T. J. (1992). PA-C vs. OPA-C . . . "Physician Assistant-Certified" . . . American Society of Orthopaedic Physician Assistants. *Journal of the American Academy of Physician Assistants, 5*(1), 70–71.

Kark, S. L. (1981). *The Practice of Community-Oriented Primary Health Care.* New York: Appleton-Century-Crofts.

Katterjohn, K. R. (1982). Dermatologic physician assistants [Letter]. *Journal of the American Academy of Dermatology, 6,* 950–951.

Katz, H. P., Cushman, I., Brooks, W., Peterson, M., Nicklas, R., Gemma, S., et al. (1994). A physician assistant laceration management program. *HMO Practice, 8,* 187–189.

Kaups, K. L., Parks, S. N., & Morris, C. L. (1998). Intracranial pressure monitor placement by midlevel practitioners. *Journal of Trauma, 45*(5), 884–886.

Keahey, D., & Goldgar, C. (2004). An integrated evidence-based medicine curriculum in physician assistant training: From undergraduate to postgraduate. *Perspective on Physician Assistant Education, 15*(2), 91–98.

Kearns, P. J., Wang, C. C., Morris, W. J., Low, D. G., Deacon, A. S., Chan, S. Y., & Jensen, W. A. (2001). Hospital care by hospital-based and clinic-based faculty: A prospective, controlled trial. *Archives of Internal Medicine, 161*(2), 235–241.

Keith, C. (1974). Auxillary utilization in dentistry. *PA Journal, 4,* 14–20.

Keith, D. E., & Doerr, R. J. (1987). Survey of a physician assistant internship concerning practice characteristics and adequacy of training. *Journal of Medical Education, 62*(6), 517–519.

Kelly, P. (2000). *Determining the influence of pre-admission health care experience on measures of entry-level clinical competence in a cohort of physician assistant graduates* [Dissertation]. Nova Southeastern University, Fort Lauderdale, FL.

Kenyon, V. A. (1985). Feldshers and health promotion in the USSR. *Physician Assistant, 9,* 25–29.

Kessler, R., & Berlin, A. (1999). Physician assistants as inpatient caregivers. A new role for mid-level practitioners. *Cost Quality, 5,* 32–33.

Kiernan, B., & Rosenbaum, H. D. (1977). The impact of a physician assistant in diagnostic radiology [PA-DR] on the delivery of diagnostic radiologic clinical services. *Investigative Radiology, 12*(1), 7–14.

Kimmos, B. (2005). A day in the life. How PAs live and work. *Journal of the American Academy of Physician Assistants, 18*(12), 28–30.

Kindman, L. A. (2006). Medical education after the Flexner report. *New England Journal of Medicine, 356*(1), 90.

Kirk, L. M. (2006). Who will provide health care for you and me? Facing the crisis in primary care. *ACP Observer.* Retrieved November 5, 2007, from http://www.acponline.org/journals/news/july06/president.htm

Kirz, H. L., & Larsen, C. (1986). Costs and benefits of medical student training to a health maintenance organization. *Journal of the American Medical Association, 256*(6), 734–739.

Kleinpell, R. M., Ely, E. W., & Grabenkort, R. (2008). Nurse practitioners and physician assistants in the intensive care unit: An evidence-based review. *Critical Care Medicine, 36*(10), 2888–2897.

Knaus, W. A. (1981). *Inside Russian Medicine: An American Doctor's First Hand Report.* New York: Everst House.

Knickman, J. R., Lipkin, M., Jr., Finkler, S. A., Thompson, W. G., & Kiel, J. (1992). The potential for using non-physicians to compensate for the reduced availability of residents. *Academic Medicine, 67*(7), 429–438.

Knott, P. (2008). Postgraduate education for the physician assistant: Where are we heading? *Journal of Physician Assistant Education, 19*(3), 6–7.

Kohlhepp, B. (2006). *Chairman's speech at the House of Delegates, Monday, May 29, 2006.* Retrieved July 5, 2008, from https://www.nccpa.net/News_06AAPAConfAnnouncement.aspx

Kohlhepp, B., Rohrs, R., & Robinson, P. (2005). Charting a course to competency. *Journal of the American Academy of Physician Assistants, 18*(7), 14–15, 18.

Koperski, M., & Rodnick, J. E. (1999). Recent developments in primary care in the United Kingdom: From competition to community-oriented primary care. *Journal of Family Practice, 48*(2), 140–145.

Krasner, M., Ramsay, D. L., Weary, P. E., & Johnson, M. L. (1977). New health practitioners and dermatology manpower planning. *Archives of Dermatology, 113*(9), 1280–1282.

Krasuski, R. A., Wang, A., Ross, C., Bolles, J. F., Moloney, E. L., Kelly, L. P., et al. (2003). Trained and supervised physician assistants can safely perform diagnostic cardiac catheterization with coronary angiography. *Catheterization and Cardiovascular Interventions, 59*(2), 157–160.

Krein, S. L. (1997a). The employment and use of nurse practitioners and physician assistants by rural hospitals. *Journal of Rural Health, 13*(1), 45–58.

Krein, S. L. (1997b). Rural hospitals and provider-based rural health clinics: The influence of market and institutional forces (nurse practitioner, physician assistant). *Dissertation Abstracts International, 58*(05b), 2381.

Krein, S. L. (1999). The adoption of provider-based rural health clinics by rural hospitals: A study of market and institutional forces. *Health Services Research, 34*(1), 33–60.

Kuhns, D. H. (2002). Globalizing the PA profession. *Journal of the American Academy of Physician Assistants, 15*(10), 45–50.

Kuttler, H. (2007a). From PAs in urgent care to chief executive officer. *AAPA News, 28*(28), 8.

Kuttler, H. (2007b). Placing students with preceptors a "scramble" for PA programs. *AAPA News, 28*(16), 1–6.

Kuttler, H. (2007c). International medical graduates included in Ontario PA initiative. *AAPA News, 11*(3), 207–219.

Kuttler, H., & American Academy of Physician Assistants. (2006). Government official to PAs: "Ontario is open for business." *AAPA News, 27*(11), 6.

Lairson, P. D., Record, J. C., & James, J. C. (1974). Physician assistants at Kaiser: Distinctive patterns of practice. *Inquiry, 11*(3), 207–219.

Landon, B., Loudon, J., Selle, M., & Doucette, S. (2004). Factors influencing the retention and attrition of community health aides/practitioners in Alaska. *Journal of Rural Health, 20*(3), 221–230.

Lane, S., & Jones, P. E. (2009). Overcoming barriers to publication. *Journal of the Physician Assistant Education, 20*(1), 4–5.

Lantos, J. D. (1997). *Do We Still Need Doctors?* New York: Routledge.

Lapius, S. K. (1983). Physicians and midlevel practitioners. Can the conflict be resolved? *Postgraduate Medicine, 73*(3), 94–95.

Larson, E. H., Hart, L. G., & Ballweg, R. M. (2001). National estimates of physician assistant productivity. *Journal of Allied Health, 30*(3), 146–152.

Larson, E. H., Hart, L. G., Goodwin, M. K., Geller, J., & Andrilla, C. (1999). Dimensions of retention: A national study of the locational histories of physician assistants. *Journal of Rural Health, 15*(4), 391–402.

Larson, E. H., Hart, L .G., & Hummel, J. (1994). Rural physician assistants: A survey of graduates of MEDEX Northwest. *Public Health Report, 109,* 266–274.

Larson, E. H., Palazzo L., Berkowitz, B., Pirani, M. J., & Hart, L. G. (2003). The contribution of nurse practitioners and physician assistants to generalist care in Washington state. *Health Services Research, 38*(4), 1033–1050.

Larson, L. W., Gerbert, D. A., Herman, L. M., Leger, M. M., McNellis, R., O'Donoghue, D. L., et al. (2009). ACC/AHA 2005 guideline update: Chronic heart failure in the adult. *Journal of the American Academy of Physician Assistants, 19*(4), 53–57.

Larson, M. S. (1977). *The Rise of Professionalism.* Berkley, CA: University of California Press.

Laur, W. E., Posey, R. E., & Waller, J. D. (1981). The dermatologic physician's assistant: An overview of one year's experience. *Journal of the American Academy of Dermatology, 5,* 367–372.

Lawrence, D. (1978). Physician assistants and nurse practitioners: Their impact on health care access, costs, and quality. *Health & Medical Care Services Review, 1*(2), 1, 3–12.

Lee, J., Cooper, J., Lopez, E. C., King, B., & Duhaylongsod, F. (2000). Survey on utilization of nonsurgeon practitioners in cardiothoracic surgery (SUNPICS). *Surgical Physician Assistant, 6*(12), 14–21.

Legler, C. F. (1983). A survey of physician attitudes toward the PA. *Physician Assistant*, 7(5), 98, 101–104, 109.

Legler, C. F., Cawley, J. F., & Fenn, W. H. (2007). Physician assistants: Education, practice and global interest. *Medical Teacher*, 29(1), 22–25.

Legler C. F., Pedersen K. J., Bensulock, M. M., & Kennedy W. W. (2005). *The global applicability of physician assistants*. Poster session. Retrieved April 12, 2007, from http://www.paeaonline.org/iacpage.html

Lennox, K. P. (2008). Expanding PAs' roles in aesthetic practices. *ADVANCE for Physician Assistants*, 16(1–2), 30.

LeRoy, L. (1981). *The Implications of Cost-Effectiveness Analysis of Medical Technology, Background Paper # 2 Case Studies of Medical Technologies, Case Study # 16: The Costs and Effectiveness of Nurse Practitioners*. Washington, DC: Office of Technology Assessment.

Lewis, D. E. (1975). *The physician's assistant concept.* Unpublished doctoral dissertation, Department of Education in the Graduate School of Duke University.

Lewit, E. M., Bentkover, J. D., Bentkover, S. H., Watkins, R. N., & Hughes, E. F. (1980). A comparison of surgical assisting in a prepaid group practice and a community hospital. *Medical Care*, 18(9), 916–929.

Li, L. B., Williams, S. D., & Scammon, S. L. (1995). Practicing with the urban underserved. A qualitative analysis of motivations, incentives, and disincentives. *Archives of Family Medicine*, 4(2), 124–133.

Liaison Committee on Medical Education. (2001). Medical schools in the United States. *Journal of the American Medical Association*, 286(9), 1085–1093.

Lichter, P. R. (1995). Confusing licensure with education: Medicine's slippery slope. *Federal Bulletin*, 82(1), 16–20.

Lieberman, D., & Lalwani, A. (1994). Physician-only and physician assistant statutes: A case of perceived but unfounded conflict. *Journal of American Medical Women's Association*, 49, 146–149.

Lieberman, D. A., & Ghormley, J. M. (1992). Physician assistants in gastroenterology: Should they perform endoscopy? *American Journal of Gastroenterology*, 87(8), 940–943.

Lin, S. X., Hooker, R. S., Lenz, E. R., & Hopkins, S. C. (2002). Nurse practitioners and physician assistants in hospital outpatient departments, 1997–1999. *Nursing Economic$*, 20(4), 174–179.

Lindenauer, P. K., Rothberg, M. B., Pekow, P. S., Kenwood, C., Benjamin, E. M., & Auerbach, A. D. (2007). Outcomes of care by hospitalists, general internists, and family physicians. *New England Journal of Medicine*, 357(25), 2589–2600.

Liptak, A. (2005, March 6). Go ahead. Test a lawyer's ingenuity. Try to limit damages. *The New York Times*, section 4, p. 5.

Little, G. A., & Buus-Frank, M. E. (1996). Transition from housestaff in the neonatal intensive care unit: A time to review, revise, and reconfirm [Editorial]. *American Journal of Perinatology*, 13(2), 127–129.

Liu, C., Chien, C., Chou, P., Liu, J., Chen, V. T., Wei, J., et al. (2005). An analysis of job satisfaction among physician assistants in Taiwan. *Health Policy*, 73(1), 66–77.

Loblolly boys. (February 2004). *The Bosun's Chronicle*, 4(2). Retrieved May 11, 2008, from http://www.julianstockwin.com/Newsletter/Newsletter%20Feb%202004.txt

Loera, J. A., Kuo, Y. F., & Rahr, R. R. (2007). Telehealth distance mentoring of students. *Telemedicine Journal and E-Health*, 13(1), 45–50.

Lohr, S. (2005, February 27). Bush's next target: Malpractice lawyers. *The New York Times*, section 3, p. 1.

Lurie, N., Rank, B., Parenti, C., Woolley, T., & Snoke, W. (1989). How do house officers spend their nights? A time study of internal medicine house staff on call. *New England Journal of Medicine*, 320(25), 1673–1677.

Lyman, P., Elli, L., & Gebhart, R. (1999). Physician assistants in the Department of Veterans Affairs. *Veterans Health System Journal*, 4(3), 25–29.

Lynge, D. C., Larson, E. H., Thompson, M. J., Rosenblatt, R. A., & Hart, L. G. (2008). A longitudinal analysis of the general surgery workforce in the United States, 1981–2005. *Archives of Surgery*, 143(4), 345–350.

Machotka, P., Ott, J. E., Moon, J. B., & Silver, H. K. (1973). Competence of child health associates. I. Comparison of their basic science and clinical knowledge with that of medical students and pediatric residents. *American Journal of Diseases of Children (1960)*, 125(2), 199–203.

Magnus, B. (2007). Foreign-trained doctors dominate pilot project. *Canadian Medical Association Journal*, 178(11), 1411.

Makinde, J. F., & Hooker, R. S. (2009). PA doctoral degree debt. *ADVANCE for Physician Assistants*, 17(3), 30–31.

Mainous, A. G., III, Bertolino, J. G., & Harrell, P. L. (1992). Physician extenders: Who is using them? *Family Medicine*, 24(3), 201–204.

Marsters, C. E. (2000). Pneumothorax as a complication of central venous cannulation performed by physician assistants. *Surgical Physician Assistant*, 6(3), 18–24.

Martin, K .E. (2000). A rural-urban comparison of patterns of physician assistant practice. *Journal of the American Academy of Physician Assistants*, 13(7), 49–50, 56, 59, 63–66, 72 passim.

Martin, D. (2007). Perfected and strengthened through trials and suffering. *Journal of the American Academy of Physician Assistants*, 20(1), 52–53.

Marvelle, K., & Kraditor, K. (1999). Do PAs in clinical practice find their work satisfying? *Journal of the American Academy of Physician Assistants*, 12(11), 43–50.

Mastrangelo, R. (1993). The name game. *ADVANCE for Physician Assistants*, 1(3), 13.

Mathew, M. S., & Stevens, R. (1982). Medical evaluation of CMHC patients by a physician's assistant. *Hospital & Community Psychiatry, 33*(3), 224–225.

Mathur, M., Rampersad, A., Howard, K., & Goldman, G. M. (2005). Physician assistants as physician extenders in the pediatric intensive care unit setting—A 5-year experience. *Pediatric Critical Care Medicine, 6*(1), 14–19.

Matthews, W. A., & Yohe, C. D. (1984). PAs in psychiatry: Filling the gap. *Physician Assistant, 8,* 26.

Mattingly, D. E., & Curtis, L. G. (1996). Physician assistant impairment. A peer review program for North Carolina. *North Carolina Medical Journal, 57*(4), 233–235.

Maxfield, R. G., Lemire, M. D., Thomas, M., & Wansleben, O. (1975). Utilization of supervised physician's assistants in emergency room coverage in a small rural community hospital. *Journal of Trauma, 15*(9), 795–799.

May, F. L. (1988). It's a fact: PAs and NPs help ensure cost-conscious quality. *Provider, 14*(4), 42.

Mayes, J. R. (1991). Reader disputes "Legislation" column [Letter]. *AORN Journal, 53*(1) 13–14.

McCabe, D. (2007). The next wave: "Physician extenders." *Canadian Medical Association Journal, 177*(5), 477.

McCaig, L. F., Besser, R. E., & Hughes, J. M. (2002). Trends in antimicrobial prescribing rates for children and adolescents. *Journal of the American Medical Association, 287*(23), 3096–3102.

McCaig, L. F. & Burt, C. W. (2005). National hospital ambulatory medical care survey (NHAMCS): 2003 emergency department summary. *Vital and Health Statistics, 358.*

McCaig, L. F., Hooker, R. S., Sekscenski, E. S., & Woodwell, D. A. (1998). Physician assistants and nurse practitioners in hospital outpatient departments, 1993–1994. *Public Health Reports (Washington, DC: 1974), 113*(1), 75–82.

McCarty, J. E., Stuetzer, L., & Somers, J. E. (2001). Physician assistant program accreditation—History in the making. *Perspective on Physician Assistant Education, 12*(1), 24–38.

McCowan, T. C., Goertzen, T. C., Lieberman, R. P., LeVeen, R. F., & Martin, V. A. (1992). Physician's assistants in vascular and interventional radiology [Letter; Comment]. *Radiology, 184*(2), 582.

McDaniel, M. J. (2008, November). *CASPA The Applicant Pool—2007 Cycle 7 Report.* Savannah, GA: CASPA Advisory Committee, Physician Assistant Education Association.

McDowell, L., Clemens, D., & Frosch, D. (1999). Analysis of physician assistant program performance on the PANCE based on degree granted, length of curriculum, and duration of accreditation. *Perspective on Physician Assistant Education, 10*(4), 180–184.

McKelvey, P. A., Oliver, D. R., & Conboy, J. E. (1986). PA roles in a tertiary medical center. *Physician Assistant, 10*(1), 149–152, 159.

McKibbin, R. C. (1978). Cost-effectiveness of physician assistants: A review of recent evidence. *PA Journal, 8*(2), 110–115.

Mechanic, D., McAlpine, D. D., & Rosenthal, M. (2001). Are patients' office visits with physicians getting shorter? *New England Journal of Medicine, 344*(3), 198–204.

Medical Group Management Association. (2005). *Physician Compensation and Production Survey: 2005 Report Based on 2004 Survey.* Englewood, CO: Medical Group Management Association.

Medical Group Management Association. (2006). *Physician Compensation and Production Survey: 2006 Report Based on 2005 Survey.* Englewood, CO: Medical Group Management Association.

Meikle, T. H. (1992). *An Expanded Role for the Physician Assistant.* Washington, DC: Association of Academic Health Centers.

Mendenhall, R. C., Repicky, P. A., & Neville, R. E. (1980). Assessing the utilization and productivity of nurse practitioners and physician's assistants: Methodology and findings on productivity. *Medical Care, 18*(6), 609–623.

Merritt, Hawkins, & Associates. (2006). *Summary report: 2006 review of physician recruitment incentives.* Retrieved June 24, 2008, from http://www.merritthawkins.com/pdf/2006_incentive_survey.pdf

Miles, D. L., & Rushing, W. A. (1976). A study of physicians' assistants in a rural setting. *Medical Care, 14*(12), 987–995.

Miller, A. A., Allison, L., Asprey, D., et al. (2001). Programs degree task force final paper, September 28, 2000. *Perspective on Physician Assistant Education, 11,* 157–160.

Miller, J. I., Craver, J. M., & Hatcher, C. R. (1978). Use of physicians' assistants in thoracic and cardiovascular surgery in the community hospital. *American Surgeon, 44*(3), 162–164.

Miller, J. I., & Hatcher, C. R. (1978). Physicians' assistants on a university cardiothoracic surgical service. A five-year update. *Journal of Thoracic and Cardiovascular Surgery, 76*(5), 639–642.

Miller, W., Riehl, E., Napier, M., Barber, K., & Dabideen, H. (1998). Use of physician assistants as surgery/trauma house staff at an American College of Surgeons–verified level II trauma center. *Journal of Trauma, 44*(2), 372–376.

Millis, J., & Council on Medical Education. (1966). *Citizen's Commission on Graduate Medical Education, The Graduate Education of Physicians.* Chicago: American Medical Association.

Mills, A. C., & McSweeney, M. (2002). Nurse practitioners and physician assistants revisited: Do their practice patterns differ in ambulatory care? *Journal of Professional Nursing, 18*(1), 36–46.

Mishel, M. H. (1998). Uncertainty in illness. *Image Journal of Nursing Scholarship, 20,* 225–232.

Mitchell, J., Hayhurst, C., & Robinson, S. M. (2004). Can a senior house officer's time be used more effectively? *Emergency Medicine Journal, 21*(5), 545–547.

Mittman, D. (1995) Physician's assistant (PA) and CNS [Letter]. *Clinical Nurse Specialist, 9*(2), 121.

Monroe, J. R. (2001). PAs and dermatology. Good times, nice work, and a special issue. *Journal of the American Academy of Physician Assistants, 14*(4), 4–10.

Moore, G. T. (1994). Will the power of the marketplace produce the workforce we need? *Inquiry, 31*(3), 276–282.

Moore, G., & Showstack, J. (2003). Primary care medicine in crisis: Toward reconstruction and renewal. *Annals of Internal Medicine, 138*(3), 244–247.

Morgan, P., & Hooker, R. S. (2009, in press). Choice of specialty among physician assistants in the U.S. *Health Affairs.*

Morgan, P. A., Shah, N. D., Kaufman, J. S., & Albanese, M. A. (2008). Impact of physician assistant care on office visit resource used in the United States. *Health Services Research, 43*(5), 1906–1922.

Morgan, P. A., Strand, J., Østbye, T., & Albanese, M. A. (2007). Missing in action: Care by physician assistants and nurse practitioners in national health surveys. *Health Services Research, 42*(5), 2022–2037.

Morian, J. P., Jr. (1986). The PA's role in medical research: Implications for PA education. *Physician Assistant, 10*(3), 141–142, 146, 161.

Morreale, J., & Chitradon, R. (1977). *A cost analysis of the use of physician's assistants providing primary medical care in a psychiatric setting.* Pittsburgh, PA: Western Psychiatric Institute and Clinic and the University Center for Urban Research, University of Pittsburgh.

Morton-Rias, D., & Hammond, J. (2008). Education. In R. M. Ballweg, E. M. Sullivan, D. Brown, & D. Vetroskly (Eds.), *Physician Assistant: A Guide to Clinical Practice* (4th ed.). Philadelphia: Elsevier/Saunders.

Moses, R. E., & Feld, A. D. (2007). Physician liability for medical errors of nonphysician clinicians: Nurse practitioners and physician assistants. *American Journal of Gastroenterology, 102*, 6–9.

Mott, J. S., & Borden S. L. (1994). The impaired PA. *Journal of the American Academy of Physician Assistants, 7*(9), 682–684

Mueller, K. J., Patil, K., & Boilesen, E. (1998). The role of uninsurance and race in healthcare utilization by rural minorities. *Health Service Research, 33*(3, pt 1), 597–610.

Mullan, F. (1989). *Plagues and Politics: The Story of the United States Public Health Service.* New York: Basic Books.

Mullan, F. (2002). *Big Doctoring in America.* Berkeley, CA: University of California Press.

Mullan, F. (2005). The metrics of the physician brain drain. *New England Journal of Medicine, 353*(1), 1810–1818.

Mullan, F., & Epstein, L. (2002). Community-oriented primary care: New relevance in a changing world. *American Journal of Public Health, 92*(11), 1748–1755.

Mullan, F., & Frehywot, S. (2007). Non-physician clinicians in 47 sub-Saharan African countries. *Lancet, 370*(9605), 2158–2163.

Mullan, F., Rivo, M. L., & Politzer, R. M. (1993). Doctors, dollars, and determination: Making physician workforce policy. *Health Affairs (Milwood), 12*(suppl), 138–151.

Mundinger, M. O. (2004). *Advanced Practice Nurses: The Preferred Primary Care Provider for the Twenty-First Century.* San Francisco: Jossey-Bass.

Murray, R. B., & Wronski, I. (2006). When the tide goes out: Health workforce in rural, remote and indigenous communities. *Medical Journal of Australia, 185*(1), 37–38.

Myers, H. C. (1978). *The Physician's Assistant: A Baccalaureate Curriculum.* Philippi, WV: Aldersonson-Broaddus College.

Nasca, T. J., Veloski, J. J., Monnier, J. A., Cunninghan, J. P., Valerio, S., Lewis, T. J., et al. (2001). Minimum instructional and program-specific administrative costs of educating residents in internal medicine. *Archives of Internal Medicine, 161*(5), 760–766.

National Advisory Commission on Health Manpower. (1967). *Report of the National Advisory Commission on Health Manpower* (Vols. I and II). Washington, DC: U.S. Government Printing Office.

National Commission on Certification of Physician Assistants. (1995). *Report on the Content of the Physician Assistant National Certifying Examination and the Physician Assistant National Recertifying Examination.* Atlanta, GA: Author.

National Council of State Boards of Nursing. (2006). *Vision Paper: The Future Regulation of Advanced Practice Nursing.* Chicago: Author.

National Rural Health Association. (2007). *What's different about rural health care?* Retrieved June 22, 2008, from http://www.ruralhealthweb.org/go/left/about-rural-health/what-s-different-about-rural-health-care

Neighbors, J. (2007). The diagnosis and management of hepatitis C: The role of the physician assistant. *Internet Journal of Academic Physician Assistants, 5*(2), 16.

Nelson, E. C., Jacobs, A. R., Breer, P. E., & Johnson, K. G. (1975). Impact of physician's assistants on patient visits in ambulatory care practices. *Annals of Internal Medicine, 82*(5), 608–612.

Nelson, E. C., Jacobs, A. R., Cordner, K., & Johnson, K. G. (1975). Financial impact of physician assistants on medical practice. *New England Journal of Medicine, 293*(11), 527–530.

Nelson, E. C., Jacobs, A. R., & Johnson, K. G. (1974). Patients' acceptance of physician's assistants. *Journal of the American Medical Association, 228*(1), 63–67.

Nelson, E. C., Johnson, K. G., & Jacobs, A. R. (1977). Impact of Medex on physician activities: Redistribution of physician time after incorporating a Medex into the practice. *Journal of Family Practice, 5*(4), 607–612.

Nelson, L. B. (1982). New Jersey physician assistant graduates are successful practitioners. *Journal of the Medical Society of New Jersey, 79*, 829–833.

Nestor, M. S. (2005). The use of mid-level providers in dermatology: A liability risk? *Seminars in Cutaneous Medicine and Surgery, 24*(3), 148–151.

Nicholson, J. G. (2008). *Physician ssistant Medical Practice in the Health Care Workforce: A Retrospective Study of Medical Malpractice and Safety Comparing Physician Assistants to Physicians and Advanced Practice Nurses.* Unpublished dissertation, University of Wisconsin, Madison.

Nora, L. M., Poreroy, C., Curry, T. E., Jr., Hill, N. S., Tibbs, P. A., & Wilson, E. A. (2000). Revising appointment, promotion, and tenure procedures to incorporate an expanded definition of scholarship: The University of Kentucky College of Medicine experience. *Academic Medicine, 75*(9), 913–924.

Nyberg, S. M., Waswick,W., Wynn, T., & Keuter, K. (2007). Midlevel providers in a Level I trauma service: Experience at Wesley Medical Center. *Journal of Trauma, 63*(1), 128–134.

Oakes, D. L., MacLaren, L. M., Gorie, C. T., & Finstuen, K. (1999). Predicting success on the physician assistant national certifying examination. *Perspective on Physician Assistant Education, 10*(2), 63–69.

O'Callaghan, N. (2007). Addressing clinical preceptorship teaching development. *Journal of Physician Assistant Education, 18*(4), 37–39.

O'Connor, T. M., & Hooker, R. S. (2007). Extending rural and remote medicine with a new type of health worker: Physician assistants. *Australian Journal of Rural Health, 15*(6), 346–351.

Odom, G. L. (1975). Over-all view of neurosurgical manpower and training. Clinical Neurosurgery, 22, 59–66.

Office of Inspector General, Office of Enhancement and Inspection. (1993). *Enhancing the utilization of nonphysician services.* New York: Department of Health and Human Services.

Office of Inspector General (OIG). (2001). *Medicare coverage of non-physician practitioner services.* New York (OEI New York Regional Office): Office of Evaluations and Inspections, OIG, Department of Health and Human Services.

Office of Technology Assessment. (1986). *Nurse Practitioners, Physician Assistants, and Certified Nurse-midwives: An Analysis [Case Study 37].* Washington, DC: Government Printing Office.

Office of Technology Assessment. (1990). *Health Care in Rural America.* Washington, DC: Government Printing Office.

O'Hearn, C. J. (1991). Physician assistants' role in combat medicine [Letter]. *Postgraduate Medicine, 90*(3), 48.

Ohman-Strickland, P. A., Orzano, A. J., Solberg, L. I., DiCiccio-Bloom, B., O'Malley, D., Tallia, A. F., Balasubramanian. B. A. et al. (2008). Quality of diabetes care in family medicine practices: Influence of nurse-practitioners and physician's assistants. *Annals of Family Medicine, 6*(1), 14–22.

Oliver, D. R. (1993). Physician assistant education: A review of program characteristics by sponsoring institution. In D. K. Clawson & M. Osterweis (Eds.), *The Roles of Physician Assistants and Nurse Practitioners in Primary Care.* Washington, DC: Association of Academic Health Centers.

Oliver, D. R., Conboy, J. E., Donahue, W. J., Daniels, M. A., & McKelvey, P. A. (1986). Patients' satisfaction with physician assistant services. *Physician Assistant, 10*(7), 51–60.

Olsen, D.M.; Kane, R.L.; Manson, J.; Newman, J. (1978). Measuring impact of Medex using third-party payer claims. *Inquiry, 15* (2), 160–165.

Orcutt, V. L. (2008). The supply and demand of physician assistants in the United States: A trend analysis. *Dissertation Abstracts International: Section B: The Sciences and Engineering, 68*(8), 5118.

Orcutt, V. L., Hildebrand, A., & Jones, P. E. (2006). The doctoral pipeline in physician assistant education. *Journal of Physician Assistant Education, 17*(1), 6–9.

Organisation for Economic Co-operation and Development (OECD). (2008). *OECD health data 2008: Statistics and indicators for 30 countries.* Retrieved April 13, 2007, from http://www.oecd.org/document/30/0,2340,en_2649_37407_12968734_1_1_1_37407,00.html

Ormond, B. A., Wallin, S., & Goldenson, S. M. (2000). *Supporting the Rural Health Care Safety Net.* Washington, DC: Urban Institute.

O'Rourke, R. A. (1987). The specialized physician assistant: An alternative to the clinical cardiology trainee [Editorial]. *American Journal of Cardiology, 60*(10), 901–902.

Ortiz, D., Addari, G., Hastings-Schmidt, V., Mead, K., & Tobojka, D. (2000, May 29). *Factors Affecting Physicians Decisions to Hire Physician Assistants.* Poster session Ppesented at the American Academy of Physician Assistants 28th Annual Conference, Chicago.

Østbye, T., Yarnall, K. S., Krause, K. M., Pollak, K., Gradison, M., & Michener, J. L. (2005). Is there time for management of patients with chronic diseases in primary care? *Annals of Family Medicine, 3*(3), 209–214.

Osterweis, M., & Garfinkel, S. (1993). Roles and functions of non-physician practitioners in primary care. In D. K. Clawson & M. Osterweis (Eds.), *The Roles of Physician Assistants and Nurse Practitioners in Primary Care.* Washington, DC: Association of Academic Health Centers.

Oswanski, M. F., Sharma, O. P., & Shekhar, S. R. (2004). Comparative review of use of physician assistants in a level I trauma center. *American Surgeon, 70*(3), 272–279.

Ott, J. E., Bellaire, J., Machotka, P., & Moon, J. B. (1974). Patient management by telephone by child health associates and pediatric house officers. *Journal of Medical Education, 49*(6), 596–600.

Otterbourg, E. J. (1986). The expanding role of physician assistants in neonatology. *Physician Assistant, 10*(4), 116–121.

Ottley, R. G., Agbontaen, J. X., & Wilkow, B. R. (2000). Pulse of the profession. The hospitalist PA: An emerging opportunity. *Journal of the American Academy of Physician Assistants, 13*(11), 21–22.

Ouslander, J. G., & Osterweil, D. (1994). Physician evaluation and management of nursing home residents. *Annals of Internal Medicine, 120*(7), 584–592.

Page, R. R. (1975). *The Military Physician's Assistant. Study File 7.4.5 DASD (HA)*. Pentagon City, VA: Office of the Assistant Secretary of Defense (Health and Environment).

Paine, S. J. (1996). Legal issues surrounding professional impairment. *Journal of the American Academy of Physician Assistants, 9*(12), 16–19.

Palmer, P. N. (1990). Latest expansion of physician assistants' scope of practice raises questions [Editorial]. *AORN Journal, 51*(3), 671–672.

Pan, S., Geller, J. M., Muus, K. J., & Hart, L. G. (1996). Predicting the degree of rurality of physician assistant practice location. *Hospital Health & Services Administration, 41*(1), 105–119.

Pantell, R. H., Reilly, T., & Liang, M. H. (1980). Analysis of the reasons for the high turnover of clinicians in neighborhood health centers. *Public Health Report, 95*, 344–350.

Parker, H. J., McCoy, J. F., & Connor, R. B. (1972). Delegation of tasks in radiology to allied health personnel. Reaction of radiologists. *Radiology, 103*(2), 257–261.

Parkhurst, D. C., & Ramsery, C. M. (2006). The marriage of problem-based learning with standardized patients: An evaluation of physician assistant students' cultural competency in communication. *Journal of Physician Assistant Education, 17*(1), 58–62.

Parle, J. V., Ross, N. M., & Doe, W. F. (2006). The medical care practitioner: Developing a physician assistant equivalent for the United Kingdom. *Medical Journal of Australia, 185*(1), 13–17.

Parrish, T. G. (2004). Cultural perspectives. The story catches you and you begin to understand. *Perspective on Physician Assistant Education, 14*(2), 131–134.

Parse, R. R. (1992). Human becoming: Parse's theory of nursing. *Nursing Science Quarterly, 5*(1), 35–42.

Pathman, D. E., Fryer, G. E., Jr., Phillips, R. L., Smucny, J., Miyoshi, T., & Green, L. A. (2006). National Health Service Corps staffing and the growth of the local rural non-NHSC primary care physician workforce. *Journal of Rural Health, 22*(4), 285–293.

Patterson, P. K. (1969). Parent reaction to the concept of pediatric assistants. *Pediatrics, 44*, 69–75.

Pedersen, D. M., Chappell, B., Elison, G., & Bunnell, R. (2008). The productivity of PAs, APRNs, and physicians in Utah. *Journal of the American Academy of Physician Assistants, 21*(1), 42–47.

Pedersen, D. M., Houchins, J., Pedersen, K. J., & Aldrich, T. (1998). A three-year retrospective analysis of the economic impact on clinical practice sites involved in training second-year physician assistant students. *Perspective on Physician Assistant Education, 9*(1), 8–13.

Pedersen, K. J., Hooker, R. S., Legler, C. F., Kortyna, D. E., Harbert, K. R., Eisenhauer, W. A., & Baggett, A. (2003). Report on the findings of the Ad Hoc Committee on International Physician Assistant Education. *Perspective on Physician Assistant Education, 14*(4), 220–232.

Pelligrino, E. D. (1976). Prescribing and drug ingestion symbols and substances. *Drug Intelligence and Clinical Pharmacy, 10*(11), 624–630.

Pender, N., & Pender, A. R. (1996). *Health Promotion in Nursing Practice*. Norwalk, CT: Appleton & Lange.

Pereira, C., Bugalho, A., Bergstrom, S., Vaz, F., & Cotiro, M. (1996). A comparative study of caesarean deliveries by assistant medical officers and obstetricians in Mozambique. *British Journal of Obstetrics and Gynaecology, 103*(6), 508–512.

Perkins, J. E., Rahr, R. R., & Kurial, M. (2001). Health promotion and wellness in physician assistant programs. *Perspective on Physician Assistant Education, 12*(1), 5–12.

Perlman, F. (1976). Physicians' assistants in allergy-merits and demerits. *Annals of Allergy, 37*(2), 114–118.

Perry, H. B., III. (1977). Physician assistants: An overview of an emerging health profession. *Medical Care, 15*(12), 982–990.

Perry, H. B., III. (1978a). The job satisfaction of physician assistants: A causal analysis. *Social Science & Medicine, 12*(5A), 377–385.

Perry, H. B., III. (1978b). An analysis of the specialty and geographic location of physician assistants in the United States. *American Journal of Public Health, 68*(10), 1019–1021.

Perry, H. B., III. (1980). An analysis of the effects of personal background and work setting variables upon selected job characteristics of physician assistants. *Journal of Community Health, 5*, 228–243.

Perry, H. B., III. (1989). Role satisfaction: An important and neglected subject. *Journal of the American Academy of Physician Assistants, 2*(6), 427–428.

Perry, H. B., & Breitner, B. (1982). *Physician Assistants: Their Contribution to Health Care*. New York: Springer.

Perry, H. B., III, & Redmond, E. L. (1984). Career trends and attrition among PAs. *Physician Assistant, 8*(6), 121–129.

Peterson, M .L. (1980). The Institute of Medicine report, "A manpower policy for primary health care": A commentary from the American College of Physicians. *Annals of Internal Medicine, 92*(6), 843–851.

Pew Health Professions Commission. (1993). *Health Professions Education in the Future: Schools in Service to the Nation*. San Francisco: Center for the Health Professions.

Peysner, J. (1996). Physicians' assistants: Legal implications of the extended role [Editorial]. *British Journal of Nursing, 5*, 592.

Phelps, P. B., & Lyons, G. G. (2000). Emphasizing domestic violence prevention in the physician assistant curriculum. *Perspective on Physician Assistant Education, 11*(1), 43–44.

Phillips, R. L., Dodoo, M. S., Petterson, S., Bazemore, A., Teevan, B., Bennett, K., et al. (2009). Specialty and Geographic Distribution of the Physician Workforce: What Influences Medical Student and Resident Choices? Washington, DC: Policy Studies in Family Medicine and Primary Care, Robert Graham Center. .

Philpot, R. J. (2005). *Financial returns to society by National Health Service corps scholars who receive training as physician assistants and nurse practitioners.* Unpublished doctoral dissertation, University of Florida.

Physician Assistant Education Association. (2007). *Twenty-Second Annual Report on Physician Assistant Educational Programs in the United States, 2005–2006.* Alexandria, VA: Author.

Physician Assistant Education Association. (2008a). *Twenty-Third Annual Report on Physician Assistant Educational Programs in the United States, 2006–2007.* Alexandria, VA: Author.

Physician Assistant Education Association. (2008b). *PA Programs' Purchasing Power Survey.* Alexandria, VA: Author.

Physician Assistant Education Association. (2008c). *Twenty-Fourth Annual Report on Physician Assistant Educational Programs in the United States, 2007–2008.* Alexandria, VA: Author.

Physician Assistant History Center. (2008a). *Biographies: Richard A. Smith, MD, MPH.* Retrieved February 9, 2008, from http://pahx.org/smithBio.html.

Physician Assistant History Center. (2008b). *Biographies: Henry K. Silver, MD (1918–1991).* Retrieved February 9, 2008, from http://pahx.org/silverBio.htm

Physician Assistant History Center. (2008c). *Biographies: John Webster Kirklin, MD (1917–2004).* Retrieved February 9, 20008, from http://pahx.org/kriklinBio.htm

Physician Payment Review Commission. (1994). *Nonphysician practitioners.* Washington, DC: Author.

Picot, S .J., Zauszniewski, F., Debanne, S. M., & Holston, E. C. (1999). Mood and blood pressure responses in black female caregivers and non caregivers. *Nursing Research, 48*(3), 150–161.

Pohutsky, L. C. (1982, March 22). *The Origin and Development of the Physician's (sic) Assistant Programs in the United States, 1960–79.* Doctoral thesis, Teachers College, Columbia University, New York.

Polansky, M. (2003). A primer on oncology for the primary care PA. *Journal of the American Academy of Physician Assistants, 16*(10), 8–11.

Polansky, M. (2007). A historical perspective on postgraduate physician assistant education and the association of postgraduate physician assistant programs. *Journal of Physician Assistant Education, 18*(3), 100–108.

Pondy, L. R., Jones, J. M., & Braun, J. A. (1973). Utilization and productivity of the Duke Physician's Associate. *Socio-economic Planning Sciences, 7*(4), 327–352.

Poppen, C. F. (1996). Physician assistants in otorhinolaryngology—Head and neck surgery. *NEWS-Line for Physician Assistants, 5*(9), 8.

Power, L., Bakker, D. L., & Cooper, M. I. (1973). *Diabetes Outpatient Care Through Physician Assistants—A Model for Health Maintenance Organizations.* Springfield, IL: Thomas Publishing.

Probst, J. C., Moore, C. G., Baxley, E. G., & Lammie, J. J. (2002). Rural-urban differences in visits to primary care physicians. *Family Medicine, 34*(8), 609–615.

Pucillo, J. M. (2000). Welcome to the jungle: The Bolivia diaries. *PA Today, 8*(5), 34–38.

Rada-Sidinger, P., & Connor, P. (1992). Profiles in caring: PAs as primary care providers for poor and underserved children. *Journal of the American Academy of Physician Assistants, 5*(10), 784–789.

Ramer, S. C. (1996). *The Medical Professions.* Armonk, NY: M. E. Sharpe.

Ramos, M. (1989). Occupational medicine. An overview for physician assistants. *Physician Assistant, 13*(2), 79–86.

Ramos, M. (2003). Occupational and environmental medicine. In R. M. Ballweg, S. Stolberg, & E. Sullivan (Eds.), *Physician Assistant: A Guide to Clinical Practice.* (2nd ed.). Philadelphia: W.B. Saunders.

Record, J. C. (1981a). Staffing primary care in 1990: The findings and policy implications. *Springer Series on Health Care and Society, 6,* 131–153.

Record, J. C. (1981b). The productivity of new health practitioners. *Springer Series on Health Care and Society, 6,* 37–52.

Record, J. C., Blomquist, R. H., McCabe, M. A., McCally, M., & Berger, B. D. (1981). Delegation in adult primary care: The generalizability of HMO data. *Springer Series on Health Care and Society, 6,* 68–83.

Record, J. C., & Greenlick, M. R. (1975). New health professionals and the physician role: A hypothesis from Kaiser experience. *Public Health Reports, 90*(3), 241–246.

Record, J. C., McCally, M., Schweitzer, S. O., Blomquist, R. M., & Berger, B. D. (1980). New health professions after a decade and a half: Delegation, productivity and costs in primary care. *Journal of Health Politics, Policy & Law, 5*(3), 470–497.

Record, J. C., & Schweitzer, S. O. (1981a). Staffing primary care in 1990: Effects of national health insurance on staffing and costs. *Springer Series on Health Care and Society, 6,* 115–127.

Record, J. C., & Schweitzer, S. O. (1981b). Staffing primary care in 1990—Potential effects on staffing and costs: Estimates from the model. *Springer Series on Health Care and Society, 6,* 87–114.

Reed, L. (2006). Determinants of faculty job satisfaction and potential implications for physician assistant program personnel. *Journal of Physician Assistant Education, 17*(1), 30–35.

Regan, D. M., & Harbert, K. R. (1991). Measuring the financial productivity of physician assistants. *Medical Group Management Journal, 38*(6), 46, 48, 50–52.

Reines, H. D., Robinson, L., Duggan, M., O'Brien, B. M., & Aulenbach, K. (2006). Integrating midlevel practitioners into a teaching service. *American Journal of Surgery, 192*(1), 119–124.

Reinhardt, U. E. (1972). A production function for physician services. *Review of Economics and Statistics, 54*(1), 55–66.

Repicky, P. A., Mendenhall, R. C., & Neville, R. E. (1982). The professional role of physician's assistants in adult ambulatory care practices. *Evaluation & Health Professions, 5*(3), 283–301.

Resneck J. S., Jr. & Kimball, A. B. (2008). Who else is providing care in dermatology practices? Trends in the use of nonphysician clinicians. *Journal of the American Academy of Dermatology, 58*(2), 211–216.

Resnick, A. S., Todd, B. A., Mullen, J. L., & Morris, J. B. (2006). How do surgical residents and non-physician practitioners play together in the sandbox? *Current Surgery, 63*(2), 155–164.

Reynolds, E. W., & Bricker, J. T. (2007). Nonphysician clinicians in the neonatal intensive care unit: Meeting the needs of our smallest patients. *Pediatrics, 119*(2), 361–369.

Ricketts, T. C. (1999). The changing nature of rural health care. *Annual Review of Public Health, 21*(1), 639–657.

Ricketts, T. C., Hart, L. G., & Pirani, M. (2000). How many rural doctors do we have? *Journal of Rural Health, 16*(3), 198–207.

Riess, J., & Lawrence, D. (1976). *Practitioners in Remote Practices: Summary of a Study of Training, Utilization, Financing and Provider Satisfaction.* Washington, DC: Division of Medicine, Bureau of Health Manpower; Department of Health, Education and Welfare.

Riportella-Muller, R., Libby, D., & Kindig, D. (1995). The substitution of physician assistants and nurse practitioners for physician residents in teaching hospitals. *Health Affairs, 14*(2), 181–191.

Roblin, D. W., Becker, E. R., Adams, E. K., Howard, D. H., & Roberts, M. H. (2004). Patient satisfaction with primary care: Does type of practitioner matter? *Medical Care, 42*(6), 579–590.

Roblin, D. W., Howard, D. H., Becker, E. R., Adams, E. K., & Roberts, M. H. (2004). Use of midlevel practitioners to achieve labor cost savings in the primary care practice of an MCO. *Health Services Research, 39*(3), 607–626.

Roemer, M. I. (1977). Primary care and physician extenders in affluent countries. *International Journal of Health Services, 7*(4), 545–555.

Roemer, M. I. (1977). Primary care and physician extenders in affluent countries. International Journal of Health Services. 7 (4), 545-555.

Rogers, C. (1994). Nonphysician providers and limited-license practitioners: Scope-of-practice issues. *Bulletin of the American College of Surgeons, 79*(2), 12–17.

Rogers, B. (2000). Physician assistants in nonclinical roles put medical knowledge to work on a broader scale. *AAPA News 6,* 8–9.

Rogers, S. E. (2002). *Physician assistants working and volunteering abroad: A survey.* Unpublished doctoral dissertation, Arizona School of Health Sciences Physician Assistant School, Mesa, AZ.

Romm, J., Berkowitz, A., Cahn, M. A., Cornely, P. B., Kerlin, B., & Morris, S. B. (1979). The physician extender reimbursement experiment. *Journal of Ambulatory Care Management, 2*(2), 1–12.

Rose, C. (2001). PA devotes career to psychiatric care. *NEWS-Line for Physician Assistants, 10*(3), 4–7.

Rosen, R. G. (1986). The Montefiore Medical Center experience. In S. F. Zarbock & K. Harbert (Eds.), *Physician Assistants: Present and Future Models of Utilization.* New York: Praeger.

Rosenblatt, R. A., Andrilla, C., Holly, A., Curtin, T., & Hart, L. G. (2006). Shortages of medical personnel at community health centers: Implications for planned expansion. *Journal of the American Medical Association, 295*(9), 1042–1049.

Rosenblum, A., Nuttbrock, L., McQuistion, H., Magura, S., & Joseph, H. (2002). Medical outreach to homeless substance users in New York City: Preliminary results. *Substance Use & Misuse, 37*(8–10), 1269–1273.

Rosenfeld, J. C. (1997). Integration of physician assistants and surgical residents in a general surgery residency. *Current Surgery, 54,* 556–558.

Rosinski, E. F. (1971). Physician's assistants. A review of their status. *Israel Journal of Medical Sciences, 7*(5), 697–700.

Rosinski, E. F. (1972). Education and role of the physician. A redefinition. *Journal of the American Medical Association, 222*(4), 473–475.

Rosinski, E .F., & Spencer, F. J. (1967). The training and duties of the medical auxiliary known as the assistant medical officer. *American Journal of Public Health, 57*(9), 1663–1669.

Ross A. C. (2008). The role of physician assistants in oncology. *ADVANCE for Physician Assistants, 12*(3), 46–49.

Ross, N., & Parle, J. (2008). Physician assistants: A UK perspective on clinical need, education and regulation. *Clinical Teacher, 5*(1), 28–32.

Rothwell, W. (1993). PAs in cardiothoracic surgery. *Journal of the American Academy of Physician Assistants, 6*(2), 150–157.

Rourke, L. L., Rourke, J., & Brown, J. B. (1996). Women family physicians and rural medicine. Can the grass be greener in the country? *Canadian Family Physician, 42,* 1063–1067.

Rousselot, L. M., Beard, S. E., & Berrey, B. H. (1971). The evolution of the physician's assistant: Brownian movement or coordinated progress. *Bulleting of the New York Academy of Medicine, 47*(12), 1473–1500.

Roy, S. C., & Andrews, H. A. (1998). *The Roy Adaptation Model.* Norwalk, CT: Appleton & Lange.

Rubeck, T. J., Coombs, J., Keck, M., McDaniel, J., Agar Barwick, T., Kang, S., et al. (2007). Central application service for physician assistants: Five-year report. *Journal of Physician Assistant Education, 18*(3), 52–59.

Rubenstein, E. B., Fender, A., Rolston, K. V., Elting, L. S., Prasco, P. J., Palmer, I., et al. (1995). Vascular access by physician assistants: Evaluation of an implantable peripheral port system in cancer patients. *Journal of Clinical Oncology: Official Journal of the American Society of Clinical Oncology 13*(6), 1513–1519.

Rudy, E. B., Davidson, L. J., Daly, B., Clochesy, J. M., Sereika, S., Baldisseri, M., et al. (1998). Care activities and outcomes of patients cared for by acute care nurse practitioners, physician assistants, and resident physicians: A comparison. *American Journal of Critical Care, 7*(4), 267–281.

Ruff, C. C., Gray, J., Arthur, M., & Merenstein, G. (2006). Development and outcomes of a rural track within a primary care physician assistant program. *Journal of Physician Assistant Education, 17*(4), 37–41.

Russell, J. C., Kaplowe, J., & Heinrich, J. J. (1999). One hospital's successful 20-year experience with physician assistants in graduate medical education. *Academic Medicine, 74*(6), 641–645.

Sadler, A. M., Jr. (1975). New health practitioner education: Problems and issues. *Journal of Medical Education, 50*(12 pt 2), 67–73.

Sadler, A. M., Jr., Sadler, B. L., & Bliss, A.A. (1972). *The Physician's Assistant: Today and Tomorrow.* New Haven, CT: Yale University Press.

Sadler, A. M., Jr., Sadler, B. L., & Bliss, A. A. (1975). *The Physician's Assistant: Today and Tomorrow* (2nd ed.). Cambridge, MA: Ballinger.

Safriet, B. J. (1994). Impediments to progress in health care workforce policy: License and practice laws. *Inquiry, 31*(3): 310–317.

Salmon, M. A., & Stein, J. (1986). Distribution of nurse practitioners and physician assistants: Are they meeting the need for primary care? *North Carolina Medical Journal, 47*(3), 147–148.

Salyer, S. W. (2002). Continued growth for military PAs. *Journal of the American Academy of Physician Assistants, 15*(10), 35–39.

Salyer, S. W. (2008). A clinical doctorate in emergency medicine for physician assistants: Postgraduate education. *Journal of Physician Assistant Education, 19*(3), 53–56.

Salzberg, E., & Grover, A. (2006). Physician workforce shortages: Implications and issues for academic health centers and policymakers. *Academic Medicine, 81*(9), 782–787.

Samarel, N., Fawcett, J., Krippendorf, K., Piacentino, J. C., Eliasof, B., Hughes, P., et al. (1998). Women's perceptions of group support and adaptation to breast cancer. *Journal of Advanced Nursing, 28,* 1259–1268.

Samsot, M. (1998). Innovations in dermatology. *NEWS-line for Physician Assistants, 7,* 4–7.

Samsot, M., & Heinlein, M. (1996). Orthopaedic PA duties: Extensive and on the increase. *NEWS-Line for Physician Assistants, 5*(4), 4–7.

Samuels, R. C., Chi, G. W., Rauch, D. A., Palfrey, J. S., & Shelov, S. P. (2005). Lessons from pediatrics residency program directors' experience with work hour limitations in New York state. *Academic Medicine, 80*(5), 467–471.

Schaefer, K. M., & Potylycki, M. J. S. (1993). Fatigue associated with congestive heart failure. *Journal of Advanced Nursing, 18,* 260–268.

Schafft, G. E., & Cawley, J. F. (1987). Geriatric care and the physician assistant. *The Physician Assistant in a Changing Health Care Environment.* Rockville, MD: Aspen Publishers.

Schectman, J. M., Elinsky, E. G., & Pawlson, L. G. (1991). Effect of education and feedback on thyroid function testing strategies of primary care clinicians. *Archives of Internal Medicine, 151*(11), 2163–2166.

Scheffler, R. M. (1977). The employment, utilization, and earnings of physician extenders. *Social Science & Medicine (1982), 11*(17–18), 785–791.

Scheffler, R. M. (1979). The productivity of new health practitioners: Physician assistants and Medex. *Research in Health Economics, 1*(1), 37–56.

Scheffler, R. M. (2008). *Is There a Doctor in the House? Market Signals and Tomorrow's Supply of Doctors.* Berekley, CA: Stanford University Press.

Scheffler, R. M., Waitzman, N. J., & Hillman, J. M. (1996). The productivity of physician assistants and nurse practitioners and health work force policy in the era of managed health care. *Journal of Allied Health, 25*(3), 207–217.

Schmittou, E. V. (1977). Cadaver kidney procurement: A unique role for a physician assistant. *PA Journal, 7*(1), 23–28.

Schneider, D. P., & Foley, W. J. (1977). A systems analysis of the impact of physician extenders on medical cost and manpower requirements. *Medical Care, 15*(4), 277–297.

Schneller, E. S. (1978). *The Physician's Assistant: Innovation in the Medical Division of Labor.* Lexington, MA: Lexington Books.

Schneller, E. S. (1994). A PA by any other name. *Journal of the American Academy of Physician Assistants, 7,* 689–692.

Schneller, E. S., & Simon, J. A. (1977). A profile of the backgrounds and expectations of the class of 1977. *PA Journal, 7,* 67–72.

Schneller, E. S., & Weiner, T. S. (1978). The black physician's assistant: Problems and prospects. *Journal of Medical Education, 53,* 661–666.

Schroeder, S. A. (1992). Must America look to non-doctors for primary care? [interview by Mark Holoweiko]. *Medical Economics, 69*(24), 82–87.

Schroy, P.C., Wiggins, T., Winawer, S. J., Diaz, B., & Lightdale, C. J. (1988). Video endoscopy by nurse practitioners: A model for colorectal cancer screening. *Gastrointestinal Endoscopy, 34*(5), 390–394.

Schulman, M., Lucchese, K. R., & Sullivan, A. C. (1995). Transition from housestaff to nonphysicians as neonatal intensive care providers: Cost, impact on revenue, and quality of care. *American Journal of Perinatology, 12*(6), 442–446.

Searle, N. S., Haidet, P., Kelly, P. A., Schneider, V. F., Seidel, C. L., & Richards, B. F. (2003). Team learning in medical education: Initial experiences at ten institutions. *Academic Medicine, 78*(10), S55.

Segal-Gidan, F. (2002). Who will care for the aging American population? *Journal of the American Academy of Physician Assistants, 15*(12), 4, 7.

Sekscenski, E. S., Sansom, S., Bazell, C., Salmon, M. E., & Mullan, F. (1994). State practice environments and the supply of physician assistants, nurse practitioners, and certified nurse-midwives. *New England Journal of Medicine, 331*(19), 1266–1271.

Sells, C. J., & Herdener, R. S. (1975). Medex: A time-motion study. *Pediatrics, 56*(2), 255–261.

Seto, T. B., Taira, D. A., Davis, R. B., Safran, C., & Phillips, R. S. (1996). Effect of physician gender on the prescription of estrogen replacement therapy. *Journal of General Internal Medicine, 11*(4), 197–203.

Shi, L., & Samuels, M. E. (1997). Practice environment and the employment of nurse practitioners, physician assistants, and certified nurse midwives by community health centers. *Journal of Allied Health, 26*(3), 105–111.

Shi, L., Samuels, M. E., Konrad, T. R., Ricketts, T. C, Stoskopt, C. H., & Richter, D. L. (1993). The determinants of utilization of nonphysician providers in rural community and migrant health centers. *Journal of Rural Health, 9*(1), 27–39.

Shi, L., Samuels, M. E., Ricketts, T. C., & Konrad, T. R. (1994). A rural-urban comparative study of non-physician providers in community and migrant health centers. *Public Health Reports, 109*(6), 809–815.

Shi, L., & Singh, D. A. (2008). *Delivering Health Care in America.* Sudbury, MA: Jones & Bartlett.

Shortell, S. M. (1974). Occupational prestige differences within the medical and allied health professions. *Social Sciences & Medicine, 8,* 1–9.

Sidel, V. W. (1968). Feldshers and "feldsherism": The role and training of the feldsher in the USSR [Review]. *New England Journal of Medicine, 278*(17), 934–939.

Sidel, V. W. (1969). Lessons from abroad: The feldsher in the USSR. *Annals of the New York Academy of Sciences, 166*(3), 957–966.

Sidel, V. W. (1972). The barefoot doctors of the People's Republic of China. *New England Journal of Medicine, 286*(24), 1292–1300.

Sigurdson, L. (2007). Meeting challenges in the delivery of surgical care. Clinical & Investigative Medicine, 30(Suppl. 4), S35–S36.

Silver, H. K. (1971a). New allied health professionals: Implications of the Colorado child health associate law. *New England Journal of Medicine, 284*(6), 304–307.

Silver, H. K. (1971b). The syniatrist. A suggested nomenclature and classification for allied health professionals. *Journal of the American Medical Association, 217*(10), 1368–1370.

Silver, H. K. (1973a). A blueprint for pediatric health manpower for the 1970's. The 1972 George Armstrong lecture. *Journal of Pediatrics, 82*(1), 149–156.

Silver, H. K. (1973b). A new primary-care medical practitioner. *American Journal of Diseases of Children (1960), 126*(3), 324–327.

Silver, H. K., & McAtee, P. A. (1984). On the use of nonphysician "associate residents" in overcrowded specialty-training programs. *New England Journal of Medicine, 311*(5), 326–328.

Silver, H. K., & McAtee, P. A. (1988). Additions to departments of medicine [Letter]. *New England Journal of Medicine, 318*(10), 645–646.

Silver, H. K., & Ott, J. E. (1973). The child health associate: A new professional to provide comprehensive health care to children. *Physician Assistant, 3*(2), 21–26.

Silver, H. K., Ott, J. E., Dungy, C. I., Fine, L .L., Moore, V. M., & Krugman, R. D. (1981). Assessment and evaluation of child health associates. *Pediatrics, 67*(1), 47–52.

Simkens, A. B. M., van Baar, M. E., van Balen, F. A. M., Verheij, R. A., van den Hoogen, H. J. M., & Schrijvers, A. J. P. (2009). The physician assistant in general practice in the Netherlands. *Journal of Physician Assistant Education, 20*(1), 30–38.

Simmer, T. L., Nerenz, D. R., Rutt, W. M., Newcomb, C. S., & Benfer, D. W. (1991). A randomized, controlled trial of an attending staff service in general internal medicine. *Medical Care, 29*(7), JS31–JS40.

Simmons, J. (2000). PAs become part of political process by running for public office. *AAPA News, 21*(1), 14.

Simon, A. F., Link, M.S., & Miko, A.S. (2001). *Seventeenth Annual Report on Physician Assistant Education in the United States, 2000–2001.* Alexandria, VA: Association of Physician Assistant Programs.

Singer, A. J., Hollander, J. E., Cassara, G., Valentine, S. M., Thode, H. C., Jr., & Henry, M. C. (1995). Level of training, wound care practices, and infection rates. *American Journal of Emergency Medicine, 13*(3), 265–268.

Singer, A. M., & Hooker, R. S. (1996). Determinants of specialty choice of physician assistants. *Academic Medicine, 71*(8), 917–919.

Skinner, A .L. (1968). Parental acceptance of delegated pediatric services. *Pediatrics, 41*(5), 1003–1004.

Smith, C. W., Jr. (1981). Patient attitudes toward physicians' assistants. *Journal of Family Practice, 13*(2), 201–204.

Smith, J. L. (1992). Physicians' assistants doing endoscopy? [Editorial]. *American Journal of Gastroenterology, 87*(8), 937–939.

Smith, M. K., & Hendersen-Andrade, N. (2006). Facing the health worker crisis in developing countries: A call for global solidarity. *Bulletin of the World Health Organization, 84,* 426.

Smith, M. O. (1996). Correctional medicine: An outstanding setting for the PA. *Physician Assistant, 20*(7), 103–104.

Smith, R. A. (1969). Medex: A demonstration program in primary medical care. *Northwest Medicine, 68*(11), 1023–1030.

Smith, R. A. (1974). The medical assistant. Discussion on assurance of qulaity, competence and accountability. *Public Health Papers,* (60), 142–152.

Smith, R. A. (1978). *Manpower and Primary Health Care: Guidelines for Improving/Expanding Health Services Coverage in Developing Countries.* Honolulu, HI: The University Press of Hawaii.

Smith, R. A., Bassett, G. R, Markarian, C. A., Vath, R. E., Freeman, W. L., & Dunn, G. F. (1971). A strategy for health manpower. Reflections on an experience called MEDEX. *Journal of the American Medical Association, 217*(10), 1362–1367.

Society of Physician Assistants in Otorhinolaryngology/Head & Neck Surgery. (2003). SPAO 2003: ENT PA productivity survey. Retrieved June 6, 2008, from http://www.entpa.org/scope_of_practice.html

Sonntag, V. K., Steiner, S., & Stein, B. M. (1977). Neurosurgery and the physician assistant. *Surgical Neurology, 8*(3), 207–208.

Sox, H. C., Jr. (1979). Quality of patient care by nurse practitioners and physician's assistants: A ten-year perspective. *Annals of Internal Medicine, 91*(3), 459–468.

Sox, H. C. (2003). The future of primary care. *Annals of Internal Medicine, 138*(3), 230–232.

Sox, H. C., Jr., Sox, C. H., & Tompkins, R. K. (1973). The training of physician's assistants. The use of a clinical algorithm system for patient care, audit of performance and education. *New England Journal of Medicine, 288*(16), 818–824.

Spenkelink-Schut, G., Koch, R. P. P., & Kort, H. S. M. (2006). De physician assistant: Een nieuwe masteropleiding binnen het medisch domein van de gezondheidszorg in Nederland. [The physician assistant in the Dutch health care]. *Dutch Journal of Education and Health Care, 5,* 18–22.

Spitzer, W. O. (1984). The nurse practitioner revisited: Slow death of a good idea. *New England Journal of Medicine, 310*(16), 1049–1051.

Stahlfeld, K. R., Robinson, J. M., & Burton, E. C. (2008). What do physician extenders in a general surgery residency really do? *Journal of Surgical Education, 65*(5), 354–358.

Stanhope, W. (1991). Postgraduate training: Who needs it? *Physician Assistant, 15*(11), 14–16.

Stanhope, W. D., Fasser, C. E., & Cawley, J. F. (1992). The FMG debate continues . . . Foreign medical graduate. *Journal of the American Academy of Physician Assistants, 5*(8), 612–614.

Staton, F. S., Bhosele, M. J., Camacho, F. T., Feldman, S. R., & Balkrishnan, R. (2007). How PAs improve access to care for the underserved. *Journal of the American Academy of Physician Assistants, 20*(6), 32–36.

Starfield, B. H. (1993). Roles and functions of non-physician practitioners in primary care. In D. K. Clawson & M. Osterweis (Eds.), *The Roles of Physician Assistants and Nurse Practitioners in Primary Care.* Washington, DC: Association of Academic Health Centers.

Starfield, B. (1994). Is primary care essential? *Lancet, 344*(8930), 1129–1133.

Starr, P. (1982). *The Social Transformation of American Medicine.* New York: Basic Books.

Staton, F. S., Bhosle, M. J., Camacho, F. T., Feldman, S. R., & Balkrishnan, R. (2007). How PAs improve access to care for the underserved. *Journal of the American Academy of Physician Assistants, 20*(6), 32–36.

Stead, E. A., Jr. (1966). Conserving costly talents—Providing physicians' new assistants. *Journal of the American Medical Association, 198*(10), 1108–1109.

Stead, E. A., Jr. (1967). The Duke plan for physician's assistants. *Medical Times, 95,* 40–48.

Stead, E. A., Jr. (1968a). A college-based physician's assistant program. *Medical Times, 96,* 847–850.

Stead, E. A., Jr. (1968b). Educational programs and manpower. *Bulletin of the New York Academy of Medicine, 44,* 204–213.

Stead, E. A., Jr. (1969). The physician's assistant—Job description and licensing. *Medical Times, 97,* 246–247.

Stead, E. A., Jr. (1971). Use of physicians' assistants in the delivery of medical care. *Annual Review of Medicine, 22,* 273–282.

Stead, E. A., Jr. (2001). A new way of making doctors: Distance learning for nontraditional students. *North Carolina Medical Journal, 62*(6), 326–327.

Stecker, M. S., Armenoff, D., & Johnson, M. S. (2004). Physician assistants in interventional radiology practice. *Journal of Vascular and Interventional Radiology, 15*(3), 221–227.

Steiner, S. (2008). One day in the life. *Journal of the American Academy of Physician Assistants, 21*(43), 22–24.

Steinwachs, D. M., Weiner, J. P., Shapiro, S., Batalden, P., Coltin, K., & Wasserman, F. (1986). A comparison of the requirements for primary care physicians in HMOs with projections made by the GMENAC. *New England Journal of Medicine, 314*(4), 217–222.

Storey, P. B., & Roth, R. B. (1971). Emergency medical care in the Soviet Union. A study of the Skoraya. *Journal of the American Medical Association, 217*(5), 588–592.

Storms, D. M., & Fox, J. G. (1979). The public's view of physicians' assistants and nurse practitioners: A survey of Baltimore urban residents. *Medical Care, 17*(5), 526–535.

Stradtman, J. C. (1989). Utilizing physician's assistants in the medical intensive care unit: A pilot project. *Hospital Topics, 67*(2), 24–25.

Straker, H., & LeLacheur, S. (2007). Integrating cultural competency across the curriculum. *Journal of Physician Assistant Education, 18*(2), 60–63.

Strand, J. (2006). The practicante: Puerto Rico physician assistant prototype. *Journal of Physician Assistant Education, 17*(2), 60–62.

Strand J., & Carter, R. (2003). Primary care training grants through Title VII, section 747: The Duke experience. *Perspective on Physician Assistant Education,14*(1), 25–30.

Strickland, W. J., Strickland, D. L., & Garretson, C. (1998). Rural and urban nonphysician providers in Georgia. *Journal of Rural Health, 14*(2), 109–120.

Strunk, H. K. (1973). Patient attitudes toward physician's assistants. *California Medicine, 118*(6), 73–77.

Stuart, R. B., & Blair, J. H. (1974). Army physicians' attitudes about physicians' assistants. *Military Medicine, 141*(6), 470–472.

Stuart, R. B., Robinson, H. A., Jr., & Reed, R. F. (1973). The training and role of physicians' assistants in the Army Medical Department. *Military Medicine, 138*(4), 227–230.

Sturmann, K. M., Ehrenberg, K., & Salzberg, M. R. (1990). Physician assistants in emergency medicine. *Annals of Emergency Medicine, 19*(3), 304–308.

Sullivan, S. (2000). Nutrition education in physician assistant programs: A national survey. *Perspective on Physician Assistant Education, 11*(1), 18–24.

Swann, K. (2000). Las Vegas company makes house calls. *AAPA News, 6*(21), 11.

Sweet, M. (2008, April). Side by side: Can physician assistants help rural doctors? *Australian Rural Doctor,* 6–14.

Sylvester, P. A. (1996). Forensic medicine. *Journal of the American Academy of Physician Assistants, 9,* 53–65.

Synowiez, P.M. (1986). Utilization of physician assistants in group practice. *College Review* (Denver, CO), *3*(2), 57-67.

Synowiez, P. M., Fisher, R. L., & Royer, T. C. (1984). PAs in a tertiary medical center: A ten-year experience. *Physician Assistant, 8,* 63–64, 69, 75.

Tabachnick, D. (2006). The role of the physician assistant in the psycho-oncology team. *Psycho-oncology, 15*(1), S63–S64.

Talbot, M. (1994). Canadian Forces physician assistants [Letter]. *Canadian Medical Association Journal, 150,* 1058–1059.

Taft, J. M., & Hooker, R. S. (1999). Physician assistants in neurology practice. *Neurology, 52*(7), 1513.

Taylor, L. G. (2000). Nurse practitioners' impact on primary health care outcomes in rural clients. *Dissertation Abstracts International, 61*(11b), 5804.

Ten Cate, O. (2007). Medical education in the Netherlands. *Medical Teacher, 29*(8), 752–757.

Terris, M. (1977). Issues in primary care: False starts and lesser alternatives. *Bulletin of the New York Academy of Medicine, 53*(1), 129–140.

Thomas, C. (1997). *Partners of the Heart: Vivien Thomas and His Work with Alfred Blalock: An Autobiography.* Philadelphia: University of Pennsylvania Press.

Thomas, G. P., McNellis, R. J., & Ortiz, G.R. (2003). Physician assistants enhance quality of care in asthma patients. *Journal of Allergy and Clinical Immunology, 111*(Abstract Supplement), S71–S440.

Thompson, T. (1972). Utilization of specialty-trained physician's associates. *Physician's Associate, 2,* 153–156.

Thompson, T. T. (1971). Radiologists look at physician's assistants in radiology. *Radiology, 100*(1), 199–202.

Thompson, T. T. (1974). The evaluation of physician's assistants in radiology. *Radiology, 111,* 603–606.

Thorpe, K. E. (1990). House staff supervision and working hours. Implications of regulatory change in New York State. *Journal of the American Medical Association, 263*(23), 3177–3181.

Tideiksaar, R. (1986). Models of physician assistant utilization in geriatrics. In S. F. Zarbock & K. Harbert (Eds.), *Physician Assistants: Present and Future Models of Utilization.* New York: Praeger.

Tiger, S. (1982). PAs and publishing. *Physician Assistant/Health Practitioner, 6*(10), 13-4.

Tiger, S. (1992). A brief history of *Physician Assistant*: An editor's retrospective. *Physician Assistant, 15,* 54–55.

Tiger, S. (1993) Roots and radicals [Editorial]. *Physician Assistant, 17*(8), 11.

Timmer, S. (1991). Call for uniform guidelines for postgraduate surgical residency programs. *Journal of the American Academy of Physician Assistants, 4*(6), 453–454.

Todd, B. A., Resnick, A., Stuhlemmer, R., Morris, J. B., & Mullen, J. (2004). Challenges of the 80-hour resident work rules: Collaboration between surgeons and nonphysician practitioners. *Surgical Clinics of North America, 84*(6), 1573–1586.

Toth, P. S., Pickrell, K. L., & Thompson, L. K., III. (1978). Role of physician's assistant and the plastic surgeon. *Southern Medical Journal, 71*(4), 430–431.

Trigg, M. E. (1990). PA utilization on a pediatric bone marrow transplant unit. *Physician Assistant, 14*(3), 64, 67–68, 70.

Turner, J. G., Clark, A. J., Gauthier, D. K., & Williams, M. (1998). The effect of therapeutic touch on pain and anxiety in burn patients. *Journal of Advanced Nursing, 28,* 10–20.

United Nations, Department of Economic and Social Affairs, Population Division. (Eds.) (2004). *World Population to 2300.* New York: Author.

U.S. Department of Agriculture. (2004). *Measuring rurality: Rural-urban continuum codes.* Retrieved June 22, 2008, from http://www.ers.usda.gov/ Briefing/Rurality/RuralUrbCon/

U.S. Department of Health & Human Services. Health Resources Services Administration. (2006). *The registered nurse population: Findings from the 2004 national sample survey of registered nurses.* Retrieved August 19, 2008, from http://bhpr.hrsa.gov/healthworkforce/ reports/rnpopulation/preliminaryfindings.htm

U.S. Department of Labor, Bureau of Labor Statistics (2008). *Occupational Outlook Handbook. Physicians and Surgeons.* Retrieved February 29, 2008, from http://www.bls.gov/oco/ocos074.htm#projections _data

Vangsnes, E. H. (2005). A policy and program analysis of federal support for physician assistant education: Title VII, Section 747 of the Public Health Act. *Perspective on Physician Assistant Education, 16*(2), 79–83.

van Everdinck, I., den Hollander E., van der Lecq A., & Reiter L. (2006). *Physician assistants: Leiden University Medical Center, the Netherlands.* Presented at the American Academy of Physician Assistants Annual PA Conference, San Francisco.

van Leeuwen, D. J. (2002). Liver biopsy: Who should do it . . . and who will show up in court? *American Journal of Gastroenterology, 97*(6), 1285–1288.

Van Rhee, J., Ritchie, J., & Eward, A. M. (2002). Resource use by physician assistant services versus teaching services. *Journal of the American Academy of Physician Assistants, 15*(1) 33–38, 40, 42 passim.

Van Valkenburg, J., Ralph, B., Lopatofsky, L., Campbell, M., & Brown, D. (2000). The role of the physician extender in radiology. *Radiologic Technology, 72*(1), 45–50.

Vause, R. C., Beeler, A., & Miller-Blanks, M. (1997). Seeking a practice challenge? PAs in federal prisons. *Journal of the American Academy of Physician Assistants, 10*(2), 59–62.

Vaz, F., Bergstrom, S., Vaz, M., Langa, J., & Bugalho, A. (1999). Training medical assistants for surgery. *Bulletin of the World Health Organization, 77*(8), 688–691.

Velie, L. (1965, August). Where the jobs are—Health careers unlimited. *Reader's Digest,* 108–112.

Verboon, E. M. (2005). The development of physician assistant education in the Netherlands. *Perspective on Physician Assistant Education, 16*(2), 108–109.

Wachter, R., & Goldman, L. (1996). The emerging role of "hospitalists" in the American health care system. *New England Journal of Medicine, 335*(7), 514–517.

Wakerlin, G. E., Stoneman, W., III, & Rikli, A. E. (1972). Physician's assistants—Nurse associates. An overview. *Missouri Medicine, 69*(10), 779–785.

Wallen, J., Davidson, S. M., Epstein, D., &, Connelly. J. P. (1982). Nonphysician health care providers in pediatrics. *Paediatrician, 11*(3–4), 225–239.

Walters, R. (1986). Geisinger Medical Center tertiary care perspectives. In S. F. Zarbock & K. Harbert (Eds.), *Physician Assistants: Present and Future Models of Utilization.* Praeger, New York.

Webster, B. S., & Snook, S. H. (1990). The cost of compensable low back pain. *Journal of Occupational Medicine, 32,* 13–15.

Weiner, J. D. (2006). *History of the navy corpsman.* Retrieved February 1, 2008, from http://www.jeffreywiener.com/pamphlet.htm

Weiner, J. P. (1994). Forecasting the effects of health reform on U.S. physician workforce requirement. Evidence from HMO staffing patterns. *Journal of the American Medical Association, 272*(3), 222–230.

Weiner, J. P. (2002). A shortage of physicians or a surplus of assumptions? *Health Affairs, 21*(1), 160.

Weiner, J. P., Steinwachs, D. M., & Williamson, J. W. (1986). Nurse practitioner and physician assistant practices in three HMOs: Implications for future U.S. health manpower needs. *American Journal of Public Health, 76*(5), 507–511.

Weisman, G. S., Winawer, S. J., Baldwin, M. P., Miller, C. H., Cummins, R. L., Ephraim, R., et al. (1987). Multicenter evaluation of training of non-endoscopists in 30-cm flexible sigmoidoscopy. *Ca: A Cancer Journal for Clinicians, 37*(1), 26–30.

Wen, C. P., & Hays, C. W. (1975). Medical education in China in the postcultural Revolution era. *New England Journal of Medicine, 292*(19), 998–1005.

Weston, J. L. (1980). Distribution of nurse practitioners and physician assistants: Implications of legal constraints and reimbursement. *Public Health Reports, 95,* 253–256.

Westwood, O. M., & Richardson, L. (2005). Developing a medical care practitioner to meet the needs of England. *Perspective on Physician Assistant Education, 16*(11), 51–54.

Whitcomb, M. E. (2006). The shortage of physicians and the future role of nurses. *Academic Medicine, 81*(9), 779–780.

Whitcomb, M. E. (2007a). Who will lead? *Academic Medicine, 82*(2), 115–116.

Whitcomb, M. E. (2007b). The shortage of physicians: A challenge for the physician assistant profession. *Journal of Physician Assistant Education, 18*(1), 5–6.

White, G. L. (1992). *The Medical School's Mission and the Population's Health.* New York: Springer-Verlag.

White, R. I., Jr., Denny, D. F., Jr., Osterman, F. A., Greenwood, L. H., & Wilkinson, L. A. (1989). Logistics of a university interventional radiology practice. *Radiology, 170*(3, Pt 2), 951–954.

White, R. I., Jr., Rizer, D. M., Shuman, K. R., White, E. J., Adams, P. E., Kinnison, M. L., et al. (1988). Streamlining operation of an admitting service for interventional radiology. *Radiology, 168*(1), 127–130.

White, S. M., & Geronemus, R. (2002). Should non-physicians perform cosmetic procedures? *Dermatologic Surgery, 28*(9), 856–859.

White, K., Williams, T. F., & Greenberg, B. (1961). The ecology of medical care. *New England Journal of Medicine, 265,* 885–892.

Whitman, N. A. (2000). Whitman sampler. Is teaching a certifiable profession? *Perspective on Physician Assistant Education, 11*(2), 136.

Whitman, N. A., & Pedersen, D. (1998). The use of standardized patients to evaluate a physician assistant program curriculum. *Perspective on Physician Assistant Education, 9*(2), 93–96.

Wiemiller, M. J. P. M., Somers, K. K., & Adams, M. B. (2008). Postgraduate physician assistant training programs in the United States: emerging trends and opportunities. *Journal of Physician Assistant Education, 19*(4), 58–63.

Willams, W. H., Kopchak, J., Yearby, L. G., & Hatcher, C. R. (1984). The surgical physician assistant as a member of the cardiovascular surgical team in the academic medical center. In R. D. Carter & H. H. Perry, III (Eds.), *Alternatives in Health Care Delivery.* St. Louis: Warren Green.

Willis, J. B. (1990). Prescriptive practice patterns of physician assistants. *Journal of the American Academy of Physician Assistants, 3,* 39–56.

Willis, J. B. (1993). Barriers to PA practice in primary care and rural medically underserved areas. *Journal of the American Academy of Physician Assistants, 6*(6), 418–422.

Willis, J. B., Cyr, B., Schafft, G., & Steinbrueck, S. P. (1986). 1985 physician assistant role delineation study: Ten years later. *Physician Assistant, 10*(12), 33–38, 80–81.

Willis, J. B., & Reid J. (1990). Montana physician's survey. *Journal of the American Academy of Physician Assistants, 3*(1), 57–60.

Wilson, I. B., Landon, B. E., Hirschhorn, L. R., McInnes, K., Ding, L., Marsden, P. V., et al. (2005). Quality of HIV care provided by nurse practitioners, physician assistants, and physicians. *Annals of Internal Medicine, 143*(10), 729–736.

Wilson, W. M., White, G. L., Jr., & Murdock, R. T. (1990). Physician assistants in ophthalmology: A national survey. *Physician Assistant, 14*(1), 57–59.

Wing, P., Langlier, M. H., Salsberg, E., & Hooker, R. S. (2004). The changing professional practice of physician assistants, 1992–2000. *Journal of the American Academy of Physician Assistants, 17*, 37–49.

Wong, R. C. K. (1999). Screening flexible sigmoidoscopy by nonphysician endoscopists: It's here to stay, but is it the right test to do? [Editorial]. *Gastrointestinal Endoscopy, 49*(2), 262–264.

Woodin, J., McLeod, H., McManus, R., & Jelphs, K. (2005a, March 20). Evaluation of U.S.-trained physician assistants working in the NHS in England: The introduction of U.S.-trained physician assistants to primary care and accident and emergency departments in Sandwell and Birmingham. *BMJ News*, p. 14.

Woodin, J., Mcleod, H., McManus, R., & Jelphs, K. (2005b). *Evaluation of U.S.-trained PAs Working in the NHS in England. Final Report.* Birmingham: Health Services Management Centre, Department of Primary Care and General Practice, University of Birmingham.

Woolsey, L. J. (2005). Geriatric medicine and the future of the physician assistant profession. *Perspective on Physician Assistant Education, 16*(1), 24–28.

World Health Organization. (1980). *The Primary Health Worker.* Geneva, Switzerland: Author.

World Health Organization. (1987a). *Report on the Community-Based Education of Health Personnel.* Geneva, Switzerland: Author.

World Health Organization. (1987b). *The Primary Care Worker.* Geneva, Switzerland: Author.

Wright, D. D., Kane, R. L., Snell, G. F., & Woolley, F. R. (1977). Costs and outcomes for different primary care providers. *Journal of the American Medical Association, 238*(1), 46–50.

Wright, W. K., & Hirsch, C. S. (1987). The physician assistant as forensic investigator. *Journal of Forensic Science, 32*(4), 1059–1061.

Wright, K., Cawley, J. F., Ahuja, M., & Hooker, R. S. (2008, Fall). *Sponsorship of PA educational programs.* Presented to the Physician Assistant Education Association, Alexandria, VA.

Yanni, F., Backman, P. F., & Potash, J. (1972). Physician's attitudes on the physician's assistant. *Physician's Associate, 2*(1), 6–10.

Young, G. P. (1993). Status of clinical and academic emergency medicine at 111 Veterans Affairs medical centers. *Annals of Emergency Medicine, 22*(8), 1304–1309.

Yturri-Byrd, K., & Glazer-Waldman, H. (1984). The physician assistant and care of the geriatric patient. *Gerontology & Geriatrics Education, 5*(1), 33–41.

Yuanli, L., Hsiao, W. C. L., Qing, L., Xingzhu, L., & Ren, M. (1995). Transformation of China's rural health care financing. *Social Science & Medicine, 41*, 1085–1093.

Zarychta, W. A., Milner, M. R., & Hunter-Buskey, R. N. (2008). PAs in the U.S. public health service. (2008). *ADVANCE for Physician Assistants, 16*(5–6), 52–54.

Zayas, T. T. (1999). Qualities of effective preceptors on physician assistant students: Third place award J. Peter Nyquist student writing competition. *Perspective on Physician Assistant Education, 10*(1), 7–11.

Zeckhauser, R., & Eliastam, M. (1974). The productivity potential of the physician assistant. *Journal of Human Resources, 9*(1), 95–116.

Zellmer, M. R. (1992). A survey of Minnesota physicians regarding delegation of prescriptive practice to PAs. *Journal of the American Academy of Physician Assistants, 5*(8), 582–586.

Zellmer, M., & Hadley, R. (2004). A descriptive analysis of capstone projects requirements in physician assistant academic and professional master's degree programs. *Perspective on Physician Assistant Education, 15*, 82–87.

Zimmerly, J. G., & Norman, J. C. (1985). Physician assistants and malpractice liability. *Physician Assistant Consultant, 5*, 11–13.

INDEX